a LANGE medical book

CURRENT Geriatric Diagnosis & Treatment

Edited by

C. Seth Landefeld, MD
Professor of Medicine and Chief, Division of Geriatrics
University of California, San Francisco
San Francisco, California
Associate Chief of Staff, Geriatrics
& Extended Care
VA Medical Center
San Francisco, California

Robert M. Palmer, MD, MPH
Head
Section of Geriatric Medicine
Cleveland Clinic Foundation
Cleveland, Ohio

Mary Anne G. Johnson, MD
Director, Geriatrics & Extended Care Service Line
VA Medical Center
San Francisco, California
Professor of Medicine
Division of Geriatrics
University of California, San Francisco
San Francisco, California

C. Bree Johnston, MD, MPH
Associate Professor of Medicine
Division of Geriatrics
University of California, San Francisco
San Francisco, California
Division of Geriatrics
Director, Geriatrics Fellowship Program
VA Medical Center
San Francisco, California

William L. Lyons, MD
Assistant Professor
Section of Geriatrics & Gerontology
Department of Internal Medicine
Nebraska Medical Center
Omaha, Nebraska

Lange Medical Books/McGraw-Hill
Medical Publishing Division

New York   Chicago   San Francisco   Lisbon   London   Madrid   Mexico City   Milan   New Delhi   San Juan   Seoul
Singapore   Sydney   Toronto

Current Geriatric Diagnosis & Treatment

5 6 7 8 9 0 DOCDOC 0 9 8 7

ISBN: 0-07-139924-0
ISSN: 1549-5736

Notice

Medicine is an ever-changing science. As new research and clinical experience broaden our knowledge, changes in treatment and drug therapy are required. The authors and the publisher of this work have checked with sources believed to be reliable in their efforts to provide information that is complete and generally in accord with the standards accepted at the time of publication. However, in view of the possibility of human error or changes in medical sciences, neither the authors nor the publisher nor any other party who has been involved in the preparation or publication of this work warrants that the information contained herein is in every respect accurate or complete, and they disclaim all responsibility for any errors or omissions or for the results obtained from use of the information contained in this work. Readers are encouraged to confirm the information contained herein with other sources. For example and in particular, readers are advised to check the product information sheet included in the package of each drug they plan to administer to be certain that the information contained in this work is accurate and that changes have not been made in the recommended dose or in the contraindications for administration. This recommendation is of particular importance in connection with new or infrequently used drugs.

This book was set in Adobe Garamond by Pine Tree Composition, Inc.
The editors were Catherine A. Johnson and Peter J. Boyle.
The production supervisor was Richard Ruzycka.
The text was designed by Eve Siegel.
R.R. Donnelly was printer and binder.

This book is printed on acid-free paper.

Contents

Authors

Norman Adair, MD
Assistant Professor
Department of Pulmonary & Critical Care Medicine
Wake Forest University School of Medicine
Winston-Salem, North Carolina
Respiratory Diseases

Harold P. Adams, Jr., MD
Professor
Division of Cerebrovascular Diseases
Department of Neurology
Carver College of Medicine
University of Iowa
Iowa City, Iowa
Cerebrovascular Disease

Joshua Adler, MD
Associate Professor of Clinical Medicine
Division of General Internal Medicine
Director, Ambulatory Practices
Department of Medicine
University of California, San Francisco
San Francisco, California
Parkinson's Disease & Essential Tremor

Cathy A. Alessi, MD
Associate Professor
University of California, Los Angeles School of Medicine
Los Angeles, California
VA Geriatric Research, Education & Clinical Center
Sepulveda, California
Sleep Disorders

M. Aamir Ali, MD
The Marvin M. Schuster Center for Digestive
    & Motility Disorders
The Johns Hopkins Bayview Medical Center
Baltimore, Maryland
Abdominal Complaints & Gastrointestinal Disorders

David C. Aron, MD, MS
Professor of Medicine
Division of Clinical & Molecular Endocrinology
Case Western Reserve University School of Medicine
Cleveland, Ohio
Director, VA HSR&D Center for Quality
    Improvement Research
Louis Stokes Cleveland DVA Medical Center
Cleveland, Ohio
Diabetes in the Elderly

Laurence H. Beck, MD
Chairman
Division of Medicine
Cleveland Clinic Florida
Weston, Florida
Renal System, Fluid & Electrolytes

Susan M. Begelman, MD, RVT
Medical Director, Noninvasive Vascular Laboratory
Section of Vascular Medicine
Department of Cardiovascular Medicine
The Cleveland Clinic Foundation
Cleveland, Ohio
Peripheral Vascular & Thromboembolic Disease

David E. Blumenthal, MD
Department of Rheumatology
Cleveland Clinic Foundation
Cleveland, Ohio
Geriatric Rheumatology

Robert Bonomo, MD
Infectious Diseases Section
    and Geriatrics & Extended Care
Louis Stokes Veterans Affairs Medical Center
Associate Professor
Division of Infectious Disease
Case Western Reserve–University Hospitals
    of Cleveland
Cleveland, Ohio
Common Infections

Rebecca Boxer, MD
Geriatric Fellow
Center on Aging
University of Connecticut
Farmington, Connecticut
Principles of Drug Therapy

James Campbell, MD, MS
Professor and Chairperson,
Department of Family Practice/Geriatrics
Case Western Reserve University School of Medicine
MetroHealth Medical Center
Cleveland, Ohio
Use of Alcohol, Tobacco, & Non-prescribed Drugs

Elise C. Carey, MD
Geriatrics Postdoctoral Fellow
Division of Geriatrics
University of California, San Francisco
San Francisco, California
Parkinson's Disease & Essential Tremor

Daisy G. Ciocon, PhD
Associate Professor
Florida International University
North Miami, Florida
Common Pain Syndromes & Management of Pain

Jerry O. Ciocon, MD
Chairman
Department of Geriatric Medicine
Cleveland Clinic Florida
Weston, Florida
Common Pain Syndromes & Management of Pain

Elizabeth L. Cobbs, MD
Associate Professor of Medicine
Department of Health Care Sciences
The George Washington University Medical Center
Washington, District of Columbia
Office Practice

Rossana D. Danese, MD
Assistant Professor of Medicine
Division of Clinical and Molecular Endocrinology
Case Western Reserve University School of Medicine
Cleveland, Ohio
Diabetes in the Elderly

Chad Deal, MD
Head
Center for Osteoporosis and Metabolic Bone Disease
Cleveland Clinic Foundation
Cleveland, Ohio
Osteoporosis & Hip Fractures

Laurie Dornbrand, MD
Associate Clinical Professor of Medicine
University of California, San Francisco
Health Issues of the Aging Male

Catherine E. DuBeau, MD
Associate Professor of Medicine
Section of Geriatrics
University of Chicago
Chicago, Illinois
Urinary Incontinence

Carmel Bitondo Dyer, MD
Associate Professor of Medicine
Baylor College of Medicine
Director, Geriatrics Program
Harris County Hospital District
Quentin Mease Hospital
Houston, Texas
Elder Mistreatment

Julie A. Elder, DO
Associate Staff, Women's Health
General Internal Medicine
Cleveland Clinic Foundation
Cleveland, Ohio
Speical Issues in Women's Health

Alfred L. Fisher, MD, PhD
Geriatrics and Molecular Medicine Fellow
University of California, San Francisco
Department of Medicine
Division of Geriatrics
San Francisco VA Medical Center
San Francisco, California
Anti-Aging and Complementary Therapies

Diana J. Galindo, MD
Internal Medicine/Geriatrics
Cleveland Clinic Florida
Weston, Florida
Common Pain Syndromes & Management of Pain

Steven R. Gambert, MD
Professor of Medicine
Johns Hopkins University School of Medicine
Baltimore, Maryland
Chairman and Physician-in-Chief
Department of Medicine
Sinai Hospital of Baltimore
Baltimore, Maryland
Endocrine Disorders

Barbara A. Gilchrest, MD
Professor and Chairman
Department of Dermatology
Boston University School of Medicine
Chief of Dermatology
Boston Medical Center
Boston, Massachusetts
Common Skin Disorders

Sharon K. Inouye, MD, MPH
Professor of Medicine, Department of Internal
   Medicine
Director, Mentored Clinical Research Scholar Program
Co-Director, Program on Aging
Yale University School of Medicine
New Haven, Connecticut
Delirium

Diana V. Jao, MD
On Lok Senior Health
San Francisco, California
Sleep Disorders

Larry E. Johnson, MD, PhD
Associate Professor of Geriatrics, and Family and
   Preventive Medicine
University of Arkansas for Medical Sciences
Little Rock, Arkansas
 Medical Director, Extended Care
Central Arkansas Veterans Healthcare System
North Little Rock, Arkansas
Nutrition & Failure to Thrive

Mary Anne G. Johnson, MD
Director, Geriatrics & Extended Care Service Line
VA Medical Center
San Francisco, California
Professor of Medicine
Division of Geriatrics
University of California, San Francisco
San Francisco, California
Community-Based & Nursing Home Long-Term Care;
   Common Infections

C. Bree Johnston, MD, MPH
Associate Professor of Medicine
Division of Geriatrics
University of California, San Francisco
San Francisco, California
Director, Geriatrics Fellowship Program
Division of Geriatrics
VA Medical Center
San Francisco, California
Geriatric Assessment

Hosam Kamel, MD
Assistant Professor of Medicine
Division of Geriatrics & Gerontology
Medical College of Wisconsin
Milwaukee, Wisconsin
Health Issues of the Aging Male

Marshall B. Kapp, JD, MPH
Professor and Director
Office of Geriatric Medicine & Gerontology
Department of Community Health
Wright State University School of Medicine
Dayton, Ohio
Common Legal & Ethical Issues

Lucia C. Kim, MD, MPH
Assistant Professor of Medicine
Baylor College of Medicine
Houston, Texas
Principles of Drug Therapy

Brian E. Lacy, MD, PhD
Assistant Professor of Medicine
The Marvin M. Schuster Center for Digestive and
   Motility Disorders
The Johns Hopkins Bayview Medical Center
Baltimore, Maryland
Abdominal Complaints & Gastrointestinal Disorders

C. Seth Landefeld, MD
Professor of Medicine and Chief, Division of Geriatrics
University of California, San Francisco
Associate Chief of Staff, Geriatrics & Extended Care
VA Medical Center
San Francisco, California
The Need for Expertise in Geriatric Medicine in the Care
   of Older Patients; Hospital Care

Chinh D. Le, MD
Assistant Clinical Professor of Medicine
University of California, Irvine
College of Medicine
Irvine, California
Principles of Rehabilitation

Kewchang Lee, MD
Chief, Psychiatry Consult Service
VA Medical Center
Assistant Clinical Professor
Department of Psychiatry
University of California, San Francisco
San Francisco, California
Depression & Other Mental Health Issues

Bruce Leff, MD
Associate Professor of Medicine
Johns Hopkins University School of Medicine and
    School of Hygiene and Public Health
Baltimore, Maryland
Home Care

Enrique C. Leira, MD
Assistant Professor and Co-director
Souers Stroke Institute
Department of Neurology
Saint Louis University
St. Louis, Missouri
Cerebrovascular Disease

Timothy Lewis, MD
Instructor of Clinical Medicine
Division of General Internal Medicine
University of Cincinnati Medical Center
Cincinnati, Ohio
Visual and Hearing Impairment

Daniel Loo, MD
Assistant Professor
Residency Program Director
Department of Dermatology
Boston University School of Medicine
Boston, Massachusetts
Common Skin Disorders

William L. Lyons, MD
Assistant Professor
Section of Geriatrics & Gerontology
Department of Internal Medicine
Nebraska Medical Center
Omaha, Nebraska
*The Need for Expertise in Geriatric Medicine in the Care
    of Older Patients; Palliative Care*

Jane Mahoney, MD
Assistant Professor of Medicine, Geriatrics
University of Wisconsin Medical School
Madison, Wisconsin
Falls & Mobility Disorders

Janet McElhaney, MD
Associate Professor
Division of Geriatrics
University of Connecticut Health Center
Farmington, Connecticut
Cancers in the Geriatric Population

Lynn McNicoll, MD, FRCPC
Assistant Professor of Medicine
Brown University School of Medicine
Providence, Rhode Island
Geriatrician
The Miriam Hospital
Providence, Rhode Island
Delirium

David R. Mehr, MD, MS
Associate Professor
Department of Family and Community Medicine
University of Missouri-Columbia School of Medicine
Columbia, Missouri
Prevention and Health Promotion

Barbara J. Messinger-Rapport, MD, PhD
Assistant Professor
Department of Medicine
Case Western Reserve University
Cleveland, Ohio
Attending Physician
Section of Geriatric Medicine
Cleveland Clinic Foundation
Cleveland, Ohio
Hypertension; Special Issues in Women's Health

Swarna Meyyazhagan, MD
Fellow, Section of Geriatric Medicine
Cleveland Clinic Foundation
Cleveland, Ohio
Hypertension

Myron Miller, MD
Professor
Department of Medicine
Division of Endocrinology and Division of Geriatric
    Medicine and Gerontology
Johns Hopkins University School of Medicine
Baltimore, Maryland
Academic Director
Division of Geriatric Medicine
Department of Medicine
Sinai Hospital of Baltimore
Baltimore, Maryland
Endocrine Disorders

John E. Morley, MB, BCh
Dammert Professor of Gerontology
St Louis University Medical School
Director, Geriatric Research Education & Clinical
    Center
St Louis VA Medical Center
St Louis, Missouri
Anti-Aging & Complementary Therapies

Joanne E. Mortimer, MD
Professor of Medicine
Head, Division of Medical Oncology and Hematology
Eastern Virginia Medical School
Medical Director, Sentara Cancer Institute
Norfolk, Virginia
Cancers in the Geriatric Population

Laura Mosqueda, MD
Director of Geriatrics
    and Associate Professor of
    Clinical Family Medicine
University of California, Irvine
College of Medicine
Irvine, California
Principles of Rehabilitation

Mary Norman, MD
Baylor Senior Health Network
Addison, Texas
San Francisco, California
Depression & Other Mental Health Issues

Robert M. Palmer, MD, MPH
Head, Section of Geriatric Medicine
Cleveland Clinic Foundation
Cleveland, Ohio
Continuity of Care

Steven Z. Pantilat, MD
Associate Professor of Medicine
University of California, San Francisco
San Francisco, California
Palliative Care

Peter Pompei, MD
Associate Professor of Medicine
Department of Medicine
Stanford University School of Medicine
Stanford, California
Surgical & Perioperative Care

Michael W. Rich, MD
Associate Professor of Medicine
Washington University School of Medicine
Director, Cardiac Rapid Evaluation Unit
Barnes-Jewish Hospital
St. Louis, Missouri
Cardiac Disease

Richard W. Rissmiller, Jr. MD
Fellow in Pulmonary/Critical Care Medicine
Wake Forest University School of Medicine
Winston-Salem, North Carolina
Respiratory Diseases

David Sengstock, MD
Resident
Geriatric Research Education and Clinical Center
Ann Arbor Veterans Affairs Health System
Ann Arbor, Michigan
Syncope and Dizziness

Ronald I. Shorr, MD, MS
Associate Professor of Preventive Medicine,
University of Tennessee Health Science Center
Memphis, Tennessee
Associate Director, Internal Medicine & Transitional
    Residency Programs
Methodist Healthcare
Memphis, Tennessee
Principles of Drug Therapy

Kaycee M. Sink, MD
Geriatrics Research Fellow
Division of Geriatrics
VA Medical Center
San Francisco, California
Cognitive Impairment & Dementia

Manish Srivastava, MD
Fellow, Section of Geriatric Medicine
Cleveland Clinic Foundation
Cleveland, Ohio
Osteoporosis & Hip Fractures

Stephanie Studenski, MD, MPH
Professor
Division of Geriatrics
Department of Medicine
University of Pittsburgh School of Medicine
Staff Physician, VA Pittsburgh GRECC
Pittsburgh, Pennsylvania
Exercise

Dennis H. Sullivan MD
Director, Geriatric Research Education & Clinical
    Center
Central Arkansas Veterans Health Care System
Professor of Geriatrics & Internal Medicine
University of Arkansas
Little Rock, Arkansas
Nutrition & Failure to Thrive

Mark A. Supiano, MD
Professor of Medicine
Division of Geriatrics
University of Michigan
Director, Geriatric Research Education and Clinical
    Center
Ann Arbor Veterans Affairs Health System
Ann Arbor, Michigan
Syncope and Dizziness

Paul E. Tatum, III, MD
Department of Family and Community Medicine
University of Missouri-Columbia School of Medicine
Columbia, Missouri
Prevention and Health Promotion

Holly L. Thacker, MD, FACP
Director of the Women's Health Center
    at the Gault Women's Health and Breast Pavilion
Departments of Internal Medicine and Obstetrics
    & Gynecology
Cleveland Clinic Foundation
Cleveland, Ohio
Special Issues in Women's Health

David R. Thomas, MD, FAGS, FACP
Division of Geriatric Medicine
Saint Louis University Health Sciences Center
St. Louis, Missouri
Pressure Ulcers

Pearl Toy, MD
Professor
Department of Laboratory Medicine
University of California San Francisco
San Francisco, California
Anemia

Gregg Warshaw, MD
Martha Betty Semmons Professor of Geriatric
    Medicine
Professor of Family Medicine
Director, Office of Geriatric Medicine
University of Cincinnati Medical Cetner
Cincinnati, Ohio
Visual & Hearing Impairment

Mary E. Whooley, MD
Associate Professor
Department of Medicine
University of California, San Francisco
San Francisco, California
Depression & Other Mental Health Issues

B. Gwen Windham, MD
Fellow, Geriatric Medicine & Gerontology
Johns Hopkins University School of Medicine
Baltimore, Maryland
Home Care

Kristine Yaffe, MD
Associate Professor
Departments of Psychiatry, Neurology, and
    Epidemiology
University of California, San Francisco
Chief, Geriatric Psychiatry
San Francisco VA Medical Center
San Francisco, California
Cognitive Impairment and Dementia

Preface

Current Geriatric Diagnosis and Treatment addresses the medical problems that are most common, most serious, or most troublesome to older adults. With the explosion in the number of older adults, especially those age 85 years or older, this information is especially important because most physicians and nurses will spend most of their professional lives caring for older adults. Thus, *Current Geriatrics* presents critical information about cancers, coronary artery disease, and other common diseases as well as the geriatric syndromes such as dementia, delirium, and falls.

Current Geriatrics pays special attention to fundamental principles of late life:

- The physiologic reserve of organ systems diminishes with age.
- Age-related decrease in physiologic reserve has consequences, including: The ability to meet physical, mental, and social challenges often diminishes with age; acute insults to one organ system may precipitate problematic decline in the function of other organ systems; geriatric syndromes such as falls or delirium become more common.
- Neuropsychiatric effects and manifestations of disease often become prominent in older adults, sometimes precipitated by difficult social circumstances and often exacerbating difficulties in social function and living independently.
- Older persons are closer to the end of life than to its beginning, and the goals of care will differ according to personal values and preferences, often focusing more on caring than on cure.
- Care for older persons is provided in several settings from home to long-term care to acute hospital.

Current Geriatrics provides up-to-date, accessible information for patient management that will be useful to those providing medical care to older adults:

- House officers and medical students will find the information they need on call and before rounds for diagnosis and treatment;
- Internists and family physicians will find state-of-the-art reviews and references;
- Nurse practitioners, physician assistants, and nurses will find concise discussions of the broad range of topics they will encounter.

Diagnostic and therapeutic strategies are based on current evidence, with references to recent key articles.

We thank our associate authors for their ground-breaking contributions to this first edition of *Current Geriatrics*. We welcome comments and recommendations for future editions and look forward to advancing medical practice in caring for older adults.

C. Seth Landefeld, MD
Robert M. Palmer, MD, MPH
Mary Anne G. Johnson, MD
C. Bree Johnston, MD, MPH
William Lyons, MD

SECTION I
Approach to the Geriatric Patient

The Need for Expertise in Geriatric Medicine in the Care of Older Patients

1

William L. Lyons, MD, & C. Seth Landefeld, MD

The discipline of geriatric medicine arose in part because aged patients are more complex than they were in middle age, with some extra decades under their belt. Many persons who live long enough become as qualitatively different from younger adults as children are. Yet most health care providers are not taught the principles and perspectives that come into play when caring for the aged.

DIMINISHED PHYSIOLOGICAL RESERVE

The connection between old age and frailty—in its popularly understood sense—is ancient. Older people are predisposed to suffering bad health outcomes, including bothersome symptoms, diminished ability to perform desired tasks and roles, and death. For some, these outcomes result from recurrences or exacerbations of diseases that plagued them earlier in life. For others, they result from serious diseases, such as cancer or cardiovascular disease, which increase in incidence with age. For many older people, the years take a more global toll in reduced vitality and resilience. This reduction in vitality and resilience results in part from a gradual diminution in the maximum capacity of physiological systems: cardiovascular, pulmonary, renal, musculoskeletal, neurological, endocrine, and immune. The rate of decrease in physiological capacity and its time of onset differ among persons, but a decrease is universal at some point after the age of 30. The decrease in physiological capacity may be imperceptible throughout life,

but often physiological capacity falls below a threshold that is noticed. As a result, simple activities of everyday living, such as walking to mail a letter or shopping for groceries, may slow, then become difficult, and eventually require assistance of a device or another person.

One common manifestation of this diminished reserve is the appearance of well-described geriatric syndromes. Because many elders are operating near the capacity of one or more of their weakened physiological systems, even a small event (such as initiation of a new medication or an otherwise mild illness or injury) can generate a system failure. A number of such failures seem to be particularly prevalent—syncope, falls, delirium—perhaps reflecting the systems (cardiovascular, musculoskeletal, and cerebral, respectively) in which humans most commonly run out of reserve.

There are several clinically important consequences of geriatric patients' diminished physiological reserve.

1. Disease presentation in older persons is often atypical. Whereas a 45-year-old with pneumococcal pneumonia may present with complaints of fever, productive cough, and pleurisy, an 85-year-old may, with the same infection, present with acute confusion, or light-headedness and new urinary incontinence.

2. Occam's razor, or the law of diagnostic parsimony, may not apply. The old adage that a single unifying diagnosis will explain all of a patient's clinical findings works much better in the care of

young or middle-aged patients than in the care of frail elders. With many older patients, symptoms and findings precede the crisis that leads to the physician's visit or they coincide in time and are unrelated. Often a crisis is precipitated by an event largely because of the context of contributing comorbid conditions and diminished physiological capacity; for example, a viral upper respiratory infection that would hardly slow a 30-year-old might precipitate ventilatory failure and delirium in an 80-year-old with chronic obstructive pulmonary disease and mild cognitive impairment who lives alone. Clinicians treating elders need to become comfortable with the notion of not "making the diagnosis" and selecting a single therapeutic "magic bullet." Often, when a reasonable search for a single cause has not turned up a clear cause for a new illness episode, it is necessary instead to direct attention and treatment to multiple potential contributing factors. At the risk of overgeneralizing, a provider caring for an elder with syncope is more likely to benefit her by attending to issues of dehydration, polypharmacy, and posture (patterns of assuming upright position) than by ruling out the elusive pulmonary embolus and failing to consider these common issues.

3. Diminished physiological reserve produces weakened compensatory mechanisms, which may otherwise allow a disease to present at an earlier, less severe stage in elders. A case of Graves' disease, which would have produced only mild nervousness in a middle-aged woman, may cause an 80-year-old to become profoundly confused and incapable of caring for herself.

4. Weakened compensatory mechanisms contribute to the slowed recovery from illness seen in many elders.

5. Certain preventive measures (eg, vaccines for influenza or pneumococcal pneumonia or exercise training to prevent falls) are beneficial in many elders because they support focal areas of diminished reserve.

6. Beyond the fact that older patients have more interactions with the health care system (more drugs, more procedures), their weakened reserve puts them at greater risk of iatrogenic injury.

NEUROPSYCHIATRIC CHANGES & THE MIND–BODY INTERACTION

Aging is associated with an increase in the prevalence of serious brain diseases, such as dementia and stroke. More subtle changes in cognition, personality, or mood also seem to occur with the passage of time. Taken together, all of these effects mean the elderly population has a broad spectrum in intellect, outlook, and vitality. The interaction between neuropsychiatric deficits and physical health and function is intrinsic to geriatric practice and is an area of intense gerontological research. A few phenomena seem to be clear. Neuropsychiatric problems are generally associated with (and are probable contributors to) both physical frailty and social isolation, and neuropsychiatric deficits and medical comorbidities have a potent, negative interaction. A demented elder with pneumonia has a far graver prognosis than one with either dementia or pneumonia alone. A reciprocal dynamic of body–mind frailty is at play as well. Mood and cognition are both influenced by physical illness (eg, depression arises commonly in the wake of myocardial infarction), and the strength of the interaction may be greater in the older population.

CLOSER TO THE END THAN THE BEGINNING

The fact that elderly persons are closer to the end of life than are the young has several implications for providers of geriatric care. At a practical level, this influences medical decisions, such as whether to replace a native cardiac valve with a bioprosthetic or a longer lived mechanical valve and when to cease screening for colon cancer. More broadly, the later stages of life may bring with them a change in a patient's goals for health care. Younger patients usually seek cure of disease and prolongation of life. Many elders seek the same, but a substantial number place greater emphasis on comfort, function, and the ability to live independently. Experienced providers of geriatric care learn to engage their patients in goals-of-care discussions, a skill less called for in the care of younger individuals.

MULTIPLE VENUES OF HEALTH CARE

Because of the great variety of elders' health needs, functional deficits, social supports, and goals of care, professional services for this group are provided in more settings than with any other population. Familiarity with the capabilities, characteristics, strengths, and weaknesses of local clinics, acute hospitals, rehabilitation hospitals, skilled nursing facilities, residential care facilities, geropsychiatric units, hospices, and home care agencies will assist the clinician in caring for older patients. It is not unusual for a frail elder to pass through a number of these venues during a single illness episode. Negotiating the transitions between venues of care is an essential part of geriatric health care.

THE IMPORTANCE OF MONEY & FAMILY

Finally, although everybody needs financial reserves and a loving family or friends, these are particularly precious resources for the health of elders. Many elders come to medical attention because of some combination of economic constraints and social isolation. The cost of medications, professional services, and personal help increases with age for many people, whereas incomes do not, leading to a financial imbalance that impoverishes some older persons and forces many to neglect some needs to pay for others. Without assistance from concerned others, getting to grocery stores, pharmacies, and physician appointments may become impossible. With older patients, the key to diagnosis and treatment in a difficult situation often lies in the social history.

Covinsky KE et al: Relation between symptoms of depression and health status outcomes in acutely ill hospitalized older persons. Ann Intern Med 1997;126:417. [PMID: 9072926] (Depressive symptoms slowed functional recovery from an acute illness, illustrating the synergistic effects of neuropsychiatric impairment and medical illness.)

Mahoney JE et al: Problems of older adults living alone after hospitalization. J Gen Intern Med 2000;15:611. [PMID: 11029674] (Older persons who live alone and receive home nursing after hospitalization were less likely to improve in function, and more likely to be institutionalized, than those who live with others.)

Resnick NM, Marcantonio ER: How should clinical care of the aged differ? Lancet 1997;350:1157. [PMID: 9343575] (Overview of differences required in approaching the elderly patient.)

Rosenfeld KE et al: End-of-life decision making: A qualitative study of elderly individuals. J Gen Intern Med 2000;15:620. [PMID: not available] (Discussions with elderly about advance directives and goals of care should focus on valued life activities and acceptable health status rather than specific medical interventions.)

Sands LP et al: Cognitive screening identifies trajectories of functional recovery from admission to three months after discharge in hospitalized elders. J Gerontol A Biol Sci Med Sci 2003;58:37. [PMID: 12560409] (Cognitive impairment slowed functional recovery from an acute illness, illustrating the synergistic effects of neuropsychiatric impairment and medical illness.)

Tinetti ME et al: Dizziness among older patients: A possible geriatric syndrome. Ann Intern Med 2000;132:337. [PMID: 10691583] (Dizziness was associated with predisposing characteristics and precipitating situational factors and is illustrative of other multifactorial geriatric syndromes.)

Continuity of Care

Robert M. Palmer, MD, MPH

The plan of care provided by primary care physicians and practitioners (PCPs) is becoming more challenging as the population ages and patients move across living situations, ranging from independent living to nursing home residence. Currently, about 13% of the American population is 65 years of age and older. By 2030 that percentage is expected to approach 22%. Primary care practice will be increasingly geriatric practice.

By convention, *elderly* is defined as being 65 years of age or older. However, this definition encompasses a range of ages spanning 5 decades and fails to consider the heterogeneity in the rate of aging and the incidence of chronic age-related diseases in the elderly population. PCPs who guide older patients through the process of care need to appreciate the differences in goals of medical therapy as elderly patients age and their site of care changes. Even as patients receive the medical care of specialists in outpatient or hospital settings, the PCP remains at the center of the care plan, helping to coordinate the complex, often conflicting recommendations of medical and other health professionals. The PCP helps sort out the major issues confronting the patient, helps the patient and family make important decisions about the scope and aggressiveness of medical care, and offers supportive reassurance to patients and their families through frequent office or hospital visits or telephone communication.

THE CARE PROCESS

The care process begins with the first encounter between the PCP and the older patient, most often in the outpatient setting. The first encounter establishes the rapport between physician and patient, creating a sense of trust and confidence on the part of the patient. That rapport is strengthened by the continuity of care provided by the PCP, who helps the older patient adapt to chronic illness, recover from acute and curable diseases, or move to a new living situation.

Manton KG, Gu X: Changes in the prevalence of chronic disability in the United States black and nonblack population above age 65 from 1982 to 1999. Proc Natl Acad Sci USA 2001;98:6354. [PMID: 11344275] (National surveys conducted over the past 3 decades show that the rate of physical disability measured in terms of independent performance of ADL is gradually decreasing.)

HEALTH CARE-RELATED CHOICES

As patients age, there is a transition in the health care, from primary prevention and curative interventions to secondary prevention and chronic disease management. However, the opportunities to delay or prevent physical disability, illness, and functional decline (loss of independent performance of ADLs), through detection of risk and implementation of effective interventions, never cease. Greater collaboration with allied health professionals and family caregivers is justified.

Personal Values

To establish goals of medical care with older patients, PCPs should understand the patient's personal values, health care expectations, and priorities. Discussions with family members, at the discretion of the patient, can be the source of substantial enlightenment regarding the patient's values.

Although the fear of death may be great, some older persons have a greater fear of loss of autonomy resulting from physical disability and of becoming a financial, emotional, or physical burden to their families. Others, however, may value life extension at any cost, even over quality of life and degree of suffering. Insight into the patients' values is gained through discussion regarding patients' perceptions about the quality of life they have and seek. For example, what priorities do they hold most dear? How important are religious beliefs in the decision to pursue or forgo medical care? How important are the wishes and interests of family members or close friends? Older patients will often define their values primarily in the context of what is perceived to be the best decisions for their family members, especially when issues of finances or caregiving are involved.

Values change over time, so periodic discussions with the patient are advisable. Even when it appears that patients lack specific goals for medical care, they can be asked what events or activities make living important or worthwhile, thereby serving as incentives for recovery and living.

Patients' values extend to their expectations for each health care encounter. Open-ended questions directed to patients give them license to discuss nonmedical issues such as personal losses or worries that might be of a sensitive nature and otherwise left unrevealed.

Physician Recommendations

The PCP needs to update medical information to make the most accurate diagnoses and to offer the soundest advice. Laboratory and diagnostic studies are obtained and reviewed, and recommendations made in the context of each patient's value system.

A geriatric assessment should be performed so that the physician can objectively evaluate the patient. A geriatric assessment helps to catalogue the medical, psychosocial, and environmental factors that affect health and level of functioning. Medical diagnoses are catalogued and updated on the patient's problem list.

In the care process, periodic review of the patient's functional status is useful, with a focus on changes in domains of health: performance of basic ADLs and IADLs; cognition; gait and mobility, including recent falls; nutritional status (weight loss of > 10 lb in 6 mo); social supports; and living situation. A change in functional status indicates a significant decline in general health or the potential for further decline and signifies the need for further investigation and perhaps closer medical follow-up. Diagnostic investigations must be undertaken in consideration of the patient's ability and willingness to undergo difficult or discomforting diagnostic studies. For example, in pursuing a workup for gastrointestinal bleeding, the patient might be too physically frail to undergo colonoscopy. A more cautious course of evaluation is justified. In contrast, when an otherwise high-functioning patient expresses a desire for an aggressive evaluation, the PCP again serves as a patient advocate to pursue the subspecialty consultation.

Negotiating Choices

Patients' judgments regarding whether to proceed with interventions are based on the degree of accurate information they receive and are often influenced by the opinions of their family members. Differences in opinions among patients, families, and physicians are common and can be resolved through a process of negotiation. Contingencies are created with explicit time frames for assessing the patient's decision. For example, if the patient refuses colonoscopy for evaluation of occult blood loss, the option of a less invasive procedure is given (eg, checking for occult blood on several more samples of stool and performing frequent blood counts to detect anemia). The overall strategy is reviewed and modified. If the reluctant patient continues to have occult gastrointestinal bleeding, the contingency plan might change to include colonoscopy without proceeding to more invasive therapies unless there is a risk of bowel obstruction resulting from carcinoma. This decision is documented in the PCP's record and is transmitted to specialists involved in the patient's care. The outcome (eg, a negative colonoscopy) is reviewed and issues of further evaluation (upper endoscopy) are considered. Although this process of recommending a course of diagnosis, negotiation, and agreement on strategy is lengthy, it can be carried out over the course of several office visits and reviewed and updated during office visits scheduled for other purposes (eg, blood pressure checks or immunizations).

CHANGING GOALS & OBJECTIVES

The goal of patient care is to prevent disease and disability and help aging patients enjoy optimal quality of life. The objectives of patient care change with advancing age. In part, they are influenced by the patient's additional years of life expectancy, functional status and level of physical disability, and presence of ultimately fatal diseases.

Young–Old

For the young–old, the goals of therapy are somewhat similar to those for middle-aged patients. For example, the average 65-year-old American woman has an additional life expectancy of about 19 years, thereby justifying a medical approach that focuses on primary prevention of diseases, screening, and detection of diseases in early and treatable stages. Because the young–old have a low rate of disability, the preservation of physical independence is given a high priority. Hence, medical priorities include weight loss for overweight patients, especially those with cardiovascular risk factors, and regular and sustained programs of endurance and resistive exercises. Aggressive diagnostic investigations and interventions are offered to older patients as they would be to middle-aged patients.

Old–Old

As patients' age, additional years of life expectancy decline and influence the degree of aggressiveness of diagnostic and therapeutic actions and hence the goals of therapy. For the old–old, the goals of therapy become influenced by the occurrence of chronic and ultimately disabling or fatal diseases, such as Alzheimer's disease. Increasingly, more consideration is given to quality of life issues (largely determined by functional status) in the finite remaining years. However, aggressive efforts are warranted to prevent functional disability and treat chronic diseases. Evidence is growing that the old–old benefit from medical treatments for hypertension, coronary artery disease, and osteoporosis. Falls are potentially preventable for these at-risk patients.

Very–Old

For the very old, a more cautious approach is best considered before embarking on extensive testing or aggressive interventions. Decisions must weigh the benefits against the discomforts or harm of diagnostic studies and therapies. For example, chronic hemodialysis and renal transplantation are increasingly being offered to elderly patients. These approaches might be appropriate for older patients whose functional status would be greatly improved with the therapy but not for those with a guarded prognosis as a result of severe comorbid conditions (eg, advanced Alzheimer's disease). By age 85 the average woman has an additional life expectancy of ~6 more years, the average man 5 years. It becomes more difficult for the PCP to justify screening tests and therapeutic interventions that might have limited use. One analysis that examined the role of cancer screening in older patients found substantial variability in the likelihood of benefit for patients of similar ages with varying life expectancies. Those with life expectancies of < 5 years are unlikely to derive any survival benefit from cancer screening. In fact, there is a likelihood of potential harm (ie, by detecting cancers that would never have become clinically significant and implementing treatment).

Walter LC, Covinsky KE: Cancer screening in elderly patients: A framework for individualized decision making. JAMA 2001; 285:2750. [PMID: 11386931] (Framework for guiding physicians and elderly patients to more informed cancer screening decisions by detailing the benefits and harms that need to be weighed when making screening decisions.)

ADVANCE CARE PLANNING

The PCP is in the pivotal position of helping patients plan their future care. In particular, physicians can promote earlier patient–physician discussions about end-of-life care preferences and the completion of advance directives. The discussions, often held before or during a patient's transition in living situation or general health, include sensitive issues such as the patient's wishes for end-of-life care (eg, cardiopulmonary resuscitation, intensive care, ventilator support) and nutritional support during acute or end-stage illness. In the event of end-of-life care, one should review the goals of continuing care, including palliation, comfort measures, and the role of hospice.

Advance directives, health care proxies, and living wills permit patients to make decisions regarding their health care, to be implemented when the patient becomes incapacitated. A living will explicitly addresses the actual treatment preferences of a competent adult. It specifies the use, withholding, or withdrawal of life-sustaining treatments if the individual loses the capacity to make such decisions because of terminal illness or permanently unconscious state. Comfort care measures are continued in these states. The durable power of attorney for health care designates surrogate health care decision-makers if the person becomes incapacitated. The designated agent is allowed to act on the person's behalf in making decisions regarding medical care, including the withdrawal of nutritional support or other treatments in the event of a terminal illness or permanently unconscious state. State laws vary in terms of content and portability of the durable power of attorney for health care. Incompetent patients who lack next of kin or power of attorney for health care require guardianship.

Advance directives, although desirable, do not always reflect the wishes of the patient during a moment of crisis. Even in the face of terminal illness, many patients, their families, or physicians insist on aggressive interventions for critical illness, suggesting that these decisions need to be decided before the incident critical illness or at least early in the course of the illness.

Miller DL, Bolla LR: Patient values: the guide to medical decision making. Clin Geriatr Med 1998;14:813. [PMID: 9799481] (Advance directives express a patient's preferences regarding end-of-life care and are used to guide medical treatment. Patients who lack decision-making capacity require appropriate surrogate involvement.)

Crawley LM et al: Strategies for culturally effective end-of-life care. Ann Intern Med 2002;136:673. [PMID: 11992303] (Physicians should assess the cultural background of each patient and inquire about values that may affect end-of-life care.)

Hruby M et al: How do patients view the role of the primary care physician in inpatient care? Am J Med 2001;111:21S. [PMID: 11790364] (Patients under the care of an inpatient physician desire contact with their PCP and good communication between the PCP and hospital physicians.)

RELEVANT WORLD WIDE WEB SITES

Alzheimer's Association: www.alz.org

Caregiver resources: www.caregiver911.com

National Association of Area Agency on Aging: www.n4a.org

National Family Caregivers Association: www.nfcacares.org

National Safety Council: www.nsc.org

Senior Scope: www.seniorscope.com

U.S. Department of Health and Human Services, Administration on Aging: www.aoa.dhhs.gov

Prevention & Health Promotion

Paul E. Tatum III, MD, & David R. Mehr, MD, MS

■ PREVENTIVE SERVICES

Even in the very elderly, preventive interventions can limit disease and disability. However, selecting appropriate interventions requires consideration of life expectancy and care goals. Preventive interventions are typically categorized as primary, secondary, or tertiary. Primary prevention refers to prevention of disease (eg, immunizations); secondary prevention is the early detection of disease before it becomes symptomatic (eg, mammography to detect early breast cancer); and tertiary prevention refers to activities to optimize health once disease is already detected.

Since the 1980s both the U.S. Preventive Services Task Force (USPSTF) and the Canadian Task Force on Preventive Health Care have provided evidence-based scientific reviews of preventive health services to guide primary care decision making. The fundamental standard applied by the task force is whether the intervention leads to improved health outcomes (eg, reduced disease-specific morbidity or mortality). For screening, tests must be able to detect the condition or risk factor earlier than without screening and without excessive false-positive or false-negative results, and early intervention must be superior to waiting until patients manifest signs or symptoms of disease. For counseling interventions, there must be evidence that changing behavior reduces risk and that counseling to reduce risk is effective in changing behavior. Immunizations must exhibit biologic efficacy, and chemoprophylactic agents must demonstrate both biological efficacy and evidence that patients will comply with use of the drug. For each proposed preventive service, the USPSTF rates the evidence for and against the intervention and provides recommendations based on the weight of the evidence (Table 3–1). In its current approach, the USPSTF separates insufficient evidence from a rating of small benefit. High-quality evidence is very limited for interventions in the elderly population.

Harris RP et al: Current methods of the U.S. Preventive Services Task Force: A review of the process. Am J Prev Med 2001; 20(3S):21. [PMID: 11306229]

Canadian Task Force on Preventive Health Care: Evidence-Based Clinical Prevention. http://www.ctfphc.org

Centers for Disease Control: National Prevention Information Network. http://www.cdcnpin.org

U.S. Preventive Services Task Force: www.ahrq.gov/clinic/uspstfix.htm

■ SCREENING ISSUES FOR THE GERIATRIC PATIENT

The standard approach to evaluating preventive services is more difficult for older people. Many important screening studies have excluded those older than 65 or 70. However, beyond the standard evaluation of preventive services, 2 additional issues assume major importance in evaluating preventive interventions for elderly persons: (1) individual and family values regarding the value of life extension in old age and (2) the effect of limited life expectancy on the usual risk–benefit considerations. Many recommendations concerning preventive geriatrics have suffered from lumping together all elderly people instead of recognizing their distinctions. As individuals move from health to disability, the goals of prevention in many cases will change from life extension to improving quality of life in the near term.

A framework for individualized decision making for cancer screening in elderly patients is shown in Table 3–2. This framework applies more generally to screening when life extension is the primary outcome of interest. The framework can be applied after the individual's life expectancy is estimated. Rather than using the average life expectancy for a given age, the patient's health status should also be incorporated into the prediction (Figure 3–1). Patients with a number of comorbid conditions or functional impairments may have a life expectancy that is lower than average for their age, whereas those without any significant comorbidity or functional impairment may live longer than average. The risk of experiencing the condition and the potential benefit from screening can be weighed against the potential harms.

Table 3–1. Strength of recommendation from the USPSTF.

Evidence quality	Net benefit			
	Substantial	Moderate	Small	Zero/negative
Good	A	B	C	D
Fair	B	B	C	D
Poor	I	I	I	I

A: strong recommendation to provide service; B: recommendation to provide service; C: no recommendation for or against provision of service; D: recommendation against providing service; I: insufficient evidence to make recommendation.
Adapted from U.S. Preventive Services Task Force: Current Methods of the U.S. Preventive Services Task Force: A review of the process. Am J Prev Med 2001;20(3S):21.

Screening decisions need to incorporate patients' values and preferences. In general, prevention efforts should be aimed at increasing the percentage of life that is lived in good health rather than prolonging time spent in poor health. However, individual values will differ regarding the extent to which these considerations apply. Therefore, deciding when to discontinue specific interventions, such as cancer screening, requires individual discussion of potential benefits and risks, including the possibility of invasive follow-up tests and treatment-related morbidity or even mortality. The Ethics Committee of the American Geriatric Society (AGS) has issued useful guidelines that highlight the importance of individualizing care decisions.

Walter LC, Covinsky KE: Cancer screening in elderly patients: a framework for individualized decision making. JAMA 2001;285:2750. [PMID: 11386931]

American Geriatric Society Ethics Committee: Health Screening Decisions for Older Adults. http://www.americangeriatrics .org/products/positionpapers/stopscreening.shtml

Table 3–2. Steps to individualize decision making for screening tests.

1. Estimate the individual's life expectancy.
2. Estimate the risk of dying from the condition.
3. Determine the potential benefit of screening.
4. Weigh the direct and indirect harms of screening.
5. Assess the patient's values and preferences.

Adapted from Walter LC, Covinsky KE: Cancer screening in elderly patients: A framework for individualized decision making. JAMA 2001;285:2750. Used with permission.

■ SCREENING & TREATMENT

CARDIOVASCULAR DISEASE

Modifiable risk factors for cardiovascular disease include cholesterol levels, hypertension, tobacco use, diabetes, obesity, and physical inactivity.

Hyperlipidemia

As with younger patients, excellent evidence supports treating hyperlipidemia in even very elderly patients with known coronary disease. Systematic reviews of secondary prevention trials have shown 25–30% reductions in 5-year coronary disease outcomes in elderly patients. Although the evidence for specific treatment goals is much less robust, the Third Report of the National Cholesterol Education Program (ATP III) recommends that the goal for patients with coronary artery disease should be a low-density lipoprotein (LDL) cholesterol level < 100 mg/dL.

Limited direct evidence exists regarding the benefits and disadvantages of screening and treating patients older than 65 years who do not have coronary artery disease. The ATP III states that older persons who are at higher risk but otherwise in good health are candidates for cholesterol-lowering therapy. The USPSTF indicated that evidence favors continued screening in older persons. The USPSTF recommended that screening incorporate some assessment of overall coronary disease risk (eg, Framingham or ATP III risk models) and that treatment be based on at least 2 measurements. This recommendation appears sound at least for those 65–75 years old and even older individuals with reasonable life expectancy at higher risk for coronary disease (eg, smokers, hypertensives, diabetics). Examination of cholesterol levels every 5 years may be reasonable if the patient desires. For very elderly individuals, physicians will need to carefully weigh life expectancy and care goals in deciding whether dietary or drug treatment for hyperlipidemia outweighs potential risks. Dietary restriction should be avoided in those at risk for undernutrition.

Statin drugs are generally well tolerated. However, rhabdomyolysis, the most serious side effect of statins, is commonly the result of drug interactions rather than a specific response to the drug itself. Therefore, care must be exercised when prescribing statins for elderly patients taking multiple drugs.

LaRosa JC et al: Effect of statins on risk of coronary disease: A meta-analysis of randomized controlled trials. JAMA 1999; 282:2340. [PMID: 10612322]

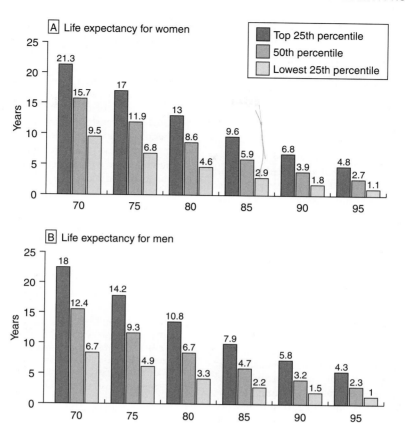

Figure 3–1. Life expectancy by age. From Walter LC, Covinsky KE: Cancer screening in elderly patients: a framework for individualized decision making. JAMA 2001;285:2750. Used with permission.

Pignone MP et al: Screening and treating adults for lipid disorders. Am J Prev Med 2001;20(3S):77. [PMID: 113-6236]

Hypertension

A systematic review demonstrated the benefits of detecting and treating systolic and diastolic hypertension in individuals 60–80 years of age. One cardiovascular death was prevented for every 50 hypertensive elders treated over 5 years, and total cardiovascular morbidity and mortality was reduced 5.2% (number needed to treat = 19). Although the specific data supported treatment of blood pressures above 90 mm Hg diastolic and 160 mm Hg systolic, risk from hypertension at all ages is probably continuous. In view of this, Report 7 of the Joint National Commission on Detection, Evaluation, and Treatment of High Blood Pressure recommends that the upper limit of 140 mm Hg for systolic blood pressure be used for the elderly. Little evidence exists regarding treatment of hypertension in those older than 80. Some observational data even suggest that high blood pressures may be better than low blood pressures in the very old. Clearly, in the very old, particularly those with multiple comorbidities, hypertension should be treated cautiously to avoid such complications as orthostatic hypertension, which may contribute to falls. Nonetheless, all elders who are candidates for active medical treatment should undergo periodic screening for hypertension. The optimal interval for screening has not been determined.

Mulrow C et al: Pharmacotherapy for hypertension in the elderly (Cochrane Review). In: The Cochrane Library, Issue 2 ed. Update Software, 2003.

Satish S et al: The relationship between blood pressure and mortality in the oldest old. J Am Geriatr Soc 2001;49:367. [PMID: 11347778]

CANCER

Breast Cancer

Strategies to prevent breast cancer include self-breast exam, clinical breast exam, and screening mammography. The USPSTF gives both self-breast examination and clinical breast examination alone an "I" rating (see Table 3–1) and mammogram screening for women older than 40 a "B" rating. The USPSTF concluded that, because the risk of breast cancer was high after age 70, the evidence from randomized controlled trials was generalizable to older women. Others have suggested that women with 5 years of life expectancy may be reasonable candidates for continued screening. However, patients' preferences, physicians' judgment, and concurrent illnesses should be major considerations in determining whether or not to screen. Elderly women in whom breast cancer develops and who have 3 or more comorbid conditions, such as cancer, hypertension, diabetes, stroke, or coronary artery disease, are 20 times more likely to die from a cause other than breast cancer over a 3-year period. Screening elderly women with multiple comorbidities may thus cause an undue burden.

Women who have moderate to high risk factors or who are very concerned about the development of breast cancer may choose to continue screening after age 75 or 80. Those who are unwilling to suffer the potential negative consequences might choose to stop screening earlier despite a possibly increased risk of dying from breast cancer.

Parnes BL et al: When should we stop mammography screening for breast cancer in elderly women? J Fam Pract 2001;50:110. [PMID: 11219555]

U.S. Preventive Services Task Force: Screening for breast cancer: recommendations and rationale: http://www.ahrq.gov/clinic/3rduspstf/breastcancer/brcanrr.htm

Colorectal Carcinoma

Colorectal cancer incidence approximately doubles each decade from age 40 to 80, thereby justifying screening considerations in older patients. Consensus favors colorectal cancer screening beginning at age 50 for average-risk individuals, although there is less agreement on when to conclude screening. The USPSTF strongly recommends some form of colorectal cancer but does not make a firm recommendation on the specific approach. The American Cancer Society (ACS) has endorsed guidelines recommending either of the following for average-risk patients: (1) total colon examinations (air-contrast barium enema or colonoscopy) every 10 years or (2) annual fecal occult blood tests and flexible sigmoidoscopy every 5 years.

Strong evidence supports fecal occult blood testing's effectiveness in preventing colorectal cancer mortality. Annual examinations provide higher rates of detection but also more false positives. Weaker evidence (several case-controlled studies) supports sigmoidoscopy, and a single case-control study and indirect evidence suggest the effectiveness of colonoscopy. Taking into account the usual slow transformation of polyps into cancers, elderly adults may not live long enough to achieve any screening benefits. Therefore, unless there is a history of carcinoma, those with several endoscopic examinations may be able to discontinue screening between ages 75 and 80 unless they are unusually healthy.

Risks of screening include discomfort and complications from endoscopic examinations (eg, perforation or hemorrhage). These may also occur from follow-up of the many false-positive results of fecal occult blood testing.

Rudy DR, Zdon MJ: Update on colorectal cancer. Am Fam Phys 2000;61:1759. [10750881]

Tatum P, Mehr D: At what age can colorectal cancer screening stop? J Fam Pract 2001;50:575. [PMID: 11485702]

Towler BP et al: Screening for colorectal cancer using the faecal occult blood test, Hemoccult (Cochrane Review). In: The Cochrane Library, Issue 2 ed. Update Software, 2003.

U.S. Preventive Services Task Force: Screening for colorectal cancer: recommendations and rationale: www.ahrq.gov/clinic/3rduspstf/colorr.htm.

Cervical Cancer

Most cervical cancer in the elderly occurs because of inadequate screening. For that reason, most women who have had repeatedly normal smears probably do not need to continue Pap smears indefinitely. The USPSTF recommends ceasing screening at age 65 in women who have had adequate recent screening with pap smears and are otherwise not at high risk for cervical cancer. The AGS recommends screening until at least age 70 but indicates that little evidence exists for or against screening after this age. However, the AGS does recommend that any older woman of any age who has never had a Pap smear be screened until she has 2 negative pap smears 1 year apart. Additionally, a history of multiple sexual partners presumably remains a risk factor in old age. Older women who begin new sexual relationships might benefit from at least temporary resumption of screening. Women who had a hysterectomy for a nonmalignant indication may also stop having Pap smears if no cervical tissue remains.

The follow-up of an abnormal Pap smear is an area of some controversy, but the American Society for Colposcopy and Cervical Pathology 2001 Consensus Guidelines for the management of women with cervical cytologic abnormalities serves as a useful reference. Postmenopausal women with atypical squamous cells of uncertain significance (ASC-US) have a lower incidence of cervical intraepithelial neoplasia grades 2 and 3 than younger women. Providing a course of intravaginal estrogen and repeating a Pap smear 1 week after completing the estrogen is a reasonable option for ASC-US follow-up, with a repeat test at 4–6 mo. Negative Pap smears may indicate that normal surveillance can be resumed, but if the repeat screen remains ASC-US colposcopy should be performed. A course of intravaginal estrogen followed by a repeat Pap smear is also a reasonable approach to treatment of postmenopausal women with a low-grade squamous intraepithelial lesion. In contrast, women with atypical glandular cells not otherwise specified (AGC-NOS) have a substantial risk for cervical neoplasia, and colposcopy with endocervical sampling is recommended. If atypical endometrial cells are present, the patient should have endometrial biopsy. Women with high-grade squamous intraepithelial lesions should have colposcopy and endocervical sampling.

American Geriatric Society: Screening for cervical carcinoma in older women. J Am Geriatr Soc 2001;49:655. [11380762]

Sawaya GF: Positive predictive value of cervical smears in previously screened postmenopausal women: The Heart and Estrogen/Progestin Replacement Study (HERS). Ann Intern Med 2000;133:942. [PMID: 11119395]

Videlefsky A et al: Routine vaginal cuff smear testing in post-hysterectomy patients with benign uterine conditions: When is it indicated? J Am Board Fam Pract 2000;13(4):233. [PMID: 10933286]

Wright TC et al: Consensus statement: 2001 consensus guidelines for the management of women with cervical cytological abnormalities. JAMA 2002;287:2120. [PMID: 11966387]

U.S. Preventive Services Task Force: Screening for cervical cancer: www.ahrq.gov/clinic/3rduspstf/cervicalcan/cervcanrr.htm

Prostate Cancer

Screening tests for prostate cancer are among the most controversial potential preventive services. Prostate-specific antigen (PSA) testing can detect early-stage cancers, but whether a screening program will result in better or worse overall health outcomes is not clear. Furthermore, screening for prostate cancer is associated with important harms, including frequent false-positive results and complications of treatment for some cancers that might never have affected a patient's health. Although no major organization recommends universal screening, there are clearly marked differences in enthusiasm. The USPSTF in its most recent recommendations (2002) states that information is insufficient to recommend for or against routine screening (Recommendation I). They further indicate, "Given the uncertainties and controversy surrounding prostate cancer screening, clinicians should not order the PSA test without first discussing with the patient the potential but uncertain benefits and the possible harms of prostate cancer screening." In contrast, the ACS recommends offering screening with digital rectal exam and PSA testing. They recommend discussion about the "benefits and limitations of testing. In elderly men, the screening controversy is particularly important because of both the smaller potential time of life remaining to benefit and the increased prevalence of histological cancer of the prostate with age. Furthermore, prostate cancer screening is associated with significant risks to quality of life in older men. For every 100 men undergoing a PSA, 10 will have an abnormal result, but only 3 of the 10 will actually have cancer. For those undergoing treatment for prostate cancer, about 50% will have significant side effects, including impotence, urinary incontinence, and rectal injury.

Since 1997, the ACS has recommended that screening be continued annually as long as men have a 10-year life expectancy. The 10-year life expectancy is a reasonable time to stop screening if one chooses to screen at all. For many men, this will occur by age 75 (see Figure 3–1). Because of the uncertainty, the importance of shared decision making between patients and physicians has been emphasized to enable patients to make informed decisions about screening based on the risks and benefits. A discussion tool kit available from the American Academy of Family Physicians (AAFP) may be a useful adjunct.

Gambert SR: Prostate cancer: when to offer screening in the primary care setting. Geriatrics 2000;56:22. [PMID: 11196336]

Smith RA: American Cancer Society guidelines for the early detection of cancer: Update of early detection guidelines for prostate, colorectal, and endometrial cancers. CA Cancer J Clin 2001;51:38. [PMID: 11577479]

American Academy of Family Physicians: Prostate cancer screening counseling tools: www.aafp.org/x19519.xml

U.S. Preventive Services Task Force: Screening for prostate cancer: recommendations and rationale: www.ahrq.gov/clinic/3rduspstf/prostatescr/prostaterr.htm

Lung Cancer

The USPSTF, ACS, and AAFP recommend against screening for lung cancer with routine chest radiographs or sputum cytologies. Low-dose computed tomography screening can identify smaller nodules than routine chest radiographs; however, as with prior screening interventions, the key issue is whether screening will reduce mortality. For that reason, the Society of Thoracic Radiology does not recommend mass screening for lung cancer. Prevention efforts should still focus on encouraging older smokers to quit.

Aberle DR et al: A consensus statement of the Society of Thoracic Radiology: Screening for lung cancer with helical computed tomography. J Thorac Imaging 2001;16:65. [PMID: 11149694]

Patz EF et al: Current concepts: Screening for lung cancer. N Engl J Med 2000;343:1627. [PMID: 11096172]

Skin Cancer

The ACS recommends an annual total body skin examination for all individuals older than 40. Alternatively, the USPSTF concluded that there is insufficient evidence for or against routine screening for skin cancer (Recommendation I) but urges clinicians to remain alert for skin lesions with malignant features: rapidly changing lesions and those with asymmetry, border irregularity, color variability, or a diameter > 6 mm.

Helfand M et al: Screening for skin cancer. Am J Prev Med 2001; 20(3S):47. [PMID: not available]

Jerant AF et al: Early detection and treatment of skin cancer. Am Fam Physician 2000;62:357. [PMID: 10929700]

Ovarian Cancer

The ACS recommends annual pelvic examinations to screen for ovarian cancer despite a lack of evidence of any improvement in outcome with any screening method (pelvic examination, ultrasonogram, or serum tumor markers). The American College of Obstetrics and Gynecology Committee on Gynecologic Practice makes no specific recommendations for ovarian cancer screening. Even in the elderly, most women with positive screening tests will not have ovarian cancer but will require invasive studies (eg, laparoscopy) for confirmation. The USPSTF and several other organizations recommend against screening. Routine screening for ovarian cancer in an asymptomatic population is not recommended.

American College of Obstetricians and Gynecologists Committee on Gynecologic Practice: Routine cancer screening. ACOG Committee Opinion 2000;247:1. [PMID: not available]

DIABETES MELLITUS

Despite the known complications of diabetes and the proven benefits of interventions to control blood sugar, there is no direct evidence of the benefit of early identification of diabetes in elderly people. The American Diabetes Association recommends screening every 3 years with a fasting blood sugar in all patients older than 45 and suggests a fasting sugar of 126 as the threshold for a diagnosis of diabetes. A 1998 cost-effectiveness analysis from the Centers for Disease Control estimated potential screening benefits. For those older than 65, earlier identification had minimal effect on reducing renal disease or blindness and produced no increase in life years or quality-adjusted life years. According to the USPSTF, insufficient evidence exists to recommend for or against screening the general population. However, in a recent update, the USPSTF recommends screening for diabetes mellitus in adults with hypertension or hyperlipidemia because treatment goals for those conditions might be altered with the additional diagnosis. Clinicians additionally might choose to screen older individuals at particularly high risk for diabetes mellitus, notably obese patients, with a fasting serum glucose. Potential benefits will clearly decline with age; thus, screening those older than 75 or 80 years has very limited potential for benefit.

THYROID DISORDERS

Hypothyroidism may be difficult to detect clinically in older people and is common in older women. It may cause significant functional impairment, such as fatigue and constipation, as well as elevations in cholesterol and weight gain. In 1998, the American College of Physicians issued a clinical guideline that recommended screening asymptomatic women older than 50 for occult thyroid disease. The authors of the evidence review concluded that 1 case of overt thyroid disease is found for every 71 women screened who are older than 60. The preferred screening test is a sensitive thyroid-stimulating hormone (TSH) level. Follow-up free thyroxine (free T_4) is indicated when the TSH is undetectable or > 10 mU/L. For older men and women, a wide range of problems should prompt diagnostic testing, but this is a separate issue from routinely screening asymptomatic patients.

Insufficient data exist to recommend for or against treatment of subclinical hypothyroidism (elevated TSH with normal free T_4) or subclinical hyperthyroidism (undetectable TSH with normal free T_4 and normal triiodothyronine [T_3]). In general, subclinical hypothyroidism progresses to overt hypothyroidism at the rate of about 2–3% per year. Treating subclinical hypothyroidism may prevent this progression, reduce serum lipids, and reverse subtle symptoms of mild hypothyroidism. However, treatment requires continued medication at some cost and may cause iatrogenic hyperthyroidism. Treating subclinical hyperthyroidism may reduce atrial fibrillation and osteoporosis; however, over a 10-year period only one third of patients will experience atrial fibrillation, whereas two thirds will remain in sinus rhythm.

Cooper DS: Clinical practice. Subclinical hypothyroidism. N Engl J Med 2001;345:260. [PMID: 21342639]

Toft AD: Clinical practice. Subclinical hyperthyroidism. N Engl J Med 2001;345:512. [PMID: 21396742]

SENSORY DISORDERS

Vision Impairment

The USPSTF recommends visual acuity screening with a Snellen chart or other method for all elderly people; however, they conclude that there is insufficient evidence to recommend for or against routine fundoscopy or glaucoma screening by primary physicians. Primary physicians may want to consider periodic referral to vision care specialists for glaucoma screening.

Hearing Impairment

Elderly people should be questioned about their hearing; otoscopy and audiometric testing should be performed on those who indicate problems. Alternatives include structured questionnaires and screening audiometry with an instrument such as the Welch Allyn AudioScope. Although it is clear that physicians should do some form of hearing screening, the optimum approach is unsettled.

■ HEALTH PROMOTION

Common behavioral activities that relate to health include smoking cessation, healthy diet, regular physical activity, and appropriate alcohol use. Appropriate behavioral counseling interventions to cover these issues differ from screening interventions because they address complex behavior related to daily living; require repeated action; need to be modified over time; and are influenced by multiple spheres of influence, including family, peers, and community. However, many barriers prevent effective delivery of behavioral interventions, including focus on medically urgent issues, lack of time, inadequate training, low patient demand, and lack of supportive resources. Furthermore, clinicians may not notice health benefits, even though they may be substantial. For example, a group for tobacco cessation might achieve 30% quit rates, whereas primary care may only achieve a 5–10% success rate. However, the group may reach only a small proportion of smokers, whereas individual counseling might reach 70% of smokers and, therefore, have greater impact.

One useful approach to counseling is known as the "Five As" (Table 3–3) and involves minimal contact interventions that can be used in a brief encounter.

Stone EG et al: Interventions that increase use of adult immunization and cancer screening services: A meta-analysis. Ann Intern Med 2002;136:641. [PMID: 21987734]

Table 3–3. The five A's of behavioral change.

Assess: Ask about health risks and factors affecting choice of behavior change.

Advise: Provide behavior change advice that is clear, specific, and personalized.

Agree: Select treatment goals and methods based on patient's interest and willingness to change.

Assist: Use behavior change techniques such as self-help and counseling combined with medical treatment when appropriate.

Arrange: Schedule follow-up contacts to assist/support and adjust treatment plan as needed.

Modified from Evaluating Primary Care Behavioral Counseling Interventions: An evidence-based approach. Am J Prev Med 2002; 22:267. Used with permission.

PHYSICAL ACTIVITY

To assess and motivate the sedentary older patient to exercise, a detailed exercise history should include lifelong patterns of activity, activity in the last 2–3 mo, patient concerns about exercise, level of interest, and social preferences regarding exercise. An exercise prescription on a prescription pad is useful to encourage activity and should be personalized to include time for exercise, type of activity, and frequency. In addition, it should take into consideration the facilities available and comorbidities of each patient. At follow-up, progress should be monitored and care taken to address any pain and monitor for injury.

Christmas C, Andersen RA: Exercise and older patients: Guidelines for the clinician. J Am Geriatr Soc 2000;48:318. [PMID: 20195199]

Singh MA: Exercise comes of age: Rationale and recommendations for a geriatric exercise prescription. J Gerontol A Biol Sci Med Sci 2002;57:M262. [PMID: 21979673]

SMOKING CESSATION

Counseling and provision of assistance (eg, nicotine patch or bupropion) by health care providers significantly improve abstinence rates over at least 1 year. Offices and clinics should establish routine procedures to regularly question patients about whether they have smoked in the last 3 months, a more sensitive approach than simply than asking whether patients are current smokers. Advice to quit is an important motivator in tobacco cessation. Smokers who are identified should be counseled about the benefits of quitting and encouraged to set a date for quitting. Because tobacco use is a chronic condition, repeated efforts are warranted, and there is a strong relationship between intensity of tobacco dependency counseling and its effectiveness. Ongoing support after quitting is also important. The U.S. surgeon general's guideline is a helpful resource.

U.S. Public Health Service Tobacco Use and Dependence Clinical Practice Guideline Panel, Staff, and Consortium Representatives: A clinical practice guideline for treating tobacco use and dependence. JAMA 2000;283:3244. [PMID: 20325308]

NUTRITION

For the general population, the USPSTF recommends counseling to reduce fats and increase fruits, vegetables, and grain products containing fiber in the diet. In patients older than 75 or 80, protein-calorie malnutrition becomes an important concern. Some elderly people remain on restrictive diets despite weight loss. Certainly in those at significant risk for malnutrition, restrictive diets should be avoided if possible.

Suboptimal levels of vitamins may be risk factors for chronic disease such as cardiovascular disease, cancer, and osteoporosis. For most individuals, a single multivitamin should provide adequate levels. Because the recommended intake of vitamins B_{12} and D is closer to twice the recommended dairy intake, it is reasonable to recommend multivitamin supplements with additional vitamin D and B_{12}.

Fairfield KM, Fletcher RH: Vitamins for chronic disease prevention in adults: Scientific review. JAMA 2002;287:3116. [PMID: 12069675]

Fletcher RH, Fairfield KM: Vitamins for chronic disease prevention in adults: Clinical applications. JAMA 2002;287:3127. [PMID: 12069676]

INJURY PREVENTION

Falls

Risk of recurrent falls can be predicted by asking all older persons about falls in the past year. Those who report a fall should have a test of functional gait. Persons with abnormal gait may require further assessment and intervention.

Burns & Automobile Accidents

The USPSTF recommends that elderly drivers be counseled to wear seat belts and avoid alcohol use when driving. All older people should be counseled to use smoke detectors, avoid hazardous use of cigarettes (eg, in bed), and reduce tap water temperature to 120–130°F.

American Geriatrics Society, British Geriatrics Society, and American Academy of Orthopaedic Surgeons Panel on Falls Prevention: Guideline for the prevention of falls in older persons. J Am Geriatr Soc 2001;49:664. [PMID: 21275673]

■ IMMUNIZATIONS & CHEMOPROPHYLAXIS

IMMUNIZATIONS

Both influenza and pneumococcal vaccination are widely recommended and important preventive strategies for general health in the elderly.

Influenza Vaccine

The effectiveness of the influenza vaccination depends on the recipient's age and immunocompetence. Among community-dwelling adults older than 60, the vaccine has been 56% effective in reducing influenza-related illness, although efficacy may be lower among those older than 70. Among elderly long-term care residents, vaccine effectiveness in preventing influenza may only be 30–40%; however, it may be 50–60% effective in preventing pneumonia and hospitalization and 80% effective in preventing death. Several studies suggested that vaccinating health care workers may be as or even more important than vaccinating residents in preventing deaths.

Healthy People 2010 set a goal of 90% vaccination coverage for all persons older than 65. The optimal time to receive the vaccine is October or November; however, given the potential for shortage of vaccines, elderly patients should be given the vaccine in October. Side effects are typically minor and last less than 2 days. Major side effects are generally related to hypersensitivity in patients with egg allergy, because the vaccine comes from highly purified inactivated flu virus grown in eggs.

U.S. Department of Health and Human Services, Office of Disease Prevention and Health Promotion: Health People 2010.

U.S. Department of Health and Human Services, 2000.

Pneumococcal Vaccine

The 23-valent pneumococcal vaccine represents 85–90% of the serotypes that cause invasive disease in the United States and has been shown to be 56–81% effective in preventing invasive bacteremia. The Advisory Committee on Immunization Practices (ACIP) recommends that persons aged 65 or older who were vaccinated before age 65 should receive 1 revaccination 5 years after the initial vaccination and that previously unvaccinated individuals should receive 1 dose at age 65. Whether repeated pneumococcal vaccinations should be given and at what interval remain unclear. The vaccine has rarely been associated with major side effects, although up to half of vaccine recipients will have a mild local reaction that persists for 48 h.

Tetanus Immunization

Most cases of tetanus in the United States occur in un-vaccinated older people. If an adult has never had a primary series of tetanus, then 3 doses are required; otherwise, the ACIP recommends a booster dose of tetanus-diphtheria toxoid vaccine every 10 years. However, the USPSTF and others have noted that far fewer immunizations may be sufficient to maintain immunity. A realistic and important goal, nonetheless, is for older individuals who received a primary immunization series to receive at least 1 additional booster.

Bridges C et al: Prevention and control of influenza: Recommendations and Reports. MMWR Morb Mortal Wkly Rep 2002;51:1. [PMID: not available]

Zimmerman RK: Adult vaccination: Part 1. Vaccines indicated by age. Teaching Immunization for Medical Education (TIME) Project. J Fam Pract 2000;49(suppl):S41. (PMID: not available]

CHEMOPROPHYLAXIS

Hormone Replacement

Although evidence from observational studies supported hormone replacement therapy, randomized trials have shown smaller benefits and increased risks. The Heart and Estrogen/Progestin Replacement Study trial found an increased risk of mortality from coronary artery disease in women using hormone replacement after myocardial infarction. The conjugated estrogen/medroxyprogesterone acetate arm of the Women's Health Initiative was terminated early because of excess risk of breast cancer and evidence that overall risks exceeded benefits (rates of coronary artery disease, stroke, and pulmonary embolism were also higher than in the control group). The role of estrogen replacement alone in those who have had a hysterectomy remains to be determined; however, long-term combined therapy for prevention of cardiovascular disease and fractures seems imprudent.

Grady D et al: Cardiovascular disease outcomes during 6.8 years of hormone therapy: Heart and Estrogen/Progestin Replacement Study Follow-Up (HERS II). JAMA 2002;288:49. [PMID: 12090862]

Writing Group for the Women's Health Initiative Investigators: Risks and benefits of estrogen plus progestin in health postmenopausal women: Principal results from the Women's Health Initiative randomized controlled trial. JAMA 2002; 288:321. [PMID: not available]

Aspirin

Aspirin reduces the risk of death and infarction in patients with established heart disease and should be considered for primary prevention as well.

The use of aspirin may reduce the risk of CHD but not total mortality and stroke. In addition, the benefit of its use may increase substantially with increasing cardiac risk. The risk of GI bleeding is higher in the elderly.

The USPSTF strongly recommends (Recommendation A) that clinicians discuss aspirin chemoprevention with adults at increased risk for CHD, concluding that the benefit of aspirin outweighs the risk of bleeding in patients who have a 5-year risk of heart disease of at least 3%. Because most elderly patients will have a risk greater than 3%, it may be reasonable to limit aspirin for prevention to those with a life expectancy of 5 years or more. Clinical calculators are now available to help accurately predict cardiac risk, and an estimate of 5-year mortality may be gained by halving the 10-year estimate of risk.

Hayden M et al: Aspirin for the primary prevention of cardiovascular events: Summary of the evidence. Ann Intern Med 2002;11136(2):161. [PMID: 11790072]

Lauer MS: Clinical practice. Aspirin for primary prevention of coronary events. N Engl J Med 2002;346:1468. [PMID: 12000818]

U.S. Preventive Services Task Force: Aspirin for the primary prevention of cardiovascular events: recommendations and rationale:http://www.ahrq.gov/clinic/3rduspstf/aspirin/asprr.htm

Geriatric Assessment

Bree Johnston, MD, MPH

The term *geriatric assessment* is generally used to describe a clinical approach to older patients that goes beyond a traditional medical history and physical. Although geriatric assessment may encompass many different settings, structures, and models of care, a unifying feature of all types of geriatric assessment is the clinical application of the biopsychosocial model to older patients.

The rationale of geriatric assessment is to better recognize common geriatric disorders in order to improve functional outcomes and quality of life for older adults. The elderly are heterogeneous in function; thus, the approach to geriatric assessment depends in part on the patient being assessed and the site of assessment.

Although this chapter is primarily geared toward the outpatient setting, many of the principles can be applied to patients in inpatient, home, and long-term care settings as well.

TEAMS IN GERIATRIC ASSESSMENT

Although geriatric assessment may be comprehensive and interdisciplinary and involve multiple team members (eg, social services, nursing, medical, physical therapy, occupational therapy, psychology, audiology, dentistry, pharmacy, nutrition, speech therapy), it may also involve just 2 or 3 informal team members and be much more simple in approach. An interdisciplinary team is one in which multiple disciplines meet together to develop a single treatment plan for a patient, whereas for a multidisciplinary team individual members perform separate assessments, notes, and treatment plans. In general, the extra work involved with an interdisciplinary team process is most justifiable in settings that serve primarily frail, complex patients. For patients in nursing homes or rehabilitation facilities, a treating team may consist of 5 or more disciplines with an interdisciplinary structure and use extensive assessment tools, whereas a geriatric outpatient practice may use an ad hoc team, brief screening tools, and follow-up with more extensive tests or team management only when indicated. Regardless, many of the principles of assessment are the same.

FUNCTIONAL ASSESSMENT

Functional impairment is common in the elderly and has many potential causes, including age-related changes, social factors, and disease. About 25% of patients older than 65 need the help of another person to perform activities of daily living (ADLs; bathing, dressing, eating, transferring, continence, toileting) or instrumental ADLs (IADLs; transportation, shopping, cooking, using the telephone, managing money, taking medications, cleaning, laundry). Fifty percent of individuals older than 85 need the help of another person to perform ADLs. Functional information should be included in the assessment of all older people.

Direct observation of function is the most accurate method of functional assessment but is impractical in most health care settings. Self-report of ADLs and IADLs is usually accurate but should be corroborated when possible, especially when the information is suspect.

Functional information can be used as a baseline to measure future declines in function and to determine the need for support services or placement, medical or surgical interventions (eg, need for knee replacement surgery), or rehabilitative therapies.

Subtle or new declines in IADL function may be an early sign of depression, dementia, fear of falling, worsening incontinence, loss of vision, or other disease, such as coronary artery disease. If no reversible cause of IADL decline is found after a reasonable medical search, the physician should focus on supportive services. Likewise, loss of ADL function often signals a worsening disease process or a combined impact of multiple comorbidities but at a more advanced stage. Although most persons with ADL impairments are able to stay home with appropriate services, a nursing home level of care may be necessary if persons with ADL impairments require placement.

Screening Measures

For highly functional independent elders, standard functional screening measures will not be useful in capturing subtle functional impairments. One technique that may be useful for these elders is to identify and regularly query about a target activity, such as playing bridge, golf, fishing, or practicing law, that the patient enjoys and regularly participates in (advanced ADLs). If the patient begins to drop the activity, it may indicate an early impairment, such as dementia, incontinence, or worsening hearing loss.

Combined Screening Instrument

A number of simple geriatric screening instruments have been published for the purpose of increasing the detection of common geriatric conditions. The rationale of these instruments is to use a number of sensitive prescreening questions or instruments for common conditions and to follow up abnormal responses with further testing or interventions. At University of California, San Francisco, we adapted the screening instruments developed by Lachs et al and later modified by Moore et al (Figure 4–1). Our screening instrument is easy to use, well accepted by practitioners and patients, and relatively quick to administer. The tool could be even more efficient if parts of it were administered by nonphysician personnel. Although it has not been proved that the use of such instruments improves outcomes, it stands to reason that increased detection of common geriatric problems would result in improved outcomes if detection is linked to interventions that are proved to be effective in the literature.

GERIATRIC ASSESSMENT EFFICIENCY

Geriatric assessment can be time consuming. A number of strategies can help make the process more efficient, such as using sensitive, brief assessment instruments, and following up with more in-depth instruments when necessary, using nonphysician personnel to help perform standard geriatric assessments, and using observations to help make diagnoses (observing gait as part of physical examination).

SPECIFIC DIAGNOSES

Falls & Gait Impairment

Falls are the leading cause of nonfatal injuries and unintentional injury and death in older persons. Every older person should be asked about falls because many will not routinely volunteer such information. In addition, persons should be asked about perceived home hazards that might be remediable. Because gait impairments commonly coexist with falls, a gait assessment is important to perform in older people and is likely to be more sensitive for abnormalities (which are commonly multifactorial because of muscular weakness, arthritis, as well as specific neurological impairments) than other components of the neurological examination.

A number of techniques for gait assessment are available to the primary care practitioner. The first, the "Get Up and Go" test, involves asking a patient to get up from a chair without using arms, walk 10 ft, and turn around and sit down. The observer can look for problems with strength (inability to get up without using the hands), gait, balance, judgment, and use of adaptive devices. When the "Get Up and Go" test is timed ("Timed Up and Go"), performance in 15 s or longer is correlated with impairments in ADLs and falls. The Tinetti Gait and Balance Evaluation (see Appendix) provides a structured framework for assessing specific components of gait and balance. Poorer performance on this instrument is associated with an increased risk of falling. Many practitioners find this scale useful for refining diagnostic acumen for specific pattern recognition, monitoring changes over time, and providing more interrater reliability between exams than with more subjective examinations.

Vision Impairment

Recommendations regarding assessment of vision impairment by primary care physicians vary. Given the commonness of eye problems in older people and the inability of most primary care physician's offices to perform high-quality, comprehensive eye examinations, periodic examinations by an optometrist or ophthalmologist are reasonable for most older people. Periodic examinations by an optometrist or ophthalmologist are especially important for patients at high risk of glaucoma or with diabetes.

Vision screening in the primary care setting with a Snellen eye chart for far vision and a Jaeger card for near vision is relatively easy to perform and may provide valuable on-the-spot information for the practitioner. Although some authors have advocated using vision screening questions, it is not clear whether such questions are sensitive enough to be useful screening tools.

Hearing Impairment

More than 33% of individuals older than 65 and 50% of those older than 85 have some hearing loss. Hearing loss is correlated with social and emotional isolation, clinical depression, and limited activity.

The optimal screening method for hearing loss in the elderly is undetermined. The whispered voice test is easy to perform; sensitivities and specificities range from 70–100%. Hand-held audiometry is also available, but performance probably depends on the skill of the operator and the environment in which it is performed. The U.S. Screening and Prevention Task Force recommends using screening questions about hearing loss in the elderly. Structured questionnaires such as the Hearing Handicap Inventory for Elderly-Screening (see Appendix) are most useful for assessing the degree to which hearing loss interferes with functioning.

Source: Pt _____ Other _____   Patient name _____   Date _____

History items	Abnormal	Action	Result and comments
Have you had any falls in the last year?	Yes	Tinetti or other gait assessment Further exam, home eval & PT Consider osteoporosis risk	_____
Do you have trouble with stairs, lighting, bathroom, or other home hazards?	Yes to any	Home eval &/or PT	_____
Do you have a problem with urine leaks or accidents?	Yes	Rule out reversible (DIAPPERS) _____ History (stress, urge), exam, PVR	
Over the past month, have you often been bothered by feeling sad, depressed, or hopeless? During the past month, have you often been bothered by little interest or pleasure in doing things?	Yes	GDS or other depression assessment	_____
Do you ever feel unsafe where you live? Does anyone threaten you or hurt you?	Yes	Explore further, social work, APS	_____
Is pain a problem for you?	Yes	Comment	_____

Do you have any problems with any of the following areas? Who assists? Do you use any devices? (For "Yes" answers, consider causes, social services and/or home eval/PT/OT.)

Doing strenuous activities like fast walking/bicycling?	Yes___ No ___	_____
Cook	Yes___ No ___	_____
Shop	Yes___ No ___	_____
Do heavy housework like washing windows	Yes___ No ___	_____
Do laundry	Yes___ No ___	_____
Get to a place beyond walking distance by driving or bus	Yes___ No ___	_____
Manage finances	Yes___ No ___	_____
Get out of bed/transfer	Yes___ No ___	_____
Dress	Yes___ No ___	_____
Toilet	Yes___ No ___	_____
Eat	Yes___ No ___	_____
Walk	Yes___ No ___	_____
Bathe (sponge bath, tub, or shower)	Yes___ No ___	_____

Figure 4–1. Two-page simple geriatric screen (PT, physical therapy; DIAPPERS, *D*elirium, *I*nfection, *A*trophic urethritis and vaginitis; *P*harmaceuticals, *P*sychological disorders, *E*xcessive urinary output, *R*estricted mobility, *S*tool impaction; PVR, postvoid residual urine test; GDS, Geriatric Depression Scale; APS, Adult Protective Services; OT, occupational therapy; BMI, body mass index; MMSE, Mini-Mental State Exam.) Adapted from Lachs M et al: A simple procedure for general screening for functional disability in elderly patients. Ann Intern Med 1990;112:699; Moore A: Screening for common problems in ambulatory elderly: Clinical confirmation of a screening instrument. Am J Med 1996;100: 438; Podsiallo D et al: The timed up and go: A test of basic functional mobility for frail elderly persons. J Am Geriatr Soc 1991;39:142; Whooley MA: Case-finding instruments for depression. J Geriatr Intern Med 1997;12:439.

Dementia

Dementia is common in the elderly but is commonly missed by primary care practitioners. As treatments become more effective for Alzheimer's disease and related disorders, early diagnosis becomes more important. The Mini-Mental State Exam (see Appendix) is a useful screening test, but it often takes 10 min or longer to complete in persons with cognitive impairment. The 3-item recall, in combination with the clock draw, is briefer and has reasonable test characteristics. When the patient is able to remember all 3 items and can draw a completely normal clock, dementia is unlikely. If the patient is unable to perform either task correctly, further evaluation is indicated.

Scanlan J, Borson S: The Mini-Cog: Receiver operating characteristics with expert and naïve raters. Int J Geriatr Psychiatry 2001;16:216. (The combination of the 3-item recall and the clock draw test was highly sensitive and specific for dementia. Validation in other populations is needed before this test is widely implemented as a screening test.)

Review medications that patient brought in	Abnormal Confusion about meds > 5 meds Doesn't bring in	Action Consider simplification Medi-set or other aid Consider	Comments _____

PHYSICAL EXAM ITEMS
(The next few items will be performed by nursing staff in some settings)

Weight/BMI And ask "have you lost weight?" If so, how much?	BMI <21 Loss of 5%	Alert provider Or nutrition eval Consider medical, dental, social	_____
Jaeger Card or Snellen eye chart Test each eye (with glasses)	Can't read 20/40	Alert provider or refer	_____
Whisper short sentences @ 6–12 inches (Out of visual view) or audioscopy	Unable to hear Retest/refer/ Hearing handicap inventory	Cerumen check	_____
Name 3 objects/re-ask in 5 min Ask patient to draw a clock face inside a 8-in circle that you draw	Remember <3 Clock draw abnormal	MMSE or other	_____
Rise from your chair (do not use arms to get up), walk 10 ft, turn, walk back to the chair and sit down	Observed problem or unable in <15 seconds	Tinetti and/or further exam Home eval & PT	_____
Touch the back of your head with your hands. Pick up the pencil.	Unable to do either	Further exam Consider OT	_____

(Remember to ask about the 3 items!)

Additional comments & other areas of concern: Caregiver stress, poverty and financial resources, alcohol, social isolation, advance directives and health care wishes.

Figure 4–1. *(Continued)*

Incontinence

Incontinence in the elderly is common but often goes unmentioned. Women are twice as likely as older men to be incontinent; overall, ~6–14% of older women experience incontinence daily. A simple question about involuntary leakage of urine is a reasonable screen. Some authors advocate following up a single screening question with "Have you lost your urine on at least 5 different occasions?," but it is equally reasonable to ask patients whether they perceive incontinence to be a problem or have to wear pads, diapers, or briefs because of urine leakage.

Depression

Depression is commonly missed in primary care. Although major depression is no more common in the elderly than in younger populations, depressive symptoms are. In ill and hospitalized elders, the prevalence of depression is ≥ 25%. A positive response to either of 2 questions is sensitive for depression:

Over the past month, have you often been bothered by feeling sad, depressed, or hopeless?

During the past month, have you often been bothered by little interest or pleasure in doing things?

Positive responses should be followed up with more comprehensive interviews because the specificity of a positive response is not high.

Malnutrition

Weight loss or poor nutritional status may be an indicator of functional decline, dementia, or medical illness. Although there is no agreement how or who to screen, checking for weight loss, body mass index, and physical signs of malnutrition (eg, temporal wasting, loss of muscle mass) and weight loss is easy and reasonable in a primary care setting. Unintentional loss of > 5% of body weight should trigger further evaluation. Loss of 5% of body weight in 1 mo or 10% of body weight over 6 mo is associated with increased morbidity and mortality.

OTHER ISSUES

Caregiver Support

Providing primary care for a frail elder requires that attention be paid to the caregiver as well as the patient because the health and well-being of the patient and caregiver are intricately linked. High levels of functional dependence place an enormous burden on a caregiver. Burnout, neglect, and abuse are possible consequences of high caregiver loads. Asking the caregiver about stress, burnout, anger, and guilt is often instructive. For the stressed caregiver, a social worker can often identify helpful programs such as caregiver support groups, respite programs, adult day care, and hired home health aids.

Abuse

Because of the possibility of abuse, vulnerable elders should have the opportunity to be interviewed alone. Direct questioning about abuse and neglect is wise, particularly under circumstances of high caregiver load. Clues to the possibility of elder abuse include observation of behavioral changes in the presence of the caregiver, delays between injuries and treatment, inconsistencies between an observed injury and an associated explanation, lack of appropriate clothing or hygiene, and unfilled prescriptions. A simple question—"Do you ever feel unsafe or threatened?"—is a reasonable initial screen.

Financial & Emotional Resources

Old age can be a time of reduced resources, both emotional and financial. The old–old are at particular risk of social isolation and poverty. Screening questions about social contacts and financial resources are often helpful in guiding providers in designing realistic treatment and social service planning.

EVIDENCE-BASED POINTS

- *Many (but not all) articles examining the impact of geriatric assessment have shown an improve-* ment in functional outcomes and reduced nursing home placement.
- *Those interventions showing the greatest impact tend to be associated with provision of care over time, and primary, rather than consultative, care.*
- *How geriatric assessment can best be incorporated into primary care has not yet been determined, particularly within the constraints of current reimbursement schedules and productivity standards.*

REFERENCES

Cohen HJ et al: A controlled trial of inpatient and outpatient geriatric evaluation and management. N Engl J Med 2002; 346:905. (Assessment conducted at 11 Veteran's Affairs Medical Centers showed significant reductions in functional decline with inpatient geriatric evaluation and management and significant improvements in mental health with outpatient geriatric evaluation and management with no increase in costs.)

Campion E: Specialized care for elderly patients. N Engl J Med 2002;346:874. (Review of the history of geriatric assessment.)

Stuck AE et al: Home visits to prevent nursing home admission and functional decline in elderly people. Systematic review and meta-regression analysis. JAMA 2002;287:1022. (Preventive home visit programs had no overall impact on mortality or other outcomes. However, programs that had more than 9 follow-up visits showed a 34% reduction in nursing home visits, and those that had multidimensional geriatric assessment and follow-up were associated with a 24% reduction in functional decline.)

SECTION II

Environments of Care

Office Practice

Elizabeth L. Cobbs, MD

With market forces encouraging the decentralization of health service delivery to the outpatient arena, the office practice serves as the backbone of health care for older adults. The elderly visit outpatient physicians at least 150% more frequently than the general population. This trend is expected to continue in the coming decades, especially in those older than 75, whose visit volume is expected to quadruple. The office practice must be prepared to address multiple aspects affecting the health of older persons, from prevention to end-of-life care (Table 5–1).

FINANCIAL ISSUES

A successful outpatient practice must have a sound financial basis, be able to manage costs and produce adequate revenues, and achieve improvements in value over time as market forces continue to shape the external practice environment. Most physicians accept Medicare assignment, which limits revenue reimbursement for "cognitive" practices. Billing evaluation and management codes should reflect the time and effort given by the clinician in the process of evaluation and care of multiple and complex medical problems that are addressed at frequent intervals.

Fee-for-Service Reimbursement

Although current systems for compensating physicians do not directly reward quality and service, practices can achieve financial rewards while maximizing quality and service. Fee-for-service (FFS) reimbursement (as in traditional Medicare) pays for traditional office visits but may not compensate providers for other forms of care (eg, group visits, nonvisit care). The complexity of the visit determines the relative value units (RVUs) and, in turn, determines the level of provider reimbursement for the visit. Financial success is achieved when providers maximize complexity of visit billing in adequate volume. Internal systems for scheduling (eg, open access or same-day scheduling methods) may reduce no-show rates and achieve higher visit volumes. Managing uncomplicated matters without an office visit may pay off in the long term, saving valuable office time to be used for visits that generate a higher level of reimbursement. Providers should seek to do as much as possible for each patient during a visit, thus maximizing the RVU and increasing efficiency of the visit.

Group visits (including several patients, the physician, and other members of the health care team) may be useful even under the FFS model for reimbursement. Group visits, typically lasting 2 h, should always be voluntary and might increase the patient's satisfaction with care as well as quality of care outcomes. Physicians save time by delivering patient education to multiple patients at once. Group visits emphasize self-management of the chronic condition and enhance opportunities for peer support and regular contact with the clinical team. Patients have opportunities to ask questions and gain information in the setting of a supportive peer group. Group visits have been reported to reduce emergency department visits and to improve access to certain aspects of care.

Capitated Reimbursement

Capitated reimbursement encourages providers to develop innovative and potentially non-visit-based services to meet their patients' needs. Providers are motivated to increase their panel size (or number of capitated patients) while minimizing overhead costs. Capitated systems of reimbursement provide incentives

Table 5–1. Scope of services in office practice for older adults.

Advance care planning
Advocacy for patients and families
Behavioral modification (smoking cessation, increasing physical activity)
Bereavement and grief counseling
Care management
Caregiver support
Chronic disease management
Comprehensive geriatric assessment
Diagnosis and treatment of medical problems
Driving safety management
Education of patients, caregivers, and families
Elder mistreatment recognition, assessment, and referral
End-of-life care
Interdisciplinary team management
Pain management
Palliative care
Prevention and screening
Preoperative assessment
Medication management
Rehabilitation
Specialty referral
Urgent care

to providers to manage their panel of patients more effectively, whereas FFS systems provide incentives to increase the number of complex visits in caring for their patients.

Health Maintenance Organizations

The financial incentives for providers will necessarily have an impact on the kinds of services offered. Health maintenance organizations (HMOs) have provided care for older adults in many regions throughout the United States for the past 2 decades. One managed-care model serving older adults uses nurse practitioners as care managers to integrate social and medical services and provide comprehensive after-hours coverage for urgent-care needs. Providers have a strong incentive to avoid hospitalization if possible and to address geriatric issues (eg, falls, depression, incontinence, exercise, hearing loss, medication use, advance directives).

COMMUNICATION

Most clinicians believe that the quality of care for the elderly is strongly influenced by the communication between patient and clinician.

Communication with old–old patients can be enhanced in the office by using some practical techniques:

1. Speak directly to the patient to enable lip reading.
2. Close shades and curtains if glare is present.
3. Reduce extraneous background noise (eg, by closing doors) to reduce difficulty with speech discrimination and hearing.
4. Position caregivers, if present, behind the patient to prevent talking to them and not the patient.
5. For hearing-impaired patients without hearing aids, use an assistive hearing device such as a headphone and amplifier set.
6. Speak slowly in a moderate tone of voice.
7. Provide written or printed summary of diagnoses and recommendations.

Computer use is increasing among older adults and their caregivers and offers a viable tool for enhancing health outcomes. Computer technologies assist providers and patients in the management of chronic diseases by educating providers and patients, identifying nonadherence, and monitoring individual and population outcomes. However, computer use may be deterred by losses in manual dexterity and visual function.

INITIAL VISIT

General Considerations

The patient's primary caregiver should be asked to accompany the patient to the office for the first visit so that the main reason for the visit can be identified and quality of care assessed. When the frail patient has difficulty communicating and appears without the family member or friend who scheduled the appointment, the reason for the office visit may remain unclear.

The role of the physician needs to be clarified with the patient and caregiver. Some patients may prefer a brief opinion regarding their health problems in the form of a consultation, whereas others are interested in establishing a primary care relationship.

The patient's living arrangement (nursing home, assisted-living facility, or private residence) and modes of transportation available (and impediments to follow-up office visits) need to be documented. The patient's other family caregivers should be identified and a guardian, power of attorney, or health care advocate should be assigned. Prescription and nonprescription medications as well as alternative treatments should be reviewed; patients should be instructed to bring all their medications with them on the first visit. All of this information can be obtained by asking the patient or caregiver to complete a questionnaire in advance of the patient's initial appointment.

A screening office assessment streamlines the evaluation (Appendix). Trained office staff can complete the

10-min screen before the physical examination. For further initial evaluation, several efficient techniques are available.

Hearing & Visual Impairments

Screening can be done with written and verbal instructions. To check visual acuity, ask the patient to read a few lines from a newspaper or read numbers on a hand-held chart. To check for significant hearing impairment, perform the whisper test by asking the patient to repeat a short list of numbers whispered by an examiner positioned 2 ft behind. The degree of hearing impairment can be quantified with a hand-held audioscope.

Cognitive Function

The Clock Drawing Test can be used to screen for memory impairment. Patients are asked to draw the face of a clock with hour and minute hands to a specific time.

If cognitive impairment is suspected, document the magnitude and area of impairment using the Mini-Mental State Exam (Appendix).

Mobility

Balance and gait disorders are common and are associated with an increased risk of falling. The Up and Go Test assesses balance and gait by having the patient stand up from a chair, walk a short distance, turn around, and sit down again. A Timed Up and Go Test, > 20 s, may predict the risk of falls in the next year. The Functional Reach Test measures balance. Have the patient stand next to a wall, with feet stationary and 1 arm outstretched, and lean forward as far as possible without stepping. A reach distance of < 6 in. is considered abnormal and warrants further evaluation.

Arm & Hand Function

Upper extremity dysfunction can easily interfere with self-care activities. Assess arm and shoulder function by asking the patient to place both hands behind the midback and raise them above the head. Evaluate hand and finger dexterity by having the patient pick up small objects, such as coins, from a flat table surface. Consider referral to physical or occupational therapy if the patient has difficulty with these activities.

Bladder Continence

Urinary incontinence is an often underreported symptom that can jeopardize older persons' independent living. Ask patients whether they have "lost urine and gotten wet." If yes, further office evaluation or referral to a specialist is warranted.

Emotional Status

Anxiety and depressive disorders affect many older adults. Ask the patients whether they often feel sad (possible depression). If yes, quantify the extent of depressive symptoms with a questionnaire such as the Geriatric Depression Scale.

Physical Examination

A targeted physical examination saves time on the initial office visit by deferring certain parts of the customary examination (eg, funduscopic examination) that are not immediately necessary. Check for orthostatic hypotension, pressure ulcers, signs of malnutrition, and signs of physical abuse. Perform brief neurological (gait, muscle strength, balance), cardiovascular (pulses, murmurs, heart rhythm), and abdominal (bruits, masses) examinations.

FOLLOW-UP VISITS

Brief assessments can identify patients with new or potential medical problems that warrant further evaluation:

- Change in basic activities of daily living since last visit.
- Change in weight or appetite.
- Change in memory.
- Change in mood.
- New falls (or problems with walking).
- Problems with bowels or bladder.

GERIATRIC SYNDROMES, CHRONIC DISEASES, & CONDITIONS

Many of the most common chronic conditions (Table 5–2) and their associated disabilities are preventable. Disease management guidelines and targets for diseases (eg, hypertension, diabetes) are increasingly available. Information systems that provide clinical reminders are effective in improving long-term selected outcomes. The office practice should maintain a system of clinician reminders and tracking of select outcomes. Patient educational materials for common diseases and conditions should be on hand.

Specialty care has been shown to improve outcomes in some instances and should always be considered when conditions become progressive and difficult to treat. Other disciplines (eg, physical, occupational, and speech therapy) are helpful adjuncts to care. Selected complementary and alternative medicine should be considered.

Table 5–2. Aging and chronic diseases.

Heart disease[a]
COPD[a]
Dementia[a]
Vision loss[a]
Hearing loss[a]
Musculoskeletal diseases[a]
Osteoarthritis[a]
Diabetes[a]
Cancer[a]
Neurological diseases[a]
Parkinson's disease[a]

COPD, chronic obstructive pulmonary disease.
[a]Often disabling.

Clinicians must periodically screen for geriatric syndromes and chronic conditions because they often go unreported (eg, urinary incontinence). Such syndromes may also be correlated with others (eg, depression).

The use of practice guidelines and consensus statements for various chronic diseases presents challenges. Guidelines for prevalent conditions (eg, dementia) frequently differ in content, methodology, and recommendations. Clinicians must be continually evaluating new evidence guiding various aspects of screening, diagnosis, and treatment.

Safety Issues

A. Elder Mistreatment

The phenomenon of elder mistreatment has become increasingly recognized. Although evidence is lacking for screening effectiveness, clinicians should maintain an awareness of risk factors for elder mistreatment and local resources for referral.

B. Driving Skill

Although most geriatricians acknowledge that physicians are responsible for reporting patients who are potentially dangerous drivers and are willing to take action, many do not know how to do so. Clinicians should be aware of their state laws governing reporting of driving safety concerns.

C. Substance Abuse

Many problems that are common in younger adults persist into late life and respond to similar interventions. Older persons benefit from substance abuse screening and intervention to prevent and reverse morbidity. Although alcohol is the substance most frequently abused, prescription sedative abuse and narcotic abuse also occur.

INTERDISCIPLINARY COLLABORATION & CARE COORDINATION

An interdisciplinary, comprehensive approach to patient care is the hallmark of geriatric medicine. It is necessary to collaborate with other health care professionals (eg, therapists, specialists, nutritionists, social workers), other professionals (eg, financial advisors, lawyers, pastors) who may aid comprehensive planning, local (eg, Offices on Aging and the Area Agency on Aging) and national (eg, Alzheimer's Association, adult day health programs, Meals on Wheels, senior nutrition programs) resources, care management services to coordinate interdisciplinary care.

Integrated systems of care promote comprehensive geriatric management and goal-directed service coordination. Collaboration with community service organizations eases the patient's transition from hospital to home or through short-term skilled nursing care. The primary physician serves as the patient's advocate through the system of health services by integrating recommendations and treatments into a coherent plan that serves the patient's best interests. Continuity of care is enhanced by involvement of the primary care clinician (eg, communicating key information to other health professionals about the patient's history, values and preferences for care, and previous functional status). The records of outside providers are incorporated into the patient's office record.

PHYSICAL ENVIRONMENT OF THE OFFICE

The physical environment of the office practice influences accessibility, effectiveness, efficiency, safety, and patient and family satisfaction. Ease of access depends on, among other factors, the availability of transportation, parking, and wheelchair accessibility.

Patients with functional deficits may need assistance in moving to the examination room, undressing, and climbing onto the examination table. An adjustable electric examination tables save time and enhance comfort.

Extra space is needed in examination rooms to accommodate caregivers and wheelchair-bound patients and their families. A handicap accessible bathroom must be available. Good lighting and contrasting colors in signs and interior design are helpful for visually impaired patients.

PREVENTION

Preventive care is a major focus of office practice. Substantial variation exists among practice sites in the provision of preventive health services, suggesting that there are opportunities for many practices to improve preventive care.

Immunization

Immunizations are widely underused. Immunization recommendation by a health care provider appears to be a key factor in whether an adult will be vaccinated. Adults who are medically underserved are at particular risk for underimmunization.

Cancer Screening

Decisions about cancer screening for older adults must be individualized to integrate quantitative concerns (risk of cancer death, benefit of outcomes) and qualitative factors (patient preferences). Cancer screening recommendations vary by guideline source and fail to incorporate burdens of other disease states that older persons often have. Various strategies may be used to promote screening practices. The frequency and continuity of office visits are linked to the provision of preventive services such that more, not fewer, office visits are needed to achieve preventive health services targets.

SYMPTOM MANAGEMENT, PALLIATIVE CARE, & END-OF-LIFE CARE

The management of pain and other adverse symptoms associated with chronic disease (eg, dyspnea and chronic obstructive pulmonary disease) is an important aspect of geriatric office practice. Recognition of pain as the fifth vital sign has resulted in the availability of a number of tools for assessing and monitoring relief.

Interdisciplinary care is helpful to develop comprehensive care plans and identify additional resources to help patients and families. Palliative care may accompany treatments aimed at cure or disease modification.

Hospice consultation should be considered when serious conditions progress and when death would not be unexpected.

Patients who wish to be at home through end of life need coordinated services to ensure the delivery of appropriate and timely services, support families and caregivers, and achieve effective end-of-life care (eg, symptom management, death pronouncement, family bereavement).

Goals of Care & Advance Care Planning

The office practice is the natural locus for advance care planning. The process of developing goals of care extends throughout the course of care. For those patients who have the capacity to make health decisions, clinicians provide information about treatment choices with the attendant risks, benefits, and burdens and counsel patients on medical choices. If the patient has an impaired capacity to make health care decisions, a surrogate decision maker should be identified and counseled. Health decision aids may facilitate shared decision making, but the key element is the ongoing dialogue and understanding between the patient and clinician.

Role of Caregivers & Families

Older patients are often accompanied to the office visit by a third person (eg, spouse, adult child, caregiver, or friend), who may be an advocate, a passive participant, or even an antagonist.

Ask the patient in private whether permission is granted for the third person to be present in the examination room. Even with permission granted, it is a good idea for the practitioner to spend some time alone with the patient during each visit.

Medication Management

Accurate assessment of medication use is problematic. Even when patients are asked to bring in all their medications, the list of medications generated is in accord with the lists generated during a visit to the home only about 50% of the time. Vitamins, herbal remedies, and minerals are typically overlooked.

Specific prescribing problems include dosage, duplication, drug–drug interactions, and duration.

Periodic drug regimen review is recommended, especially when benzodiazepines and nonsteroidal anti-inflammatory drugs are prescribed. Communicating with the pharmacist may also be useful, depending on the practice setting. Cognitive function is linked to the ability to take medications independently. Caregivers should be asked to help monitor medication adherence.

REFERENCES

American Geriatrics Society: care management position statement. J Am Geriatr Soc 2000;48:1338. [PMID: 11037025]

Andersen-Ranberg K et al: Healthy centenarians do not exist, but autonomous centenarians do: A population-based study of morbidity among Danish centenarians. J Am Geriatr Soc 2001;49:901. [PMID: 11527481]

Bierman AS: Functional status: The sixth vital sign. J Gen Intern Med 2001;16:785. [PMID: 11722694]

Bogardus ST et al: Evaluation of a guided protocol for quality improvement in identifying common geriatric problems. J Am Geriatr Soc 2002;50:328. [PMID: 12028216]

Burton LC et al: Health outcomes and Medicaid costs for frail older individuals: A case study of a MCO versus fee-for-service care. J Am Geriatr Soc 2002;50:382. [PMID: 12028225]

Callahan EJ et al: The influence of patient age on primary care resident physician-patient interaction. J Am Geriatr Soc 2000; 48:30. [PMID: 10642018]

Chakravarthy MV et al: An obligation for primary care physicians to prescribe physical activity to sedentary patients to reduce the risk of chronic health conditions. Mayo Clin Proc 2002; 77:165. [PMID: 11838650]

Christmas C, Anderson RA: Exercise and older patients: Guidelines for the clinicians. J Am Geriatr Soc 2000;48:318. [PMID: 10733061]

Cohen HJ et al: A controlled trial of inpatient and outpatient geriatric evaluation and management. N Engl J Med 2002;346: 905. [PMID: 11907291]

Edelberg HK et al: Medication management capacity in highly functioning community-living older adults: Detection of early deficits. J Am Geriatr Soc 1999;47:592. [PMID: 10323653]

Engleman KK et al: Impact of geographic barriers on the utilization of mammograms by older rural women. J Am Geriatr Soc 2002;50:62. [PMID: 12028248]

Fischer LR et al: Geriatric depression, antidepressant treatment, and healthcare utilization in a health maintenance organization. J Am Geriatr Soc 2002;50:307. [PMID: not available]

Fried TR et al: Understanding the treatment preferences of seriously ill patients. N Engl J Med 2002;346:1061. [PMID: 11932474]

Gill TM et al: Restricted activity among community-living older persons: Incidence, precipitants, and health care utilization. Ann Intern Med 2001;135:313. [PMID: 11529694]

Goldman L: Key challenges confronting internal medicine in the early twenty-first century. Am J Med 2001;110:463. [PMID: 11331058]

Hanlon JT et al: Use of inappropriate prescription drugs by older people. J Am Geriatr Soc 2002;50:26. [PMID: 12028243]

Kizer KW: Establishing health care performance standards in an era of consumerism. JAMA 2001;286:1213. [PMID: 11559267]

McCusker J et al: Rapid emergency department intervention for older people reduces risk of functional decline: Results of a multicenter randomized trial. J Am Geriatr Soc 2001;49: 1272. [PMID: 11890484]

Morrison I: The future of physicians' time. Ann Intern Med 2000; 132:80. [PMID: 10627256]

Preston JA et al: The effect of multifaceted physician office-based intervention on older women's mammography use. J Am Geriatr Soc 2000;48:1. [PMID: not available]

Reuben DB et al: A randomized clinical trial of outpatient comprehensive geriatric assessment coupled with an intervention to increase adherence to recommendations. J Am Geriatr Soc 1999;47:269. [PMID: 10078887]

Unutzer J et al: Care for depression in HMO patients aged 65 and older. J Am Geriatr Soc 2000;48:871. [PMID: 10968289]

Walter LC, Covinsky KE: Cancer screening in elderly patients: A framework for individualized decision-making. JAMA 2001; 285:2750. [PMID: 11386931]

Wright PJ: Delivery of preventive services to older black patients using neighborhood health centers. J Am Geriatr Soc 2000; 48:124. [PMID: 10682940]

Home Care

B. Gwen Windham, MD, & Bruce Leff, MD

■ HOME CARE MODELS

Specific home care models have proved effective. These models include interdisciplinary home care programs that integrate medical and social supportive services focusing on the care of chronically disabled persons, home geriatric assessment, posthospital case management/facilitated discharge schemes, home rehabilitation, and home hospital.

INTERDISCIPLINARY HOME CARE

Interdisciplinary home care consists of a functioning multidisciplinary team of physicians and other health care professionals, including nurses, home health aides, social worker, and physical and occupational therapists. The team meets on a regular basis, manages the care of active patients carefully, and integrates medical and social supportive services. Such programs have demonstrated improvement in function, reduced costs, decreased medication use, improved satisfaction, improved end-of-life care, and fewer nursing home admissions and outpatient visits.

HOME GERIATRIC ASSESSMENT PROGRAMS

Home geriatric assessment programs work to identify patient problems in several spheres and provide targeted interventions with the aim of improving clinical outcomes for patients. Results of these studies are varied; however, some have been associated with long-term functional benefits and reductions in nursing home placement.

POSTHOSPITALIZATION CASE MANAGEMENT

Specific home-based case management strategies, especially those that are focused on conditions associated with complex management issues and high rates of early hospital readmission (eg, congestive heart failure), have been associated with a significant reduction in the number of acute hospital readmissions.

HOME REHABILITATION

Home rehabilitation (specifically after a stroke) has proved to be feasible, acceptable to patients and caregivers, and as effective as hospital-based rehabilitation.

HOME HOSPITAL

Home hospital models that provide hospital-level services in the home setting as a substitute for a needed hospital admission have been developed and have demonstrated comparable clinical outcomes, reduced length of stay, and reductions in important geriatric complications such as confusion.

■ MEDICARE HOME HEALTH SERVICES

ELIGIBILITY REQUIREMENTS

Medicare will pay for certain home care services. Physicians who care for older patients need to be familiar with the basic entry criteria for these services. Medicare was designed as an acute illness benefit rather than insurance to pay for the long-term care of older persons with chronic conditions. Thus, Medicare home health benefits are linked to transitions from acute care settings and to what Medicare refers to as a "skilled need." Home health care services for Medicare patients are covered by Medicare Part A. Physicians and approved home health agencies are reimbursed for services as long as certain criteria are met. The basic requirements for Medicare to reimburse home health expenses are as follows: The physician certifies that the patient is homebound, the patient has a skilled need, the skilled need is reasonable and necessary, the rendered service is intermittent or part time, and the physician signs Form CMS-485, which is the plan of care.

Homebound Requirement

To qualify as "homebound," a patient must have a condition resulting from illness or injury that makes it a "considerable and taxing effort to leave the home" without the aid of supportive devices such as crutches, canes, wheelchairs or walkers, special transportation, or another person or if leaving the home is medically contraindicated. However, a person does not have to be bedridden or absolutely homebound. Absences from the home must be infrequent, of short duration, or for medically relevant services. Examples of nonmedical reasons for leaving the home are attending religious services or taking a stroll or drive. No specific definition of "short duration" is provided in the Medicare guidelines. Illnesses or injuries that result in a person's confinement to the home include stroke, blindness, dementia, amputation, or a psychiatric problem in which the patient refuses to leave the home or would be unsafe leaving the home unattended.

Skilled Need Requirement

A skilled need is required to receive reimbursement from Medicare for home health services. Skilled needs are those that require special training and certification to administer to be safe and effective, such as those provided by nurses or therapists. An example of a skilled need is the monitoring of a patient with a complex medical condition that requires readjustment of medicines and reevaluation by a skilled nurse. Examples include wound care treatment, catheter care, physical therapy, and training of patients or caregivers to manage medical conditions such as diabetes or wound treatment. Single home visits by a skilled nurse for the sole purpose of obtaining a blood specimen do not qualify as a skilled need. Once a person has home health services for a skilled need, other covered Medicare home health services such as social work, occupational therapy, and home health aide can also be obtained. Thus, the skilled nursing or physical therapy need unlocks the Medicare home health benefit for the patient, and a broad range of services may be used as appropriate for the care of the patient. Services can be provided as long as the skilled need exists.

All skilled needs are not reimbursable. For example, if a patient has been managing his or her diabetes with injections without difficulty and the glucose is well controlled, training would not be appropriate, and payment would be denied. If the patient had been taking oral medications, however, and the physician adds insulin to the medical regimen, it would be appropriate to request nursing services to train the patient to manage diabetes on the new insulin regimen.

Reasonable & Necessary Skilled Need

Skilled needs must be reasonable and necessary. Documentation should be provided on the plan of care (Form CMS-485) and any supplementary forms. If appropriate medical information is not present, the med-ical record will be reviewed by a regional intermediary designated by the Center for Medicare and Medicaid Services (CMS, formerly the Health Care Financing Administration [HCFA]) to determine whether the services are reasonable and necessary. One example of a reasonable and necessary skilled need is that of the patient discharged home after hospitalization with heart failure. However, this person's need would not qualify as reasonable and necessary if there was no documentation of changes to the medical regimen and Form CMS-485 documented the patient as having stable vital signs and no functional impairments. Another example provided in the *Home Health Agency Manual* is a patient who was discharged from the hospital after a hip fracture, and home health services were requested for monthly vitamin B_{12} injections. Although the injection is a skilled need, if there is no documentation of approved conditions for the administration of vitamin B_{12}, there is no evidence that the injection is medically necessary or reasonable, and the claim would be denied.

Centers for Medicare & Medicaid Services: Home Health Agency manual: cms.hhs.gov/manuals/11_hha/HH00.asp

Part-Time or Intermittent Service

According to the 1997 BBA, "intermittent" means skilled nursing care that is provided fewer than 7 days per week or less than 8 h per day for 21 days or less for a medical condition that is expected to require skilled services for treatment at least once every 60 days. Therefore, a one-time intravenous infusion (eg, the condition is not expected to recur and will not require intermittent service) would not qualify for reimbursement. Exceptions to the time limit may be made on an individual basis if appropriate documentation is provided.

Plan of Care

Form CMS-485 is the comprehensive plan of care for each patient. This form lists diagnoses, medications, diet, activities, and services needed, such as wound treatments, in addition to other information. The patient must be under the care of a physician qualified to sign the physician certification at the time of enrollment into home health, and the physician must review and sign the form at least every 60 days. Additional state requirements regarding timing of signatures may also exist. Physicians can bill Medicare for certifying the plan of care.

BILLING FOR CARE PLAN OVERSIGHT

Medicare Part B pays for care plan oversight (CPO) using CMS common practice coding system code G0181. Separate codes must be used for initial certification, recertification, and CPO. CPO responsibilities include time spent in discussion with members of the home care team or pharmacists. It may also include time spent reviewing records or coordinating care with other disciplines. CPO does not include time spent in discussion with pharmacists for the purpose of calling in prescriptions, nor does it include time spent in discussions with patients or family members. CPO billing information is provided in Table 6–1.

PAYMENT DENIALS

Single visits are common reasons for payment denial, even if the visit resulted in administering a skilled need. If a patient complained of urinary symptoms, Medicare would not pay for a home health nurse to make a single visit to obtain a urinary specimen, even if the patient was diagnosed and treated with antibiotics for an infection. The patient would need to be hospitalized, placed in hospice, or die as a result of the presenting problem to receive reimbursement for that home visit.

Another common reason for denial is the determination of nonacute events (eg, when physical therapy is ordered for frail patients with medically stable diseases or with gradual progressive disability). Since its inception, Medicare has operated based on an acute care model, and reimbursements are primarily for acute events with a foreseeable period of recovery. In most cases, there must be a clear end point before services will be approved. Before home health services are requested, the physician should consider whether the service is expected to improve the patient's condition.

Table 6–1. Care plan oversight (CPO) billing information.

Medicare beneficiary is receiving Medicare-covered home health services.

30 minutes physician supervision per patient per calendar month.

Physician face-to-face encounter within 6 months before the month for which CPO is billed.

No financial or contractual relationship with the home health agency.

Only 1 attending physician bills during the calendar month.

If billing for CPO services during postoperative period, CPO services must not be related to the surgery.

Must have the provider number of the home health agency.

Physician who bills must also sign plan of care and furnish services.

Physician is not billing for Medicare ESRD capitation payment and CPO for the same beneficiary during the same month.

One of the most common reasons for denial is failure of physicians to sign Form CMS-485. The plan of care should be reviewed at least every 60 days, updated, if needed, and signed.

■ ADDITIONAL RESOURCES

MEDICAID

Medicare recipients may also receive Medicaid ("dual eligible") if they meet the income and wealth requirements.

Medicaid provides reimbursement for many home health services for which Medicare does not. In addition, several states have launched Medicaid waiver programs to provide home care services for Medicare patients who are Medicaid and nursing home eligible in hopes of reducing nursing home admissions. States must assure CMS that the cost of providing these services in the home or community will not exceed that of placing individuals in an institution. Some of the services provided include personal care, respite care, and other needed assistance in the home.

AREA AGENCIES ON AGING

Area Agencies on Aging (AAAs) were established in 1973 under the Older Americans Act to provide resources for older adults. Local AAAs provide several types of assistance: information and access services, community-based services, in-home services, housing services, and elder rights services.

Information and access services include providing information and referrals for services outside the AAA, caregiver support, and retirement planning and education. Community-based services include employment services such as skill assessment, testing, and job placement. They also offer information on senior centers, congregate meals, adult day care, and volunteer opportunities. In-home services consist of Meals on Wheels, assistance with personal care, shopping and housekeeping, telephone calls and personal visits for homebound adults, personal emergency response devices, financial assistance with gas and electric bills for low-income individuals, and respite care for caregivers. AAAs help older adults find alternative housing as they transition from independent living to varying levels of need for assistance, usually in an attempt to avoid nursing home placement. Senior housing facilities, group homes, assisted-living facilities, and adult foster care are options that AAAs help individuals to explore. AAAs can also provide information on nursing home placement. Finally, AAAs provide legal assistance and investigate elder abuse charges and neglect, including self-neglect both in the community and within long-term care facilities.

HOSPICE

Medicare recipients may elect to use the Medicare hospice benefit in cases of terminal illness. Terminal illness is defined as a condition from which the person is expected to die within 6 mo if the condition runs its normal course. Patients who decide to use the hospice benefit must be eligible for Medicare Part A, be certified by their physician and the hospice medical director as terminally ill, sign a statement choosing hospice care instead of routine Medicare benefits for the specified illness, and receive care of their terminal illness through a Medicare-approved hospice program. Hospice care is provided in hospice facilities, nursing homes, and residences.

The focus of hospice is comfort care rather than treatment with intent to cure. Certified staff members have special training in hospice care work. They include physicians, nurses, counselors (including those for family members after the death of their loved one), dietitians, speech therapists, physical and occupational therapists, clergy, social workers, and volunteers, who help with daily tasks such as shopping and personal care. Hospice benefits also include provision of medical supplies and equipment and medications for symptom control and pain relief.

Although cancer is the most common diagnosis in the hospice program, nontraditional terminal illnesses such as dementia, cardiac disease, and neurologic diseases are eligible for hospice. Physicians must certify that the expected life expectancy is less than 6 mo. However, patients who outlive the 6-mo expectancy may remain in the hospice program if their condition is believed to be terminal and the physician certifies their terminal status. Forms are available through hospice programs and home health agencies to help physicians and other providers determine whether a patient meets requirements for hospice benefits.

Some physicians and hospice programs are reluctant to provide hospice care if they are not certain of the patient's actual life expectancy or if the person has lived beyond the initial 6-mo period within the hospice program for fear of fraud and abuse charges. This fear is unfounded. In fact, the benefit appears to be underused; physicians tend to refer patients to hospice at the very end of their lives. According to the National Hospice and Palliative Care Organization, 33% of hospice patients died within 1 week of admission to hospice, whereas only 6% lived for more than 6 mo.

■ THE PHYSICIAN'S ROLE IN HOME CARE

A physician may provide home care at several distinct levels: community-based long-term care, posthospitalization and rehabilitation care, acute home care, and assessment visits. In providing such care, the physician often works in conjunction with the resources of a home health agency, including skilled nursing care, home health aide care, physical and occupational therapists, and social workers. A review of these types of care, the physician's role, and the key advantages and disadvantages of each is provided in Table 6–2.

One inference to be drawn from the description of these categories is the importance of selecting appropriate patients for home care. Patient selection requires an understanding of the patient's medical condition; suitability of the patient's environment, including the level of available caregiver support; and ability of the home health agency to support the patient's particular needs.

LONG-TERM CARE

The focus of the physician's role varies, to some extent, depending on the patient's circumstances and the level of home care. In long-term care, the physician provides ongoing medical services, coordinates activities of the interdisciplinary team when skilled services are involved, and serves as an advocate for patients, referring them to appropriate community services to foster continued independence.

POSTACUTE HOSPITALIZATION & HOME REHABILITATION CARE

In posthospitalization care and home rehabilitation care, the focus is on restoring function and completing the management of medical problems. The interdisciplinary care team provides much of the care in this setting.

HOME CARE & ASSESSMENTS

In acute home care, the physician is actively involved in management of acute illness. Physician home visits and close coordination of the interdisciplinary care team are crucial to assess and manage the patient. In addition, assessment home visits, which may be performed on a one-time basis, allow a physician to evaluate the impact of the home environment, caregiver, or functional disability on the patient's health, including nonadherence, difficult diagnoses, and excessive use of health services.

Table 6-2. Types of physician home care.

Type of care	Focus	Who is in charge	Level of care	Advantages	Main services	Disadvantages
Acute home care	Management of acute illness	Physician	May be similar to hospital level of care	Patient at home; avoid iatrogenic illness; efficient comprehensive assessment	Physician, nursing	Health care system may not be able to deliver care of this nature.
Postacute/ rehabilitation	Complete hospital treatment; restoration of function	Home health agency staff	Less than acute	Continue care in home environment; ease transition from hospital to home	Occupational and physical therapy, nurse, nurse aide, physician	
Community-based long-term care	Alternative to nursing home care or assisted-living facility care	Often informal family caregivers with intermittent formal home health agency staff	Less intensive than acute or postacute/ rehabilitation focused home care	Long-term management of medical problems	Physician, case manager, home health agency resources on intermittent basis	Careful balance between autonomy and risk; must address social issues
Assessment	Investigational	Physician	Similar to community-based long-term care	Direct observational assessment of environment, caregiver, functional disability	Physician	

Table 6–3. Home care equipment.

Essential
Sphygmomanometer
Stethoscope
Phlebotomy equipment
Thermometer
Specimen cups for urine, sputum
Gloves
Ear wax removal equipment
Reflex hammer
Vibration fork
Occult blood cards and developer
Lubricating jelly
Toenail clippers
Tongue depressors
Prescription pad
Sharps container

Optional
Dictaphone
Glucometer
Digital camera
Laptop computer
Blood analyzers
Pulse oximeter
Wound care kit
Gynecological speculum
Peak flowmeter
Scale

HOUSE CALLS

In addition to the usual components of a patient encounter (ie, the history and physical examination and counseling), the house call permits and encourages functional, caregiver, and environmental assessments. Inspecting the home environment (eg, rooms and ob-

stacles, lighting, bathroom setup, kitchen setup, refrigerator contents, medication setup [with patient and caregiver permission]) can help the physician understand functional and medical issues. Also, observations of patient–caregiver interactions in the home are often remarkably different from those observed in the office setting and can provide valuable insight into management issues. Recommended equipment for house calls is listed in Table 6–3.

Binstock RH, Cluff LE (editors): Home Care Advances. Springer, 2000.

Calkins E et al (editors): New Ways to Care for Older People—Building Systems Based on Evidence. Springer, 1999.

Oldenquist GW et al: Home care: What a physician needs to know. Cleve Clin J Med 2001;68:433. [PMID 11352323]

Leff B, Burton JR: The future history of home care and physician house calls in the United States. J Gerontol A Biol Sci Med Sci 2001;56:M603. [PMID 11584032]

McCall N et al: Medicare home health before and after the BBA. Health Aff (Millwood) 2001;20:189. [PMID 11585166]

Stuck AE et al: Home visits to prevent nursing home admission and functional decline in elderly people. Systematic review and meta-regression analysis. JAMA 2002;287:1022. [PMID 11866651]

van Haastregt et al: Effects of preventive home visits to elderly people living in the community: A systematic review. BMJ 2000; 320:754. [PMID 10720360]

American Academy of Homecare Physicians: http://aahcp.org (This organization is an excellent source of information on home care as it relates to physician practice in home care.)

Center for Medicare and Medicaid Services: http://www.cms.hhs.gov (Various sites have excellent information on the Medicare home health and hospice program.)

National Association of Area Agencies on Aging: http://www.n4a.org (This site has a number of helpful links to find local services.)

National Association for Home Care: http://www.nahc.org (This site—for a trade group that represents home care agencies, hospices, home care aide organizations, and medical equipment suppliers—provides general information and links related to the home care industry.)

Hospital Care

C. Seth Landefeld, MD

Hospital care is a critical issue for older patients, and hospitalization heralds a period of high risk that extends beyond discharge, especially for the frail and the very old. In addition, older patients are the lifeblood of every hospital, except those limited to obstetrics and pediatrics. These points are illustrated by the following observations:

- Persons age 65 years or older account for 36% of hospitalizations and nearly 50% of hospital revenues, even though they comprise only 13% of the population.
- Nearly 66% of Americans die in a hospital, and > 80% of deaths occur in persons 65 years of age or older. In the year before death, nearly all older Americans are hospitalized, accounting for ~20% of all Medicare expenditures.
- Adverse outcomes of hospitalization are directly related to age: Loss of ability to care for oneself increases with age (occurring in 15%, 30%, and 45% of medical patients in their 70s, 80s, and 90s, respectively), as do hospital mortality rates.

Hospital care can be improved in older patients, and it is likely that such improvements would lessen suffering and save lives and money. Preventable adverse events occur in 5% of persons age 65 years and older compared with 2% of younger patients. Opportunities to administer preventive maneuvers, such as pneumococcal and influenza vaccination, are frequently missed. Focused efforts have improved treatment of specific conditions such as myocardial infarction, congestive heart failure, and pneumonia. Moreover, reengineering the microsystem of care (eg, how care is delivered on a hospital ward or how hospital care is linked to posthospital care) can improve the outcomes of older patients.

Efforts to improve hospital care for older persons may prove especially high yield because of their high risk for adverse outcomes. An intervention that reduces hospital mortality 20% in terms of relative risk might reduce hospital mortality from 10% to 8% in 80-year-olds but only from 2% to 1.6% in 50-year-olds. Thus, such an intervention would prevent the deaths of 20 of every 1000 hospitalized 80-year-olds compared with 4 of every 1000 hospitalized 50-year-olds.

Bird CE et al: Age and gender differences in health care utilization and spending for Medicare beneficiaries in their last years of life. J Palliat Med 2002;5:705. [PMID: not available] (During the last year of life, most older Americans are hospitalized, accounting for > 66% of Medicare expenditures for these persons.)

Brennan TA et al: Incidence of adverse events and negligence in hospitalized patients. Results of the Harvard Medical Practice Study I. N Engl J Med 1991;324:370. [PMID: 1987460] (Adverse events occurred in 4% of hospitalizations, and 25% were due to negligence. Adverse events were twice as common in patients age 65 years and older.)

Fried TR et al: Older persons' preferences for site of terminal care. Ann Intern Med 1999;131:109. [PMID: 10419426] (Far more people prefer terminal care at home than receive it.)

GENERAL APPROACH

Two general issues should be considered in caring for older persons in the hospital: determining the goals of care and designing and implementing strategies to achieve those goals. Failure to consider both these issues explicitly is common, often leading to a disconnect between hospital care and the hopes and expectations of those involved. Such disconnects lead to frustration and dissatisfaction on the parts of patients, family members, and caregivers.

The goals of hospital care for older persons vary widely. For patients, for example, the goals may include prolonging survival, relieving specific symptoms, maintaining or regaining ability to walk or care for oneself, getting help taking care of oneself, being reassured during a frightful experience, and providing comfort and peace while dying. Family members may share these goals but may also have additional goals, such as getting help caring for the patient, facilitating a transition in care from home to long-term care, or being protected from a frightening situation. Physicians and other professionals involved in the care of the patient may share some of these goals and also aim to reduce the pathophysiological manifestations of disease (such as hypoxia) or to get the patient out of the hospital in a certain amount of time to reduce work and hospital costs.

At the time of admission, the physician should attempt to define the major goals of care of each patient and of other involved parties, including key family members and professionals. Assumptions that a patient wants "everything" or wants "comfort care" will often be incorrect. The discussion of goals of care should be tailored to the situation; it may be brief or postponed in a life-threatening situation, and it may be a major focus of the admission evaluation in other patients with worsening of a chronic condition. Such discussions may be initiated with open-ended requests, such as "Different patients have different goals when they are admitted to the hospital. Can you tell me about what you would like us to accomplish while you are in the hospital?" Discussions of goals of care will be more broad ranging than simply cataloging do-not-resuscitate (DNR) decisions or reviewing options for specific therapeutic interventions. In fact, DNR and other decisions may be ill-informed without discussion of the goals of care.

Explicit articulation of goals of care will sometimes identify disagreements or unreasonable expectations, which should be recognized and usually addressed. Also, some goals may conflict with specific duties (eg, the physician's primary duty to act in the patient's interest) and should not be pursued. In general, a physician responsible for a patient should not act on goals of reducing lengths of stay or limiting therapy when those actions are not in the patient's interest.

Designing and implementing strategies to achieve the goals of care will require the physician's expertise and will often involve teamwork with other experts. For example, consider the situation of an 83-year-old widow with chronic obstructive pulmonary disease (COPD) and mild cognitive impairment who lives alone, has declined over the past month in her ability to take care of her home and her affairs, is admitted with hypoxia and hypercarbia attributed to a COPD exacerbation, and wishes to live in her home until she dies. Although the physician may have the expertise to treat the COPD exacerbation, he or she may want to involve nursing, social work, and occupational therapy in rehabilitative and adaptive efforts to promote the patient's independent function at home after discharge. To achieve the patient's goals of care, the physician's time may be spent better on involving and coordinating these other expert professionals than in "fine-tuning the numbers" beyond that necessary for the patient's function.

Fried TR et al: Understanding the treatment preferences of seriously ill patients. N Engl J Med 2002;346:1061. [PMID: 11932474] (Seriously ill patients differed in their choices and attitudes about the burdens of treatment, possible outcomes, and their likelihood.)

Tsevat J et al: Health values of hospitalized patients 80 years or older. HELP Investigators. Hospitalized Elderly Longitudinal Project. JAMA 1998;279:371. [PMID: 9459470] (Most patients were unwilling to trade survival for quality of life, but preferences varied greatly. Proxies and multivariable analyses could not gauge health values of patients accurately, indicating that health values should be elicited directly from the patient.)

ADMISSION ASSESSMENT

Assessment of complementary clinical domains should be performed on admission in each older patient. Problem-focused assessment will identify and address the reason for admission. In addition, a geriatric assessment tailored to the hospitalized patient will improve the care of most older patients.

Geriatric assessment of the hospitalized patient focuses on assessment of the patient's neuropsychiatric and functional status and of the social context of the patient's life and illness.

Neuropsychiatric assessment should include assessment of mental status, affect, and mobility. Among hospitalized older medical patients, ≥ 20% have dementia, ≥ 10% are delirious on admission, and another 15% experience delirium during hospitalization. Symptoms of depression are common, and 33% of hospitalized older medical patients have major or minor depression.

Neuropsychiatric assessment begins on meeting the patient. Stop to consider the possibility of dementia, delirium, depression, and impaired mobility: They are frequently present but infrequently reported. To whom are you speaking? If you are obtaining the history from a surrogate rather than the patient, cognitive impairment from dementia or delirium or both is likely. Look for impaired consciousness or attention. Listen for evidence of any change in mental status or behavior, and watch for signs of impaired thinking, speech, judgment, or function in performing activities of daily living (ADLs). Mental status can be further assessed by the Mini-Mental Status Examination or by shorter tests. Serious cognitive impairment is indicated by failure to know the year or by inability to recall any of 3 items; it is largely ruled out by orientation to date or by recall of 3 items and ability to draw the face of a clock (see Chapter 4). Ask the patient whether he or she has felt sad, depressed, or hopeless over the last month.

Functional assessment determines the patient's ability to walk and to perform basic ADLs (eg, bathing, dressing, transferring from a bed to a chair, using the toilet) both on admission and at baseline before onset of the acute illness. Patients who are dependent on admission (ie, they require the help of another person in performing 1 or more ADLs) have longer hospitalizations on average than otherwise similar patients who are not dependent. They are at higher risk for death in the hospital. If they survive, they are at high risk for remaining dependent on discharge. Patients dependent in ADLs at discharge are at increased risk for nursing home placement and for death during the next year.

The patient's social context is critical to care and recovery, especially after hospitalization, and this domain falls within the responsibilities of the physician as well as the social worker. Ask where the patient lives and with whom, whether he or she feels safe there, and whether he or she wishes to return to that place when leaving the hospital. Determine who assists, or would be available to assist, the patient with ADLs and instrumental ADLs, such as shopping, performing household chores, using transportation, and handling medicines and money. Will these persons be able to provide the care needed after hospitalization? These persons will be important factors in continuing medical care outside the hospital as well as in other aspects of the patient's well-being.

Neuropsychiatric and functional assessment and a geriatrically focused review of systems may identify conditions that are commonly considered geriatric syndromes, including dementia, delirium, functional decline, incontinence, falls, sensory impairment, and social isolation. Each of these conditions can and should be addressed specifically. In addition, however, it is important to recognize that frequently 2 or more geriatric syndromes occur synchronously in frail patients, and that the burden of this frailty on patients, families, and professionals is substantial.

Bierman AS: Functional status. The sixth vital sign. J Gen Intern Med 2001;16:785. [PMID: 11722694] (An appeal for systematic assessment of functional status in hospitalized elders.)

Covinsky KE et al: Measuring prognosis and case-mix in hospitalized elders: The importance of functional status. J Gen Intern Med 1997;12:203. [PMID: 9127223] (Ability to perform ADLs on admission is a strong predictor of survival and lower hospital costs.)

Lachs MS et al: A simple procedure for general screening for functional disability in elderly patients. Ann Intern Med 1990;112:699. [PMID: 2334082] (A reasonable approach that can be adapted to hospitalized older patients.)

THERAPY

In general, the treatment of disease should not differ according to age. Treatment should be selected on the basis of the goals of care for a particular patient and on the basis of evidence that a particular treatment regimen will achieve the specified goal.

Older patients may differ from younger patients according to their goals. For example, treatment directed primarily at amelioration of symptoms and dysfunction rather than prolongation of survival may be desired more often by patients in their 90s than by those in their 60s. Also, insofar as these choices are influenced by prognosis, which is determined in part by age, patients should be informed accurately when they desire this information. Nonetheless, the goals of care differ between patients of the same age and should be determined individually.

Evidence of the efficacy of a treatment regimen in achieving a specific goal should be sought. In some situations, treatment efficacy may differ by age. For example, thrombolytic therapy of acute myocardial infarction is less efficacious in prolonging survival in persons age 75 years and older than in younger persons, and acute coronary revascularization may be more efficacious in these patients. Doses of therapies often need to be titrated to reflect renal or hepatic function, which often decline with age. The risk of side effects from many drugs and procedures also increases with age, and these risks should be considered in estimating the net benefit of a specific treatment strategy.

Unfortunately, most evidence about the efficacy of many therapies is based on studies of younger persons, and specific evidence about the efficacy of those therapies in persons age 75 years or older is inadequate. In these situations, it is reasonable to extrapolate from evidence in younger patients, taking into account age-related differences in hepatic and renal function and risks of side effects when deciding on and implementing a specific treatment regimen.

Thiemann DR et al: Lack of benefit for intravenous thrombolysis in patients with myocardial infarction who are older than 75 years. Circulation 2000;101:2239. [PMID: 10811589] (Thrombolytic therapy for patients > 75 years old is unlikely to confer survival benefit and may have a significant survival disadvantage in contrast to the benefit of therapy in younger patients.)

Hutchins LF et al: Underrepresentation of patients 65 years of age or older in cancer-treatment trials. N Engl J Med 1999; 341:2061. [PMID: 10615079] (A total of 63% of cancer patients are 65 years of age and older, but only 25% of patients enrolled in cancer-treatment trials are 65 years or older.)

PREVENTION

Hospitalization provides an opportunity for the assessment and implementation of routine preventive maneuvers in older patients: In the hospital, patients receive far more medical care and attention than they do outside the hospital, and they are more available for and adherent to preventive maneuvers. Maneuvers that should be considered in every older hospitalized patient include

- Influenza vaccination.
- Pneumococcal vaccination.
- Testing and treatment for systolic hypertension, atrial fibrillation, and hypercholesterolemia.
- Determination of smoking status and counseling about smoking cessation.

- Screening for alcoholism and seeking counseling when indicated.
- Screening for dementia and depression and providing referral when indicated.

Screening for treatable cancer is usually not considered during hospitalization. Nonetheless, it is reasonable to implement otherwise indicated screening for breast or colorectal cancer during hospitalization.

For most patients, optimization of their daily function, including prevention of functional decline or return to baseline function, is an important goal during hospitalization. Functional decline may be prevented, and functional recovery promoted, by multicomponent strategies incorporating comprehensive geriatric assessment and management and principles of health care improvement. These strategies are exemplified by Geriatric Evaluation and Management (GEM), Acute Care for Elders (ACE), and the Hospital Elder Life Program (HELP). ACE has 4 key elements:

- A physical environment designed to facilitate independent function comfortably. Illustrative features include carpeting, uncluttered halls, and handrails to help walking.
- Patient-centered care tailored to each patient to maintain and promote independent function. Protocols are implemented by the primary nurse and based on a daily assessment to improve self-care, continence, nutrition, mobility, sleep, skin care, mood, and cognition.
- Planning to ease the return to home and to focus patient, family, and clinicians on this goal. The primary nurse assesses plans and needs on admission, and family members and a social worker are involved in planning early on.
- Medical care review avoids unnecessary procedures and medicines.

ACE is implemented on a hospital ward, the ACE Unit, to promote team function of the full array of clinicians caring for each patient and to enhance the potency of the intervention. ACE differs from GEM in that it is designed to be feasible for all hospitalized older patients from the time of hospital admission. Thus, ACE provides the opportunity to prevent further functional decline and rapidly ameliorate decline that occurred before admission.

HELP focuses on prevention of delirium. This intervention targets specific risk factors for delirium: cognitive impairment, hearing or visual impairment, sleep deprivation, immobility, and dehydration. HELP is implemented by an interdisciplinary team incorporating extensively trained volunteers.

Cohen HJ et al: A controlled trial of inpatient and outpatient geriatric evaluation and management. N Engl J Med 2002; 346:905. [PMID: 11907291] (Inpatient geriatric evaluation and management reduced functional decline with affecting survival or costs.)

Counsell SR et al: Effects of a multicomponent intervention on functional outcomes and process of care in hospitalized older patients: a randomized controlled trial of Acute Care for Elders (ACE) in a community hospital. J Am Geriatr Soc 2000;48:1572. [PMID: 11129745] (ACE improved process of care measures and satisfaction of patients, families, and providers.)

Inouye SK et al: A multicomponent intervention to prevent delirium in hospitalized older patients. N Engl J Med 1999; 340:669. [PMID: 100533175] (The Hospital Elder Life Program [HELP] reduced the incidence of delirium from 15% to 10%.)

Jencks SF et al: Change in the quality of care delivered to Medicare beneficiaries, 1998–1999 to 2000–2001. JAMA 2003;289: 305. [PMID: 12525231] (Measures of the process of hospital and outpatient care have improved for older Americans, and there is much room for further improvement.)

Landefeld CS: Improving care for older persons across the continuum of care: beyond ACE and GEM. Ann Intern Med 2003; 139:421. [PMID: not available] (Overview of comprehensive approaches to improving care of hospitalized older persons.)

Landefeld CS et al: A randomized trial of care in a hospital medical unit especially designed to improve the functional outcomes of acutely ill older patients. N Engl J Med 1995;332:1338. [PMID: 7715644] (Acute Care for Elders [ACE] improved functional outcomes at discharge and reduced nursing home admissions.)

Nichol KL et al: Influenza vaccination and reduction in hospitalizations for cardiac disease and stroke among the elderly. N Engl J Med 2003;348:1322. [PMID: 12672859] (In patients aged 65 years or older, vaccination against influenza was associated with reductions in the risk of hospitalization for heart disease, cerebrovascular disease, and pneumonia or influenza as well as the risk of death from all causes during influenza seasons.)

Stuck AE et al: Comprehensive geriatric assessment: A meta-analysis of controlled trials. Lancet 1993;342:1032. [PMID: 8105269] (Comprehensive geriatric assessment and management was associated with improved survival and health outcomes.)

MONITORING

In addition to monitoring the response to therapy of the primary manifestations of the reason for admission, neuropsychiatric and functional status should be monitored during hospitalization. Delirium develops in ~15% of hospitalized older medical patients and decline in ADL function occurs in 17%. Each of these events is associated with worse patient outcomes, longer hospital length of stay, and increased costs. There is little evidence about the efficacy of acute rehabilitation on delirium or functional decline once they have developed during hospitalization. Nonetheless, delirium and functional decline should be recognized as signs of the failure or side effects of the treatment regimen and of inadequate efforts to maintain function, and both should be reconsidered. For example, is delirium related to sleep deprivation or to a sedative–hypnotic? Is functional decline related to delirium, to poor nutrition, or to bed rest and insufficient exercise and physical therapy?

PLANNING TO GO HOME

Planning to go home, or to another setting, from the hospital should begin on admission. Moreover, this planning process should focus on defining and achieving the patient's goal of living in a particular setting. By defining this goal and beginning to work toward it early in hospitalization, planning to go home will facilitate the patient's leaving the hospital at the appropriate time. Planning to go home may differ in its focus from conventional "discharge planning," which sometimes seems aimed at getting patients out of the hospital with the connotation that they have worn their welcome thin and passed their expected length of stay. Also, by focusing on a desired goal of hospitalization, planning to go home provides a positive focus that may counter the negative expectations many older patients and their families have about the outcome of hospitalization.

Planning to go home is a joint responsibility of the patient and family, the patient's physicians and nurses, and the hospital social worker. The physician should inquire on admission or shortly thereafter about the patient's goal and the resources that may be necessary to achieve that goal. This information should be discussed with the social worker, who can collect further information and coordinate the needed resources.

Community-Based & Nursing Home Long-Term Care

8

Mary Anne Johnson, MD

■ COMMUNITY-BASED LONG-TERM CARE

ADULT DAY HEALTH CARE

Ninety percent of adult day health care (ADHC) centers are nonprofit or government programs. ADHC programs provide nursing, social service, rehabilitation, nutrition services, and transportation along with social and therapeutic activities to frail individuals living at home who might otherwise require institutional care. Through structured rehabilitation and activity programs, social support, and monitoring of health status, such programs allow elderly patients to remain at home and provide daytime respite to home caregivers. Typically, a participant attends the program several days a week.

State regulations for ADHC programs vary considerably, but the National Adult Day Services Association has set voluntary standards. Funding may come from Medicaid or other government sources (eg, Veterans Administration contracts), foundations, long-term care insurance, or participants' own resources, often on a sliding-scale basis (Table 8–1). Medicare does not pay for these services.

The Program for All Inclusive Care for the Elderly (PACE) model is centered on ADHC programs but also includes all needed health and social services. In this capitated model, Medicare and Medicaid allocations are combined for each enrollee to cover all services, including physician and hospital services. Some PACE programs also work with government agencies to provide low-income assisted-living housing for frail seniors close to or in the same building as the ADHC program.

Participants in the PACE program must be sufficiently frail to qualify for nursing home care. PACE programs use an interdisciplinary team model to manage and coordinate care across the care continuum. The hospitalization rate for PACE participants is less than half that of elderly persons with similar needs who are not enrolled in a PACE program. Such a finding sup-

ports the idea that comprehensive medical and social care programs may be more appropriate models for frail elders than traditionally funded services, which have little care coordination.

Bodenheimer T: Long-term care for frail elderly people—the On Lok model. N Engl J Med 1999;341:1324. [PMID: 10528046]

Center for Medicare and Medicaid Services: www.cms.hhs.gov/ pace (This web site provides information about the Program of All Inclusive Care for the Elderly, funding, and regulations.)

National Adult Day Services Association: www.nadsa.org (This web site provides general information, a guide to selecting an ADHC program, and a directory of programs by location.)

ASSISTED-LIVING FACILITIES

Assisted-living facilities (often referred to as board and care homes, foster homes, domiciliary care, residential care facilities) can be small, private homes with only a few residents or large complexes built specifically for this purpose. State regulations vary widely on what services can be provided and the types of residents who can be cared for in this setting. Some states are still in the process of developing regulations. In many facilities, residents must be ambulatory and continent, although some homes accept residents with more functional impairment or keep existing residents who become more functionally impaired, depending on state regulations.

Facility staff provide supervision and monitoring for health and safety, assistance with activities of daily living (ADLs) and instrumental ADLs (IADLs), medication administration, transportation to medical appointments, and coordination of services with outside agencies. Licensed nurses are usually not present on site, depending on services provided and state law. Home care agencies may provide on-site skilled nursing services, and residents usually go to the physician's office for medical care.

Generally, residents pay privately for assisted living, but many states provide some Medicaid reimbursement when the assisted-living setting is an alternative to nursing home care for Medicaid recipients. Because personal funds are used most often for this level of care,

Table 8–1. Long-term care services & financing.

Services	Source of Funding
Attendant care (ADL, IADL assistance)	Medicaid home and community based services waiver in some states; Medicare only if also receiving skilled care; personal funds; state or county funds for low-income clients; VA for eligible veterans; some long-term care insurance
Homemaker services (meal preparation, cleaning, shopping)	Personal funds; state or county funds for low-income clients; VA for eligible veterans; some long-term care insurance
Home-delivered meals	Personal funds; county funds in some counties for low-income clients; programs subsidized by OAA funds
Nonurgent transportation	Personal funds; local government subsidies for low-income clients; Medicaid for medical need
Financial management	Personal funds
Assisted living	Personal funds; Medicaid in some states for low-income clients if substitutes for nursing home care; some long-term care insurance
Adult day health care	Personal funds; Medicaid; local government funds; some long-term care insurance; government block grants
Program of all-inclusive care for elderly	Medicare and medicaid; some programs accept those who pay privately when not eligible for medicaid
Skilled home care	Medicare; personal funds; medical insurance; long-term care insurance
Hospice	Medicare; personal funds; medical insurance; long-term care insurance
Nursing home care	Medicaid; personal funds medicare for skilled need; long-term care insurance

ADL, activities of daily living; IADL, instrumental ADL, VA, Veteran's Administration; OAA, Office of Affirmative Action.

there is much more market competition than for other long-term care services, and facilities are quite diverse in terms of amenities.

The Joint Commission on Accreditation of Healthcare Organizations (JCAHO) offers accreditation for assisted-living facilities, but there are no governing federal regulations. However, assisted-living facilities are now receiving closer scrutiny by regulators. A coalition of organizations involved in assisted living has developed guidelines for assisted-living facilities that may impact any future federal regulatory process.

National Center for Assisted Living: www.ncal.org (This web site provides a history of the assisted-living movement, general information about programs and residents, and current topics of interest.)

CASE MANAGEMENT & CONTINUING CARE COMMUNITIES

In most states and communities, there is no single point of access for long-term care services and no coordination between the various programs. Case management or care management programs, which can be either government-sponsored or private, oversee the care of functionally impaired individuals living in the community to ensure that those individuals receive all needed medical and social services and to prevent nursing home placement whenever possible. Care or case management is most needed when elderly individuals

are not connected to a strong interdisciplinary team site such as a nursing home, home care program, or ADHC center.

An array of long-term care services may be available as part of a life care or continuing care retirement community where individuals can purchase or rent an apartment while independent and then move, as needed, to higher levels of care such as assisted-living and nursing home care. Meals and social and recreational opportunities are available. Such communities generally require significant financial resources to "buy in" on the part of the applicant.

■ INSTITUTIONAL LONG-TERM CARE

COMMUNITY & HOSPITAL-BASED NURSING HOMES

Almost 50% of individuals reaching age 65 will spend some time in a nursing home during their lifetime. Much regulatory attention has been paid to nursing home care, and nursing homes are subject to very strict regulatory compliance, with standards set by the federal government and surveyed by state licensing agencies.

Many hospitals operate skilled nursing units within their facilities to provide ongoing care for patients recently discharged. Hospital-based units are typically staffed at a higher nurse–patient ratio and have more licensed staff than community facilities. In these hospital-based facilities, stays are relatively short; care is focused on rehabilitation and discharge to home or a lower level of care.

The typical community nursing home is a 100-bed facility run as part of a proprietary (for profit) chain. Sixty-seven percent of facilities are proprietary, 27% are nonprofit, and 6% are government or other facilities. In community-based facilities, the population is generally very heterogeneous, requiring services ranging from restorative care and rehabilitation to hospice and long-term care.

The degree of medical complexity in nursing homes has increased dramatically because patients are being discharged from the hospital with more unresolved problems and there are other long-term care options for those with fewer care needs, creating major challenges for nursing homes.

Harrington C: Regulating nursing homes. Residential nursing facilities in the United States. BMJ 2001;323:507. [PMID: 11532849]

American Association of Retired Persons: www.aarp.org/confacts/health/choosingnh.html (This site contains the AARP's guide to choosing a nursing home.)

American Health Care Association: www.ahca.org (Web site provides general information and links to other sites.)

National Citizens' Coalition for Nursing Home Reform: www.nccnhr.org (This web site provides consumers with information about policies, quality of care, the ombudsman program, and advocacy groups.)

National Library of Medicine Medline Plus: http://www.medlineplus.gov/nursinghomes.html (This health information page provides links to organizations, consumer guides to nursing homes, information about nursing home regulations and inspections, alternatives to nursing homes, and research studies about nursing homes.)

FUNDING

Medicare will pay for nursing home care only when the patient has had a previous acute hospital admission and meets criteria for skilled care requiring treatment by a registered nurse or rehabilitation therapist (see Table 8–1). Medicare will pay for 20 days of nursing home care and part of the cost for an additional 80 days per episode of illness.

Individuals who do not qualify for Medicare payment for nursing home care because they do not have coverage, do not have a defined skilled need, or have exhausted their benefits must use personal assets for payment. Once personal assets have been spent down to a predetermined level, individuals are eligible for Medicaid nursing home benefits. This requires that many older persons become impoverished to qualify. At an average daily cost of $116, even short stays can be financially catastrophic.

States vary in their clinical eligibility criteria for Medicaid payment of nursing home care. However, in general, Medicaid covers a broader array of care needs than Medicare. Long-term care insurance is available, but many elderly people are unfamiliar with the policies or with the need for long-term care insurance, and less than 20% of the elderly can afford it.

CARE GUIDELINES

Minimum Data Set

For each person admitted to a nursing home, the interdisciplinary team must complete a federally mandated minimum data set (MDS) based on a comprehensive resident assessment. Information in the physician's admission note and progress notes is used by other disciplines to complete the MDS. The MDS is extremely important because it leads to development of the care plan and determines Medicare reimbursement. In addition, facilities and regulatory agencies use the data to monitor quality of care.

Admission Evaluation

The physician's admission evaluation should include a detailed history, with emphasis not only on recent and chronic medical conditions but also on past and present functional status, medications, immunizations, sensory impairments, pain, symptoms of depression, social support, and presence of an advance directive. The admission physical examination should be complete, with a focus on the conditions leading to nursing home admission. The examination should include, in particular, assessment of functional abilities (ADLs, IADLs), cognitive status, affect, ability to make health care decisions, condition of the skin and feet, vision and hearing deficits, orthostatic hypotension, and nutritional status. A problem list should be generated with individualized goals of care, and a medical care plan should be developed in concert with the interdisciplinary team, the resident, and the resident's family.

Medicare-Mandated Physician Visits

Medicare regulations require that the physician make monthly visits for the first 90 days of a resident's nursing home stay and then every 60 days thereafter. Depending on the state, Medicaid regulations may require more frequent, usually monthly, visits. Medicare has clearly articulated that all medically necessary visits to nursing home residents will be reimbursed. Thus, if a resident requires daily or weekly visits, appropriate documentation by the physician of the medical need for the visit should be sufficient to ensure reimbursement.

Interim visits to the postacute nursing home resident can focus on the most acute problems and monitor progress toward discharge. In the long-term resident, interim visits could focus on a particular issue (eg, discussion of an advance directive or management of a particular chronic problem). Each visit should include a discussion with the nursing staff and review of interdisciplinary notes, laboratory studies, and consultation reports as well as a review of any new problems, progress of chronic problems, and responses to any previously initiated treatments. This should include, in particular, assessment of response to pain medication, psychoactive medications of any kind, and any medication changes. During the interim visits, relevant physical examinations should be done and appropriate health maintenance and screening activities addressed, such as vaccines and cancer screening, as appropriate for the resident.

Annual Resident Assessments

The physician should perform a comprehensive assessment of the resident at the annual MDS review, contributing to the interdisciplinary team's assessment. This yearly assessment should include a problem-oriented note with updates for history and physical examination, summaries of laboratory tests and other interventions, and responses to treatments.

The physician should also perform a comprehensive review of symptoms, especially looking for those that may go unreported, such as constipation, incontinence, insomnia, and depression. Assessments of pain, weight, and functional status should be part of the annual assessment, and evaluations should be completed and documented for any significant changes.

Health maintenance and screening activities that need to be done annually should be reassessed at this time. Based on the high risk of tuberculosis (TB) in nursing home residents, purified protein derivative testing should be done annually. The Centers for Disease Control recommends influenza vaccine for all nursing home residents annually before the influenza season and pneumococcal vaccine at least once. Routine annual laboratory studies are generally not indicated, although some nursing home physicians recommend annual hematocrit, electrolytes, renal function studies, thyroid function studies, and urinalysis.

At the annual review, it is also important for the physician to review and update the goals of care, advance directives, and the interdisciplinary care plan. Ideally, the physician should attend interdisciplinary team care planning conferences, which are held within 14 days of admission, quarterly, and annually.

Emergencies

Federal regulations require the nursing home to notify the resident's physician of any significant injury or change in condition. Some facilities and physician groups have developed guidelines for when to call the physician, based on a common understanding of how quickly a resident with particular signs or symptoms needs to be evaluated. However, nursing judgment about the need to call should always supersede any written guidelines.

Most physicians who care for nursing home residents are unable to respond personally to calls regarding a change in a resident's condition. Thus, many nursing home problems are handled over the telephone, and in many instances nursing home residents are transferred to an emergency room for evaluation. These practices often result in administration of inappropriate medications such as antibiotics, unnecessary transfers to emergency rooms, and failure to follow a resident's advance directives. Implementation of a nurse practitioner/physician team approach has been demonstrated to improve care and reduce emergency room visits and hospitalizations for nursing home residents; in this model, the nurse practitioner responds to calls and performs on-site evaluations.

If a resident is transferred to an emergency room, it is essential for the physician to communicate directly with the emergency room physician to ensure continuity of care and respect for the resident's wishes and advance directives. In addition, the transfer of medical information from nursing home to hospital and from hospital to nursing home must be complete to maintain continuity of care and provide optimal care in both settings.

Mehr DR et al: Predicting mortality in nursing home residents with lower respiratory tract infection: The Missouri LRI study. JAMA 2001;286:2427. [PMID: 11712938]

Center for Aging Practices at University of Medicine and Dentistry of New Jersey: www.umdnj.edu/nhweb (This is a web-based course for health professionals regarding nursing home regulations, quality indicators, and funding.)

SPECIFIC CLINICAL ISSUES
Falls & Restraint Use

When a resident falls, a medical evaluation may identify a cause such as orthostatic hypotension, medication side effect, loss of functional status, or sensory deficits. Environmental or situational causes can often be ameliorated by providing residents with appropriate footwear, modifying floor coverings, improving access to a toilet or commode, and improving staff supervision of the resident.

In the past, restraints were used very frequently in nursing homes and were prescribed primarily to prevent falls. However, restraints can cause serious injuries and death, facilitate deconditioning, increase residents' dependence on others, and increase agitation. In addition, because residents are not mobile in restraints, there is an increased risk of pneumonia, constipation, incontinence, and pressure ulcers.

Probably one of the most important consequences of restraint use is loss of resident dignity. Restraints also demoralize staff; facilities that have reduced or eliminated restraints have experienced a significant decrease in staff turnover. Regulatory agencies carefully monitor the use of restraints in nursing homes. Regulations require documentation of need for restraints, use of nonrestraint alternatives as a first step, careful monitoring of residents during restraint use, and attempts to reduce restraint use. Physicians' responsibilities regarding restraint use include ensuring that medical causes for falls have been evaluated and eliminated, that symptoms leading to agitation have been evaluated and treated (eg, pain), and that a care plan has been developed to address the condition for which restraints are being considered or used.

In many instances, administrative policies and family requests actually promote the use of restraints; therefore, it is essential that the nursing home administration and staff, as well as residents and families, are educated in the use of, and risks associated with, restraints. This education should include the fact that all falls are not preventable.

Because not all falls are preventable and they may increase with restraint reduction, the physician should ensure that efforts are instituted to decrease injuries should falls occur. These measures may include calcium and vitamin D supplementation, exercise programs, and use of hip pads.

Neufeld RR et al: Restraint reduction reduces serious injuries among nursing home residents. J Am Geriatr Soc 1999; 47:1202. [PMID: 10522953]

Ooi WL et al: The association between orthostatic hypotension and recurrent falls in nursing home residents. Am J Med 2000; 108:106.

Ray WA et al: Benzodiazepines and the risk of falls in nursing home residents. J Am Geriatr Soc 2000;48:682. [PMID: 11126303]

Schoenfelder DP: A fall prevention program for elderly individuals. Exercise in long-term care settings. J Gerontol Nurs 2001; 26:43. [PMID: 11111630]

Incontinence

The physician must work with the nursing staff in evaluating possible causes of incontinence and in developing a plan to reduce incontinence or manage it in a way that is appropriate for the individual patient.

Catheters should never be used to manage incontinence except if needed in the short term for wound healing. Prompted voiding and timed toileting have been successful in reducing incontinence episodes.

Weight Loss

Weight loss is common in nursing home residents and is a predictor of mortality. Weight loss can be related to medical conditions, including swallowing difficulties, medications, pain, dental problems, functional impairment, depression, or chronic medical conditions. In addition, restricted and unpalatable diets are often prescribed for nursing home residents and may contribute to decreased intake. If a reversible cause of weight loss is not found, the physician can educate the resident, if possible, and the family, and jointly assess whether tube feeding is medically appropriate and consistent with the resident's desires and goals of care. Many interventions have been shown to forestall or eliminate the need for tube feeding, even in very demented patients, such as offering favorite foods, changing food consistency, and ensuring that adequate staff is available to assist the resident with eating.

Dehydration in cognitively and physically impaired nursing home residents occurs frequently. Although acute medical illnesses and the use of diuretics may contribute to dehydration, adequate fluid provision by staff will prevent most cases of dehydration.

The Council on Nutritional Clinical Strategies in Long-Term Care has published a useful interdisciplinary clinical guideline for nutritional management in long-term care based on the literature and consensus.

Gessert CE et al: Tube feeding in nursing home residents with severe and irreversible cognitive impairment. J Am Geriatr Soc 2000;48:1593. [PMID: 1129748]

Kayser-Jones J et al: Factors contributing to dehydration in nursing homes: Inadequate staffing and lack of professional supervision. J Am Geriatr Soc 1999;47:1187. [PMID: 10522951]

Thomas DR et al: Nutritional management in long-term care: Development of a clinical guideline. J Gerontol A Biol Sci Med Sci 2000;55A:M725. [PMID: 11129394]

Pressure Ulcers

Pressure ulcers occur among patients in all institutional settings. Generally, the rate of pressure ulcer development in nursing homes is a good indicator of overall quality of care. However, pressure ulcers may be present in a high percentage of residents in facilities that care for many patients at the end of life and in those that provide postacute care. Physicians should assess nursing home residents for pressure ulcers and pressure ulcer risk at admission and examine the resident frequently. If a resident develops a pressure ulcer, the physician should complete a full medical assessment, request a nutritional assessment, and consult with appropriate staff to develop a plan for healing.

Berlowitz DR et al: Are we improving the quality of nursing home care: The case of pressure ulcers. J Am Geriatr Soc 2000; 48:59.

Infections

Infections are common as a result of chronic medical conditions, age-related organ deficits, age-related decline in immune function, use of procedures and invasive devices, and congregate living. The most common infections are pneumonia, urinary tract infections, gastroenteritis, and skin and soft tissue infections.

Any change in a resident's condition, particularly one who is unable to articulate symptoms, should prompt a careful evaluation for infection. The physician can work to prevent infections by ensuring that nursing home residents receive an influenza vaccine annually, a pneumococcal vaccine once, TB screening on admission and annually, and appropriate treatment of latent TB. Indwelling catheters increase the risk of urinary tract infections; thus, efforts should be made to avoid these unless absolutely essential (eg, for wound healing). The presence of pressure ulcers increases the risk of skin and soft tissue infection; efforts to prevent pressure ulcers should reduce infection rate. All nursing home staff and physicians should use good infection control practices.

Inappropriate antibiotic use in nursing homes is common and has led to an increase in antibiotic resistance. For example, *Clostridium difficile* is a major problem in many nursing homes, and antibiotic-resistant staphylococci and enterococci are being seen more frequently. Physicians can reduce inappropriate antibiotic use by carefully assessing the need for antibiotics in febrile nursing home residents and, when needed, using the narrowest spectrum antibiotic for the shortest period of time.

Bentley DW et al: Practice guidelines for evaluation of fever in long-term care facilities. Clin Infect Dis 2000;31:148. [PMID: 11017809]

Loeb M et al: Development of minimum criteria for the initiation of antibiotics in residents of long-term care facilities: Results of a consensus conference. Infect Control Hosp Epidemiol 2001;22:120. [PMID: 11232875]

Nicolle LE et al: Antimicrobial use in long-term care facilities. Infect Control Hosp Epidemiol 2000;21:537. [PMID: 10968734]

Adverse Drug Reactions

Adverse drug reactions are common among nursing home residents and are more likely to occur with increasing numbers of comorbid conditions; with increasing numbers of medications; in newly admitted residents; and with use of opioids, antidepressants, antipsychotic medications, and antibiotics. Many of these adverse drug reactions are potentially preventable, and physician vigilance is required.

Field TS et al: Risk factors for adverse drug events among nursing home residents. Arch Intern Med 2001;161:1629. [PMID: 11434795]

BEHAVIORAL PROBLEMS

Behavioral problems (eg, aggression, agitation, inappropriate sexual behavior, wandering, persistent calling out) are very common, especially among cognitively impaired residents. Medical causes include hypoglycemia, hypoxia, medication side effect, infection, pain, sleep deprivation, and depression.

Management of behavioral problems for which there is no reversible cause is often difficult. Involvement of mental health professionals and trained nursing staff may be helpful.

Physicians who work in nursing homes should be familiar with the regulations governing the use of psychoactive medication for behavior management. These regulations require that the use of psychoactive medications be supported by excellent documentation of the clinical need. Antipsychotic medication use, in particular, is carefully reviewed by state licensing agencies, and requirements call for a tapering off of these medications when they are not being used for a primary psychiatric problem. Observational studies indicate that psychoactive medication use decreased after implementation of the federal regulations regarding use of these medications (part of OBRA 87). However, it is not clear that resident outcomes are improved.

Hughes CM et al: The impact of legislation on psychotropic drug use in nursing homes: A cross-national perspective. J Am Geriatr Soc 2000;48:931. [PMID: 10968297]

Ruby CM, Kennedy DH: Psychopharmacologic medication use in nursing home care. Indicators for survey assessment of the drug regimen reviews, recommendations for monitoring, and non-pharmacologic alternatives. Clin Fam Pract 2001;3:577.

End-of-Life Care

One in 5 deaths in the United States occurs in the nursing home, making end-of-life care an important priority in resident care. If the resident's goals of care are clearly documented in an advance directive, it will be easier for the physician and the team to make the transition from aggressive intervention to palliative care. The focus of palliative care in the nursing home is on symptom management, family support, bereavement counseling, and management of the physical, psychological, and spiritual needs of the resident. Attention is paid particularly to pain but also to dyspnea, constipation, anxiety, agitation, fear, and loneliness. Pain assessment may be difficult in the cognitively impaired resident, but guidelines have been published to help in this assessment. Residents who are dying require intensive medical, psychosocial, and spiritual interventions.

Community hospice organizations may offer services within nursing homes, and some nursing homes have developed their own hospice programs. In nursing homes where there is a specific hospice or palliative care presence, end-of-life hospitalizations are decreased.

Baer WM, Hanson LC: Families' perception of the added value of hospice in the nursing home. J Am Geriatr Soc 2000;48:879. [PMID: 10968290]

Gillick M et al: A patient-centered approach to advance medical planning in the nursing home. J Am Geriatr Soc 2001; 47:227. [PMID: 9988295]

Hanson LC: Care of the dying in long-term care settings. Clin Geriatr Med 2000;16:225. [PMID: 10783426]

Levin JR et al: Life-sustaining treatment decisions for nursing home residents: Who discusses, who decides and what is decided? J Am Geriatr Soc 1999;47:82. [PMID: 9920234]

Miller SC et al: Hospice enrollment and hospitalization of dying nursing home residents. Am J Med 2001;111;38. [PMID: 11448659]

Molloy DW et al: Systematic implementation of an advance directive program in nursing homes: A randomized controlled trial. JAMA 2000;283:1437. [PMID: 10732933]

Stein W: Pain management in the elderly. Pain in the nursing home. Clin Geriatr Med 2001;17:575. [PMID: 11459722]

Surgical & Perioperative Care

Peter Pompei, MD

■ ASSESSING & MANAGING PREOPERATIVE RISK FACTORS

Cardiovascular problems, respiratory compromise, and neuropsychiatric changes are among the most common and serious complications of operative therapies in older patients.

CARDIAC RISK

A number of different cardiac risk indexes have been developed for patients undergoing noncardiac surgery. These have been useful for stratifying patients according to their risk of cardiac complications based on information gathered preoperatively from their history, physical examination, and laboratory test results. Although quantifying the likelihood of cardiac complications can be useful to the physician by focusing attention on those patients at highest risk, it may be even more useful to have evidence-based direction on the optimal management of the identified problems.

A practice guideline has been developed by the American College of Cardiology and the American Heart Association (Figure 9–1). Step 1 asks the clinician to clarify the urgency of the procedure. Step 2 calls for knowledge of any previous coronary revascularization. In Step 3, clinical predictors culled from many studies have been divided into 3 levels of importance: minor, intermediate, and major. Advanced age is only a minor clinical predictor; rather, the presence of accumulated medical problems more strongly increases operative risk among older persons. For patients who have intermediate or minor clinical predictors, it is important to consider functional capacity (Steps 6 and 7). Patients should be asked whether they can do more than light household work (dusting or washing dishes), such as climbing a flight of stairs, walking up a hill, and walking on level ground at 4 mph (6.4 km/h). These activities are associated with more than 4 metabolic equivalents, and patients who can exert themselves to this degree are judged to have at least a moderately good functional capacity. As also shown in Steps 6 and 7, the assessment of intrinsic procedural risk will influence recommendations regarding preoperative management.

High-risk procedures include emergent major operations, aortic and other vascular surgery, and prolonged procedures with large fluid shifts or blood loss. Examples of intermediate risk procedures are carotid endarterectomy, head and neck surgery, and intraperitoneal, thoracic, orthopedic, and prostate operations. Common low-risk procedures are cataract and breast surgery and endoscopic procedures.

Additional evaluation and management are recommended for all patients with major clinical predictors before operative therapy. Noninvasive cardiac testing is recommended before operative therapy for patients with intermediate clinical predictors and poor functional status or moderate to excellent functional status if the planned procedure is high risk. Noninvasive cardiac testing is also recommended for patients with no or minor clinical predictors who have a poor functional status and are scheduled for a high-risk procedure. Like other practice guidelines, this one is intended to assist physicians in meeting the needs of most patients in the majority of circumstances, and final decisions regarding an individual patient should be made jointly by the treating physician and the patient.

PULMONARY RISK

Pulmonary complications are also common among older persons undergoing operative therapies. This is due to age-related changes in the respiratory system and to the effects of anesthesia and surgery on the lungs. Advancing age is associated with reduced alveolar elasticity and increased chest wall stiffness, changes that can predispose to atelectasis and decreased expiratory flow rates. The supine position, general anesthetic agents, and abdominal incisions contribute to reduced functional residual capacity and increased airway resistance. Resultant hypoventilation and atelectasis may cause hypoxemia and infection. Identifying patients at high risk for respiratory decompensation is a first step in attempting to reduce the complication rate.

Several characteristics identify patients at increased risk for pulmonary complications: impaired cognitive function, body mass index of ≥ 27 kg/m^2, chest wall or upper abdomen incision, smoking within the past 8 weeks, age ≥ 60 years, a history of cancer, a history of angina, an incision length ≥ 30 cm, and an American

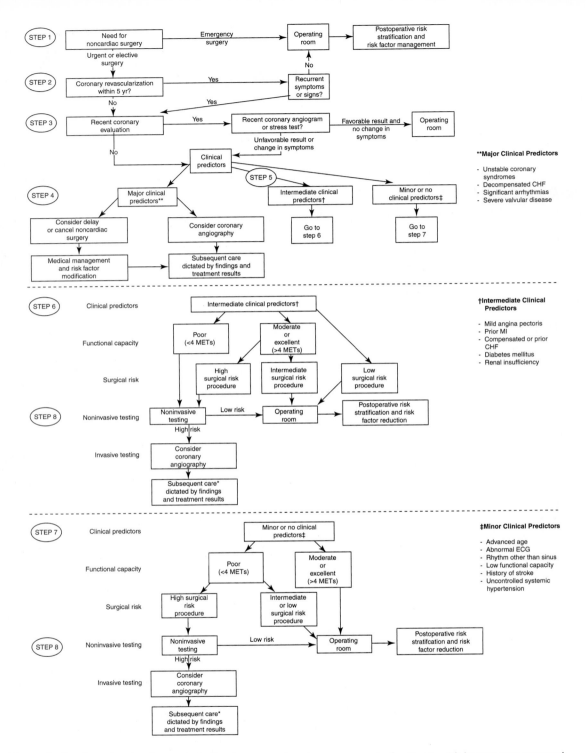

Figure 9–1. Algorithm for the preoperative assessment and management of patients with known or suspected cardiac disease. CHF, congestive heart failure; ECG, electrocardiogram; MET, metabolic equivalent; MI, myocardial infarction. From Eagle KA et al: ACC/AHA guideline update for perioperative cardiovascular evaluation for noncardiac surgery: A report of the American College of Cardiology/American Heart Association Task Force on Practice Guidelines. American College of Cardiology, 2002. Used with permission.

Society of Anesthesiologists rating of class III or greater. More work is needed to establish a valid risk index that can serve as the basis for a practice guideline. Beyond identifying those patients at greatest risk for pulmonary complications, the physician has an important role to play in encouraging coughing, deep breathing exercises, incentive spirometry, and early mobility to further reduce the risk of respiratory problems.

NEUROPSYCHIATRIC RISK

Neuropsychiatric problems such as dementia and depression are common among older patients and can contribute to poor outcomes after surgery. The most common postoperative neuropsychiatric complication is delirium. Both preoperative and intraoperative factors have been evaluated as risk factors for delirium. Factors that predispose an individual to postoperative delirium after noncardiac surgery are age ≥ 70 years; cognitive impairment; limited physical function; history of alcohol abuse; abnormal serum sodium, potassium, or glucose; intrathoracic surgery; and abdominal aneurysm surgery. Type of anesthesia and intraoperative hypotension, bradycardia, and tachycardia are not associated with delirium. Patients with a postoperative hematocrit < 30% have an increased risk of delirium. Clinicians caring for patients at greatest risk of delirium should focus management on correcting fluid, electrolyte, and metabolic derangements and optimizing replacement of blood loss.

Brooks-Brunn JA: Validation of a predictive model for postoperative pulmonary complications. Heart Lung 1998;27:151.

Gilbert K et al: Prospective evaluation of cardiac risk indices for patients undergoing noncardiac surgery. Ann Intern Med 2000; 133:356.

Marcantonio ER et al: The association of intraoperative factors with the development of postoperative delirium. Am J Med 1998;105:380.

Eagle KA et al: ACC/AHA guideline update for perioperative cardiovascular evaluation for noncardiac surgery: A report of the American College of Cardiology/American Heart Association Task Force on Practice Guidelines (Committee to update the 1996 guidelines on perioperative cardiovascular evaluation for noncardiac surgery): www.acc.org/clinical/guidelines/perio/clean/perio_index.htm

■ PERIOPERATIVE MANAGEMENT OF SELECTED MEDICAL PROBLEMS

Several medical conditions commonly encountered in older persons deserve special attention during the perioperative period. For some of these, changes in therapy are warranted preoperatively; for others, aggressive perioperative management is critical to reduce the risk of complications.

CARDIOVASCULAR PROBLEMS

Hypertension

Hypertension is among the most common chronic medical problems among older persons and is associated with an increased risk of stroke, myocardial infarction, and renal insufficiency. Perioperative myocardial ischemia is related not only to uncontrolled preoperative hypertension but also to major fluctuations in blood pressure during the procedure. This variability can be related to the effects of anesthetic agents, stimulation of the sympathetic and parasympathetic pathways, and changes in intravascular volume. Patients with chronic hypertension should have their blood pressure well controlled before any procedure, and elective procedures should be postponed if the preoperative blood pressure is > 180/110 mm Hg. Oral antihypertensives should be given with a sip of water on the day of operation and restarted as soon as possible postoperatively. When the blood pressure is elevated postoperatively, secondary causes such as pain or a distended bladder should first be investigated. Parenteral medications that are useful in controlling essential hypertension in older persons after operations include β-blockers, calcium channel blockers, angiotensin-converting enzyme (ACE) inhibitors, and drugs that block both α- and β-adrenergic receptors. Vasodilators such as hydralazine should be used with caution because of the risk of compromising diastolic filling if there is hypertrophic cardiomyopathy related to chronic hypertension.

Atherosclerosis

The administration of β-blockers perioperatively to patients with known or suspected coronary artery disease has been shown to reduce the risk of cardiac complications.

Stroke

Patients at increased risk for stroke are those with known cerebral or peripheral vascular disease and chronic obstructive pulmonary disease. Patients who have experienced transient ischemic attacks should be evaluated for carotid stenosis. If a carotid endarterectomy is indicated, this should be done before elective noncardiac surgery.

Congestive Heart Failure

Patients in decompensated heart failure should have elective procedures postponed. Drug regimens that should be continued perioperatively generally include β-blockers, ACE inhibitors, and diuretics. Optimizing ventricular filling pressures is key, and it is often difficult to accurately assess volume status in older persons by physical examination and standard laboratory parameters. Swan-Ganz catheters and transesophageal echocardiography have substantially improved our ability to monitor cardiac output and optimize volume management.

Valvular Heart Disease

The greatest risks associated with valvular heart disease include congestive heart failure and endocarditis. Asymptomatic aortic stenosis leading to myocardial ischemia or congestive heart failure can be difficult to distinguish from the more benign aortic sclerosis common in older persons. A bedside prediction rule to identify moderate or severe aortic stenosis is to listen for a systolic murmur over the right clavicle. If absent, significant aortic stenosis is unlikely; if present, the patient should be examined for reduced carotid artery volume, slow carotid artery upstroke, reduced intensity of the second heart sound, and maximum intensity of the murmur over the second right intercostal space. If 3 of these 4 findings are present, there is a significant risk of aortic stenosis, which can be confirmed by echocardiogram. Selected valvular and other cardiac conditions predispose patients to the risk of endocarditis, for which prophylactic antibiotics are indicated. Patients with prosthetic cardiac valves, complex congenital heart disease, and surgically constructed systemic-pulmonary shunts or conduits or a history of endocarditis are at highest risk. Patients at moderate risk are those with other congenital cardiac malformations, acquired valvular dysfunction, hypertrophic cardiomyopathy, mitral valve prolapse with regurgitation, or thickened leaflets. Patients undergoing procedures that involve the respiratory, biliary, or intestinal mucosa, prostate surgery, cystoscopy, or urethral dilation should be given endocarditis prophylaxis. Recommended antibiotic regimens according to procedure and patient risk category are shown in Table 9–1.

Cardiac Rhythm Disturbances

Cardiac rhythm disturbances can increase the risk of myocardial ischemia and congestive heart failure. Older persons are at increased risk for supraventricular tachycardias, especially those with a history of a supraventricular dysrhythmia, asthma, congestive heart failure, and premature atrial complexes on a preoperative electrocardiogram and those undergoing vascular, abdominal, or thoracic procedures.

It is important to try to restore sinus rhythm with infusions of adenosine or to control ventricular rate with a β-blocker or a calcium channel blocker. Atrial fibrillation is especially common after cardiac surgery, and prophylactic β-blockers should be used in all patients unless contraindicated. When atrial fibrillation develops postoperatively, conversion to sinus rhythm can be attempted with electrical cardioversion or amiodarone. Otherwise, the rate can be controlled with β-blockers or calcium channel blockers, and spontaneous reversion to sinus rhythm often occurs within 6 weeks. Patients with atrial fibrillation for more than 24–48 h should be treated with anticoagulation therapy to reduce the risk of stroke.

PULMONARY DISEASE

Smoking

Smoking cessation is a key intervention in reducing the risk of postoperative pulmonary complications. Unfortunately, abstinence for several weeks may be necessary to see significant improvements in small airway disease, hypersecretion of mucus, and tracheobronchial clearance. Other interventions, such as antibiotics, chest physiotherapy, incentive spirometry, and supplemental oxygen have been reported to improve selected outcomes. No evidence-based guideline is available to direct management of patients at risk for pulmonary complications. Expert consensus is to encourage smoking cessation, consider adjunctive chest physiotherapy (deep-breathing exercises, chest percussion, and incentive spirometry), and use antibiotics for patients with infected sputum and bronchodilators and steroids for those with bronchospasm.

Thromboembolic Complications

Thromboembolic complications are common during the perioperative period, the most serious of which is pulmonary embolism. Venous thrombosis and pulmonary emboli can be difficult to treat effectively, and attention is focused on prophylaxis. For patients older than 60 who are undergoing general surgery, current recommendations are for thrombosis prophylaxis with low-dose unfractionated heparin, low-molecular-weight heparin, or intermittent pneumatic compression devices. For patients undergoing elective hip or knee replacement or hip fracture surgery, low-molecular-weight heparin or adjusted-dose coumadin (INR target 2.5, range 2–3) are acceptable alternatives.

RENAL & ELECTROLYTE DISORDERS

Renal Failure

Impaired renal function increases the risk of postoperative renal failure. This can be due to compromised cardiac output and exposure to nephrotoxic medications. The early signs of acute renal failure are oliguria, isos-

Table 9–1. Prophylactic antibiotic regimens for patients at risk for bacterial endocarditis.

Drug	Dosing Regimen
Dental, oral, respiratory tract, or esophageal procedures	
Standard regimen	
Amoxicillin	2 g PO 1 h before procedure
Amoxicillin/penicillin-allergic patients	
Clindamycin	600 mg PO 1 h before procedure
or	
Cephalexin or cefadroxil	2 g PO 1 h before procedure
or	
Azithromycin or clarithromycin	500 mg PO 1 h before procedure
Patients unable to take oral medications	
Ampicillin	2 g IV or IM within 30 min before procedure
Penicillin-allergic patients unable to take oral medications	
Clindamycin	600 mg IV within 30 min before procedure
or	
Cefazolin	1 g IV or IM within 30 min before procedure
Genitourinary & gastrointestinal (excluding esophageal) procedures	
High-risk patients	
Ampicillin and gentamicin	IV or IM administration of ampicillin 2 g, plus gentamicin 1.5 mg/kg (not to exceed 120 mg) 30 min before the procedure; followed by ampicillin 1 g IM/IV or amoxicillin 1 g, PO 6 h after initial dose
High-risk patients allergic to ampicillin/amoxicillin	
Vancomycin and gentamicin	IV administration of vancomycin 1 g over 1–2 h plus gentamicin 1.5 mg/kg IM/IV (not to exceed 120 mg); complete injection/infusion within 30 min of starting procedure
Moderate-risk patients[a]	
Amoxicillin or ampicillin	Amoxicillin 2 g PO 1 h before procedure or ampicillin 3g IM/IV within 30 min of starting procedure
Moderate-risk patients allergic to ampicillin/amoxicillin	
Vancomycin	1 g IV over 1–2 h; complete infusion within 30 min of starting procedure

IV, intravascular; IM, intramuscular; PO, orally.
[a]Patients with prosthetic heart valves and those with a history of endocarditis are considered to be in a high-risk category and should not be considered for this regimen. Adapted from Dajani AS et al: Prevention of bacterial endocarditis: recommendations of the American Heart Association. JAMA 1997; 277:1794. Used with permission.

thenuria, and a rising serum creatinine. If the cause of the renal failure is impaired renal blood flow, the urine sodium will typically be < 40 mEq/L, and the urine–plasma creatinine ratio will be > 10:1. In contrast, if acute tubular necrosis is present, there may be granular or epithelial cell casts in the urine sediment, the urine sodium will be > 40 mEq/L, and the urine–plasma creatinine ratio will be < 10:1.

This syndrome requires aggressive management, including holding all nephrotoxic medications and meticulously maintaining a euvolemic state. Occasionally, dialysis may be necessary if hypervolemia, hyperkalemia, metabolic acidosis, or encephalopathy develops.

Obstructive Nephropathy

Obstructive nephropathy is a concern, especially in older men. Medications with anticholinergic effects may compromise detrusor function so that acute urinary retention develops.

ENDOCRINE DISORDERS

Type 2 diabetes

Type 2 diabetes is prevalent among older persons and predisposes them to conditions for which operative interventions may be necessary. Patients with diabetes are at increased risk for infections and cardiovascular complications related to surgical procedures. The stress and tissue injury associated with surgery result in release of insulin counterregulatory factors such as epinephrine, glucagon, cortisol, and growth hormone. These stimulate gluconeogenesis or blunt insulin release or insulin action, resulting in hyperglycemia. In addition, the metabolism and clearance of insulin may be altered, and nutritional intake can be quite variable during the perioperative period. All of these factors complicate the management of patients with diabetes whose glucose levels may vary widely.

Because the greatest risk of serious complications is from hypoglycemia, many clinicians accept a target blood sugar in the range of 150–200 mg/dL. Frequent monitoring of blood sugars is key in any management strategy; the blood sugar should be measured before administration of the anesthetic, during the procedure, and in the recovery room. The frequency of subsequent measures will depend in part on the level of control and the management strategy. If the patient has diet-controlled diabetes, no special preoperative interventions are required.

Perioperative hyperglycemia can be effectively managed with short-acting insulin administered subcutaneously. Patients treated with oral hypoglycemic agents should have the medication held on the day of operation, and hyperglycemia can be managed with short-acting insulin until the oral agent can be resumed. For patients receiving once-daily insulin injections, one half to two thirds the daily dose should be administered on the morning of surgery, and glucose-containing intravenous solutions should be administered at a rate delivering 5–10 g of glucose per hour. If multiple insulin injections are used to manage a patient's diabetes, one half to one third of the morning dose should be administered preoperatively, and glucose-containing intravenous solutions should be run at a constant rate. Fluctuations in blood sugar can continue for several days postoperatively, and patients must be instructed in adjusting their regimens at home as hospital stays have shortened.

Thyroidal Diseases

Thyroidal diseases are not as common as diabetes but, if unrecognized and untreated, can result in significant postoperative complications.

Hypothyroidism

Hypothyroidism is present in about 10% of hospitalized older patients. Because nonspecific and atypical manifestations are so common in older persons, it is important to maintain a high index of suspicion. Untreated hypothyroidism can slow drug metabolism and contribute to central nervous system depression and respiratory insufficiency. If rapid correction of hypothyroidism is indicated because of trauma or other emergency operations, one can safely administer 300–500 μg of L-thyroxine intravenously to improve the metabolic rate within 6 h. Stress-dose corticosteroids are commonly administered simultaneously to avoid depletion of adrenal reserves with a rapid increase in the basal metabolic rate.

Hyperthyroidism

Hyperthyroidism is much less common and occurs in fewer than 1% of hospitalized older patients. As with hypothyroidism, nonspecific and atypical clinical manifestations are common. If untreated, complications of fever, tachyarrhythmias, and congestive heart failure can result. Older patients may become hyperthyroid after nonionic contrast radiography. Restoration of a euthyroid state should be achieved before elective procedures. Emergency treatment with 1000 mg of propylthiouracil by mouth and a β-blocker to manage catecholamine surges is an option when an urgent operation is required. Again, stress-dose steroids are often given simultaneously to avoid cortisol depletion and to lower serum thyroxine and thyroid-stimulating hormone levels.

FLUID & NUTRITION MANAGEMENT
Body Composition & Fluid Regulation

Changes in body composition and fluid regulation complicate the management of older persons in the perioperative period. With aging, there is a relative increase in body fat and a reduction in muscle, total body water, and intracellular water. Thirst is blunted. The ability of the kidneys to concentrate the urine and conserve water may also decline. During the perioperative period, hormonal changes in response to the trauma of tissue injury predispose to extravascular fluid accumulation, and there is a risk of iatrogenic injury related to the administration of intravenous fluids.

The following recommendations guide calculation of fluid requirements. First, estimate the intracellular volume as percentage of body weight: 25–30% for men aged 65–85 and weighing 40–80 kg and 20–25% for women of the same age and weight ranges. Next, estimate the daily metabolic requirements per liter of intracellular volume (in the absence of acute stress and conditions that will affect salt and water balance) as follows: water, 100 mL; energy, 100 kcal; protein, 3 g; sodium, 3 mmol; potassium, 2 mmol. For example, a 75-year-old woman who weighs 60 kg has an estimated intracellular volume of 12 L. Her daily maintenance requirement for water would be 1.2 L or an administration rate of 50 mL/h. Careful monitoring of volume status is essential so that appropriate adjustments can be made based on patient response and changing conditions.

Nutrition

Nutritional issues are also important during the perioperative period when the demand for energy is increased as a result of wound healing. Optimizing preoperative nutritional status is important, although the benefits of parenteral nutrition to achieve this goal have not been consistently demonstrated. A low serum albumin is an important marker for poor postoperative patient outcomes such as prolonged hospitalization and increased morbidity and mortality.

It is accepted practice to provide supplemental enteral nutrition to malnourished patients with a functioning gastrointestinal tract and to reserve parenteral nutrition for those patients in whom enteral feedings are not possible.

CHALLENGING POSTOPERATIVE SYNDROMES

Many of the conditions previously discussed require management throughout the perioperative period. After the operation, one important goal is to restore the patient to an optimal level of functioning. This will involve, among other things, early mobilization and resumption of as many self-care activities as possible. Avoiding prolonged bed rest will reduce the risk of thromboembolism, improve the respiratory mechanics, minimize cardiovascular deconditioning, and reduce muscle loss. Managing pain and cognitive impairment are other specific tasks during the postoperative period.

PAIN MANAGEMENT

Postoperative pain is generally acute and time limited. Patient-controlled analgesic systems are now widely used. The degree of pain varies with the procedure and according to patient-specific factors. Each analgesic regimen must be tailored to the individual needs of the patient by frequently asking about pain and adjusting the pain regimen as necessary.

Not all patients will require narcotic analgesics. When narcotics are used, it is important to anticipate common adverse effects such as excessive sedation, fall risk, and constipation.

COGNITIVE DECLINE

Older patients should be monitored postoperatively for at least 2 important syndromes of brain dysfunction: delirium and postoperative cognitive decline.

Delirium

Delirium is a transient disorder characterized by abrupt onset, inattention, and altered consciousness. It occurs in 10–50% of older patients who undergo surgery and is associated with increased morbidity and mortality. Causes are varied, although metabolic derangements, drugs, infections, and cardiorespiratory disorders are commonly implicated.

Treatment is directed at correcting the underlying cause and supporting the patient through what can be a frightening experience. Drugs can be used when patients are at risk for harm as a result of the delirium. Low doses of major tranquilizers or atypical antipsychotics can be effective but should be used sparingly.

Postoperative Cognitive Decline

Postoperative cognitive decline is a separate, often subtle syndrome in which patients experience abnormalities in learning and memory. It is especially common after cardiac surgery and may persist for many months in 10–30% of patients. The cause is unknown; studies have not been able to demonstrate links with hypotension, hypoxemia, or type of anesthesia. Treatment is supportive until we have a better understanding of the causes this syndrome.

Doyle RL: Assessing and modifying the risk of postoperative pulmonary complications. Chest 1999;115:77S.

Etchells et al: A bedside clinical prediction rule for detecting moderate or severe aortic stenosis. J Gen Intern Med 1998; 13:699.

Geerts WH et al: Prevention of venous thromboembolism. Chest 2001;119:132S.

Jacober SJ, Sowers JR: An update on perioperative management of diabetes. Arch Intern Med 1999;159:2405.

Limberg et al: Ischemic stroke after surgical procedures: Clinical features, neuroimaging, and risk factors. Neurology 1998; 50:895.

Maisel WH et al: Atrial fibrillation after cardiac surgery. Ann Intern Med 2001;135:1061.

Moller JT et al: Long-term postoperative cognitive dysfunction in the elderly ISPOCD1 study. Lancet 1998;351:857.

SECTION III
Common Disorders in the Elderly

Delirium

10

Lynn McNicoll, MD, FRCPC, & Sharon K. Inouye, MD, MPH

DELIRIUM

ESSENTIALS OF DIAGNOSIS

- *Clinical diagnosis based on detailed history, cognitive assessment, and physical and neurological examination.*
- *The pathognomonic feature is an acute change in baseline mental status developing over hours to days.*
- *Fluctuating course with an increase or decrease in symptoms over a 24-h period; inattention, with difficulty focusing attention; disorganized thinking, such as rambling or incoherent speech; and altered level of consciousness (vigilant or lethargic).*
- *Perceptual disturbances, such as hallucinations, or paranoid delusions.*
- *Organic or physiological cause (eg, illness, drug related, or metabolic derangement).*
- *Delirium is often misdiagnosed as dementia, depression, or psychosis.*
- *Accepted delirium criteria provided by* Diagnostic and Statistical Manual of Mental Disorders *(fourth edition) as well as* Confusion Assessment Method.

General Considerations

Delirium is an acute disorder of attention and cognitive function that may arise at any point in the course of an illness. It is often the only sign of a serious underlying medical condition, especially in frail older persons with underlying dementia.

The prevalence of delirium on admission can range from 10–40%. During hospitalization, it may affect an additional 25–50%. The rates of postoperative delirium are estimated at 10–52%. Even higher rates (70–87%) are seen in intensive care units (ICUs). In addition, 80% of terminally ill patients become delirious before death.

Three forms of delirium have been recognized: the hyperactive, hyperalert form; the hypoactive, hypoalert, lethargic form; and the mixed form, which combines elements of both. The hypoactive form is often unrecognized and is associated with a poorer overall prognosis. It is also the more common form in older hospitalized patients. The hyperactive, agitated, combative, and hallucinating delirious patient is rarely missed.

Delirium as a geriatric syndrome is inherently multifactorial. Delirium develops as a result of the interaction between predisposing factors in vulnerable older persons and noxious insults or precipitating factors. There is rarely only 1 factor or cause, and the effects of multiple factors appear to be cumulative. Thus, clinicians should not expect to address only 1 factor and observe resolution. Rather, it is imperative to identify and address all the potential predisposing and precipitating risk factors.

A. RISK FACTORS

The major predisposing risk factor for delirium is preexisting cognitive impairment, specifically dementia, which increases the risk of delirium 2- to 5-fold. Other factors include advanced age, severe underlying illness, number and severity of comorbid conditions, functional impairment, chronic renal insufficiency, vision or hearing impairment, history of alcohol abuse, malnutrition, and dehydration. Virtually all chronic medical illnesses can predispose older persons to delirium.

B. Associated Diseases

Specific diseases associated with delirium include neurological disorders involving the central nervous system (eg, Parkinson's disease, cerebrovascular disease, trauma, infections), systemic or non-neurological infections, metabolic alterations, as well as cardiac, pulmonary, endocrine, renal, and neoplastic diseases.

C. Precipitating Factors

The foremost precipitating factors are medications, immobilization, use of indwelling bladder catheters, use of physical restraints, dehydration, malnutrition, iatrogenic complications, organ insufficiency or failure (particularly renal or hepatic), infections, metabolic derangements, and illicit drug use or withdrawal. Environmental factors (eg, noise level) and psychosocial factors (eg, depression, pain) can also precipitate delirium. Occult infections are particularly common in older persons and may present only as delirium. Metabolic disorders may also contribute to delirium, such as hyper- or hyponatremia, hyper- or hypoglycemia, hypercalcemia, thyroid or adrenal dysfunctions, and acid-base disorders.

Medications are a contributing factor in more than 40% of cases. The medications most frequently associated with delirium are those with known psychoactive effects, such as sedative-hypnotics, opiates, H_2 blockers, and drugs with anticholinergic effects (eg, antipsychotics, antihistamines, antiparkinsonian agents, antidepressants, antispasmodics). In addition, delirium risk increases in direct proportion to the number of medications prescribed. Herbal therapies have not been studied extensively with respect to delirium; however, these alternative therapies are being increasingly recognized as causing or contributing to delirium, especially when taken concurrently with a psychoactive medication. This is particularly true for psychoactive herbs, such as St. John's wort, kava kava, and valerian root.

Ely EW et al: Delirium in the intensive care unit: An under-recognized syndrome of organ dysfunction. Semin Respir Crit Care Med 2001;22:115. [PMID n/a] (Review of recent literature on delirium in critically ill patients, which presents delirium as an underrecognized form of organ dysfunction rather than an expected outcome of intensive care.)

Prevention

Risk factors and targeted preventive interventions are shown in Table 10–1. Prevention of delirium by targeting vulnerable patients with predisposing or precipitating factors has been shown to be effective. In addition, proactive geriatrics consultation (daily geriatrician visits and targeted recommendations based on a structured protocol) is effective in vulnerable patients with preexisting dementia or functional impairments.

Inouye SK et al: The Hospital Elder Life Program: A model of care to prevent cognitive and functional decline in older hospitalized patients. J Am Geriatr Soc 2000;48:1697. [PMID: 11129764] (The practical implementation of a multicomponent targeted program to improve cognitive and functional outcomes in older hospitalized patients.)

Inouye SK et al: A multicomponent intervention to prevent delirium in hospitalized older patients. N Engl J Med 1999;340:669. [PMID: 10053175] (Successful clinical trial of a multiple risk factor reduction strategy for the prevention of delirium in hospitalized older medical patients with 40% reduction in delirium.)

Table 10–1. Risk factors for delirium and targeted interventions.

Risk factor	Intervention
Sleep deprivation	Nonpharmacological sleep protocol (back massage, relaxation music, decreased noise, warm milk or caffeine-free herbal tea) Avoid using sedatives, especially diphenhydramine
Dehydration	Recognition of volume depletion and replenishment of fluids
Hearing loss	Proper hearing aids available and in use (either patient's own hearing aid or amplifier)
Vision loss	Provision of proper visual aids (patient's own glasses, magnifying lenses, or adaptive equipment)
Immobility	Ambulate as soon as possible (assistance or supervision when needed) Active range-of-motion exercises if confined to bed
Cognitive impairment	Frequent reorientation to person, place, time. A large updated board in front of the patient is useful. Avoidance of psychoactive medications.
Use of sedating or psychoactive medications	Use alternative and less harmful medications, avoid those with long half-lives, allow for impaired kidney and liver function. Use the lowest dose possible, taper and discontinue unnecessary medications.

Marcantonio ER et al: Reducing delirium after hip fracture: A randomized trial. J Am Geriatr Soc 2001;49:516. [PMID: 11380742] (Randomized controlled trial of proactive geriatric consultation, which successfully reduced occurrence of delirium in hip fracture patients by 36%.)

Clinical Findings

A. SYMPTOMS & SIGNS

The initial evaluation of delirium is largely based on establishing a patient's baseline cognitive functioning and the clinical course of any cognitive change. Thus, a detailed history from a reliable informant, such as a spouse, child, or caregiver, is most important. The history should seek to clarify the acuity of any mental status changes and seek clues to the underlying cause.

The cardinal historical features of delirium are acute onset and fluctuating course, in which symptoms tend to come and go or increase and decrease in severity over a 24-h period. This is the major feature distinguishing delirium from dementia, which usually develops gradually and progressively over months to years. To fulfill the criteria of delirium, the change must occur in the context of a medical illness, metabolic derangement, drug toxicity, or withdrawal.

1. Cognitive changes—Other features of delirium are usually determined through cognitive testing and, most importantly, close clinical observation of the quality of the patient's responses during cognitive testing. For example, a person may score correctly on the particular cognitive task, but during the task may demonstrate fluctuating attention, easy distractibility, rambling speech, or lethargy.

2. Inattention—Inattention, or the inability or decreased ability to focus, maintain, and shift one's attention, is another key clinical manifestation of delirium. Patients will demonstrate difficulty maintaining or following a conversation, becoming easily distracted, or perseverating on a previous answer. Patients may require repetition of instructions or may struggle to follow instructions on cognitive tasks, such as simple repetition, digit span, or backward recitation of the months.

3. Disorganized thinking—Disorganized thinking or speech is manifested as rambling and, at its extreme, incoherent speech. Problems with memory, disorientation, or language are frequent.

4. Altered level of consciousness——Altered level of consciousness can range from agitated, vigilant states to lethargic or stuporous states.

5. Other features—Other features commonly seen in delirious patients, but not essential for the diagnosis, are psychomotor agitation or retardation, perceptual disturbances (eg, hallucinations, illusions), paranoid delusions, emotional lability, and sleep–wake cycle disturbances.

B. PHYSICAL EXAMINATION

A detailed physical examination is essential for evaluation of delirium. Delirium may often be the initial manifestation of serious underlying disease in an older person; thus, astute attention to early localizing signs on physical examination may allow early diagnosis of a precipitating insult. Assessment of vital signs is often helpful. A careful search for evidence of occult infections should be performed, including signs of pneumonia, urinary tract infection, acute abdominal processes, joint infections, or new cardiac murmur. A detailed neurologic examination with attention to focal or lateralizing signs is also crucial.

C. SPECIAL TESTS

1. *Diagnostic and Statistical Manual of Mental Disorders–IV*—The American Psychiatric Association *Diagnostic and Statistical Manual of Mental Disorders–IV* criteria (Table 10–2) were developed based on expert opinion and remain the current standard for the definition and diagnostic criteria for delirium.

2. Confusion Assessment Method—The Confusion Assessment Method (CAM) is a simple, validated tool that is currently in widespread use (Table 10–2). It has a sensitivity of 94–100%, specificity of 90–95%, and a negative predictive value of 90–100% for delirium. It has also been validated in patients with dementia.

In the intensive care setting, it is now feasible to perform cognitive evaluation and screen for delirium using the CAM for the ICU (CAM-ICU), a modification of the CAM for use in mechanically ventilated, restrained, or nonverbal patients. The CAM-ICU has been examined in ICU patients with probable dementia and uses the same 4 key delirium features for the diagnosis.

3. Other instruments—Other instruments developed and validated for use in the identification of delirium include the Delirium Rating Scale, Delirium Severity Index, Memorial Delirium Assessment Scale, and Cognitive Test for Delirium.

D. LABORATORY FINDINGS

The algorithm in Figure 10–1 provides a systematic approach to the diagnosis and evaluation of delirium in the older person. No specific laboratory tests exist that will positively identify delirium. Current research is focusing on using serum anticholinergic activity level or neurochemical tests, such as neuron-specific enolase or protein S-100, as potential markers for the presence or severity of the syndrome.

Laboratory tests that should be considered in the evaluation of any patient with delirium include deter-

Table 10–2. Established diagnostic criteria for delirium.

DSM-IV diagnostic criteria[a]
1. There is a disturbance of consciousness (ie, reduced clarity of awareness of the environment) with reduced ability to focus, sustain, or shift attention. 2. There is a change in cognition (memory deficits, disorientation, language disturbance) or the development of perceptual disturbances that are not accounted for by preexisting dementia. 3. The disturbance develops over a short period of time (hours to days) and tends to fluctuate (during the course of the day). 4. There is evidence from the history, physical examination, or laboratory findings that the disturbance is caused by the direct physiological consequences of a general medical condition or substance (drug of abuse, medication, or toxin exposure).

CAM diagnostic criteria[b]
1. **Acute onset and fluctuating course.** This feature is based on evidence from a family member or nurse of a positive response to the following questions: Is there evidence of an acute change in mental status from the patient's baseline? Did the (abnormal) behavior fluctuate during the day, that is, tend to come and go, or increase or decrease in severity? 2. **Inattention.** This feature is based on the observation of the presence of difficulty focusing attention, (eg, being easily distracted, or having difficulty keeping track of what was being said). 3. **Disorganized thinking.** This feature is based on the observation of the presence of disorganized thinking or incoherent speech, such as rambling or irrelevant conversation, unclear or illogical flow of ideas, or unpredictable switching from subject to subject. 4. **Altered level of consciousness.** This feature is based on the observation of the presence of a level of consciousness other than "alert." This altered level of consciousness can be either vigilant (hyperalert) or various levels of hypoalert states, such as lethargy (drowsy, easily arousable), stupor (difficulty to arouse), or coma (unarousable).

[a]The diagnosis of the delirium requires the presence of features 1 and 2 and either (3 or 4). *DSM-IV, Diagnostic and Statistical Manual of Mental Disorders,* 4th edition, CAM, Confusion Assessment Method.
[b]The ratings for the CAM should be completed after review of the medical chart, discussion with a family member or nurse, and a brief cognitive assessment of the patient (eg, using the Mini-Mental State Examination and Digit Span test).

mination of complete blood count, electrolytes (including calcium), kidney and liver function, glucose, and oxygen saturation. Furthermore, in searching for an occult infection, 2 sets of blood cultures, urinalysis, and urine culture may be useful. Other laboratory tests may be pursued if specific contributing factors have not been identified in a particular patient. These include thyroid function tests, arterial blood gas, vitamin B_{12} levels, drug levels, toxicology screens, ammonia or cortisol levels, and evaluation of the cerebrospinal fluid.

E. IMAGING STUDIES

In the evaluation of delirium, a chest radiograph to rule out occult pneumonia may prove revealing. Brain imaging with computed tomography (CT) or magnetic resonance imaging are indicated if a history or signs of a recent fall or head trauma, fever of unknown origin, new focal neurological symptoms, or no obvious cause has been identified. An electroencephalogram may be indicated if there is any suggestion of seizure activity. It can also be used in differentiating delirium from a nonorganic psychiatric disorder. No definitive evidence yet exists that functional nuclear medicine scans, such as positron emission tomography or single photon emission CT scans, provide any specific data in terms of diagnosis or cause.

American Psychiatric Association: Diagnostic and statistical manual of mental disorders, 4th ed. American Psychiatric Association, 1994. (Reference standard for definition of and diagnostic criteria for delirium.)

Elie M et al: Delirium risk factors in elderly hospitalized patients. J Gen Intern Med 1998;13:204. [PMID: 9541379] (Review of delirium risk factors emphasizing that advanced age, dementia, and severity of illness are the principal risk factors for the development of delirium in the hospital.)

Ely EW et al: Delirium in mechanically ventilated patients: Validity and reliability of the Confusion Assessment Method for the intensive care unit (CAM-ICU). JAMA 2001;286:2703. [PMID: 11730446] (Validation study of a new instrument for the detection of delirium in 3 subgroups of critically ill patients: mechanically ventilated, older, and potentially demented patients.)

Inouye SK et al: Clarifying confusion: The Confusion Assessment Method. A new method for the detection of delirium. Ann Intern Med 1990;113:941. [PMID: 2240918] (Validation study for the CAM instrument in hospitalized elderly and a subset of persons with dementia.)

Differential Diagnosis

The main diagnostic dilemma facing the clinician is differentiating delirium from dementia. This is especially difficult when knowledge of baseline cognitive function is missing or when there are known cognitive

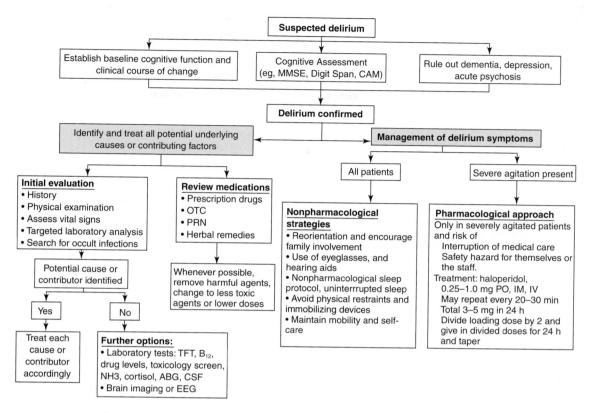

Figure 10–1. Algorithm for the evaluation of suspected delirium in the older adult. MMSE, Mini-Mental State Exam; CAM, Confusion Assessment Method; OTC, over-the-counter; PRN, as needed; TFT, thyroid function tests; B_{12}, vitamin B_{12}; NH_3, ammonia level; ABG, arterial blood gas; CSF, cerebrospinal fluid; EEG, electroencephalogram; PO, oral; IM, intramuscular; IV, intravenous. Adapted from Hazzard WR et al (editors): Principles of geriatric medicine and gerontology, fifth edition. McGraw-Hill, 2003. Used with permission.

deficits and one must determine whether the current condition is due to underlying chronic cognitive impairment or to delirium. Thus, it is crucial to obtain a reliable history about baseline status from an informant. Inattention and altered level of consciousness are usually not features of mild to moderate dementia, and their presence supports the diagnosis of delirium. In patients with known dementia, a history that includes worsening confusion over and above the baseline cognitive impairment also suggests delirium.

Other important diagnoses that must be differentiated from delirium are depression, mania, and other nonorganic psychotic disorders, such as schizophrenia. These diseases do not typically arise in the context of a medical illness. Again, the history and clinical course can assist in providing important clues in differentiating these syndromes. Altered level of consciousness is not prominent in these other diseases. At times, the differential diagnosis can be quite difficult as a result of subtle symptoms or an uncooperative patient. Because of the potential life-threatening nature of delirium, one should err on the side of treating the patient as delirious until further information is available.

Fick D, Foreman M: Consequences of not recognizing delirium superimposed on dementia in hospitalized elderly individuals. J Gerontol Nurs 2000;26:30. [PMID: 10776167] (Delirium was less likely to be recognized in patients with dementia. These cases were also more likely to be readmitted to the hospital.)

Inouye SK et al: Nurses' recognition of delirium and its symptoms: Comparison of nurse and researcher ratings. Arch Intern Med 2001;161:2467. [PMID: 11700159] (Prospective study of nurse recognition of delirium: Nurses often missed delirium when present (70% of cases missed) but rarely identified delirium when absent. The recognition was enhanced with education of delirium and cognitive impairment.)

Complications

Delirium is associated with increased morbidity, mortality, functional decline, and immobility and its attendant complications, including aspiration pneumonia, pressure ulcers, deep venous thrombosis, pulmonary emboli, and urinary tract infections. Moreover, delirium is associated with complications related to its underlying causes. All of these factors contribute to the poor long-term prognosis associated with delirium in older patients.

Inouye SK et al: Delirium: A symptom of how hospital care is failing older persons and a window to improve quality of hospital care. Am J Med 1999;106:565. [PMID: 10335730] (Considers delirium as a quality of care measure given the frequency of delirium and the correctable deficiencies in hospital care that can be implemented to reduce delirium. Provides in-depth discussion of the approaches to improving quality of care for hospitalized older persons.)

Rothschild RM et al: Preventable medical injuries in older patients. Arch Intern Med 2000;160:2717. [PMID: 11025781] (Includes delirium as one of the important preventable medical injuries in older hospitalized patients.)

Treatment

Two concurrent approaches are involved in the treatment of delirium (see Figure 10–1): (1) identification and treatment of the underlying medical cause and eradication or minimization of contributing factors of delirium; and (2) management of delirium symptoms. The first task involves the complete review of the medication history (including prescription, over-the-counter, as needed, and herbal medications) to identify potentially contributing medications that can be eliminated, converted to a less offending agent, or decreased in dosage. Drug interactions should be evaluated. Current kidney and liver function status should be assessed (eg, by estimation of the creatinine clearance) and medication dosage and frequency adjusted accordingly. A complete history and physical (including neurological) examination should be performed, along with selected laboratory and radiological screening tests. Occult infection should be evaluated. If no identifiable cause or contributor is identified, further testing should be pursued, as shown in Figure 10–1.

A. Nonpharmacological Strategies

In general, nonpharmacological strategies should be used in all delirious patients. These include reorientation (with visible and legible orientation boards updated regularly, clocks, and calendars), encouraging the presence of family members as a stabilizing presence, and transferring the patient to a private room or to a room closer to the nursing station for supervision. A skilled and sensitive staff can be vitally important in optimizing communication by using frequent verbal reorientation strategies, simple instructions and explanations, frequent eye contact, and involvement of patients in their care and in decision making. Sensory deficits should be corrected by ensuring that assistive devices (such as eyeglasses, hearing aids, listening devices) are available, functioning, and in use. All attempts should be made to minimize the use of physical restraints because they tend to worsen delirium and can aggravate or cause agitation. Instead, strategies for improving mobility, self-care, and independence should be encouraged.

Improving sleep in the delirious hospitalized older person is an important intervention. Feasible and effective nonpharmacological strategies for enhancing sleep in older people have been developed and tested and include back massage, a warm drink, relaxation techniques, soothing music, and, most importantly, uninterrupted periods of sleep with reduced light and noise level. Coordination of the timing of medications, vital signs, and procedures may be required to achieve the uninterrupted period of sleep.

B. Pharmacological Strategies

Pharmacological therapy for delirium should be reserved for severely agitated individuals whose behavior threatens to interrupt medically necessary care (such as mechanical ventilation) or poses a safety hazard. Given that all medications used in the treatment of delirium can also cause or worsen confusion, a general principle is to use the lowest dose possible and for the shortest period of time. The end point should be an awake and manageable patient, not a sedated patient. All too often, a neuroleptic is started for management of agitated delirium, but the medication is continued indefinitely, obscuring the ability to follow mental status on serial evaluation and putting the patient at significant risk for adverse drug reactions.

Neuroleptics are the preferred class of drugs in delirium management; haloperidol is the most widely used agent for agitation. It is available orally, intramuscularly, or intravenously, but the oral route remains optimal because of favorable pharmacokinetics. The parenteral routes are often medically necessary for emergent cases, but administration should be converted to oral as soon as possible. As noted in Figure 10–1, the recommended starting haloperidol dose is 0.25–1.0 mg, followed by a repeat dose every 20–30 min until the patient is manageable. The maximum dose should not exceed 3–5 mg. Vital signs should be monitored before each additional dose and frequently during active administration. Subsequently, after the loading dose, a maintenance dose is calculated by dividing the loading dose by 2 and administering this quantity in divided doses over the next 24 h and tapering over the next few days.

Common and clinically relevant adverse effects of haloperidol include sedation, hypotension, acute dystonias, extrapyramidal effects, and anticholinergic effects (eg, dry mouth, constipation, urinary retention, and increased confusion). D2-dopaminergic receptors are saturated at low doses of haloperidol. Thus, theoretically, any additional haloperidol above 5 mg over a 24-h period is only likely to increase adverse events without providing additional clinical benefit.

New, atypical neuroleptics also used in the treatment of delirium include risperidone, olanzapine, and quetiapine; however, no trials have compared these agents with placebo or haloperidol. Haloperidol is the only agent that has been shown effective in the treatment of delirium. Olanzapine has greater anticholinergic properties but fewer extrapyramidal properties than haloperidol. Although it may be beneficial for greater sedation, it poses increased risk for worsening confusion.

Benzodiazepines remain the drugs of choice for the treatment of alcohol or sedative drug withdrawal, but they are not recommended in the primary treatment of delirium in older persons because they may cause oversedation and exacerbation of confusion. Among the benzodiazepines, lorazepam is the preferred agent in geriatric practice because of its shorter half-life, lack of active metabolites, and availability in parenteral form.

American Psychiatric Association: Practice guideline for the treatment of patients with delirium. Am J Psychiatry 1999;156 (5 suppl):1. [PMID: 10327941] (Clinical practice guidelines based on review of the literature and expert opinion.)

McDowell JA et al: A non-pharmacological sleep protocol for hospitalized older patients. J Am Geriatr Soc 1998;46:700. [PMID: 9625184] (Prospective study evaluating the effectiveness of a nonpharmacological approach to improve sleep in the hospital setting.)

Milisen K et al: A nurse-led interdisciplinary intervention program for delirium in elderly hip-fracture patients. J Am Geriatr Soc 2001;49:523. [PMID: 11380743] (Intervention focused on education of nursing staff, systematic cognitive screening, and geriatric assessment reduced the duration and severity of delirium after hip fracture. No effect was noted on incidence of delirium.)

Prognosis

Delirium is independently associated with adverse hospital and long-term outcomes, including poor long-term functioning, mortality, increased length of stay, increased need for formal home health care and rehabilitation services, new institutionalization, and increased costs of care. Delirium has traditionally been described as a reversible syndrome, implying that patients invariably return to their baseline cognitive and functional state. Evidence suggests, however, that long-term cognitive and functional deficits may persist as long as 2 years posthospitalization.

Patients who experience delirium are more likely to be diagnosed with dementia at a later date.

Ely EW et al: The impact of delirium in the intensive care unit on hospital length of stay. Intensive Care Med 2001;27:1892. [PMID: 11797025] (Delirium was independently associated with increased length of stay in mechanically ventilated adult ICU patients.)

Inouye SK et al: Does delirium contribute to poor hospital outcomes? A three-site epidemiological study. J Gen Intern Med 1998;13:234. [PMID: 9565386] (Delirium was independently associated with death and new institutionalization.)

McCusker J et al: Delirium predicts 12-month mortality. Arch Intern Med 2002;162:457. [PMID: 11863480] (This prospective case-control study confirmed that delirium was an independent marker of increased mortality in older hospitalized patients.)

O'Keeffe S, Lavan J: The prognostic significance of delirium in older hospital patients. J Am Geriatr Soc 1997;45:174. [PMID: 9033515] (Even after controlling for baseline and hospital factors, delirium was independently associated with multiple negative hospital outcomes.)

RELEVANT WORLD WIDE WEB SITES

American Psychiatric Association: A Patient and Family Guide: www.psych.org/clin_res/Delirium.pdf

American Psychiatric Association guidelines: www.psych.org/clin_res/pg_delirium.cfm

Hospital Elder Life Program: www.med.yale.edu/intmed/aging/elp

Systematic Reviews of delirium studies by Martin Cole and colleagues in the Cochrane Library, Database of Abstracts of Reviews of Effectiveness: www.cochranelibrary.com

Cognitive Impairment & Dementia 11

Kaycee M. Sink, MD, & Kristine Yaffe, MD

ESSENTIALS OF DIAGNOSIS

- *Memory impairment and at least 1 or more of the following: language impairment; apraxia (inability to perform previously learned tasks); visuospatial deficits; decreased executive functioning (poor abstraction, planning, judgment).*
- *Significant impairment in social or occupational functioning.*
- *Significant decline from previous level of function.*
- *Deficits not occurring solely in the presence of delirium.*

General Considerations

The prevalence of dementia approximately doubles every 5 years after age 60. Among community-dwelling elders older than 85, the prevalence is estimated to be 25–45%. Prevalence is even higher in nursing homes (> 50%). Approximately 60–70% of dementia cases are due to Alzheimer's disease (AD); vascular dementia (VaD) and Lewy body dementia (DLB) are the other more common forms. In addition, a significant percentage of patients have mixed disease (AD and VaD or AD and DLB).

Cognitive function in the elderly ranges from cognitive changes seen in normal aging to mild cognitive impairment (MCI) to dementia. Compared with younger adults, older adults perform more slowly on timed tasks and have slower reaction times. Mild memory impairment may often present with subjective problems such as difficulty recalling names or where an object was placed. In the case of normal aging, however, the person often remembers the information later and has intact learning, and any deficits in memory function are subtle, stable over time, and do not cause functional impairment.

MCI is a cognitive impairment that is not within normal limits for that patient's age and education but is not severe enough to qualify as dementia. MCI is char-

acterized by subjective memory complaint, preferably corroborated by someone else; evidence of objective memory impairment in the context of normal abilities on most other cognitive domains (language, executive function); and intact functional status. MCI is certainly associated with an increased risk of AD and may actually represent a form of very early AD. Among patients with MCI, 10–15% per year convert to AD compared with 1–2% of age-matched controls. Although most patients with MCI will progress to AD with time, it is probably a clinically heterogeneous group, with some patients progressing to other types of dementias and others remaining cognitively stable. Donepezil and vitamin E are currently being studied in the treatment of MCI to determine whether they can prevent or delay the onset of AD.

The most severe type of cognitive impairment is dementia. This diagnosis requires deficits in multiple domains of cognitive functioning (memory plus at least 1 other) that represent a significant change from baseline and that are severe enough to cause impairment in daily functioning (Table 11–1).

Dementia often goes undiagnosed or undocumented in primary care settings, especially early in the course of the disease. Cognitive impairment and dementia should be detected as early as possible in older patients so that secondary causes of cognitive impairment can be identified. Drug therapy for AD may improve a patient's quality of life, extend the period of relatively good function, and delay nursing home placement, thereby reducing health care costs. In addition, early diagnosis allows patients and caregivers to plan future needs.

Prevention

Age, family history, female gender, and head trauma are known risk factors for AD. The risk factors for VaD are similar to those for stroke (hypertension [HTN], hyperlipidemia, diabetes mellitus, smoking, age, male gender). Prevention of VaD should be aimed at preventing and treating its modifiable risk factors. In fact, modification of these same risk factors may also be beneficial in the prevention of AD. In addition, increased education, physical activity, nonsteroidal anti-inflammatory

Table 11–1. DSM-IV diagnostic criteria for Alzheimer's Disease.

A. The development of multiple cognitive deficits manifested by both
1. Memory impairment (impaired ability to learn new information or to recall previously learned information)
2. One (or more) of the following cognitive disturbances:
   a. Aphasia (language disturbance)
   b. Apraxia (inability to carry out motor activities despite intact motor function)
   c. Agnosia (failure to recognize or identify objects despite intact sensory function)
   d. Disturbance in executive functioning (ie, planning, organizing, sequencing, abstracting)
B. The cognitive deficits in criteria A1 and A2 cause significant impairment in social or occupational functioning and represent a significant decline from a previous level of functioning.
C. The course is characterized by gradual onset and continuing cognitive decline.
D. The cognitive deficits in A1 and A2 are not due to any of the following:
1. Other central nervous system conditions that cause progressive deficits in memory and cognition (eg, cerebrovascular disease, Parkinson's disease, Huntington's disease, subdural hematoma, normal pressure hydrocephalus, brain tumor)
2. Systemic conditions that are known to cause dementia (eg, hypothyroidism, vitamin B_{12}, or folic acid deficiency, niacin deficiency, hypercalcemia, neurosyphilis, HIV infection)
3. Substance-induced conditions
E. The deficits do not occur exclusively during the course of delirium.
F. The disturbance is not better accounted for by another axis I disorder (e.g., major depressive disorder, schizophrenia).

Adapted from the American Psychiatric Association: Diagnostic and statistical manual of mental disorders, fourth edition. American Psychiatric Association, 1994. Used with permission.

drugs (NSAIDs), estrogen, statins, antioxidants (such as vitamin E), and moderate levels of alcohol intake may be associated with a decrease in the risk of AD. At this point, however, insufficient evidence exists to recommend such therapies for older patients specifically to prevent dementia.

Forette F et al: Systolic hypertension in Europe investigators. The prevention of dementia with antihypertensive treatment: New evidence from the Systolic Hypertension in Europe (Syst-Eur) study. Arch Intern Med 2002;162:2046 [PMID: 12374512]

Clinical Findings

A. Patient History

The patient history is the most important part of the evaluation of a patient with possible cognitive impairment or dementia. Although it may be unreliable, eliciting the history first from the patient can be very informative and useful. Allowing patients to give their version of the history enables assessment of recent and remote memory. The social history is particularly reliable for assessing memory and is generally nonthreatening to a patient who may feel uncomfortable having to respond to so many questions. Asking patients about their childhood, where they grew up, whether they have children and how many, any military experience, and so on helps to assess their remote memory. Questions about their medical and surgical history as well as current medications may help to assess both recent and remote memory. For example, if a patient has denied any medical or surgical history, the discovery of a large abdominal surgical scar on examination is very informative.

Because the history from a patient with cognitive impairment can be incomplete and incorrect, it is crucial to also obtain history from a family member, caregiver, or other source. The history should focus on how long the symptoms have been present, whether they began gradually or abruptly, and the rate and nature (stepwise vs. continual decline) of their progression. Specific areas on which to focus include the patient's ability to learn new things (eg, use of a microwave or a remote control), language problems (eg, word-finding difficulties or absence of content), trouble with complex tasks (eg, balancing the checkbook, preparing a meal), spatial ability (eg, getting lost in familiar places), and personality changes, behavioral problems, or psychiatric symptoms (eg, delusions, hallucinations, paranoia). Obtaining a good functional assessment will help to determine the severity of impairment and the need for caregiver support or, in patients without caregivers, the need for more supervised placement. This should include an assessment of the activities of daily living (ADLs) and instrumental ADLs (IADLs; eg, cooking, cleaning, shopping, managing finances, using the telephone, and driving or arranging transportation). In addition, the clinician should assess the patient's family and social situation because information obtained may be instrumental in developing a treatment plan.

It is important to obtain a detailed medication history and history of comorbid conditions, including symptoms of depression and alcohol and other substance use. Although potentially reversible causes of dementia account for < 5% of cases, a large part of the workup is directed toward identifying and treating these causes. Table 11–2 gives a summary of the key elements of the history and physical examination.

Roman GC: Vascular dementia revisited: Diagnosis, pathogenesis, treatment, and prevention. Med Clin North Am 2002;86: 477. [PMID: 12168556]

B. SYMPTOMS & SIGNS

Early signs and symptoms of dementia are often missed by both physicians and families, especially in AD, in which social graces are often retained until moderate stages of the disease. Subtle hints of early dementia or mild cognitive impairment may include frequent repetition of the same questions or stories, reduced activities or interests, reduced participation in former hobbies, increased accidents, and missed appointments. Poorly controlled chronic conditions may suggest lack of ad-

Table 11–2. Key elements of the history and physical examination.

History
Duration of symptoms and nature of progression of symptoms
Presence of specific symptoms related to
- ❑ Memory (recent and remote) and learning
- ❑ Language (word-finding problems, difficulty expressing self)
- ❑ Visuospatial skills (getting lost)
- ❑ Executive functioning (calculations, planning, carrying out multistep tasks)
- ❑ Apraxia (not able to do previously learned motor tasks, eg, slicing a loaf of bread)
- ❑ Behavior or personality changes
- ❑ Psychiatric symptoms (apathy, hallucinations, delusions, paranoia)
Functional assessment (ADLs and IADLs)
Social support assessment
Medical history, comorbidities
Thorough medication review, including over-the-counter medications, herbal products
Family history
Review of systems, including screening for depression and alcohol/substance abuse

Physical examination
Cognitive examination
General physical examination with special attention to
- ❑ Neurological examination, looking for focal findings, extrapyramidal signs, gait and balance assessment
- ❑ Cardiovascular examination
- ❑ Signs of abuse or neglect
Screen for impairments in hearing and vision

ADLs, activities of daily living; IADLs, instrumental ADLs.

herence to medication prescriptions because of memory problems, especially if these conditions were previously well controlled. Self-neglect, difficulty handling money, and getting lost are more obvious signs.

The current diagnostic criteria of several dementia categories need refinement and more research. With the exception of the criteria for AD (based on *Diagnostic and Statistical Manual of Mental Disorders* and NINCDS-ADRDA), the criteria for other dementia subtypes have not been rigorously validated in autopsy studies.

1. Alzheimer's disease—The classic triad of findings in AD is memory impairment manifested by difficulty learning and recalling information (especially new information), visuospatial problems, and language impairment, which, in combination, are severe enough to interfere with social or occupational functioning (see Table 11–1). Classically, AD patients have little or no insight into their deficits, which may be a result of their compromised executive functioning (planning, insight, and judgment). Early in the course of disease, patients with AD retain their social functioning and ability to accomplish overlearned, familiar tasks but often have difficulty with more complicated tasks such as balancing a checkbook or making complex decisions. Because symptoms are insidious and family members often dismiss the short-term memory loss as normal aging, 1–3 years may pass before the patient receives medical attention. Disorientation is common among patients with AD and typically begins with disorientation to time, to place, and ultimately to person. Patients develop a progressive language disorder that begins with subtle anomic aphasia and ultimately progresses to fluent aphasia and then to mutism. They have difficulty with visuospatial tasks and may be prone to getting lost, even in familiar surroundings. The disease is slowly progressive, and patients show continual decline in their ability to remain independent.

Behavioral changes are common in AD, as in all dementia subtypes, and no neuropsychiatric symptom or behavioral disturbance is pathognomonic. Early changes may be manifested by apathy and irritability (≤ 70% of patients) and depression (30–50% of patients). Agitation becomes more common as the disease progresses and may be especially notable regarding issues of grooming and dressing. Psychotic symptoms, such as delusions, hallucinations, and paranoia, are common, affecting up to 50% of patients in moderate to advanced stages.

2. Vascular dementia—The different diagnostic criteria for VaD vary in sensitivity and specificity. In general, the diagnosis is based on the presence of clinical or radiographic evidence of cerebrovascular disease in a patient with dementia. Sudden onset of dementia after a stroke or stepwise, rather than continuous, decline is supportive of the diagnosis, as are focal neurological findings on examination. However, because a considerable percentage of patients have mixed disease (VaD and AD), the course may appear to be more gradual. Mild, progressive, non-VaD may suddenly be unmasked by the occurrence of a stroke. In addition, patients with subcortical vascular disease may have a more progressive, rather than stepwise, course.

Memory impairments in VaD are often less severe than in AD. Patients with VaD have impaired recall but tend to have better recognition and benefit from cueing in contrast to AD patients. On formal neuropsychiatric testing, "patchy" deficits may be found, often with difficulty on speeded tasks and tests of executive function. As in AD, behavioral and psychological symptoms are common. Depression may be more severe in patients with VaD.

3. Dementia with Lewy bodies—The core features of DLB are parkinsonism, fluctuation in cognitive impairment, and visual hallucinations. The presence of 1 of these features suggests possible DLB, and the presence of 2–3 suggests probable DLB. These symptoms should occur in the absence of other factors that could explain them. The parkinsonism in patients with DLB generally presents after, or concurrent with, the onset of the dementia. This is in contrast to the Parkinson's disease (PD)-related dementia, which generally occurs late in the disease. Parkinsonism in DLB is manifested primarily by rigidity and bradykinesia; tremor is less common (<10–25% of patients in large series). The development of parkinsonism late in the stages of a dementia is not specific for DLB because many patients with advanced AD also develop increased tone, bradykinesia, and tremor.

Like AD, DLB is insidious in onset and progressive, although it classically has a fluctuating quality on a day-to-day basis. The fluctuation is seen in the level of alertness, cognitive functioning, and functional status. Early in the course, memory and language deficits are less prominent than in AD. In contrast, visuospatial abilities, problem solving, and processing speed are more significantly impaired than in AD at the same stage. This may be exemplified by a markedly abnormal clock drawing in the setting of a relatively good overall MMSE score.

Visual hallucinations occur in 30–60% of DLB patients compared with 5–15% of AD patients. They are classically very vivid and often are of animals, people, or mystical things. Unlike true psychosis, most patients with DLB can distinguish hallucinations from reality and, early on, tend not to be disturbed by them. Caution is advised in the use of antipsychotic medications because patients with DLB are exquisitely sensitive to neuroleptics, and a dramatic worsening of extrapyramidal symptoms may occur. Neuroleptics should not be

given as a diagnostic test because deaths have been reported among those with DLB.

4. Frontotemporal dementia—Frontotemporal dementia (FTD) is a heterogeneous syndrome within the Pick complex that also includes primary progressive aphasia and corticobasal degeneration syndrome. It is characterized by early changes in personality and behavior with relative sparing of memory. FTD develops at a relatively young age (mean age of onset in the 50s). It is estimated that FTD accounts for ~25% of presenile dementias.

FTD is often misdiagnosed as either a psychiatric disorder or AD because most patients meet the criteria for a diagnosis of AD. However, some symptoms are highly specific for FTD (97–100%; eg, hyperorality, early changes in personality and behavior, early loss of social awareness [disinhibition], compulsive or repetitive behaviors, progressive reduction in speech [early], and sparing of visuospatial abilities) and have been shown to reliably distinguish it from AD. The hyperorality may be manifested by marked changes in food preference (often toward junk food and carbohydrates) or simply excessive eating. One study showed a weight gain > 5 kg for almost 67% of patients with FTD. Another interesting phenomenon is that some patients with FTD develop new artistic talents without having had any prior interest.

Cognitive testing in patients with FTD may reveal normal MMSE scores early in the disease. More formal neuropsychiatric testing reveals deficits in frontal systems tasks such as verbal fluency, abstraction, and executive functioning, and these deficits are seen earlier than in a typical patient with AD. In contrast to patients with AD, FTD patients tend to show preserved visuospatial abilities and relatively preserved memory, especially recognition memory.

5. Other dementias—Many other diseases are associated with cognitive impairment and dementia such as PD and its related disorders, Huntington's disease (HD), HIV, and alcoholism. Approximately 30% of patients with PD develop dementia. This generally occurs late in the course of PD and is characterized by slowing of mental processing, impaired recall (but usually preserved recognition memory), executive dysfunction, and visuospatial problems. HD is a rare autosomal dominant disorder characterized by motor (chorea, dystonia), behavioral, and cognitive impairments. With the advances in HIV care and the increasing numbers of long-term survivors, HIV-associated dementia (HAD) may become more prevalent in older age groups. HAD most commonly affects patients with advanced HIV disease and is a poor prognostic sign, with median survival of 6 mo after diagnosis. Although chronic alcohol abuse impairs cognitive functioning, there is controversy as to whether a true dementia syndrome related to alcohol exists (separate from thiamine deficiency and head trauma), partly because there have been no large-scale studies.

6. Advanced & End-Stage Disease

The advanced symptoms of most dementias appear similar, and, in late stages, it is nearly impossible to distinguish between different types of dementia. In advanced dementia (typically with a score < 10 on the MMSE), language skills are significantly impaired. There may be very little meaningful speech, and comprehension is very impaired. Some patients will progress to the point of mutism. Patients with advanced dementia have progressive difficulty with even the most basic ADLs, such as feeding themselves, and may progress to the point at which they are incontinent of bowel and bladder and are completely dependent in all ADLs. Symptoms of parkinsonism such as rigidity are common. Gait is impaired and, ultimately, patients may stop walking, leading to a bed-bound state. Seizures are occasionally seen in end-stage dementia patients. Patients who do not die of other comorbidities tend to develop concomitant complications (eg, malnutrition, pressure ulcers, recurrent infections). The most common cause of death in advanced dementia is pneumonia.

C. Physical & Mental Status Examination

The physical examination of a patient with cognitive impairment or dementia focuses on identifying clues to the cause of the dementia, comorbid conditions, conditions that may exacerbate the cognitive impairment (eg, sensory impairment or alcoholism), and signs of abuse or neglect. The neurological examination should be directed at identifying evidence of prior strokes, such as focal signs, and of parkinsonism, such as rigidity, bradykinesia, or tremor, keeping in mind that late in the course of dementia increased tone and brisk reflexes are nonspecific. Gait and balance are an important part of the examination and should be assessed routinely. A careful cardiovascular evaluation, including measurement of blood pressure and examination for carotid disease and peripheral vascular disease, may help in supporting the diagnosis of VaD. Some patients without dementia who have significant hearing or visual impairments may demonstrate behavior that suggests dementia and have a low score on mental status testing. Therefore, it is important to identify and correct, if possible, sensory impairments before making a diagnosis of dementia.

D. Screening Tests

The effectiveness of screening asymptomatic patients for dementia is controversial. However, for patients with a high risk of dementia (eg, patients age 80 years and older) or for those who report memory impairment, screening with a standardized and validated tool is recommended.

1. Mini-Mental State Examination—The Mini-Mental State Examination (MMSE; see Appendix), is a 30-point tool that tests orientation, immediate recall, delayed recall, concentration/calculation, language, and visuospatial domains. However, the MMSE is a culturally and language-biased test, and adjustments should be made for age and level of education (see Appendix for median scores adjusted for age and education). When scores are adjusted for age and education, the MMSE has a high sensitivity and specificity for detecting dementia (82% and 99%, respectively). Because it is administered verbally and patients are asked to write and draw, hearing, visual, or other physical impairments may make the scoring less valid. A patient with early cognitive impairment may score within normal limits for age and education; however, if the test is repeated every 6–12 mo, the MMSE can detect cognitive decline and suggest a diagnosis of MCI or dementia. Among patients with AD, MMSE scores decline an average of 3 points per year, whereas for those with MCI, 1 point per year is more typical. In patients who are aging normally, MMSE scores should not decline much from year to year. As a general guideline, scores above 26 are normal, scores of 24–26 may indicate MCI, and a score < 24 is consistent with dementia. However, it is best to compare each patient's score with age and education adjusted median scores and to monitor for change in addition to assessing for functional decline.

2. Clock Draw Test & 3-Item Recall—Attempts have been made to create brief, focused screening tools that are less time consuming than the MMSE. Two commonly used tests are the Clock Draw Test (CDT) and the 3-Item Recall. In the CDT, the patient is asked to draw a clock face with the hands set at a designated time. Several CDTs are available, each with a different scoring system. However, evidence suggests that a simple dichotomy between normal and abnormal clocks has a relatively good sensitivity (~80%) for detecting dementia, even for inexperienced raters. Normal clocks have all the numbers in the correct position and the hands correctly placed to display the requested time. Using the CDT in combination with the 3-Item Recall is quick and easy, and if both are normal, it essentially rules out dementia. The CDT and 3-Item Recall may be particularly useful in poorly educated or non-English-speaking patients for whom the MMSE is not so helpful.

E. Cognitive Assessment

The cognitive assessment of a patient with cognitive impairment or dementia should be paired with the physical examination. Patients are less likely to be threatened or offended by questions about cognitive abilities if the questions are framed as part of the physical examination. In addition to administering a standardized assessment tool such as the MMSE, providers should also assess domains of cognitive functioning that are not well represented in the MMSE, such as judgment and insight. The diagnosis of dementia requires that, in addition to a memory deficit, there be impairment in another dimension of cognitive function such as language, motor memory (apraxia), or poor executive functioning. Language can be assessed by simply listening for a lack of content in the patient's dialogue or the use of vague terms to replace nouns, such as "thing" or "it." Asking the patient to name common things in the room may be helpful if the language seems normal. To assess the presence of apraxia, the patient can be asked to show, for example, how he would brush his teeth, blow out a match, or salute. Giving the patient a common object such as a key and asking him or her to identify it with eyes closed can test for agnosia. Evidence of impaired executive functioning is often discovered in the history and can be assessed during the examination as well. For example, if the patient is not able to describe a complex function that he or she may normally do (or used to do) in fine detail, there may be a problem with executive functioning.

Borson S et al: The Mini-Cog: A cognitive "vital signs" measure for dementia screening the multilingual elderly. Int J Geriatr Psychiatry 2000;15:1021. [PMID: 11113982]

Petersen R et al: Current concepts in mild cognitive impairment. Arch Neurol 2001;58:1985. [PMID: 11735772]

Petersen R et al: Practice parameter: Early detection of dementia: Mild cognitive impairment (an evidence-based review). Report of the Quality Standards Subcommittee of the American Academy of Neurology. Neurology 2001;56:1133. [PMID: 11342677]

F. LABORATORY FINDINGS

In the evaluation of a patient with cognitive impairment or newly diagnosed dementia, laboratory studies are generally used to rule out potentially treatable causes of dementia (Table 11–3). Vitamin B_{12} deficiency and hypothyroidism are common in the elderly and can affect cognitive functioning. Treatment of these conditions is warranted, although few cases of dementia are actually caused by (or improved with treat-

Table 11–3. Potentially "reversible"/treatable causes of cognitive impairment.

B_{12} deficiency	Subdural hematoma
Thyroid disease	Normal pressure hydrocephalus
Hypercalcemia	Central nervous system neoplasms
Depression	Drug effects
Alcoholism	Heavy metals

ment of) vitamin B_{12} deficiency or hypothyroidism. Most clinicians will also perform complete blood count, electrolytes, creatinine, glucose, calcium, and liver function tests. One should screen for latent syphilis and HIV if there is a high index of suspicion of these conditions.

G. IMAGING

Routine computed tomography (CT) or magnetic resonance imaging (MRI) scanning in the evaluation of patients with dementia remains controversial. Consensus guidelines have recommended that imaging be used only in patients with a relatively recent or rapid onset of symptoms, young age at presentation, or focal neurological signs or symptoms to rule out treatable causes of dementias such as subdural hematoma, normal pressure hydrocephalus, or tumor. However, a practice parameter of the American Academy of Neurology recommends neuroimaging with either a noncontrast CT or MRI in the routine evaluation of patients presenting with dementia. In addition to looking for structural lesions, imaging may be helpful in the diagnosis of the particular type of non-AD dementia. Neuroimaging is likely to be of low yield in patients with a typical clinical appearance of AD and symptoms that have been present for more than 1–2 years. Advantages and disadvantages of neuroimaging can be discussed with patients and families.

CT or MRI findings in AD are often nonspecific and nondiagnostic but include diffuse cerebral atrophy and ventriculomegaly disproportional to age-related norms. On MRI the hippocampus and medial temporal lobes are sometimes disproportionately affected. Imaging studies for VaD are also nonspecific. This is because many elderly patients will have some degree of small vessel ischemic disease on CT or MRI. In fact, by age 85, nearly 100% of patients will have white matter hyperintensities on imaging studies. Therefore, simply seeing evidence of vascular disease does not warrant diagnosis of VaD. If, however, there is extensive disease, multiple infarcts, or infarcts in key anatomical locations (eg, thalamus) in a patient with a history or neuropsychological findings consistent with VaD, it is probable that the imaging findings are clinically relevant. In FTD, there is classically asymmetric volume loss of the frontal or temporal lobes in comparison to the overall atrophy seen in AD.

Positron emission tomography (PET) scans measure glucose metabolism in specific areas of the brain and are currently being studied in the diagnosis of AD, especially early diagnosis. Sensitivity and specificity of the scan in diagnosing AD are reported to be 93% and 63%, respectively. Although promising, the role of PET scans in the clinical diagnosis of AD is still undetermined.

There is currently no role for single photon emission CT in either the initial or differential diagnosis of dementia because it has not shown superiority to clinical criteria.

Garde E et al: Relation between age-related decline in intelligence and cerebral white-matter hyperintensities in healthy octogenarians: A longitudinal study. Lancet 2000;356:628. [PMID: 10968435]

Gifford DR et al: Systematic review of clinical prediction rules for neuroimaging in the evaluation of dementia. Arch Intern Med 2000;160:2855. [PMID: 11025796]

Knopman DS et al: Practice parameter: Diagnosis of dementia (an evidence-based review). Report of the quality standards subcommittee of the American Academy of Neurology. Neurology 2001;56:1143. [PMID: 11342678]

H. SPECIAL TESTS/EXAMINATIONS

1. Neuropsychological testing—Neuropsychological testing is generally performed by neuropsychologists and consists of an in-depth battery of standardized examinations that test multiple cognitive domains, including intelligence, memory, language, visuospatial abilities, attention, reasoning, and problem solving as well as other measures of executive function. The diagnosis of dementia can generally be made by obtaining a detailed history and physical examination (including a brief cognitive evaluation) and does not require neuropsychological testing. However, there are instances in which referral for formal neuropsychological testing can be particularly helpful (eg, when patients have early or mild symptoms, especially if they have high premorbid intelligence and are performing "normally" on tools such as the MMSE). Neuropsychological testing can also be helpful in patients with low intelligence/education and in those with depression, schizophrenia, or other psychiatric illness in which it may be hard to determine how much the condition is contributing to the apparent cognitive deficits. Likewise, in patients with atypical features, such as early language impairment, neuropsychological testing may be helpful in the differential diagnosis of an unusual type of dementia. In addition, a more thorough cognitive battery can identify relative strengths that may be important to patients and their caregivers and may be useful for establishing a baseline from which to reassess.

2. Kohlman Evaluation of Living Skills—A Kohlman Evaluation of Living Skills (KELS), generally performed by occupational therapists, assesses a patient's ability to perform tasks required for safe independent living. For example, a patient is asked to write a check for a mock bill, make a cup of tea or coffee on the stove, use the telephone, or identify dangerous situations in pictures and state what he or she would do. This evaluation may be helpful when a patient with known or suspected dementia is living alone and there is concern about whether he or she needs to be moved to a more supervised setting such as assisted living or a board and care facility.

3. Genetic Testing—Tremendous advances have been made in elucidating the genetics of AD. Two categories of genetic defects have been defined: those that cause early-onset AD and those involved in late-onset AD. Early-onset familial AD is rare and accounts for < 5% of all AD cases. Patients with early-onset AD usually develop dementia in their 40s to 50s and almost always before age 65. Because early-onset AD is often familial, it is important to obtain a detailed family history of dementia. It is inherited in an autosomal dominant fashion. Mutations that cause early-onset AD have been identified in 3 genes thus far: presenilin 1 (*PSEN1*), presenilin 2 (*PSEN2*), and amyloid precursor protein (*APP*) on chromosomes 14, 1, and 21, respectively. A mutation in *PSEN1* is the most common. Testing for genetic mutations in a patient with early-onset AD is not clinically useful for that patient because it will not alter the management of the disease. However, if the patient has children who wish to know whether they have inherited the gene, the family should be referred for genetic counseling. In addition, genetic testing of patients with early-onset AD may be valuable for research.

In contrast to early-onset AD, late-onset AD (age > 60–65 years) is associated with genes that increase the risk of AD but not in an autosomal dominant fashion. Physicians may be asked by patients or family members for the Alzheimer's blood test, most likely referring to apolipoprotein E (*APOE*) genotyping. The association between *APOE* and risk of AD is well established. The presence of one ε4 allele increases the risk of AD by about 2–3 times, whereas the ε2 allele may be protective. It is important to keep in mind that *APOE*-ε4 is only a genetic risk factor for AD; therefore, the absence of an ε4 allele does not rule out the diagnosis nor does the presence of homozygous ε4/ε4 rule it in. In fact, most patients with AD do not carry the ε4 allele. There is broad consensus that *APOE* testing be reserved for research purposes only.

Pinsky L et al: Why should primary care physicians know about the genetics of dementia? West J Med 2001;175:412. [PMID: 11733436]

Differential Diagnosis

The differential diagnosis of dementia includes the potentially treatable causes of dementia listed in Table 11–3, among them metabolic abnormalities, structural brain lesions, medications, alcoholism, and depression. The differential diagnosis also includes delirium, uncorrected sensory deficits, amnestic disorders, and other psychiatric conditions.

A. DEPRESSION

Depression commonly coexists with dementia (up to 30–50% of patients), but it may also be the only cause for cognitive deficits and, therefore, must be ruled out or treated before a diagnosis of dementia can be made. A patient's memory complaints that are disproportional to objective deficits should alert a provider to the possibility of depression. This is in contrast to dementia, in which patients tend to minimize their deficits. It is important to keep in mind that older patients who develop reversible cognitive impairments while depressed are at high risk for dementia over the next few years.

B. DELIRIUM

Delirium is a common cause of confusion in the elderly, particularly in those who are hospitalized, and may be incorrectly labeled as dementia. In contrast to dementia, delirium is characterized by abrupt onset of altered cognition and consciousness, decreased attention, perceptual disturbances (commonly visual hallucinations), and impressive fluctuations in symptoms. Table 11–4 contrasts delirium, depression, and dementia. If delirium is suspected, underlying causes should be sought and treated. Dementia is one of the key risk factors for delirium. If cognitive deficits persist after the resolution of delirium, further workup for dementia should be pursued.

C. MEDICATIONS & SENSORY DEFICITS

Medications are commonly associated with confusion in the elderly. Many classes of drugs have been implicated, including opiates, benzodiazepines, neuroleptics, anticholinergic drugs (many unsuspected medications have significant anticholinergic properties), H_2 blockers, and corticosteroids. Clinicians should ask patients or caregivers to bring in all medications, including over-the-counter medicines, for review. Drug–drug interactions and appropriateness of doses should be assessed. In addition, any nonessential medications should be discontinued. Reassessment of the patient may reveal marked improvement in cognition and function. Similarly, correction of sensory deficits (visual or hearing impairments) in patients who have been misidentified as having dementia can be equally rewarding.

D. ALCOHOL ABUSE

Patients with cognitive impairment, disorganization, frequent accidents, or failure at home or work should be screened for alcohol abuse. Years of heavy alcohol use may contribute to permanent cognitive impairment, possibly through direct toxic effects on the brain or thiamine deficiency or from complications of alcohol abuse such as head trauma related to falls or violence. However, alcohol abuse may also be responsible for more acute declines in a patient's level of function; improvement in cognition and function may be seen on cessation of drinking.

E. OTHER PSYCHIATRIC CONDITIONS

Chronic psychiatric conditions such as schizophrenia or bipolar affective disorder may also be included in the differential diagnosis of dementia, especially when behavioral changes and psychiatric symptoms such as delusions and hallucinations predominate. In addition, elderly patients with chronic schizophrenia are more likely to develop dementia than unaffected adults. The pattern of cognitive deficits seen in geriatric schizophrenia patients is distinct from AD, and autopsy series

Table 11–4. Differentiating dementia from delirium and depression: Typical patterns.

Variable	Dementia	Delirium	Depression
Onset	Insidious/gradual	Abrupt	Fairly abrupt
Duration	Months–years	Days–weeks	Weeks–months
Source of complaint	Usually family, caregiver, friend	Providers, family	Patients themselves
Level of consciousness/alertness	Usually normal	Varies throughout the day	Usually normal
Orientation	Disoriented later in disease	Usually disoriented early	Usually normal
Attention/concentration	Good	Poor	Poor
Effort	Good	Poor or fluctuating	Poor
"Don't know" answers	Uncommon	—	Common
Memory loss for recent vs. remote information	Greater for recent	Greater for recent	~ equal for both
Loss of social skills	Late	Abrupt changes, labile	Early
Thought process/content	Impoverished	Disorganized	May be slow
Psychomotor symptoms	Normal until late in the disease	Hyper- or hypoactive	Hypoactive

confirm that AD does not account for the cognitive impairments.

Complications

A. DELIRIUM

Delirium, as well as being considered in the differential diagnosis of dementia, is also a major complication of dementia. Risk factors for delirium include cognitive impairment, severe medical illness, elevated blood urea nitrogen–creatinine ratio, and visual impairment, among others. When demented patients are hospitalized, it is critical to be aware of their high risk for delirium and take measures to avoid precipitating factors, such as the use of physical restraints and bladder catheters, malnutrition, and use of multiple new medications.

B. BEHAVIORAL & PSYCHOLOGICAL DISTURBANCES

Behavioral and psychological symptoms of dementia (BPSD) are very common, affecting up to 80% of patients with dementia. These symptoms, which are associated with worse prognosis, earlier nursing home referral, greater costs, and increased caregiver burden, include the following:

- Agitation and aggression
- Disruptive vocalizations
- Psychotic features (delusions, hallucinations, paranoia)
- Depressive symptoms
- Apathy
- Sleep disturbances
- Wandering or pacing
- Resistance to personal care (bathing and grooming)
- Incontinence

Although agitation and psychosis are common in dementia, especially as the disease progresses, any new behavioral symptoms should be evaluated before being attributed solely to the dementia. Precipitating causes of new agitation may include delirium, untreated pain, fecal impaction, urinary retention, new medications, sensory impairment, and environmental causes (eg, new environment, excessive stimulation).

The delusions seen in patients with AD are usually not as complex or bizarre as those of schizophrenia. Table 11–5 lists some common delusions of dementia. In addition, hallucinations, if present, tend to be visual compared with the auditory hallucinations common in schizophrenia. More than 50% of patients with AD will have psychosis at some point, often requiring drug therapy. However, in many patients the psychosis is self-limited. Thus, it is important to attempt periodi-

Table 11–5. Common delusions in patients with dementia.

Paranoid delusions	Misidentifications
People are stealing things	Misidentifies familiar people
Accusations of infidelity	(eg, believes daughter is wife)
Belief that someone is	Current home is not their home
trying to harm them	Impersonation (eg, spouse is an impersonator)

cally to withdraw any drug therapies being used to manage agitation or psychosis. In fact, federal regulations require an attempt to withdraw (or decrease the dose of) such medications every 6 mo in patients residing in nursing homes.

C. COMPLICATIONS RELATED TO CAREGIVER STRESS

Informal caregivers provide the majority of care to patients with dementia at considerable financial and personal costs. The risk of caregiver stress rises with the patient's advancing severity of dementia, increased dependence in ADLs, and the presence of problem behaviors. Clinicians should assess caregivers for stress because stress is associated with poor outcomes for both patients and caregivers, including increased risk of placement in a nursing home, increased risk of patient neglect or abuse, and increased risk of depression among caregivers (reported to affect 30–50%). Stress can be alleviated with therapeutic interventions.

Treatment

In the management of patients with cognitive impairment or dementia, the goals are to preserve function and autonomy for as long as possible and to maintain quality of life for both the patient and the caregivers.

A. COGNITIVE IMPAIRMENT

1. Cholinesterase inhibitors—With advances in the understanding of the pathophysiology of AD, rational drug development for treatment of AD is progressing. Currently, 4 drugs are FDA approved to treat mild to moderate AD (MMSE 10–24), all of which are acetylcholinesterase inhibitors (AChEIs): tacrine, donepezil, rivastigmine, and galantamine. All have been shown to modestly improve cognitive function and delay functional decline in mild to moderate AD. In addition, AChEIs may also be of benefit in moderate to severe dementia, but further study is needed. Although the AChEIs are FDA approved for AD, benefit has also been shown in patients with LBD and mixed AD plus VaD. All 4 AChEIs have the same relative efficacy in AD and generally differ only in their half-lives (and, therefore, dosing regimen) and specificity for receptors (rivastigmine and galantamine also inhibit butyryl-cholinesterase, but the clinical significance is still unknown). Gastrointestinal side effects, including nausea, vomiting, and diarrhea, are a class effect and are the most common reason for discontinuation. These side effects can usually be ameliorated by slow titration of the drug over 8–12 weeks. Reversible hepatotoxicity is common with tacrine, and this drug is generally not recommended for initial therapy. Table 11–6 lists the recommended initial doses and target doses for each of the AChEIs.

Assessing effectiveness of therapy with AChEIs in individual patients has not been formally standardized for clinical practice. Effect sizes are modest in clinical trials, with only 40–50% of patients showing evidence of improvement on measures of cognitive functioning, ADL scores, or subjective clinician ratings. Most experts recommend using the MMSE as well as subjective clinical impressions of the physician and caregivers to monitor effect because some of the improvements are not easily measured in clinical practice. Because MMSE scores typically decline about 3 points per year in patients with AD, monitoring MMSE scores every 6–12 mo can help providers assess effectiveness. A stable or improved MMSE score over 6–12 mo suggests the drug is effective. Although switching AChEIs because of lack of efficacy or intolerable side effects may be beneficial for some patients, there is no evidence to support doing so.

The appropriate length of treatment with AChEIs is still unknown, but some experts recommend that therapy be continued indefinitely if improvement or stabilization is noted. Clinicians and caregivers may notice a decline in function if AChEIs are discontinued.

2. Noncholinergic treatments—There has been interest in anti-oxidants, such as ginkgo biloba and vitamin E (α-tocopherol), for the treatment of dementia because they have a plausible mechanism of action. Studies of ginkgo suggest it may indeed have efficacy in mild dementia. Although few data support the use of vitamin E in the treatment of AD, many clinicians are using it given its relative safety (although it may increase the risk of bleeding) and low cost. Because of conflicting results on the benefit of selegiline, it is not currently recommended in the treatment of AD. Both vitamin E and ginkgo are being investigated in large trials for the prevention of AD.

The use of NSAIDs has been associated with a lower incidence of AD, perhaps by decreasing inflammatory processes in neuritic plaques. However, there is insufficient evidence to recommend the use of NSAIDs in the treatment of dementia, especially given their potentially dangerous side effects in the elderly.

Although estrogen has also been associated with lower risk of AD in observational studies, it was not found to be protective in a large trial. In addition, there is already good evidence from multiple trials that estrogen is not effective as a treatment for AD.

N-methyl-D-aspartate (NMDA) antagonists such as memantine are currently being used in Europe to treat dementia and may act as neuroprotectors. Secretase inhibitors are in the laboratory phases of investigation, but show promise in the potential for reducing the amyloid plaque deposition in AD.

B. VASCULAR DEMENTIA

No drug therapies have been specifically approved for the treatment of VaD. The principles of treatment of VaD rely on the treatment of stroke risk factors such as smoking and hyperlipidemia. Treatment of HTN is somewhat controversial. Although controlling HTN may help reduce the incidence of dementia, some observational data suggest that, once dementia is present, permissive mild HTN (up to systolic blood pressures in the 150s) may be better for cognitive function than lower blood pressures. Data published on the use of galantamine in VaD and mixed dementia suggest a possible benefit on cognition and function, but confirmatory studies are needed.

Table 11–6. Cholinesterase inhibitors.

Drug	Starting dosage	Target dose
Donepezil	2.5–5.0 mg qd	10 mg qd (increase q4 weeks)
Rivastigmine	1.5 mg bid	6 mg bid (increase by 1.5 mg bid q2 weeks)
Galantamine	4 mg bid	8–12 mg bid (increase q4 weeks)
Tacrine[a]	10 mg qid	20–40 mg qid (increase by 10 mg qid q4 weeks)

[a]Not generally recommended because of hepatotoxicity. If used, check liver function tests every 2 weeks for 16 weeks and then every 3 mo.

Erkinjuntti T et al: Efficacy of galantamine in probable vascular dementia and Alzheimer's disease combined with cerebrovascular disease: A randomized trial. Lancet 2002;359:1283. [PMID: 11965273]

Feldman H et al: A 24-week, randomized, double-blind study of donepezil in moderate to severe Alzheimer's disease. Neurology 2001;57:613. [PMID: 11524468]

Rapp SR et al: Effect of estrogen plus progestin on global cognitive function in postmenopausal women: the Women's Health Initiative Memory Study: a randomized controlled trial. JAMA 2003;289:2663. [PMID: 12771113]

Reisberg B et al: Memantine in moderate-to-severe Alzheimer's disease. N Engl J Med 2003;348:1333. [PMID: 12672860]

Winblad B et al: A 1-year, randomized, placebo-controlled study of donepezil in patients with mild to moderate AD. Neurology 2001;57:489. [PMID: 11502918]

C. PROBLEM BEHAVIORS

1. Nonpharmacological approaches—Because behavioral and psychological symptoms of dementia (BPSD) are common and may adversely affect both patient and caregiver quality of life, it is important to manage them as dutifully as the cognitive symptoms. Once precipitating causes (eg, delirium, pain, fecal impaction, broken hearing aids) of new behavioral problems have been ruled out, it is critical to try to identify what the behavior may represent. When patients are agitated or displaying other problem behaviors, it is generally because they do not have the language skills to express their needs. Providers and caregivers need to try to learn what the behaviors for a patient with dementia may represent and then attempt to address underlying needs. Keeping a behavior log may be useful. Federal regulation requires that the least restrictive methods for behavior problems be tried first for nursing home residents. Nonpharmacological treatments should be attempted before initiating drug therapies.

A few strategies that may be helpful in reducing agitation in patients with dementia include music, reminiscence therapy, exposure to pets, outdoor walks, and bright light exposure. One of the unifying themes in many of these strategies is that the therapy works best if it is tailored to the patient. For example, with music therapy, playing music that is consistent with patients' prior preferences seems to be superior to playing a standard tape for everyone. One study confirmed an intuitive assumption that providing intensive education and training on understanding and treating BPSD for nursing assistants or care providers also significantly decreases agitation among patients with dementia in nursing home settings.

Less evidence-based, but more practical tips for both caregivers and medical providers of patients with dementia-related difficult behaviors are presented in Table 11–7.

2. Pharmacological approaches—If nonpharmacological approaches fail, it may become necessary to add drug therapy. However, pharmacological therapies are only moderately effective at reducing BPSD and may not be more efficacious than behavioral and environmental approaches. Several classes of drugs are used for BPSD, including antipsychotics, antidepressants, mood stabilizers, and AChEIs. The first-line choice of agent is often a matter of personal choice. Although it is intuitive to assess the patient, determine the target symptoms, and select a class of drugs that is most likely to treat the target symptoms, little evidence supports this approach, except for the case of depression. Most of the drugs likely have benefits on BPSD that are not immediately obvious from their known indications. Given the absence of evidence that any one class of drugs is superior to the others, either choosing to target symptoms or choosing a drug with few side effects is a reasonable approach. Selective serotonin reuptake inhibitors, trazodone, and AChEIs are all relatively well tolerated and would be reasonable first choices. Table 11–8 lists drugs and doses commonly used to treat BPSD. Although the antipsychotics are the best studied and probably most widely used class of drugs, their side effects should be considered and weighed against potential benefits. Both low-dose traditional antipsychotics such as haloperidol and atypical antipsychotics such as risperidone and olanzapine have been shown to be effective (at about 15–25% of the dose used in young adults with schizophrenia). However, the typical neuroleptics are much more likely to cause extrapyramidal symptoms and irreversible tardive dyskinesia (TD). In 1 study, even low-dose oral haloperidol (1.5 mg/day) resulted in TD in 30% of older patients at 1 year and > 60% of patients at 3 years.

Although the incidence of EPS is lower with atypical antipsychotics, they may still occur. Other long-term side effects of atypical antipsychotics include weight gain, diabetes mellitus, and hyperprolactinemia. Although the atypical antipsychotics are clearly associated with fewer side effects, typical antipsychotics such as haloperidol may be preferable when cost is an important factor or if intravenous administration is required such as in an intensive care unit setting.

Mood stabilizers such as carbamazepine and valproic acid have shown benefit in small trials. However, because of side effects, drug–drug interactions, and necessary blood test monitoring, these agents are not recommended as first-line treatments. If attempts at nonpharmacological approaches and use of more common drug classes have failed, referral to a geriatrician or geropsychiatrist should be considered. Benzodiazepines are not recommended for the chronic management of BPSD. They have not been found to be more efficacious than other classes of drugs. In addition, adverse effects associated with benzodiazepine use, such as increased risk of falls, sedation, withdrawal, and occasionally paradoxical excitation, make them a particularly poor choice.

Carlson DL et al: Management of dementia-related behavioral disturbances: A nonpharmacologic approach. Mayo Clin Proc 1995;70:1108. [PMID: 7475342]

Doody RS et al: Practice parameter: Management of dementia (an evidence-based review). Report of the quality standards subcommittee of the American Academy of Neurology. Neurology 2001;56:1154. [PMID: 11342679]

Table 11–7. Dementia related difficult behaviors: Practical tips for caregivers and medical providers.

Maintain familiarity and routines as much as possible.
Any change in the routine can produce anxiety and distress for patients with dementia. Changes in living arrangement, going on vacation, or being hospitalized may provoke agitation and other undesirable behaviors.

Decrease number of choices.
Patients with dementia may become overwhelmed with too many choices and become frustrated by their inability to sort things out. Limiting choices may be helpful. A good example is the case of a patient who resists changing clothes or insists on wearing the same clothes every day. In this case, it might be helpful for the caregiver to lay out only 1 outfit or to give the patient 2 choices: eg, "Would you like to wear the blue blouse or the red blouse?" Similarly, simplifying conversation and environment is also important. Too much input is often overwhelming or misinterpreted.

Tell, don't ask.
At first glance, this recommendation may seem uncomfortable to some. However, with the apathy that is commonly associated with dementia, it may be a struggle to get patients with dementia to agree to do anything. Instead of asking "Do you want to go to dinner now?", which may often result in a "no" answer followed by an argument, it may be more effective to say, "It is time to go to dinner now." Similarly, patients may be more agreeable if things are framed in positive rather than negative terms. For example, use "come with me" rather then "don't go there."

Understand that they Can't, rather than they Won't.
Family members and caregivers often believe that the patient with dementia is being stubborn and willfully making things difficult. Caregivers can waste much time and energy trying to "teach" something to patients who cannot learn. Helping caregivers understand the limitations of their loved one may improve quality of life for both.

Don't' try logic or reason.
Because of the executive dysfunction that accompanies dementia, there is a relatively early loss of the ability to reason and use logic, which becomes more profound as the illness progresses. Trying to rationalize with a demented person often leads to frustration on the part of both parties. This is particularly true for delusions. If the patient has a nonthreatening delusion, arguing with him or her and trying to get him or her to see that it does not make sense is often fruitless and frustrating for both parties.

Always keep the goals in mind.
Is it really important if grandma thinks it is 1954, or that her daughter is her sorority sister? Why can't she wear that raincoat in the house if she wants to? By keeping the goals and "big picture" in mind, some conflict may be avoided. It is also important for caregivers and physicians to remember that most behaviors do not last indefinitely but are rather temporary stages.

Management

A. ADVANCE DIRECTIVES

Establishing advance directives and having the patient appoint a durable power of attorney (DPOA) for health care should be a part of the management plan of patients with dementia. It is particularly important to have this discussion as early as possible so that patients can participate in decisions to direct their end-of-life care. Even patients with moderate dementia are able to consistently state preferences and choices, including the appointment of a DPOA. In addition to preferences regarding resuscitation, specific interventions such as the use of artificial hydration and nutrition should be addressed and included. Patients may also want to appoint a DPOA for finances. Consultation with an elder law attorney or estate planner may be helpful.

B. SAFETY ISSUES

1. Driving—Cognitive impairment has been shown to adversely affect driving ability, even among patients with mild dementia. Some states require reporting of AD and "related conditions" to the department of public health or the state's department of motor vehicles. Primary care providers should familiarize themselves with their state's law on reporting. If a patient with dementia is involved in a motor vehicle accident, the physician may be held liable if required reporting has not been done.

2. Home safety—Home safety should be assessed by interviewing a reliable informant or, preferably, by a home visit from a visiting nurse or occupational therapist. Specific safety measures to consider implementing include grab bars in the bathrooms, good lighting, clear

Table 11–8. Pharmacotherapy for BPSD.

Drug	Starting dosage	Max. dosage[a]	Cost[b]
Haloperidol[c]	0.25–0.5 mg qd	2–3 mg/day	$
Risperidone[d]	0.25 mg bid	1.5 mg/day	$$$
Olanzapine[e]	2.5 mg qd	5–10 mg qd	$$$
Trazodone	25 mg qhs	50–100 mg qhs	$
SSRIs (eg, citalopram)	10 mg qd	20–40 mg qd	$$
Carbamazepine	100 mg	300–400 mg	$$
Divalproex sodium[f]	125 mg bid	~1000 mg/day	$

[a]Use the lowest dose that achieves benefit.
[b]Cost for a 30-day supply at max dose: $, < $20; $$, $20–100, $$$, > $100.
[c]Available in IV formulations.
[d]Available in liquid form; do not mix with cola or tea.
[e]Available IM and in dissolving tablets.
[f]Available in sprinkles.

pathways through the house, reducing clutter, and disabling stoves if there is a concern for potential kitchen fires. If there is any indication that a patient may not be safe in the home or there is evidence of self-neglect or concern about elder abuse by others, the provider should contact Adult Protective Services, which has a variety of resources and can quickly develop a plan for ensuring patient safety.

3. Wandering—Patients with dementia may wander and become lost. Some form of identification (eg, sewn in clothing, identification bracelet) is recommended. The Alzheimer's Association has a program called Safe Return. When registered, patients receive identification products, including wallet cards, jewelry, and clothing labels. The Safe Return program maintains a national photo/information database and 24-h toll-free emergency crisis line for help in locating missing patients. Registration can be done through the Alzheimer's Association for a nominal cost.

4. Caregiver assistance—Caring for a patient with dementia can be exhausting and stressful and can lead to physical and mental health problems in the caregiver and the risk of abuse to the patient. Immediately on making a diagnosis of dementia, the primary care provider should make a referral to a knowledgeable social worker or office on aging for a list of resources to assist the caregiver. Such resources could include provision of educational materials and referrals to the Alzheimer's Association, the Caregiver Alliance, or other support and educational organizations. Proactive use of in-home or institutional respite or adult day care services should be considered for all caregivers. In addition, the use of privately hired case managers who specialize in elder care or dementia care can be very helpful in relieving some of the caregiver burden. Primary care providers should make an assessment of caregivers at each follow-up appointment. If caregiver stress is detected, caregivers should be asked about their use of resources and provided additional referrals as needed. If caregiver stress is severe, referral to a 24-h respite program (either nursing home or assisted-living facility) may be very helpful.

Dubinsky RM et al: Practice parameter: Risk of driving and Alzheimer's disease (an evidence-based review). Neurology 2000;54(12):2205. [PMID: 10881240]

Feinberg LF, Whitlatch CJ: Are persons with cognitive impairment able to state consistent choices? Gerontologist 2001;41:374. [PMID: 11405435]

Prognosis

The prognosis of dementia is variable depending on the cause and presence of comorbid conditions. Estimates of survival from time of onset or diagnosis of AD have been broad. Median life expectancy is 3–15 years. Patients with earlier ages of onset tend to have longer survival, and patients with VaD may have slightly shorter survival. Death is commonly due to terminal pneumonia in the degenerative dementias and to cardiovascular events in VaD.

As many as 90% of patients with dementia are eventually institutionalized. The median time to nursing home placement is 3–6 years from diagnosis. Dementia severity, dependence in ADLs, difficult behaviors, and caregiver age and burden are significant risk factors for placement. Interventions that include caregiver support and education in managing difficult behaviors may extend time to nursing home placement.

Yaffe K et al: Patient and caregiver characteristics and nursing home placement in patients with dementia. JAMA 2002;287: 2090. [PMID: 11966383]

 EVIDENCE-BASED POINTS

- *AD is the most common form of dementia, accounting for approximately 66% of patients with dementia. MCI is associated with an increased risk of AD.*

- *Routine brain imaging in the diagnostic evaluation of a patient with cognitive impairment or dementia is controversial. Genetic testing, including APOE genotyping, is not indicated for clinical use.*

- Acetylcholinesterase inhibitors for treatment of AD have modest benefits on cognition, physical functioning, and behavior.
- Behavioral and psychological symptoms of dementia are associated with poor outcomes.

RELEVANT WORLD WIDE WEB SITES

Alzheimer's Association: www.alz.org (Extensive informational materials addressing issues for patients and caregivers.)

Family Caregiver Alliance: www.caregiver.org (Provides information, support, and guidance for family and professional caregivers. Includes topic specific newsletters, information on care facilities and legal issues, and online discussion lists.)

Alzheimer's Disease Education and Referral Center (of the National Institutes of Health and National Institute on Aging): www.nia.nih.gov

Falls & Mobility Disorders

12

Jane Mahoney, MD

ESSENTIALS OF DIAGNOSIS

- *Older adults who report > 1 fall in the past year or a single fall with injury or gait and balance problems are at increased risk for future falls and injuries.*
- *Falls and mobility disorders result from disease in 1 or more organ systems related to balance: sensory input (visual, vestibular, and proprioceptive), central (neurological) processing, and effector output (neuromuscular and musculoskeletal).*
- *Transient cerebral hypoperfusion may result in a syncopal fall; loss of consciousness may not be reported because of amnesia for the event.*
- *Acute factors (infectious, toxic, metabolic, ischemic, or iatrogenic) may contribute to falls and mobility disorders.*
- *Medications, particularly psychotropic drugs, increase the risk for falls.*

General Considerations

A. FALLS

Approximately 30% of people over the age of 65 fall each year. The incidence increases with age. In general, the rate of falls is higher in hospital and immediate post-hospital settings, compared to a general community setting. The incidence of falls is higher in the nursing home than in the community. Up to 50% of falls result in some injury. Approximately 10% of falls require hospitalization because of injuries sustained, including bone and hip fractures. Persistent pain and mobility limitation are common after a fall-related injury. Almost 50% of patients seen in an emergency room for a fall injury will have continued pain and mobility limitation 2 mo after the fall. In about 3% of falls, the older adult lies on the floor for at least 20 min. Falls are associated with increased risk for nursing home placement, functional decline, and fear of falling.

Risk factors include vision impairment, muscle weakness, peripheral neuropathy, balance and gait abnormalities, use of psychotropic medications, impaired cognition, foot problems, lower extremity arthritis, neurological diagnoses such as stroke and Parkinson's disease, orthostatic hypotension, and recent hospitalization. Risk factors for injury with a fall include older age, low body mass index, previous fracture, low bone mineral density, and loss of consciousness (LOC).

In the nursing home, risk factors for falls include use of psychotropic medications, a fall in the past 180 days, recent decline in function, male gender, history of wandering, use of a cane or walker, independence in transferring or wheelchair use, and impaired cognition. Patients who are nonambulatory are generally at lower risk. In the hospital setting, risk factors include impaired cognition, weakness, urinary incontinence, mobility impairment, multiple comorbidities, and use of psychotropic medications. Fall rates are highest among patients in geriatric psychiatry, rehabilitation, geriatric medical, and neurology units.

Vigorous older adults more often tend to fall as the result of environmental hazard and more often when engaged in vigorous activities, which displace the center of gravity. Frail older adults tend to fall with only minimal environmental hazard or minimal risk activities. Vigorous older adults may be at greater risk for injury, particularly if the fall is from a height or results from an activity that rapidly displaces the center of gravity, either of which may increase the momentum at impact.

B. MOBILITY DISORDERS

The onset of mobility impairment may be catastrophic (eg, after cerebrovascular accident or hip fracture) or chronic, related to progression of disease and sedentary lifestyle. In chronic progression of mobility impairment, patients report difficulty with mobility before the development of actual dependency in activities of daily living (ADLs; including bathing, toileting, dressing, transferring) and instrumental ADLs (including housework, shopping, laundry, yard work). In this preclinical stage, patients have minor abnormalities in performance tests of balance, gait, and lower extremity muscle function. Poorer performance on these tests predicts future disability.

Risk factors for impaired mobility include decreased cognition, depression, arthritis, obesity, vision impairment, and other comorbidities. Impaired cognition is associated with impaired mobility even after adjusting for comorbidities.

Blaum CS et al: Log cognitive performance, comorbid disease, and task-specific disability: findings from a nationally representative survey. J Gerontol Med Sci 2002;57A:M523. [PMID: 12110069] (This study demonstrates, in a national sample of older adults, that low cognitive performance is associated with impaired mobility, even after adjusting for multiple co-morbidities.)

Brauer et al: The interacting effects of cognitive demand and recovery on postural stability in balance-impaired elderly persons. J Gerontol Med Sci 2001;56A:M489. [PMID: 11487601] (Balance-impaired older adults had difficulty maintaining balance in response to a perturbation while simultaneously performing a cognitive task. In contrast, healthy older adults were able to maintain balance and simultaneously perform a cognitive task.)

Kannus P et al: Fall-induced injuries and deaths among older adults. JAMA 1999;281:1895. [PMID: 10349892] (This analysis of the Finnish National Hospital Discharge Register found that yearly age-adjusted fall-related injury incidence more than doubled from 1970 to 1995 for both men and women.)

Leipzig et al: Drugs and falls in older people: a systematic review and meta-analysis: I. Psychotropic drugs. J Am Geriatr Soc 1999;47:30. [PMID: 9920227] (This study provides a review and meta-analysis of data linking neuroleptics, sedative–hypnotics, and antidepressants to falls, with increased risk for those taking > 1 psychotropic drug.)

Leipzig et al: Drugs and falls in older people: a systematic review and meta-analysis: II. Cardiac and analgesic drugs. J Am Geriatr Soc 1999;47:40. [PMID: 9920228] (This review and meta-analysis shows an association of digoxin, type Ia antiarrhythmics, and diuretics with falls. The authors point out that the association is weak, and existing studies have only minimally adjusted for confounders.)

Pathogenesis

A. FALLS

Accidental falls are due to a combination of extrinsic (environmental), intrinsic (organ system abnormalities contributing to postural control), and situational (risk taking) factors. Extrinsic factors include environmental hazards, such as loose rugs, clutter, poor lighting, and improper footwear, such as loose, floppy slippers.

Intrinsic factors include abnormalities in any of the organ systems that contribute to postural control. Postural control is composed of 3 linked components: sensory input, central processing, and effector output. Sensory input for balance comes from visual, vestibular, and somatosensory input. Central nervous system movement pathways involve sensory cortex, frontal and motor cortex, brainstem, basal ganglia, and cerebellum. Effector output involves upper and lower motor neurons, muscles, and joints. Any pathology affecting any of these components of postural control will increase the risk for falls.

Approximately 10% falls are due to acute causes. These include cerebral hypoperfusion states and acute toxic, metabolic, endocrine, infectious, and ischemic changes. Psychotropic medications and alcohol may lead to transient alterations in alertness and attention and increase the risk of falls. Acute disease states increase the risk for falls, especially when they are superimposed on chronic conditions affecting postural control. Balance impairment often contributes to falls and may be acute (posterior circulation TIA or CVA), subacute (labyrinthitis, benign positional vertigo), or chronic (peripheral neuropathy, cerebellar dysfunction).

Situational factors may involve risk-taking behaviors, such as failure to use a prescribed ambulatory device or not wearing eyeglasses, and so on. All 3 types of factors are potentially remediable with intervention.

B. MOBILITY DISORDERS

The pathogenesis of mobility disorders can also be seen as extrinsic, intrinsic, and situational. Extrinsic causes include unsafe home or outdoor environment (eg, throw rugs or ice on sidewalks) that may limit mobility. Intrinsic causes include any disease that impairs balance, as described previously in the Falls section. The pathogenesis of mobility impairment is broader than that of balance impairment. A number of diseases may negatively affect mobility without impairing balance. These include any diseases causing pain or difficulty with walking, such as arthritis, claudication, lumbar spinal stenosis, and obesity. Fear of falling, anxiety, and depression may also contribute to mobility curtailment.

Situational factors include use of adaptive aids and other modifiers to enhance mobility. For example, provision of a 4-wheeled walker may allow a mobility-impaired individual to resume outdoor walking. Alternatively, lack of an appropriate adaptive aid (bath bench, walker) may lead to unnecessary curtailment of mobility.

Woolacott MH: Systems contributing to balance disorders in older adults. J Gerontol Med Sci 2000;55A:M424. [PMID: 10952363] (This brief, excellent review of research on balance control in older adults summarizes findings on changes in motor and sensory systems that contribute to balance impairment. It also summarizes recent research showing an association between attentional demands and balance.)

Prevention

An algorithm defining the guidelines issued by the American Geriatrics Society, British Geriatrics Society, and American Academy of Orthopedic Surgeons Panel on Falls Prevention is presented in Figure 12–1. Among high-risk, community-dwelling older adults, a strong, consistent reduction in rate of falls has been demonstrated from the implementation of multifactorial interventions (Table 12–1).

In nursing homes and assisted-living facilities, multidisciplinary programs comprising both facility-wide

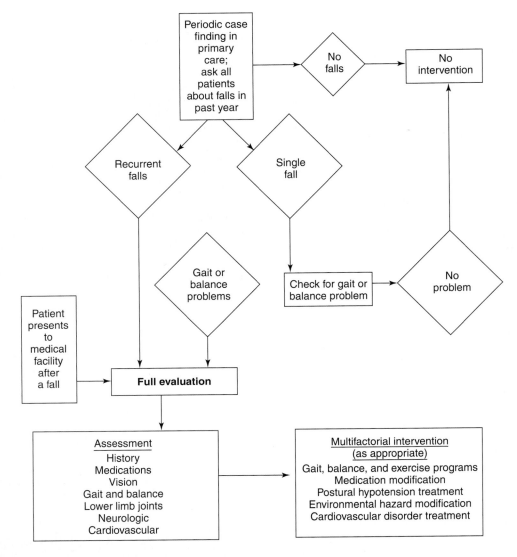

Figure 12–1. Algorithm summarizing the assessment and management of falls. From American Geriatrics Society, British Geriatrics Society, and American Academy of Orthopedic Surgeons Panel on Falls Prevention: Guideline for the prevention of falls in older persons. J Am Geriatr Soc 2002;49:666. Used with permission.

and resident-specific fall prevention strategies have been shown to reduce falls. Facility-wide strategies include staff education and environmental modifications. Individual interventions for high-risk older adults include balance and strength exercises, issuance or repair of ambulation aids, multifactorial medical interventions including medication reduction, and post-fall problem-solving conferences. Individual interventions without staff education do not appear to be successful in reducing fall in the long-term care setting. Physical therapy

as a single intervention has not been shown to prevent falls in the nursing home.

In the acute care setting, fall prevention programs have included staff education, identification of high-risk inpatients, use of bed alarms, increased toileting, medication review, and environmental modification. Uncontrolled studies of unit-based intervention programs have shown decreases in rate of falls compared with preintervention. However, randomized, controlled trials are lacking.

Table 12–1. Components of a multifactorial falls and mobility evaluation.

Evaluation domain	Specific components
History of fall	Circumstances of fall: location, time of day, activity occurring
	Situational factors: use of assistive device, glasses, risk-taking behavior, use of alcohol
	Extrinsic factors, relation to environmental hazard: trip, slip
	Associated symptoms: light-headedness, presyncope, vertigo, dysequilibrium, symptoms to suggest acute illness or neurological event
History of falls, mobility impairment	Injury, frequency, circumstances of prior falls
	Current mobility function: ability to perform ADLs, IADLs, need for assistive device, ability to walk outdoors, indoors, exercise status
Review of medical diagnoses	Chronic medical diagnoses that may impact fall risk either acutely or chronically
Medication review	Psychotropic medications: antidepressants, benzodiazepines, antipsychotics, other sedative–hypnotics
	Consider potential side effect associated with antiseizure, antihypertensive, or anticholinergic medications
Physical examination	Cardiovascular exam, including orthostatic blood pressure and pulse, heart rate and rhythm, carotid sinus testing if indicated
	Distant vision, visual fields
	Vestibular examination as appropriate
	Neurological examination, including muscle strength, prioprioception, vibratory sense, light touch, Romberg test, reflexes, tests of cortical, extrapyramidal and cerebellar function
	Lower extremity joint and foot exam
	Leg-length measurement if indicated
Cognitive screen	Mini-Mental State Examination
	Clock drawing
Performance evaluation	Rise from chair without arms, walk short distance, turn, walk back, sit down
	Turn head and look up, reach, bend
	Resist sternal nudge
	Walk over obstacles
	Ability to walk while performing other task (talking, carrying water, doing mental calculation)
Laboratory tests	Consider thyroid-stimulating hormone level
	Other laboratory tests as suggested by history and physical examination: metabolic panel, vitamin B_{12}, rapid plasma regain, complete blood count, 25-OH vitamin D, morning cortisol level
Physical therapy	Assistive devices, gait training, balance training, including gaze stabilization, strengthening, vestibular rehabilitation
Home safety evaluation	Lighting, stairs, tripping hazards, bathroom safety, floor surface, footwear, lifeline

ADLs, activities of daily living; IADLs, instrumental ADLS.

There is no evidence that restraint use decreases falls. Restraint reduction in nursing homes has not been followed by increased rates of fall injury. Use of 4 side rails should be considered a restraint, is not an effective fall reduction measure, and may increase fall-related injury because of unsafe (head-first) bed exits.

A. Correction of Vision Deficits

Correction of unilateral vision loss should be encouraged to enhance mobility, particularly if the fall is related to tripping or change in depth. Maximal lighting in the home with reduction in glare should be encouraged. Consideration should be given to switching from bifocal to distance lenses, particularly if a fall has occurred on a stair, ramp, or curb. Older adults with poor neck flexion may be more likely to have problems with inaccurate depth perception related to bifocals because they may be unable to flex the neck sufficiently to look at the feet through the upper, distant lenses.

B. Treatment of Cardiovascular Abnormalities

Consideration should be given to further evaluation and treatment for carotid sinus syndrome in the case of otherwise unexplained falls, even in the absence of a history of syncope. Use of a pacemaker in older adults with unexplained falls and cardioinhibitory carotid sinus syndrome has been shown to decrease falls. Treatment of symptomatic orthostatic hypotension should be considered when circumstances of the fall suggest this as a cause. If an asymptomatic finding of orthostasis is noted on exam, treatment is less likely to be beneficial.

C. Decreased Psychotropic Medications

As a single intervention, psychotropic medication reduction has been shown to reduce falls. Patients should be encouraged to decrease their use of sleep aids, including over-the-counter medications containing diphenhydramine or other sedating antihistamines. If a sedative–hypnotic is needed, a short-acting agent is preferred, and the dose should be started at about half of the usual starting adult dose. However, short-acting benzodiazepines, as well as the nonbenzodiazepine agent zolpidem have been associated with falls.

Antidepressants are associated with falls in a dose-dependent manner. Antidepressant and antipsychotic medication dose should be titrated downward if possible. Use of first-generation tricyclic antidepressants should be avoided.

D. Vitamin D Replacement

Vitamin D replacement for those who are deficient has been shown to decrease falls and improve body sway. Vitamin D supplementation has also been shown to improve functional status. Although a recommendation of 800 IU Vitamin D/day for older adults is reasonable, some patients may require higher doses to achieve a desired level of 25-OH vitamin D of > 32 ng/mL.

E. Implementation of Exercise Program

Exercise is efficacious in preventing falls for both high- and low-risk older adults. For high-risk older adults (those with previous falls or multiple fall risk factors), the 2 positive randomized trials of exercise as a sole intervention both used individualized, progressive exercise programs of at least 3 mo duration. In low-risk older adult, group-based rather than individualized exercise has been shown to be effective. One positive study used tai chi ch'uan, and the other positive study used weekly exercise classes incorporating balance training supplemented by daily home exercises.

A meta-analysis of the Frailty and Injuries: Cooperative Studies of Intervention Techniques (FICSIT) found an overall significant falls reduction associated with exercise; the most pronounced reduction was from those interventions that included balance exercises. The Guidelines for the Prevention of Falls in Older Persons recommends that older adults with recurrent falls be offered long-term exercise that includes balance training.

For older adults with a history of falls and specific gait and balance abnormalities on exam, a physical therapist should be consulted to establish an individualized exercise program. Although strengthening or aerobic conditioning exercises may be prescribed, therapy should also include balance exercises, which should progress over time. Sensory integration can be improved by balance exercises. Therapy of several months durations is more likely to be beneficial than therapy of shorter duration. For more fit older adults, tai chi or another group exercise program that incorporates standing balance exercises should be recommended for a goal of fall prevention. There is no evidence that exercises in the seated position will decrease falls.

Exercise treatment for mobility impairment is similar to that for falls. Exercise has been shown to reduce the progression of functional decline among older adults with moderate physical frailty. A physical therapist should be consulted if mobility impairment is severe and is associated with marked muscle weakness or aerobic deconditioning. To improve mobility, individualized treatment may focus on strengthening, aerobic training, or both. Strengthening and aerobic training have been shown to improve function and movement speed in patients with knee osteoarthritis. In the absence of cardiac signs and symptoms, a cardiac evaluation using a submaximal treadmill is generally not needed before beginning a reconditioning or strengthening program.

If mobility impairment is only mild to moderate, then patients can and should be encouraged to begin community exercise programs (either strengthening or aerobic) and do not need individualized physical therapy first. A walking program should be instituted. Walking has been shown to improve endurance and quality of life for patients with osteoarthritis and peripheral vascular disease.

F. Use of Assistive Devices

The use of an assistive device may decrease fear of falling and improve mobility. Patients who have sensory loss (visual, vestibular, or proprioceptive) as their primary cause for falls or mobility impairment may benefit from the use of a cane, which decreases sway for patients with neuropathy or vestibular loss. A cane may be particularly helpful at night, when visual cues are not available to help stabilize balance. For patients with somatosensory loss, a cane or walking stick should be used outdoors or on uneven ground.

Other ambulation aids include 4-prong canes; hemiwalkers; 2-wheeled, 3-wheeled, and 4-wheeled walkers (often with a seat); and standard walkers (4 legs, no wheels). In general, the least restrictive device that provides for safe ambulation should be used. A hemiwalker is often useful in the setting of CVA. The 3-wheeled walker provides more stability than a cane without significantly limiting dexterity of movement. However, the back wheels are out of the line of vision and may be prone to hit obstacles when used by patients with poor visuospatial skills or cognitive impairment. For patients with more marked mobility impairment, a 4-wheeled walker, which is heavier and more stable, may be preferred. A walker seat can be helpful for patients with limited endurance. Although a standard walker, with or without front wheels, is most stable, it also provides the least maneuverability. Decisions regarding the best type of walker should take into account cognitive status and in-home and out-of-home needs. Patients should be able to walk, turn, and maneuver around obstacles with the ambulation aid. Patients with severe cognitive impairment may not be able to use any assistive device appropriately. Those with severe cerebellar ataxia or brainstem CVAs may also not do well with any assistive device. For such patients, the best way to enhance mobility may be a scooter. Medicare will cover the cost of a standard walker only.

G. HOME SAFETY

Home assessment is advisable as part of a multifactorial intervention. It may be covered by Medicare in some cases and should be performed by a trained occupational or physical therapist. There are also a number of home safety checklists that patients may self-administer. The home safety assessment ideally should be tailored to match the specific deficits of the individual.

Table 12–2 provides more detailed information on matching the home safety intervention to the individual.

H. USE OF APPROPRIATE FOOTWEAR

Foot position awareness and balance improve with the use of firm, thin-soled shoes and low, rather than high, heels. Balance is also better with the use of footwear compared with going barefoot. Older adults with poor foot clearance or a history of tripping falls should avoid crepe-soled shoes (such as tennis shoes). Loose-fitting slippers or sandals should be avoided.

I. USE OF MEDICAL ALARMS & LIFELINES

Older adults at high risk for falls can be advised to use a medical alarm or lifeline bracelet or necklace when they are home alone. These systems usually work by connecting to a 24-h dispatch center that notifies a designated person or emergency medical system when activated. They are not usually covered by Medicare or supplemental insurance and cost approximately $30 or more per month. These devices do not work outside the home.

J. BEHAVIOR MODIFICATION

Patients should be informed of their specific fall risk factors and the particular types of maneuvers or activities that increase risk. In addition, patients should be

Table 12–2. Home and behavioral adaptations for specific deficits related to falls.

Adaptation	Specific deficits where adaptation likely to be of benefit
Clear floor of clutter	Decreased foot clearance
	Decreased vision, decreased depth perception
	CVA with one-sided neglect
	Dementia
Increase chair and toilet height, provide arms for chairs, rails for toilet	Muscle weakness
	Impaired balance with chair rise
	Motor apraxia
Increase lighting, decrease glare	Cataracts
	Decreased vision
	Proprioceptive loss
Increase stair safety; provide railings on both sides, mark edges of steps with contrasting tape	Decreased vision
	Proprioceptive loss
	Muscle weakness
	Decreased foot clearance
Move kitchen, bedroom, and commonly used closet items to shoulder level	Neck osteoarthritis
	Vestibular deficit
	Parkinson's disease
Avoid multitasking	Dementia
	Decreased vision
	Psychotropic medication use

CVA, cerebrovascular accident.

informed of the need for increased attention to mobility tasks. Although education alone, without multifactorial assessment and intervention, appears to be of no benefit in preventing falls, it is an important part of individualized falls prevention.

K. Use of Hip Protectors

The most cost-effective hip fracture prevention for the long-term care setting is a hip protector pad. In the nursing home setting, the risk of hip fractures is reduced by up to 60% with the use of hip protector pads. Use of hip protectors has been shown to decrease fear of falling among community-living adults. Although compliance may be problematic and may limit use, hip protectors should be offered to older adults who are at significant risk of falling. Use should be strongly encouraged for institutionalized older adults with recurrent falls or prior hip fracture.

L. Bone Mineral Density Monitoring

Older adults at high risk for falls should undergo evaluation and treatment for osteoporosis. Treatment should be strongly considered when the T score is below −1.5.

American Geriatrics Society, British Geriatrics Society, American Academy of Orthopaedic Surgeons Panel on Falls Prevention: Guideline for the prevention of falls in older persons. J Am Geriatr Soc 2001;49:179. [PMID: 11380764] (Provides recommendations for falls prevention and grades intervention strategies according to the quality of supporting evidence.)

Close J et al: Prevention of falls in the elderly trial (PROFET): A randomized controlled trial. Lancet 1999;353:93. [PMID: 10023893] (Assesses the efficacy of a multifactorial intervention to prevent falls targeted to patients aged 65 and older who had presented to an emergency room after a fall.)

Day L et al: Randomised factorial trial of falls prevention among older people living in their own homes. BMJ 2002;325:128. [PMID: 12130606] (Analyzes success of interventions, eg, exercise, home hazard management, and vision correction, in decreasing falls among primarily low-risk older adults. Although exercise alone was effective, home hazard management and vision correction provided additional benefit.)

Gill TM et al: A program to prevent functional decline in physically frail, elderly persons who live at home. N Engl J Med 2002;347:1068. [PMID: 12362007]. (Study demonstrates that intervention of home modifications plus exercise prescribed by a physical therapist reduced the progression of functional decline.)

Gillespie LD et al: Interventions for preventing falls in elderly people (Cochrane Review). Cochrane Database Syst Rev 2001;3:CD000340. [PMID: 11686957] (Review analyzed pooled odds ratios to categorize interventions that are likely to be beneficial and those that are of unknown effectiveness.)

Jensen J et al: Fall and injury prevention in older people living in residential care facilities: A cluster randomized trial. Ann Intern Med 2002;136:733. [PMID: 12020141] (A multifactorial fall prevention program was found to reduce falls and fractures among older adults living in assisted-living facilities.)

Kannus P et al: Prevention of hip fracture in elderly people with use of a hip protector. N Engl J Med 2000;343:1506. [PMID: 11087879] (Use of hip protectors was found to reduce the risk of hip fracture among ambulatory, high-risk older adults.)

Kenny RA et al: Carotid sinus syndrome: A modifiable risk factor for nonaccidental falls in older adults (SAFE PACE). J Am Coll Cardiol 2001;38:1491. [PMID: 11691528] (Use of a pacemaker was found to reduce the risk of falls among nonaccidental fallers who were found to have cardioinhibitory carotid sinus hypersensitivity on examination.)

Parker MJ et al: Hip protectors for preventing hip fractures in the elderly (Cochrane Review). Cochrane Database Syst Rev 2001;2:CD001255. [PMID:11405982]. (Review of 7 trials of hip protectors for older adults at high risk for hip fracture in nursing homes and assisted living facilities.)

Pate RR et al: Physical activity and public health. A recommendation from the Centers for Disease Control and Prevention and the American College of Sports Medicine. JAMA 1995;273:402. [PMID: 7823386] (Summary of evidence-based consensus process and statement regarding recommendations for physical activity endorsed by the Centers for Disease Control and Prevention and the American College of Sports Medicine.)

Pfeifer M et al: Effects of a short-term vitamin D and calcium supplementation on body sway and secondary hyperparathyroidism in elderly women. J Bone Miner Res 2000;15:1113. [PMID: 10841179] (Among older women with low vitamin D status, calcium plus 400 IU vitamin D daily for 8 weeks, compared with calcium alone, improved vitamin D status, decreased PTH, decreased body sway, and decreased the mean number of falls over 1 year follow-up.)

Province MA et al: The effects of exercise on falls in elderly patients. A preplanned meta-analysis of the FICSIT Trials. Frailty and Injuries: Cooperative Studies of Intervention Techniques. JAMA 1995;273:1341. [PMID: 7715058] (This preplanned meta-analysis found an adjusted significant falls incidence ratio of 0.90 for FICSIT interventions that included exercise and of 0.83 for interventions including balance exercises.)

Clinical Findings

The clinical findings for falls and mobility disorders are similar. Table 12–1 details components of falls and mobility evaluation.

A. Symptoms & Signs

Although vertigo classically corresponds to vestibular abnormalities, dysequilibrium, or sense of imbalance, is a nonspecific symptom that may indicate sensory loss or CNS abnormality. Light-headedness classically is associated with disorders relating to decreased cerebral perfusion, such as with orthostatic hypotension or other cardiovascular abnormality.

B. Patient History

Patient histories for falls and mobility disorders are similar. The history should evaluate the types of maneuvers (indoors and outdoors) that are difficult and the reason for the difficulty (eg, poor vision, pain, shortness of breath, imbalance). With mobility disorders, it is particularly important to evaluate for the presence of back or lower extremity pain with walking or other maneuvers.

The history should elicit circumstances of the fall, including environment, direction, activity engaged in at the time of the fall, time of day and relation to medications, and presence or absence of associated symptoms. Pertinent environmental circumstances include location, floor surface, lighting, and presence of environmental hazard, if any. Information about the environment can directly lead to modification of extrinsic and situational risk factors (eg, discontinued use of an unsteady chair, improving lighting).

Direction of the fall may provide a clue to the underlying pathophysiological mechanism. Forward falls typically indicate a trip. Tripping falls may be due to impaired depth perception, which may occur from either unilateral or bilateral vision loss. A tripping fall may also be due to hemineglect or poor foot clearance. Backward falls may be due to a slip. Backward falls with little or no environmental component may indicate CNS disease, including cerebellar, brainstem, or basal ganglia disease.

Activity at the time of the fall provides information about cause and prevention. For example, a fall that occurs with head turning may be related to vestibular disease, cervical arthritis, spondylosis, or a vascular cause, such as vertebrobasilar insufficiency or carotid sinus syndrome. A fall while rising from a chair may be related to muscle weakness or CNS or peripheral nervous system disease. A fall while descending or ascending stairs may be related to problems with balance, proprioception, decreased vision, muscle weakness, or orthopedic problems causing pain.

Time of day and relation to meals, medication, or alcohol is also important. For example, a fall occurring 30 min after a meal may raise suspicion of postprandial hypotension. Other situational factors about the fall are relevant because they directly lead to recommendations for behavior modification. Was the person using an assistive device at the time of the fall? What type of shoe was the patient wearing? Was the patient wearing glasses? Thick-soled, rubber or crepe-soled shoes may contribute to a trip, particularly indoors and among those with poor foot clearance. Bifocals may contribute to tripping falls, particularly for older adults who have limited neck flexion.

The history should also assess whether there were competing attentional demands at the time of the fall. Postural control worsens when a competing attentional task is given. Was the person rushing to answer the telephone or door? Was the patient carrying laundry while going upstairs?

Questions should be directed toward associated symptoms of vertigo, dysequilibrium, light-headedness, presence of other neurological symptoms, and presence of joint or leg pain or instability. Although vertigo classically corresponds to vestibular abnormalities, dysequilibrium, or sense of imbalance, is a nonspecific symptom that may indicate sensory loss or CNS abnormality. Light-headedness classically is associated with disorders relating to decreased cerebral perfusion, such as with orthostatic hypotension or other cardiovascular abnormality.

The history should also elicit any symptoms suggestive of acute contributors to the fall (eg, infectious, ischemic, toxic, metabolic, neurological). A fall may be the first sign of infection, worsened congestive heart failure, or metabolic derangement such as hypoglycemia or hyponatremia. For example, frequent falls at night in a diabetic should raise suspicion for nocturnal hypo- or hyperglycemia.

Patients should be questioned about their fear of falling. Individuals who have unnecessarily avoided or curtailed activities may benefit from a new or different assistive device or from task modification to allow resumption of the activity.

C. MEDICATION REVIEW

1. Psychotropic medications—Patients should be questioned regarding use of psychotropic medications. New medication, change in dosage, high dosage (for geriatric population), and use of > 1 psychotropic agent are associated with increased risk for hip fractures. Substantial evidence links neuroleptics, benzodiazepines, and antidepressants with falls and fractures.

a. Neuroleptics—High-potency agents may contribute to falls related to extrapyramidal side effects, whereas low-potency agents may increase fall risk as a result of sedating and anticholinergic side effects. Fall risk related to atypical antipsychotics (risperidone, olanzepine) has not been well evaluated, but it is likely that these agents also contribute to falls through extrapyramidal and anticholinergic pathways.

b. Benzodiazepines—Both long- and short-acting benzodiazepines increase the risk for falls and fractures, again in a dose-dependent manner. Zolpidem use may also be associated with hip fracture. Sedative-hypnotics may exert their effect by impairing attention or alertness. It is prudent to consider that any medication carrying a caution regarding driving may increase the risk for falls, particularly if prescribed to an older adult who is already at an increased risk for falls.

2. Antidepressants—Although first-generation tricyclic antidepressants are of particular concern, other medications such as trazadone (in doses used for antidepressant effect) and selective serotonin reuptake inhibitors have also been implicated. Newer antidepressants have not been well evaluated in regard to falls, but patients should be prescribed the lowest dose possible.

Depression itself may increase the risk for falls. A link between falls and depression is plausible because depression may lead to impaired concentration, decreased sleep, and psychomotor retardation, all of which may increase risk.

3. Cardiovascular medications—Digoxin, type IA antiarrhythmics, and diuretics may be weakly associated with falls. Other cardiac medications, including antihypertensives, angiotensin-converting enzyme inhibitors, calcium channel blockers, and nitrates, have not been linked. However, it is reasonable to evaluate antihypertensive and cardiac medications in the setting of a fall that appears related to orthostasis or postprandial hypotension.

4. Analgesics—The use of narcotic or other analgesics is not strongly linked to falls. However, new or recently increased doses of narcotics should be considered as potential contributing factors if circumstances are suggestive.

5. Other medications—Ataxia and sedation may be noted at higher doses of all antiseizure medications. It is particularly important to evaluate for cerebellar side effects when prescribing these agents for neuropathic pain. Because patients with neuropathy are already at increased risk for falls, any upward titration of neuropathic pain medications should proceed with careful monitoring to ensure that risk does not increase further.

Although support for a link between anticholinergic antihistamines (eg, diphenhydramine) and falls is not strong, use of diphenhydramine may lead to impaired driving performance and symptoms of delirium.

D. Physical Examination

Although disorders related to sensory input and CNS processing clearly affect falls and mobility, particular attention should be paid to the musculoskeletal system. The back, legs, and feet should be assessed for biomechanical, muscular, and arthritic changes affecting gait, such as decreased joint range of motion (ROM), changes in joint alignment, leg-length discrepancy, and muscle weakness.

1. Vision assessment—Specific visual deficits related to falls and mobility impairment include poor distant vision (unilateral or bilateral), reduced contrast sensitivity, decreased depth perception, decreased visual field, and posterior subcapsular cataract. The visual examination should include assessment of visual fields by confrontation, assessment of distant vision in each eye with and without distance lenses, and fundoscopic exam. Even unilateral vision impairment may affect depth perception and cause falls. If a cataract is impairing vi-

sion unilaterally, strong consideration should be given to its extraction, particularly if falls appear to be related to impaired depth perception.

2. Vestibular function assessment—Vestibular dysfunction, either peripheral or central, may be associated with classic symptoms of vertigo or with a nonspecific dizziness or dysequilibrium. Oscillopsia (a sensation that the environment is moving upon walking or moving the head) may be present. Patients may rely more on vision for maintaining balance, with increased unsteadiness in the dark. Patients may also complain of decreased balance or dizziness in crowded shopping areas or with highly patterned floor surfaces, when visual input becomes conflicting. They may also rely more on somatosensory input and display decreased balance with uneven surfaces.

Symptoms of vestibular dysfunction should prompt a more in-depth examination, including the head-thrust test, dynamic visual acuity, Dix-Hallpike maneuver, Romberg test, and march-in-place (Fukuda) test.

In the head-thrust test, the patient is instructed to look at the examiner's nose while the examiner rapidly moves the patient's head to the right and left. A positive test is noted if small, rapid eye movements are elicited.

Dynamic visual acuity assesses distant vision on the Snellen chart with slow passive head movements (2-Hz frequency). A drop of more than 3 lines in visual acuity with head movement is suggestive of dysfunction in the vestibular pathways.

The Dix-Hallpike maneuver may help with the diagnosis of benign positional vertigo. Nystagmus and vertigo that lasts for 10–30 s and is brought on within a few seconds of rapidly positioning the patient from seated to supine with the head turned 45° is a positive response.

Unilateral peripheral vestibular hypofunction is also suggested by abnormal rotation while the patient marches in place with eyes closed and arms held out straight ahead. More than 45° rotation during 30 s of marching is abnormal.

None of these tests is very sensitive for vestibular abnormality. If clinical suspicion is high, referral to an otolaryngologist for further, more sensitive testing may be warranted.

Even if no reversible cause of disease is found, most patients with vestibular dysfunction can benefit from vestibular rehabilitation exercises. They may also benefit from the use of an ambulation aid, which improves somatosensory input. Extra caution is required in the dark. In general, meclizine and sedative-hypnotics should be avoided because of the potential for adverse effects, including falls.

3. Cardiovascular assessment—The cardiovascular exam should include assessment of heart rate and rhythm as well as lying and standing (after 1 and 3 min) heart rate and blood pressure (BP). Symptoms or signs consistent with a cardiovascular cause should prompt additional evaluation. For example, presyncopal symptoms associated with prolonged standing may suggest need for delayed monitoring of standing BP. Presyncopal symptoms 30 min after a meal may suggest the need for postprandial BP monitoring. Presyncopal symptoms associated with head turning may suggest carotid sinus syndrome or vertebrobasilar insufficiency. If the history is suggestive, an electrocardiogram (ECG) may be of benefit even if the pulse is regular.

Caution should be used in ascribing orthostatic hypotension as a cause of the fall because epidemiological evidence linking orthostatic hypotension to falls is not strong. To establish orthostatic hypotension as the cause, in general, the fall should have occurred in circumstances consistent with orthostasis (eg, shortly after arising from a chair), symptoms of orthostasis should have been present at the time of the fall, and symptoms of light-headedness should be reproducible on exam.

Syncope as the cause for a fall may be underdiagnosed. Frequently with a fall there is no corroborating witness. In the absence of a witness, a patient's denial of syncope does not rule it out. In fact, a substantial proportion of patients who have syncope during carotid sinus massage will deny LOC when asked immediately afterward. Therefore, a history of multiple, otherwise unexplained falls should lead to consideration of more in-depth cardiac evaluation, including carotid sinus massage.

4. Lower extremity assessment—Varus or valgus deformities, leg-length discrepancy, and ligamentous laxity may contribute to gait impairment and falls. Arthritis may contribute to falls and impaired mobility either directly as a result of pain or indirectly because of proprioceptive loss, decreased joint ROM, or weakness in surrounding muscles. Foot deformities are associated with increased risk for falls and with gait and mobility disorders.

The lower extremity should be assessed for the presence of joint deformities, joint ROM, and pain with active and passive ROM. Feet should be examined for excess pronation or supination, painful calluses or corns, fallen metatarsals, and other biomechanical abnormalities. Orthotic devices and appropriate footwear can alleviate biomechanical deformities. The use of an assistive device may decrease joint loading. Referral to physical therapy for strengthening and endurance exercise is an integral part of treatment.

5. Neurological assessment—The neurological assessment should include light touch, joint position sense and vibration, muscle strength and tone, reflexes, and cortical, extrapyramidal, and cerebellar function.

Further diagnostic evaluation should be guided by findings from the neurological exam and the gait and balance exam (see later discussion).

6. Cognition assessment—Dementia has been strongly associated with falls through mechanisms of decreased judgment, slowed reaction time, and apraxia. Patients with Lewy body dementia have prominent extrapyramidal signs and a marked propensity to fall, which may be increased further by the use of antipsychotics. Evaluation of executive and visuospatial functioning is particularly important. The Mini-Mental State Examination and the Clock-Drawing Test are valuable in this regard.

7. Gait & balance assessment—The purposes of the gait and balance exam are 3-fold: to help determine the cause of the fall by reproducing the circumstances that evoke instability; to help determine the pathological mechanisms resulting in the gait/balance abnormality; and to help counsel patients regarding risk for falls.

The Get Up and Go Test is a simple, validated test of gait and balance. The patient is instructed to rise from a chair with armrests, walk 10 feet, turn around, walk back, and sit down using any usual ambulation aids and walking at a normal pace. The maneuver should be timed; a time of > 14 s is associated with increased risk for falls. Qualitative evaluation is also important. Imbalance, hesitancy, and lack of fluidity with chair rise, walking, turning, or sitting down are considered abnormal.

The specific gait pattern should be noted. A mildly slowed gait speed with decreased but symmetric stride length is common with older age and is not, in itself, abnormal. A broad-based gait is abnormal but nonspecific. It may be seen as an adaptation to loss of sensory input or fear of falling. It may also be seen with cerebellar disorders. A shuffling gait with decreased arm swing and tendency to festination is classic for Parkinson's disease. A related gait may be seen with frontal gait disorders, including normal pressure hydrocephalus, cerebrovascular disease, and frontal masses. There may be difficulty initiating gait, with short steps and a "magnetic gait" appearance (ie, feet appear glued to floor). Abnormally slow gait speed with short steps is also noted with high-grade cerebral white matter changes on computed tomography (CT) or magnetic resonance imaging (MRI).

A spastic gait with circumduction of the leg at the hip may be related to stroke or cervical spinal stenosis. A characteristic waddling gait and Trendelenburg's sign are seen with proximal motor weakness. Steppage gait and foot slap are seen with distal motor weakness (eg, distal motor neuropathy). Cerebellar ataxia is characterized by broad-based gait with asymmetry of step length and lack of a straight path. Irregularity of cadence and step length may be heightened with turns or rapid walking. Finally, antalgic gait is characterized by shortened stance phase on the affected side.

Gait assessment should include stepping over obstacles (eg, shoe or shoe box). Individuals with vision impairment or poor foot clearance may slow gait speed considerably when trying to step over objects, may not clear the object with the foot, or may lose balance when trying to step over. This aspect of gait testing is particularly contributory if a person has suffered a tripping fall.

It is also helpful to retest gait while diverting the person's attention, in particular when circumstances of the fall suggest the person was trying to do more than 1 task at a time. Persons with increased fall risk may perform well on gait assessment as long as their attention is focused specifically on the task, but they may show gait slowing or balance impairment when their attention is diverted. Attentional aspects can be tested in the office by asking the person to walk a short distance, turn around, and return while carrying a full glass of water, performing serial subtractions, or listing animal names. Stepping over objects can also be tested while the person does a mental task. If obvious slowing or worsening of gait or balance is noted, the individual should be cautioned regarding the need to focus attention while walking and avoid competing attentional demands.

Finally, it can be helpful to ask the person to walk as fast as possible. Patients with cerebellar ataxia may become more ataxic at rapid speed. Patients with periventricular white matter changes or other frontal gait syndromes may be unable to speed up when asked.

Other performance-based tests may help with diagnosis. Patients should be asked to rise from a chair without armrests. An inability to rise from the chair is abnormal and suggests proximal muscle weakness or impaired postural control resulting from proprioceptive, visual, or CNS abnormalities. The ability to withstand a light nudge on the sternum may be impaired with Parkinson's disease and other CNS disorders. Needing to step backward when nudged on the sternum or beginning to fall are considered abnormal and may be indicative of propensity to backward falling.

The Romberg test assesses somatosensory and vestibular input. Patients with cerebellar ataxia may be unable to put their feet together to perform the test. For those who are able to place their feet together, increased sway with the eyes closed indicates proprioceptive or vestibular abnormality. If the Romberg test is positive, the patient should be educated regarding the need for extra caution in circumstances in which visual input is limited (eg, in dim light or when the eyes are closed in the shower).

Other functional balance tests include neck turning while standing, reaching up to barely just rise on the toes, and bending over to pick up an object from the floor. Dizziness or imbalance with neck turn may indicate cervical proprioceptive loss, vestibular dysfunction, or central neurological balance disorder. Patients should be counseled regarding the need to modify head and neck movements. Difficulty reaching while on tiptoes may lead to the recommendation to move kitchen items down from top shelves. Patients with difficulty bending may benefit from the use of a reacher.

For mobility disorders, gait abnormalities associated with biomechanical, muscular, or arthritic changes include antalgic gait, decreased step length, unequal step length, and Trendelenberg gait. Adverse effects on mobility may be at least partially alleviated by appropriate orthotic devices for foot, ankle, or knee; assistive devices for ambulation; pain medication; exercise; and orthopedic surgery.

E. LABORATORY FINDINGS

No specific routine laboratory tests are indicated as part of an evaluation for falls. However, hypothyroidism may manifest as falls without other findings on history and physical exam; therefore, a thyroid-stimulating hormone test should be strongly considered.

Selection of additional laboratory tests should be directed by history and physical exam findings. A metabolic panel may be helpful when there is suspicion of acute or subacute change in health status contributing to the fall. Anemia has been noted as a risk factor for falls; a hematocrit should be obtained if there are suggestive symptoms. Falling may also be an early symptom of Addison's disease; morning cortisol testing may be considered if other signs and symptoms are suggestive. If cognitive loss or loss of proprioception and vibration is present, the vitamin B_{12} level should be obtained and a rapid plasma reagin test or Venereal Disease Research Laboratories test considered.

Vitamin D deficiency is common in frail older adults, and low 25-OH vitamin D levels are associated with decreased muscle strength and falls. Because signs and symptoms are often nonspecific, assessment of 25-OH vitamin D level should be strongly considered. A level of < 32 ng/mL is abnormal.

F. IMAGING STUDIES

Imaging studies are not considered part of the routine evaluation for falls but should be prompted by specific signs and symptoms. Head CT and MRI may be indicated if there are new or unexplained neurological findings. A rapid progression in gait impairment with a frontal gait with or without symptoms of dementia and urinary incontinence should prompt evaluation for normal pressure hydrocephalus. Slow gait speed and falls have been strongly linked with MRI findings of high-grade periventricular white matter changes, which are presumptively ischemic. Lesions have been linked to nocturnal hypotension, orthostatic hypotension, and postprandial hypotension. There is no specific treatment.

MRI of the cervical or lumbar spine is indicated if signs and symptoms suggest cervical or lumbar spinal stenosis. Findings of cervical spinal stenosis include lower extremity proprioceptive and vibratory sense loss along with lower extremity weakness, hyperreflexia, and spasticity. Upper extremity radicular symptoms and signs may be present. Lumbar spinal stenosis may produce weakness in muscles innervated by L4-S1 and classically presents with symptoms of pseudoclaudication.

G. SPECIAL TESTS

Special tests may be helpful if organ system abnormalities are found on exam. Electronystagmography and dynamic posturography may help distinguish central versus peripheral vestibular disease and its effect on balance. Sensory or motor loss in the lower extremity may indicate abnormalities in peripheral nerves, spinal cord, or brain. Electromyography, nerve conduction velocity, and somatosensory evoked potential may help delineate the specific disease.

There should be a low threshold for further cardiac testing given the overlap between syncope and falls. Carotid sinus massage should be strongly considered in the setting of unexplained recurrent falls, with or without a history of LOC, if there is no contraindication. Continuous ECG and BP monitoring is indicated. Tilt table testing may be considered, again even in the absence of history of LOC. Holter monitoring may be helpful if there are specific signs or symptoms suggesting arrhythmia as a cause. Similarly, echocardiogram may also be considered if other markers suggest that the fall is due to decreased blood flow to the brain.

More specialized balance testing may be available through physical therapy. Testing may include the sensory organization test or computerized balance platform testing, both of which help evaluate the vestibular, visual, and sensory contributions to balance. Tests of motor control, automatic postural responses, muscle activation, and dynamic weight shifting may also be performed. Although not necessary as a routine evaluation, these evaluations may help when the cause of symptoms of dizziness, dysequilibrium, or balance impairment is unclear. They also may help guide treatment by allowing prescription of specific exercises to improve sensory integration and dynamic balance.

Differential Diagnosis

A. FALLS

The first step in investigating the cause of a fall is to determine whether consciousness was maintained or lost during the event. If consciousness was lost, the differen-tial shifts to seizure and syncope; further evaluation should follow for these causes. There is growing recognition, however, that lack of patient report of LOC does not rule out syncope. Whenever possible, a witness should be interviewed to ascertain state of consciousness. In the absence of a witness, syncope must remain in the differential if a fall is otherwise unexplained.

A fall not resulting from syncope, seizure, or overwhelming environmental hazard is typically related to deficits in multiple organ systems related to balance. The evaluation should focus on the search for reversible causes; evaluation of medications; prescription for physical therapy for individualized balance and strengthening program and for evaluation for assistive device; evaluation of home safety; and patient education to modify unsafe behaviors. Table 12–3 lists reversible causes for falls.

B. MOBILITY DISORDERS

The approach to evaluation of mobility disorders is similar to that for falls. Mobility disorders are typically multifactorial, and evaluation should ascertain which factors are potentially reversible. Certain conditions may play more of a role in mobility impairment than they do in falls. Obesity, pain (particularly arthritic), decreased joint ROM, deconditioning, and depression contribute substantially to mobility impairment.

Complications

Complications of falls and mobility disorders include fear of falling, social isolation, depression, and ADL dependency. Mobility impairment may be associated with functional incontinence, accelerated deconditioning, and poor quality of sleep.

Although injuries associated with falling are most frequently minor, even minor injuries may result in further mobility restriction. Severe injury occurs infrequently but markedly increases the risk of complications. Hip fracture is associated with a sharp increase in ADL dependency, which is often permanent, and with increased risk for permanent institutionalization. Half of all hospitalizations for fall-related injury result in nursing home placement.

Treatment

Treatment of falls and mobility disorders is largely based on the detection and treatment of underlying reversible causes and on implementation of preventive measures after an event has occurred to decrease repeat incidents and fear of falling.

Prognosis

Multifactorial interventions have resulted in a 40% decrease in fall rate. Reduction in fall rates from exercise

Table 12–3. Potentially treatable causes of falls, associated falls history, and gait abnormality.

Organ system	Potentially/partially treatable causes	Associated fall history	Associated gait abnormality
Vision	Cataracts Myopia Bifocals	Tripping fall Fall on curbs or ramps or with change in depth	Often slowed gait, with decreased stride length
Proprioceptive	Vitamin B$_{12}$ deficiency Neurosyphilis Cervical spinal stenosis Some neuropathies	Worsening balance in dark or on uneven ground	Often slowed gait, decreased stride length
Vestibular	Cerumen impaction Serous otitis media Alcohol use Acoustic neuroma Benign positional vertigo Chronic vestibular disease	Worsening balance or symptoms or vertigo with head turns and movement Fall with head turn Worsening balance in the dark	Gait abnormalities with head and body turns
Cardiovascular	Orthostatic hypotension Postprandial hypotension Arrhythmia	Fall shortly after standing, typically preceded by symptoms of light-headedness Fall 30 min after meal, typically with symptoms of light-headedness Unexplained fall or reported loss of consciousness	
Central nervous system	Normal-pressure hydrocephalus Subdural hematoma Parkinson's Disease Hypothyroidism Reversible dementias Depression Psychotropic medications Alcohol	Often backward fall or fall with little or no environmental risk Fall may occur after medication, alcohol consumption	Ataxic gait (cerebellar or brainstem) Magnetic gait (poor foot clearance, frontal lobe disease or normal-pressure hydrocephalus) Shuffling, festinating gait (Parkinson's disease) Apraxia (CVA or late dementia)
Upper motor neuron	Cervical spinal stenosis	Fall in any direction	Spastic gait
Lower motor neuron	Lumbar spinal stenosis Reversible neuropathies	Fall in any direction Need to use hands to rise from chair	Often poor foot clearance Foot drop (slapping gait)
Muscular	Polymyositis Endocrinopathies Vitamin D deficiency Protein-calorie malnutrition Deconditioning, catabolic illness	Fall in any direction Need to use hands to rise from chair	May have waddling gait and Trendelenburg's sign Often poor foot clearance
Biomechanical	Leg-length discrepancy Foot deformities Joint instability, or deformity	Pain with walking Tripping fall	Often antalgic, asymmetric gait

CVA, cerebrovascular accident.

alone varies from 20–50% depending on the target population and type of exercise provided.

The prognosis for any individual patient depends on the ability to detect and treat underlying factors related to falls and on patient adherence with exercise and the use of assistive device and other behavioral modifications. Patients with cognitive impairment and a history of falls and those with certain central balance disorders (eg, Parkinson's disease, brainstem CVAs, cerebellar ataxia) have a poor prognosis because of their decreased ability to compensate.

The prognosis related to treatment of mobility disorders also depends on the ability to identify and treat reversible underlying factors. Deconditioning may be readily reversed by exercise. Both resistance and aerobic exercise increase functional ability for patients with knee osteoarthritis. Both resistance and balance exercises have been shown to increase levels of physical activity. The use of an assistive device has been shown to increase mobility. Thus, prognosis is good for gains in mobility with a multifactorial intervention strategy incorporating exercise and modification of other intrinsic and situational factors.

EVIDENCE-BASED POINTS

- *Multifactorial intervention is effective in decreasing falls in community, nursing home, and assisted-living settings.*
- *Psychotropic medication reduction is likely effective in decreasing falls among community-dwelling older adults. As part of a multicomponent intervention, it is likely effective in* decreasing falls among institutionalized older adults as well.
- *Exercise, particularly balance training, should be offered as part of a multifactorial intervention for high-risk older adults. For low-risk older adults, group-based balance exercises are likely effective as a single intervention to prevent falls.*
- *Hip protector pads are highly protective against hip fractures.*

RELEVANT WORLD WIDE WEB SITES

American Physical Therapy Association Section on Geriatrics: www.geriatricspt.org (Information and resources about physical therapy for clinicians and patients.)

Center for Injury Prevention Policy and Practice, Injury Prevention Literature Update: www.safetylit.org. (Provides weekly update with abstracts of new injury prevention literature.)

Centers for Disease Control and Prevention: www.cdc.gov. (Links to National Center for Injury Prevention, providing injury morbidity and mortality data, and National Center for Chronic Disease Prevention and Health Promotion, providing information on benefits of exercise.)

National Guideline Clearinghouse: www.guideline.gov. (Compendium of published guidelines, including guidelines on exercise and fall prevention.)

National Resource Center on Aging and Injury: www.olderadultinjury.org. (Contains resources for older adults and families on injury prevention, and has excellent links to data on unintentional injury.)

President's Council on Physical Fitness and Sports: www.fitness.gov. (Links to excellent fact sheets and reports on physical activity and health.)

Parkinson's Disease & Essential Tremor

13

Elise Carey, MD, & Josh Adler, MD

PARKINSON'S DISEASE

ESSENTIALS OF DIAGNOSIS

- *Any combination of resting tremor, bradykinesia, rigidity, and postural instability.*
- *Asymmetric onset is the norm.*
- *Responds well to levodopa in most cases.*
- *Diagnostic accuracy improves with observation over time.*

General Considerations

Parkinson's disease (PD) is a progressive neurodegenerative disorder that affects men and women equally. The prevalence is approximately 1% in the general population, with the rate rising from 0.6% for ages 60–64 to 3.5% for ages 85–89. Although PD is more frequent in older age groups, 5–10% of patients with PD acquire the disease before age 40. First-degree relatives of patients with PD are at approximately twice the risk for the disorder compared with the general population.

Pathogenesis

PD is caused by the death of dopaminergic neurons in the substantia nigra of the midbrain, which results in marked striatal dopamine deficiency. It is estimated that by the time a patient is sufficiently symptomatic to seek care 70% of the dopaminergic neurons have already died. In most patients, the specific cause of PD is unknown.

Several potential and actual genetic, environmental, and infectious causes have been identified. Genes at 3 different loci have been implicated in PD, including the alpha-synuclein gene on chromosome 4, the parkin gene on chromosome 6, and a third gene on chromosome 2. The compound, 1-methyl-4-phenyl-1,2,3, 6-tetrahydropyridine (MPTP), a by-product of metham-

phetamine production, is thought to have caused several cases in young adults in the early 1980s. Pesticides and herbicides have been associated with the development of parkinsonism as well. In the early 20th century, the von Economo encephalitis outbreak was followed by a high rate of postencephalitic parkinsonism. No other infectious agents have been clearly identified as predisposing one to parkinsonism. In addition, several medications, most notably antipsychotic agents, can cause or exacerbate parkinsonism (Table 13–1).

Clinical Findings

PD is a steadily progressive illness of insidious onset that leads to increasing disability over time (Table 13–2). The decline is not necessarily linear, and the rate of progression is variable. Many patients are first seen with stage II disease and bilateral involvement, which can make diagnosis challenging.

A. SYMPTOMS & SIGNS

The key feature of the illness is the triad of resting tremor, bradykinesia, and rigidity. Most patients will have at least 2 of these 3 features when they are first seen. Although the resting tremor is often considered the hallmark of PD, approximately 20% of patients with PD will lack tremor. Impaired postural reflexes and postural instability become evident with progression of the disease.

Several other symptoms are commonly associated with PD (Table 13–3). Masked facies, in which the patient has decreased facial expression and facial muscle movement, develops in most patients. The loss of facial expression often causes patients to appear depressed when they are not. Reduced blinking of the eye is also often noted. Slowing of speech with a decrease in volume and inflection, known as hypophonia, is a common late-stage finding. Micrographia, a reduction in the size of the written word, may become so severe that patients lose the ability to write altogether. The posture becomes stooped with generalized flexion at the trunk, hips, knees, and elbows. Postural instability is the hallmark of stage III disease, which makes patients more prone to falls when standing and often causes balance

Table 13–1. Medications associated with Parkinsonism & tremor.

Parkinsonism	Tremor
Antipsychotic medication	Amphetamines
Lithium	Antidepressants
Metoclopramide	Antipsychotic medication
	β-agonist medications
	Corticosteroids
	Lithium
	Methylxanthines (including coffee and tea)
	Thyroid hormone
	Valproic acid

difficulties of the trunk, even when the patient is seated. Gait impairment develops, marked by the loss of arm swing on the affected side and, eventually, festination. With festination, the patient's center of gravity is shifted forward by the flexed posture, and the patient's steps are too short to bring the feet back under the trunk. As a result, patients take increasingly fast but short steps in an effort to position their lower limbs under their flexed trunk.

As PD progresses, it can potentially affect many systems. Respiratory dysfunction of some degree occurs commonly; pulmonary infection is an unfortunate and frequent consequence. Gastrointestinal dysfunction, including dysphagia and constipation, is common. Autonomic dysfunction can result in postural hypotension,

Table 13–2. Hoehn & Yahr's staging of Parkinsonism.

Stage	Description
I	Unilateral involvement only; little or no functional impairment
II	Bilateral or midline involvement, no balance impairment
III	Impaired postural reflexes and difficulty with balance, still able to walk independently, mild to moderate disability, still physically capable of leading independent lives in most cases
IV	Severely disabling disease; patient cannot get out of bed or chair unassisted but is able to walk independently, however unsteadily, once up
V	Bedridden or wheelchair-bound; cannot ambulate independently

Based on Hoehn MM, Yahr MD: Parkinsonism: Onset, progression, and mortality. Neurology 1967;17:427.

bladder dysfunction, sexual dysfunction, and sweating abnormalities.

B. PATIENT EXAMINATION

The diagnosis of PD is based on the history and physical examination and often reveals itself over time. No laboratory or imaging studies exist that are diagnostic of PD, although some imaging tests are under investigation.

The physical examination should include a complete neurological examination. In addition, the patient should be carefully observed for the cardinal motor features of PD: tremor, bradykinesia, and rigidity. The characteristic tremor is a 3- to 6-Hz resting tremor of the distal extremities, commonly called a "pill-rolling" tremor because the patient appears to be rolling a pill in his fingers as the wrist cycles between pronation and supination. The tremor is most pronounced at rest and often disappears with use of the affected extremity.

Bradykinesia, or motor slowing, is not caused by weakness but by difficulty with the execution of movements. It is most prominent with repetitive activities, especially those involving change in direction, such as alternately pronating and supinating the hand. Movements become not only slower with repetition but also smaller, much like in micrographia. To elicit a decrease in movement size, the examiner asks the patient to tap the first finger and thumb together in wide taps, extending the fingers as widely as possible. Over time, the movement will become progressively smaller in a patient with PD. Another way to elicit this is to have the patient draw a series of large circles on a piece of paper, never lifting the pen from the paper. Again, the circles will become progressively smaller as the patient's efforts continue.

Rigidity can be elicited by passively moving the patient's extremities, resulting in a ratcheting motion of the extremity being manipulated, almost as though it is catching on something repeatedly as it is being moved along its course ("cogwheeling").

Gait should also be carefully observed. The gait of PD is shuffling and festinating. Loss of arm swing on the affected side is a characteristic feature of a parkinsonian gait, as is the "en bloc turn," in which the patient takes several small steps to turn him- or herself around as a unit, with the trunk and feet aligned throughout the turn.

Impaired postural reflexes can be assessed with the "pull test." The patient is asked to stand with the feet shoulder-width apart and to resist any effort at displacement. The examiner should warn the patient that he or she will be pulled from behind and should stand behind the patient to prevent falling. The examiner then pulls the patient from behind with modest effort. A positive pull test occurs when the patient takes more than 1 step

Table 13–3. Definitions.

Symptom	Definition
Bradykinesia	Motor slowing resulting from difficulty executing movements
Bradyphrenia	Slowness of thought
Cogwheeling	Occurs when an extremity rigid from parkinsonism is passively manipulated. A ratcheting motion is felt by the examiner as the extremity is moved along its course, as if caught on the cogs of a wheel
Masked facies	Decreased facial muscle movement and consequent loss of facial expression
Hypophonia	Slowed speech that is low in volume and with reduced inflection
Micrographia	Small handwriting
Festination	Gait impairment, marked by the patient's center of gravity being shifted. The patient will take increasingly rapid short steps in an effort to bring the feet under the center of gravity, leading to an accelerated, forward flexed gait, often resulting in a fall.
En bloc turn	Turn characteristic of PD gait in which the patient takes several small steps to turn the body around as a unit, with the body aligned with the feet throughout the turn. Patients with PD are often unable to make a fluid turn in one step, as with normal gait.
Dyskinesia	Involuntary, abnormal writhing and jerking movements, distinct from tremor, which usually occur with the peak effect of the levodopa dose.
Wearing off effect	Phenomenon in which the response to levodopa therapy becomes progressively shorter over time, leading to loss of mobility and function before the next dosage.
On–off effect	Unpredictable, sudden shift between periods of mobility and immobility not related to the timing of levodopa therapy.

backward to regain balance after the pull, indicating impaired postural reflexes.

C. LABORATORY FINDINGS

There are no laboratory tests that assist in the diagnosis of PD.

D. IMAGING TESTS

A number of imaging studies are currently being investigated in PD, including magnetic resonance imaging (MRI), positron emission tomography (PET), single photon emission tomography (SPECT), and proton magnetic resonance spectroscopy (MRS). MRI is most useful in distinguishing PD from other parkinsonian syndromes, but it is not used currently for monitoring disease progression. PET and SPECT may prove useful in monitoring disease progression but are still considered investigational.

Gelb DJ et al: Diagnostic criteria for Parkinson disease. Arch Neurol 1999;56:33. [PMID: 9923759]

Hely MA et al: The Sydney multicentre study of Parkinson's disease: Progression and mortality at 10 years. J Neurol Neurosurg Psychiatry 1999;67:300. [PMID: 10449550]

Hoehn MM, Yahr MD: Parkinsonism: Onset, progression, mortality. Neurology 1967;17:427. [PMID: 11775596]

Müller J et al: Progression of Hoehn and Yahr stages in parkinsonian disorders: A clinicopathologic study. Neurology 2000;55:888. [PMID: 10994019]

Differential Diagnosis

Commonly used, although not yet validated, diagnostic criteria that may aid in the diagnosis are presented in Table 13–4. Drug-induced parkinsonism, multiple system atrophy, progressive supranuclear palsy, and Lewy body dementia (LBD) should be considered in the differential diagnosis. These are considered Parkinson's plus syndromes because there is involvement of central nervous system structures outside the basal ganglia. Parkinson's plus syndromes tend to be less responsive to levodopa than PD and often progress to disability more rapidly.

Drug-induced parkinsonism is associated with medications that deplete dopamine storage or block postsynaptic dopamine receptors. Neuroleptic agents are most commonly associated with parkinsonism, although other medications have also been implicated (see Table 13–1). Drug-induced parkinsonism is indistinguishable from naturally occurring PD, except for the symmetric onset of symptoms. Recognition of drug-induced parkinsonism is extremely important because it may be partially or completely reversible with the discontinuation of the offending agent.

In multiple-system atrophy (Shy-Drager syndrome), parkinsonism is accompanied by autonomic insufficiency, leading to postural hypotension, erectile dysfunction, incontinence, and anhidrosis. There may be lower motor neuron or cerebellar abnormalities as well.

Table 13–4. Diagnostic guidelines for Parkinson's disease.

Cardinal clinical features	Frequency (%)
Resting tremor	76–100
Bradykinesia	89–99
Rigidity	77–98
Asymmetric onset	72–75

Diagnostic guidelines

Possible Parkinson's Disease

Two of 4 cardinal features present

No features suggestive of an alternative diagnosis to date, including hallucinations unrelated to medication, dementia, supranuclear gaze palsy, or severe dysautonomia.

Beneficial response to levodopa or dopamine agonist or the patient has not received an adequate trial of one of these medications.

Probable Parkinson's Disease

Three of 4 cardinal features present

No features suggestive of an alternative diagnosis in the first 3 years of parkinsonian symptoms, including hallucinations unrelated to medication, dementia, supranuclear gaze palsy, or severe dysautonomia.

A definite clinical response to levodopa or a dopamine agonist.

Adapted from Gelb DJ et al: Diagnostic criteria for Parkinson's disease. Arch Neurol 1999;56:33. Used with permission.

Progressive supranuclear palsy (PSP) presents with gait unsteadiness, bradykinesia, and rigidity, which is more severe in the axial structures than the limbs. The hallmark feature of PSP is supranuclear gaze paresis, which initially affects vertical eye movements, leading to impairment of downward gaze. Horizontal eye movements are eventually affected as well. Because of these difficulties with downward gaze, patients suffering from this illness often develop sloppiness in dress, urinating, and eating. Cognitive impairment often occurs as the illness progresses.

LBD is marked by parkinsonism, fluctuating cognitive function, and visual hallucinations. Patients with LBD will have marked visuospatial impairment and psychotic features in the setting of a relatively preserved memory initially. It can be distinguished from PD early on by the presence of cognitive dysfunction and hallucinations while the patient still has mild parkinsonism.

Other illnesses sometimes confused with PD include depression, normal pressure hydrocephalus (NPH), and essential tremor. Depression, with its associated flat affect, poorly modulated voice, and psychomotor retarda-

tion can sometimes be mistaken for parkinsonism. Indeed, the 2 illnesses may sometimes coexist, making the distinction particularly difficult. A trial of antidepressant therapy may be helpful in making the distinction. NPH is marked by the triad of urinary incontinence, gait impairment, and cognitive impairment. Symmetric bradykinesia and bradyphrenia may also be present. The gait impairment of NPH is often called a "magnetic gait," in which the patient's feet seem to cling to the floor while walking. This can be distinguished from the parkinsonian gait, which is more shuffling or festinating.

Complications

Complications in PD develop from both progression of the disease itself and medication therapy. Potential complications related to disease progression include dysphagia, defecation dysfunction, respiratory dysfunction, gait impairment, postural hypotension, sexual dysfunction, bladder dysfunction, dementia, and depression. Potential complications related to medications include drug-induced dyskinesias, hallucinations, and delirium.

Treatment

A. NONPHARMACOLOGICAL THERAPY

Patient education, addressing the support needs of the patient and caregiver, exercise, and nutrition are the most important nonpharmacological therapies (see Figure 13–1 for management algorithm). Patients and families should understand the natural history of the disease and be educated on the availability of community resources. Although exercise has not been found to diminish the cardinal symptoms of the disease, it does help to reduce the negative effects of these symptoms on mobility and functional status. Exercise has been found to improve mood, strength, flexibility, and mobility. A good program will have a blend of aerobic, strengthening, and stretching exercises and emphasizes building the extensor muscles to counteract the flexor posture that develops.

Most patients will experience constipation. Emphasizing a high-fiber diet and sufficient fluid intake will help to diminish its severity. Maintaining bone health with calcium and vitamin D supplementation is crucial in this population, which is prone to falls as a result of gait abnormalities and postural instability. In later stages of the illness and with more complicated medication regimens, some protein restriction may be necessary to reduce amino acid competition with levodopa for absorption. A consultation with a nutritionist can be helpful in addressing these issues.

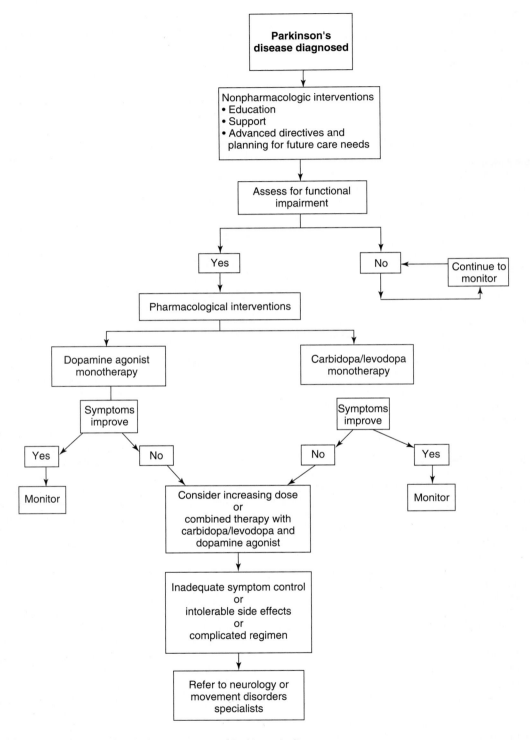

Figure 13-1. Algorithm for the management of Parkinson's disease.

B. Pharmacotherapy

Parkinson's disease is a treatable but incurable illness. Goals of pharmacotherapy are to reduce symptoms and manifestations of the illness by replacing or compensating for lost dopaminergic neuron activity. For specific dosing recommendations for each regimen, see Table 13–5.

Because none of the available medications have been shown to delay disease progression, the decision to initiate treatment is based on the severity of symptoms and the presence of functional impairment. In the case of mild disease without functional impairment, it is reasonable to delay therapy until symptomatic relief is needed. If, however, a patient is threatened with loss of employment, decrease in functional status, loss of independence, or social impairment because of symptoms, it is prudent to initiate pharmacotherapy.

1. Levodopa—Levodopa is the most effective drug in the treatment of PD. By providing dopamine replacement, levodopa ameliorates all of the major motor symptoms of Parkinson's disease, including tremor, bradykinesia, and rigidity. In so doing, it reduces morbidity and disability, and it is effective in most patients with PD. It does not, however, stop progression of the disorder. Later features of the disease are not responsive to levodopa, namely postural instability, autonomic dysfunction, freezing, speech difficulties, psychiatric problems, and dementia.

Although levodopa is clearly the most effective therapy for PD, it is associated with the eventual development of adverse symptoms in the majority of patients. As many as 50–90% of patients will experience motor complications associated with levodopa therapy after 5–10 years of treatment. These motor complications include dyskinesias and motor fluctuations. The dyskinesias may take many forms but generally manifest as abnormal twisting, turning, and jerking movements. Motor fluctuations include the "wearing-off effect" and the "on–off effect." In the wearing-off effect, the response to individual levodopa doses becomes progressively shorter, requiring increasing frequency of the dosing regimen. The on–off effect is usually a late-stage event and involves the sudden and unpredictable shift between "on" periods of mobility and "off" periods of immobility that do not seem to be related to the timing of medication therapy. The use of a long-acting carbidopa-levodopa formulation (Sinemet CR) has not been found to reduce dyskinesias compared with Sinemet. The neuropsychiatric complications of Parkinson's disease, such as psychosis, dementia, and confusion, can also be exacerbated by levodopa therapy. In addition to the adverse side effects that develop with long-term levodopa therapy, there is some concern, based on animal data, that levodopa may be neurotoxic. However, data with humans are lacking. Given its efficacy in treating the symptoms of parkinsonism, it is not reasonable to withhold levodopa based on this potential concern.

Levodopa is generally administered in combination with the dopamine decarboxylase inhibitor, carbidopa, in the form of Sinemet. Carbidopa prevents the peripheral conversion of levodopa to dopamine, which can result in nausea, vomiting, hypotension, and, rarely, cardiac irregularities. It takes approximately 75–150 mg of carbidopa per day to adequately inhibit peripheral decarboxylase activity. Thus, when lower doses of Sinemet are being given, additional carbidopa is sometimes needed to avoid peripheral side effects. Levodopa therapy should be started slowly and gradually increased to the lowest dose that provides a satisfactory clinical response. Levodopa should be taken on an empty stomach. Patients who experience nausea when taking levodopa on an empty stomach can take it with soda crackers or a similar simple carbohydrate to help diminish nausea without interfering with absorption.

The long-acting carbidopa-levodopa preparation Sinemet CR may be easier for some patients to take because less frequent dosing is required. Its bioavailability is approximately 70% of that of the regular preparation, so a higher dose is needed to achieve the same effect. The onset of action of Sinemet CR is slower, so a small amount of the immediate-release form can be coadministered if necessary.

2. Dopamine agonists—Dopamine agonists directly stimulate dopamine receptors. Two of the older agents, bromocriptine and pergolide, are ergot derivatives. The newer agents, ropinirole and pramipexole, are both nonergot dopamine agonists. They have been more extensively studied and are more currently commonly used. Dopamine agonists are approved for use as monotherapy in Parkinson's disease, although they are more commonly used as adjunctive therapy to levodopa. As monotherapy, these agents improve many of the motor symptoms of PD and reduce disability. As adjunctive therapy, dopamine agonists decrease motor fluctuations and dyskinesias by allowing for Sinemet dose reduction. When used as initial therapy for PD, the newer dopamine agonists have been found to be similar in effectiveness to levodopa for symptom control and disability reduction. In addition, the dopamine agonists have been associated with fewer motor complications than levodopa alone at 2–5 years. Dopamine agonists are considered a first-line therapy in the treatment of PD, especially in younger patients, who will likely experience motor complications from levodopa therapy during the course of their treatment. However, adverse effects appear to be more common with dopamine agonists than with carbidopa-levodopa.

Table 13–5. Pharmacological treatment of Parkinson's disease.

Medication	Recommended starting dosage	Usual dosage	Cost/mo	Comments
Carbidopa/levodopa				
Sinemet	25-mg/100-mg tablet qod. Gradually increase to the lowest dose that provides satisfactory benefit.	200–400 mg levodopa qd, divided into tid dosing	$$	Once > 600 mg levodopa per day is required, consider adding a second agent rather than further escalating the dose. Take on an empty stomach if possible. If nausea develops, take with soda crackers or other simple carbohydrate.
Sinemet CR	50 mg/200 mg bid	Titrate to effect	$$$	Sinemet CR has only 70% of the bioavailability of the shorter acting agent, so higher doses may be required.
Dopamine agonists				
Pramipexole	0.125 mg tid	0.5–1.5 mg tid	$$$	Double dose weekly during the second and third weeks of therapy. After the third week, dose can be increased at a weekly interval by 0.75 mg/day, depending on response and tolerance.
Ropinirole	0.25 mg tid	2–8 mg tid	$$–$$$	Increase daily dose by 0.75 mg each week until adequate dose response.
Amantadine	100 mg qod × 1 week	100 mg bid-tid	$	Modest therapeutic benefit and numerous side effects.
Anticholinergics				
Benztropine	0.5 mg bid	0.5–2.0 mg bid	$	Modest therapeutic benefit and numerous side effects.
Trihexyphenidyl	0.5–1.0 mg bid	2 mg tid	$	
COMT inhibitors				
Entacapone	200 mg administered with each levodopa dose	Max dose 1600 mg/day	$$–$$$	Reducing levodopa by approximately 30% after initiating COMT inhibitors can help reduce dopaminergic side effects.
Tolcapone	100 mg tid	200 mg tid	$$$	
Selegiline	5 mg qod	5 mg with breakfast and 5 mg with lunch	$	No neuroprotective effect demonstrated. Modest therapeutic benefit and numerous side effects.

$ = ≤ $30; $$ = $30–$100; $$$ = > $100. COMT, catecholamine-O-methytransferase.

Adverse effects of dopamine agonists include nausea, vomiting, orthostatic hypotension, flushing, sweating, somnolence, dizziness, and psychiatric symptoms. Psychiatric symptoms, including psychosis, may be more common in older patients. Most adverse effects occur with the initiation of the medication and will dissipate over days to weeks as tolerance develops. Starting at low doses and titrating up slowly reduces the severity of adverse effects. The ergot-derived dopamine agonists bromocriptine and pergolide are associated uncommonly with erythromelalgia, pulmonary or retroperitoneal fibrosis, and Raynaud's phenomenon.

3. Initiating pharmacotherapy with dopamine agonist and/or levodopa—Many physicians advocate initiating treatment with a dopamine agonist as a first-line agent and supplementing a dopamine with levodopa as needed. Others advocate starting with levodopa and supplementing with a dopamine agonist after a dose of 600 mg or more of levodopa is required. It seems reasonable to start pharmacotherapy with a dopamine agonist in patients with a longer life expectancy because they are at a higher risk for experiencing dyskinesias during the course of their illness. Dopamine agonist therapy can then be supplemented with levodopa to achieve the desired symptomatic benefit. On the other hand, levodopa may be the preferred agent in physiologically older patients, who have a lower risk of experiencing levodopa-related motor complications and who are at higher risk for dopamine agonist-induced psychiatric symptoms. Patients of any age with cognitive impairment are likely to tolerate levodopa better than a dopamine agonist.

When symptoms progress on monotherapy with either levodopa or a dopamine agonist, most neurologists advocate combining lower doses of the 2 agents rather than increasing a single agent to its maximal dose. This approach is thought to reduce the incidence and severity of medication side effects. Referral to a neurologist should be considered when symptoms cannot be adequately controlled using 2 agents.

4. Other agents—Other medications used in the treatment of PD include selegiline, amantadine, anticholinergic agents, and catecholamine-O-methyltransferase inhibitors (COMT inhibitors). Selegiline, amantadine, and the anticholinergic agents provide only a modest therapeutic benefit and are associated with numerous side effects, especially in the elderly population. These agents should generally be used in consultation with a neurologist.

COMT inhibitors, on the other hand, can be quite useful as adjunctive therapies in the treatment of PD. They increase the bioavailability of levodopa, thereby prolonging its duration of action. The result is often more stable symptom control. Unfortunately, COMT

inhibitors can worsen the dopaminergic side effects of levodopa, including dyskinesias and neuropsychiatric problems. To help diminish this side effect, the levodopa dose should be reduced by approximately 30% when initiating COMT inhibitors. Patients who require COMT inhibitors usually have advanced disease; therefore, it is prudent to consult a neurologist before initiating these agents.

D. Surgical Therapies

In many patients, medications become progressively less effective in relieving parkinsonian symptoms while medication side effects become more severe. Some of these patients may benefit from interventional therapies. The ideal candidate for an interventional procedure is a patient with progressive motor symptoms who still has a response to dopaminergic medications, has progressive dopaminergic side effects, and has normal cognition.

1. Pallidotomy—Pallidotomy is the surgical destruction of the globus pallidus. Pallidotomy relieves contralateral drug-induced dyskinesias in up to 90% of patients and decreases off-state symptoms in approximately 30% of patients. Pallidotomy is associated with a 10–15% incidence of persistent adverse outcomes, including intracerebral hematoma, visual changes, and cognitive decline.

2. Deep brain stimulation—Deep brain stimulation (DBS) is nondestructive and reversible. In DBS, a 4-contact lead is placed into the brain and connected to a programmable generator that is implanted in the chest, similar to a cardiac pacemaker. The frequency and amplitude of stimulation are adjusted to deliver maximum symptomatic benefit.

DBS of the globus pallidus appears to improve all motor aspects of PD, including bradykinesia, speech, gait, rigidity, dyskinesia, and tremor. DBS of the subthalamic nucleus also seems to improve virtually all of the motor symptoms of PD, decreasing dyskinesias, and even reducing medication requirements.

Complications with DBS are less common than with ablative procedures and include infections, bleeding, and stimulation of neighboring structures in the brain. Infections and bleeding are rare, occurring in < 10% of patients, and they usually do not result in serious permanent problems. Readjusting the stimulation parameters alleviates side effects resulting from stimulation of neighboring brain structures.

E. Treatment of Complications

1. Dyskinesias—Dyskinesias are a motor complication of dopaminergic therapy and can manifest as dystonia or choreiform movements. When severe, dyskinesias can be more disabling than the features of PD itself.

Dyskinesias often correspond in time with the peak blood level of levodopa. In such cases, a slight reduction in the levodopa dosage should be attempted. If a patient is on the sustained-release formulation of levodopa, changing to the short-acting formulation may allow for more predictable control over these symptoms. Adding a dopamine agonist to levodopa therapy to smooth out stimulation of dopamine receptors while simultaneously reducing the levodopa dose may also provide some relief. If the patient does not respond to the conservative measure listed previously or if the dyskinesias do not correspond to the peak dose of levodopa, referral to a neurologist is advisable.

2. Dementia—Dementia may occur in up to 30% of patients, depending on age, disease duration, and illness severity. It is usually a late development in PD and increases the likelihood of nursing home placement. If dementia is an early feature of the illness, another parkinsonian syndrome, such as LBD, should be suspected. Patients with cognitive impairment or dementia are at increased risk for delirium and psychosis and may tolerate antiparkinsonian medications poorly. Sedatives, anticholinergic medications, and amantadine should be avoided. In patients with cognitive impairment and parkinsonism, medications need to be prescribed with great care, balancing improvement of motor symptoms against adverse neuropsychiatric effects.

3. Delirium, hallucinations, & psychosis—Hallucinations are common in patients with PD. These occur both as a result of the disease itself and secondary to dopaminergic therapy. It is estimated that up to 20% of PD patients treated with dopaminergic drugs develop drug-induced hallucinations. These hallucinations are usually visual and are often not disturbing to the patient. If they are not disturbing the patient or causing behavioral problems, no specific change in pharmacotherapy is warranted. However, reassurance and education should be given to patients and their families. If the hallucinations begin to cause the patient distress, become frightening, or cause behavioral problems, dose reductions in dopaminergic medications should be attempted. If unsuccessful, antipsychotic medications may be beneficial. Typical antipsychotics, like haloperidol, should be avoided because they are likely to worsen parkinsonism. Atypical antipsychotics, however, are effective and are less likely to aggravate parkinsonism. Clozapine and quetiapine appear to be the most beneficial of the atypical antipsychotic medications in this situation. The main side effect of concern in clozapine is rare, but life-threatening, agranulocytosis (1–2%). Weekly blood count monitoring is, therefore, required in patients taking clozapine. Clozapine should be started at a low dose and titrated slowly to effect. The other atypical antipsychotics, risperidone and olanzapine, are effective against psychosis but do occasionally worsen parkinsonism.

If delirium develops, medical problems such as infection or metabolic abnormalities should be sought and treated. Unnecessary medications, including sedatives, anxiolytics, and anticholinergics, should be stopped when possible. If delirium persists, the dose of levodopa or dopamine agonists, or both, should be reduced as tolerated. Ultimately, a choice may need to be made between optimal control of parkinsonian symptoms and delirium. Sometimes, a low-dose atypical antipsychotic can be helpful in controlling delirium, but careful monitoring for worsening parkinsonism is required.

4. Depression—Depression is common in PD, occurring in up to 40% of patients at some point during their illness. Parkinsonian features such as bradykinesia, bradyphrenia, and masked facies can make it difficult to distinguish between depression and parkinsonism. PD patients with depression should be treated with antidepressant therapy and psychotherapy when appropriate. Selective serotonin reuptake inhibitors (SSRIs) are recommended as first-line therapies because they avoid the anticholinergic effects of the tricyclic antidepressants. Of the SSRIs, citalopram is associated with the fewest drug interactions. Coadministration of SSRIs with selegiline should be avoided because of the theoretical risk of inducing the serotonin syndrome.

5. Orthostatic hypotension—Orthostatic hypotension is common in late-stage PD and is thought to result from decreased intravascular volume. Medications that contribute to orthostatic hypotension, including antihypertensives and diuretics, should be reduced in dosage or discontinued. Levodopa and dopamine agonists can exacerbate postural hypotension; thus dose reduction, if feasible, may be of benefit. Sodium intake should be increased. The head of the bed should be elevated to approximately 35°. Eating small, frequent meals can help avoid exacerbation of symptoms mediated by splanchnic vasodilatation. Caffeine in the morning may be beneficial. Waist-high stockings might also provide some symptomatic relief but can be difficult for patients to tolerate. Hot weather, hot liquids, and hot showers should be avoided.

Pharmacotherapy is appropriate for symptomatic patients only when nonpharmacological interventions have not proven useful. Fludrocortisone, a mineralocorticoid, and midodrine, an α_1-agonist, are sometimes used, but both should be used with caution in medically complicated patients. Both can have adverse cardiovascular effects, and midodrine may cause urinary retention in men with benign prostatic hypertrophy.

6. Falls—Falls are of multifactorial etiology in patients with PD and are related to postural instability, impaired balance, muscle weakness, freezing, festinating gait, and orthostatic hypotension among other causes. Falls in any patient may have multiple causes, so taking a careful history is important. Postural instability may be improved with dopaminergic therapy early on, but in later stages it tends to respond less well. People who fall from freezing tend to fall forward onto their hands and knees, so wrist and knee guards may help prevent injury. Gait training and strength exercises, supervised by a physical therapist, may be the most useful fall prevention interventions available regardless of the specific cause. In addition, most patients with PD who fall will benefit from ambulatory assist devices such as front-wheeled walkers. Front-wheeled walkers are more useful than canes or walkers without wheels because patients with PD have difficulty initiating movement, which makes repeatedly lifting the assist device with each step burdensome. Moreover, providing education to patients and caregivers about the removal of throw rugs, extension cords, and other obstacles in the home may reduce the risk of falls. A home safety evaluation can be helpful in identifying factors in the home that may place a patient at increased risk for falling.

7. Gastrointestinal complications—Dysphagia, disordered salivation, constipation, and defecatory dysfunction occur much more commonly in patients with PD than in age-matched controls. The presence of these complications corresponds with the severity and duration of the disease but not with age, gender, antiparkinson therapy, activity, or diet.

Dysphagia affects more than half of patients with parkinsonism. It primarily affects the oropharyngeal phase of swallowing, although esophageal transport may be involved as well. Oropharyngeal dysphagia is a result of the effects of PD on the skeletal muscles of the oropharynx, leading to impaired pharyngeal bolus transport. Drooling occurs as a result of the inability to transfer saliva to the pharynx. Dysphagia is associated with respiratory symptoms, including coughing, choking, nocturnal dyspnea, and aspiration.

Constipation and difficult defecation affect 30–60% of patients. Constipation is the result of slowed colonic transport and can, in severe cases, lead to megacolon or volvulus. Defecatory dysfunction seems to be a result of the effects of PD on the skeletal muscles of the rectum and pelvic floor, leading to a "paradoxical" rectosphincteric reflex, in which the internal anal sphincter responds to rectal fullness with hypercontractility instead of relaxation.

a. Dysphagia—The dysphagia of parkinsonism does not respond to dopaminergic therapy or to standard promotility agents, such as metoclopramide. Consequently, treatment of dysphagia focuses on efforts to avoid aspiration. Speech therapy is invaluable in identifying the presence of moderate to severe dysphagia and in teaching maneuvers to assist in bolus transfer. When patients progress to a point at which they are unable to reliably take in proper nutrition or medications, enteral feeding may be considered if the patient so desires.

b. Constipation & defecatory dysfunction—Like dysphagia, constipation and defecatory dysfunction do not respond to dopaminergic therapies. Stool softeners, prokinetic agents, laxatives, fiber, and fluids are first-line agents, just as they are in patients without PD. Prokinetics may be particularly helpful in counteracting slowed colonic transport in parkinsonism, but this has not been well studied.

Anticholinergic medications should be discontinued whenever possible once constipation develops. In severe defecatory dysfunction, enemas and manual disimpaction may be necessary. It is important to make sure that these patients move their bowels regularly (at least once every 3 days) to avoid impaction and megacolon.

F. Referral Guidelines

In general, one should consider referring patients to a neurologist or movement disorders specialist in the following circumstances: (1) when the diagnosis of Parkinson's disease is in question; (2) when a patient is not responding to standard therapies or has unacceptable side effects; (3) when complications of PD and its treatments, such as dyskinesias and hallucinations, are a prominent feature of the disease; and (4) when surgical interventions are being considered.

G. Advance Planning

Advanced planning for long-term care needs can often give patients and their families a sense of control over their fate. An early referral to attorneys or estate planners who specialize in elder law and who are skilled in the financial and legal issues of chronic illness and disability can be crucial in relieving some of the anxieties brought on by progressive disability. It is also important to establish a power of attorney for health care and finances early on, while the patient is still able to discuss concerns and desires. Organizations such as the Caregiver Alliance can be helpful with these issues.

Hallett M et al: Evaluation of surgery for Parkinson's disease: A report of the Therapeutics and Technology Assessment Subcommittee of the American Academy of Neurology. Neurology 1999;53:1910. [PMID: 10599758]

Koller WC et al: Immediate-release and controlled-release carbidopa/levodopa in PD. Neurology 1999;53:1012. [PMID: 10496260]

Kubu CS et al: Cognitive outcome following pallidotomy: The influence of side of surgery and age of patient at disease onset. J Neurosurg 2000;92:384. [PMID: 10701523]

Olanow CW, Koller WC: An algorithm (decision tree) for the management of Parkinson's disease. Neurology 1998;50 (suppl 3):S1. [PMID: 9524552]

Parkinson Study Group: Low-dose clozapine for the treatment of drug-induced psychosis in Parkinson's disease. N Engl J Med 1999;340:757. [PMID: 10072410]

Parkinson Study Group: Pramipexole vs levodopa as initial treatment for Parkinson disease. JAMA 2000;284:1931. [PMID: 11035889]

Rascol O et al: A five-year study of the incidence of dyskinesia in patients with early Parkinson's disease who were treated with ropinirole or levodopa. N Engl J Med 2000;342:1484. [PMID: 10816186]

Targum SD, Abbott JL: Efficacy of quetiapine in Parkinson's patients with psychosis. J Clin Psychopharmacol 2000;20:54. [PMID: 10653209]

Prognosis

PD is associated with an increase in mortality; the relative risk of death ranges from 1.6–3 times that of the general population. The mean duration of illness from symptom onset to death is approximately 9 years, although there are occasional patients with slow progression who can live 20 years or more. Once patients reach Hoehn and Yahr's stage V of PD and are bed or wheelchair bound, the mean life expectancy is 9–12 months. Pneumonia is the most common cause of death in patients with PD, followed by cardiovascular disease.

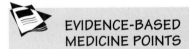

EVIDENCE-BASED MEDICINE POINTS

- *Long-acting carbidopa-levodopa has not been found to reduce dyskinesias compared with short-acting carbidopa-levodopa.*
- *When used as initial therapy for PD, the newer dopamine agonists have been found to be similar in effectiveness to levodopa for symptom control and disability reduction. In addition, the dopamine agonists have been associated with fewer motor complications than levodopa alone at 2–5 years.*
- *Low-dose clozapine has been found to be more effective than placebo against drug-induced psychosis and has not been found to worsen parkinsonism. It also had a positive effect on tremor.*

RELEVANT WORLD WIDE WEB SITES

American Parkinson Disease Association, Inc.: www.apdaparkinson.com (Provides information on educational programs, support groups, treatment options, and publications)

Family Caregiver Alliance: www.caregiver.org (Provides information on support groups, hiring caregivers, and issues of long-term care.)

National Parkinson Foundation, Inc.: www.parkinson.org (Provides information on educational programs, support groups, treatment options, and publications)

ESSENTIAL TREMOR

ESSENTIALS OF DIAGNOSIS

- *Characterized by a bilateral action tremor of the hands and forearms and possibly the head, voice, trunk, and legs.*
- *Other neurological signs are absent.*
- *Positive family history.*
- *Beneficial response to alcohol.*

General Considerations

Essential tremor (ET) is a common movement disorder with an estimated prevalence of 0.4–6%. It occurs most commonly in people older than 65. Approximately 30–50% of cases are familial with an autosomal dominant inheritance pattern. It is a progressive condition.

Differential Diagnosis

ET is a 4- to 12-Hz action tremor of the hands and forearms, with its greatest amplitude distally. It can also affect the voice, trunk, and legs, and occasionally presents as an isolated head tremor. ET tends to be most obvious during sustained extension of an extremity or during voluntary movements such as drinking or writing. It can be distinguished from an intention tremor, which is coarser and occurs as a limb approaches a target, such as in the finger-nose-finger maneuver. ET often improves with alcohol intake and is not associated with other neurological symptoms or signs.

The diagnosis of ET is made by history and physical examination. Particular emphasis is placed on an assessment of neurological symptoms and on the neurological examination. Other conditions that may be associated with tremor, including Parkinson's disease, dystonia, and Wilson's disease, should be considered. Furthermore, tobacco and caffeine use, as well as certain medications (see Table 13–1), may result in an enhanced physiological tremor that can mimic ET.

ET is usually slightly asymmetric. Having a patient bring a cup of water from an outstretched arm to the mouth to drink will demonstrate worsening of the tremor in most cases. In contrast, enhanced physiological tremor is symmetric and should not be worsened by a voluntary task. The tremor of PD is usually a resting tremor, and the neurological exam will often show other signs of parkinsonism in addition to the tremor. Action tremors are also found in dystonia and Wilson's disease, but these conditions generally are associated with other neurological abnormalities and occur in a younger population.

Complications

ET can result in significant functional impairment and social embarrassment. The tremor can render patients unable to feed themselves, drink without spilling, apply makeup, or brush their teeth. Some patients are unable to write, type, or perform other fine motor movements. This can result in early retirement, social isolation, and enhanced care needs.

Treatment

The goal of treatment is to improve function and reduce social embarrassment associated with the tremor. If the tremor is mild, treatment may not be required.

A. PHARMACOTHERAPY

1. First-line agents—Primidone and propranolol are the most effective medications for treating ET. Primidone is an anticonvulsant medication that has been found to be 40–50% effective in reducing the tremor of ET. It is most effective in treating hand tremor and has little or no efficacy in treating head or voice tremor. It can be administered as single nighttime dose or as multiple daily doses, but the former is recommended to improve compliance. The usual therapeutic dosage ranges from 50–350 mg/day. Adverse effects occur in 20–30% of patients, including vertigo, nausea, and unsteadiness. These side effects are temporary and will abate with continued use of the drug. Chronic use is rarely associated with side effects.

Propranolol is the best studied and most effective of the β-adrenergic blocking agents in the treatment of ET. Approximately 40–50% of patient with ET treated with propranolol will experience symptomatic relief. Like primidone, it is more effective in treating hand tremor than voice or head tremor. The optimal dosage ranges from 240–320 mg/day. The sustained-release preparation is equally as effective as the short-acting preparation. Potential side effects include bradycardia, hypotension, fatigue, rash, erectile dysfunction, and diarrhea.

Primidone and propranolol are both more effective than placebo; neither have a clear advantage over the other. Primidone may be better tolerated over the long

term than propranolol, so some experts favor starting with primidone.

2. Second-line agents—Gabapentin is well tolerated and has been found to be more effective than placebo (usual therapeutic dosage: 1200–3600 mg/day). Alprazolam is the only benzodiazepine that has been found to be effective in ET, and it caused sedation in half of the patients in the doses required to improve tremor (usual therapeutic dosage: 0.75–2.5 mg/day). The risk of dependence, in addition to the sedation, makes alprazolam an undesirable chronic treatment. Calcium-channel blockers and theophylline have been used but have not been adequately studied in ET and are not recommended for routine use.

B. OTHER THERAPIES

1. Interventional therapies—ET patients with severe, disabling, medication-resistant tremor may be candidates for interventional therapies. Unilateral thalamotomy and continuous deep brain stimulation (DBS) improve contralateral tremor and disability scores in > 70% of those treated. Dysarthria, dysequilibrium, cognitive impairment, and weakness occur in < 10% of patients after thalamotomy. DBS may be associated with fewer adverse events.

2. Botulinum toxin A—Intramuscular injections of botulinum toxin A into the intrinsic muscles of the dominant hand have been found to reduce tremor amplitude but not improve function.

Gorman WP et al: A comparison of primidone, propranolol, and placebo in essential tremor, using quantitative analysis. J Neurol Neurosurg Psychiatry 1986;49:64. [PMID: 3514797]

Koller WC et al: Pharmacologic treatment of essential tremor. Neurology 2000;54(suppl 4):S30. [PMID: 10854350]

Louis ED: Essential tremor. N Engl J Med 2001;345:887. [PMID: 11565522]

Pahwa R et al: Surgical treatment of essential tremor. Neurology 2000;54(suppl 4):S39. [PMID: 10854351]

Schuurman PR et al: A comparison of continuous thalamic stimulation and thalamotomy for suppression of severe tremor. N Engl J Med 2000;342:461. [PMID: 10675426]

EVIDENCE-BASED POINTS

- *Both primidone and propranolol are more effective than placebo, but neither is conclusively better than the other.*

- *Thalamotomy and DBS are equally as effective in reducing tremor, but DBS is associated with fewer adverse events.*

Depression & Other Mental Health Issues

Mary A. Norman, MD, Mary E. Whooley, MD, & Kewchang Lee, MD

DEPRESSION

ESSENTIALS OF DIAGNOSIS

- *Depressed mood.*
- *Loss of interest or pleasure in almost all activities.*
- *Unintentional weight change, lack of energy, change in sleep pattern, psychomotor retardation or agitation, excessive guilt, or poor concentration.*
- *Suicidal ideation or recurrent thoughts of death.*
- *Somatic rather than mood complaints in the elderly.*

General Considerations

The prevalence of major depression is estimated at 1–2% for elders in the community and 10–12% for those in primary care settings. However, even in the absence of major depression as defined by *Diagnostic and Statistical Manual of Mental Disorders* (fourth edition; *DSM-IV*) criteria, up to 27% of elders experience substantial depressive symptoms that may be relieved with intervention. For institutionalized elders, the rates of major depression are much higher: 12% for hospitalized elders and 43% for permanently institutionalized elders.

Women are twice as likely to experience major depression as men. Other risk factors include prior episodes or a personal family history of depression, lack of social support, use of alcohol or other substances, and a recent loss of a loved one. Several medical conditions are also associated with an increased risk of depression, including Parkinson's disease, recent myocardial infarction, and cerebrovascular accident. These conditions share common threads of loss of control of body or mind, increasing dependence on others, and increased social isolation.

Depression is associated with poorer self-care and slower recovery after acute medical illnesses. It can accelerate cognitive and physical decline and leads to an increased use and cost of health care services. Among depressed elderly who have had a stroke, rehabilitation efforts are less effective and mortality rates are significantly higher.

Clinical Findings

A. SYMPTOMS & SIGNS

Major depression is defined as depressed mood or loss of interest in nearly all activities (or both) for at least 2 weeks, accompanied by a minimum of 3 or 4 of the following symptoms (for a total of at least 5 symptoms): insomnia or hypersomnia, feelings of worthlessness or excessive guilt, fatigue or loss of energy, diminished ability to think or concentrate, substantial change in appetite or weight, psychomotor agitation or retardation, and recurrent thoughts of death or suicide (Table 14–1). Severity of depression varies and is important in determining optimal treatment and prognosis. Patients with less severe depressive symptoms who do not meet criteria for major depression may also benefit from psychotherapy and pharmacotherapy.

B. SCREENING TOOLS

Elderly patients can have fewer mood and more somatic complaints, which are often difficult to differentiate from underlying medical conditions. Special screening tools that consider this difference have been developed for the elderly population. The Geriatric Depression Scale is widely used and validated in many different languages. Its shortened 15-item scale (Table 14–2) is often used for ease of administration. A separate 2-item scale consisting of 2 questions about depressed mood and anhedonia has also been shown effective in detecting depression in the elderly (see Table 14–2). Screening alone has not been found to benefit patients with unrecognized depression, but in combination with patient support programs, such as frequent nursing follow-up and close monitoring of adherence to medication, it improves outcomes.

Table 14–1. Diagnostic criteria for depression.

Diagnostic category	Criteria[a]	Duration
Dysthymia	3 or 4 dysthymic symptoms,[b] including depressed mood	≥ 2 year
Major depression	≥ 5 depressive symptoms,[c] including depressed mood or anhedonia	≥ 2 week
Mild	Few (if any) symptoms in excess of those required for the diagnosis; minimal impairment in functioning	
Moderate	Greater number and intensity of depressive symptoms; moderate impairment in functioning	
Severe	Marked intensity and pervasiveness of depressive symptoms; substantial impairment in functioning	

[a]From the *Diagnostic and Statistical Manual of Mental Disorders,* fourth edition.
[b]Dysthymic symptoms include depressed mood, poor appetite or overeating, sleep disturbance, lack of energy, low self-esteem, poor concentration, and hopelessness.
[c]Depressive symptoms include depressed mood, enhedonia, weight change, sleep disturbance, psychomotor problems, lack of energy, excessive guilt, poor concentration, and suicidal ideation.

Differential Diagnosis

Diagnosing depression in the elderly can be challenging because of the presence of multiple comorbid conditions. Many patients with mild cognitive impairment may have predominantly depressive symptoms. With effective treatment of depression, their cognitive performance frequently improves; however, these patients still are at high risk for progression to dementia within the next 3 years. Bereavement often manifests with depressed mood, which may be appropriate given a patient's recent loss. However, if depressive symptoms

Table 14–2. Geriatric depression scale (short form).[a]

Depression Scale

1. Are you basically satisfied with your life?		Yes/**No**
2. Have you dropped many of your activities and interests?		**Yes**/No
3. Do you feel that your life is empty?		**Yes**/No
4. Do you often get bored?		**Yes**/No
5. Are you in good spirits most of the time?		Yes/**No**
6. Are you afraid that something bad is going to happen to you?		**Yes**/No
7. Do you feel happy most of the time?		Yes/**No**
8. Do you often feel helpless?		**Yes**/No
9. Do you prefer to stay at home rather than going out and doing new things?		**Yes**/No
10. Do you feel that you have more problems with memory than most?		**Yes**/No
11. Do you think it is wonderful to be alive now?		Yes/**No**
12. Do you feel pretty worthless the way you are now?		**Yes**/No
13. Do you feel full of energy?		Yes/**No**
14. Do you feel that your situation is hopeless?		**Yes**/No
15. Do you think that most people are better off than you are?		**Yes**/No
	SCORE:	_____

Directions: Score 1 point for each bolded answer. A score of 5 or more is a positive screen for depression.

Two-Question Case-Finding Instrument[b]

1. During the past month, have you often been bothered by feeling down, depressed, or hopeless?	**Yes**/No
2. During the past month, have you often been bothered by having little interest or pleasure in doing things?	**Yes**/No

Directions: Yes to either question is a positive screen for depression.

[a]From Sheikh, JI, Yesavage JA: Geriatric depression scale (GDS): Recent evidence and development of a shorter version. Clinical Gerontology 1986;5:165. Used with permission.
[b]From Whooley MA et al: Case-finding instrument for depression: Two questions are as good as many. J Gen Intern Med 1997;12:439. Used with permission.

persist longer than 2–3 months, a diagnosis of major depression should be considered.

Elderly patients who experience delirium caused by an underlying medical illness may have mood changes. Other comorbid psychiatric illnesses must also be considered, such as anxiety disorder, substance abuse disorder, or personality disorders. Patients with bipolar disorder or psychotic disorders may have depressed mood; thus, it is important to ask patients about prior manic episodes, hallucinations, or delusions.

Depression can also be confused with other medical conditions. Fatigue and weight loss, for example, may be associated with diabetes mellitus, thyroid disease, underlying malignancy, or anemia. Patients who have Parkinson's disease may first present with depressed mood or flat affect. Sleep disturbances as a result of pain, nocturia, or sleep apnea may also lead to daytime fatigue and depressed mood.

A complete history and physical examination, including assessment of cognitive status, is critical in the evaluation of depression in the elderly. Because depression is a clinical diagnosis, no routine laboratory tests are indicated. Testing may be tailored to each patient based on their underlying comorbidities and presenting symptoms. A complete review of medications, both prescription and over the counter, is essential. Medications such as benzodiazepines, narcotics, glucocorticoids, interferon, and reserpine may cause depressive symptoms. Contrary to earlier beliefs, β-blockers have not been proven to cause depression. Screening for alcohol and other substance use or addiction is another important part of the medical history. Substance use can interfere with compliance and contribute to high relapse rates, although active substance abuse should not preclude treatment for depression. For patients who struggle with addiction, "dual diagnosis" programs (alcohol or other substance dependence and psychiatric disorder) may be optimal.

Treatment

A. PATIENT & FAMILY EDUCATION/SUPPORTIVE CARE

Educating patients and families about depression is the cornerstone of successful treatment. Depression continues to carry a stigma in many communities and cultures. Appropriate education can help patients understand that their condition results from a combination of inherited factors and personal and environmental stressors. Providers should also emphasize that physical symptoms and sleep disturbances are characteristic of depression; thus, relief of depression should make other physical symptoms more bearable. Encouraging physical activity with a family member or friend can be a simple, effective step toward improving social support and overall well-being.

Involving families in the care of elderly patients is crucial for both diagnosing depression and developing an effective treatment plan. Caregivers of elderly patients, especially if impaired physically or cognitively, may be experiencing considerable stress and depression as well. Many programs are available that may alleviate stress and promote positive social interactions for patients. Adult day programs, senior centers, and senior support groups can be helpful resources for patients and their families, and geriatric social workers can assist with finding appropriate programs for each patient. Caregiver support groups and formal respite programs are also available in most communities.

B. PHARMACOTHERAPY

1. Antidepressants—

a. **Selection**—Overall, antidepressants, including tricyclic antidepressants (TCAs), selective serotonin reuptake inhibitors (SSRIs), and newer agents, are equally effective in the treatment of geriatric depression (Table 14–3). However, because of side effect profiles and propensity for drug interactions, monoamine oxidase inhibitors (eg, phenelzine and tranylcypromine) and tertiary amine TCAs (eg, amitriptyline, imipramine, and doxepin) are rarely used in the elderly. Likewise, fluoxetine is generally avoided in the elderly because of its long half-life and inhibition of the P450 system. Choice of therapy among the remaining drugs is generally determined by side effect profile and the patient's comorbid symptoms such as anxiety, insomnia, pain, and weight loss, although anxiety and insomnia do not necessarily predict a better response to more sedating medications. Renal and hepatic functions are also important considerations in the elderly and should be assessed before initiation of therapy.

SSRIs are safe in overdose and have no known adverse cardiac effects. Thus, they are a reasonable first choice in treating elderly patients with depression. Other agents also offer unique advantages: Mirtazapine stimulates appetite and can help with insomnia, and bupropion can reduce craving in smoking cessation. Secondary amine TCAs (eg, nortriptyline, desipramine) can offer beneficial effects for patients with neuropathic pain, detrusor instability, or insomnia. Venlafaxine, which has serotonergic and noradrenergic activity, is another effective alternative that is also useful in treating anxiety and neuropathic pain.

b. **Dosage**—In general, elderly patients should begin an antidepressant by taking half of the manufacturer-recommended starting dose (to minimize side effects), but the medication should be titrated to the recommended target dose in weekly increments (see Table 14–3). Elderly patients are frequently undertreated because the provider fails to adequately titrate the dose to a therapeu-

Table 14–3. Selected antidepressants for use in elderly patients.[a]

Generic name	Trade name	Initial dose	Target dose[b]	Cost per month[c]	Other indications
Serotonin-norepinephrine reuptake inhibitors:					
Citalopram	Celexa	10 mg qd	20–40 mg qd	$$	OCD; diabetic neuropathy; poststroke depression[d]; panic disorder
Escitalopram	Lexapro	5–10 mg QD	10–20 mg QD	$$	
Fluoxetine	Prozac	10 mg qAM	20–40 mg qAM	$$	Bulimia; OCS[d]
Paroxetine	Paxil	10 mg qd or qhs	10–40 mg qd/qhs	$$	OCD[d]; panic disorders,[d] migraine, social phobias[d] PTSD, premature, ejaculation
Sertraline	Zoloft	25 mg qAM	50–200 mg qAM	$$$	OCD; panic disorders[d], PTSD[d]; premature ejaculation
Secondary amines:					
Tricyclic:					
Desipramine	Norpramin	10 mg qd or qhs	20–150 mg qd/qhs	$	Attention deficit disorder (ADD),[d] bulimia neuropathic pain; postherpetic neuralgia; panic disorder; PTSD
Nortriptyline	Aventyl, Pamelor	10 mg qhs	20–100 mg qhs	$	ADD; chronic low back pain; irritable bowel syndrome; neuropathic pain; panic disorder
Bicyclic:					
Venlafaxine	Effexor	12.5 mg bid	75 mg bid	$$$	Generalized anxiety disorder (XR formulation only)[d]; neuropathic pain; OCD
	Effexor XR	37.5 mg qd	75–150 mg qd	$$	
Serotonin antagonist:					
mirtazapine	Remeron	7.5 mg qhs	15–45 mg qhs	$$$	Anxiety; insomnia; weight loss
Norepinephrine-dopamine reuptake inhibitor:					
bupropion	Wellbutrin	75 mg bid	100 mg tid	$$$	ADD; anorgasmia; smoking cessation (SR form only)[d]
	Wellbutrin SR	75 mg qAM	150 mg bid	$$$	
Serotonin antagonist and reuptake inhibitor:					
Nefazodone	Serzone	50 mg bid	150 mg bid	$$	Panic disorder; PTSD
Trazodone[e]	Desyrel	25–50 mg qhs	50–200 mg qhs	$	Insomnia
Psychostimulants:					
Methylphenidate	Ritalin	2.5–5 mg at 7 AM and noon	5–10 mg at 7 AM and noon	$	ADD[d]
Dextroamphetamine	Dexedrine	2.5–5 mg qAM	2.5–5 mg at 7 AM and noon	$	ADD[d]

[a]The information provided is intended only as a guide for the treatment of depression in medical outpatients. Providers should refer to the package inserts or consult with a pharmacist for individual dosing recommendations, precautions, and drug interactions.
[b]The target dose is the dose likely to be effective for a typical geriatric patient.
[c]Average wholesale price range in U.S. dollars for a 30-day supply of usual target dose. $, $30–$50; $$, $51–$80; $$$, ≥ $80.
[d]Approved by the U.S. Food and Drug Administration for this indication.
[e]Trazodone is too sedating at therapeutic doses for depression; it is best used in lower doses (50–100 mg) as an adjunctive therapy for patients with insomnia.
Adapted from Whooley MA, Simon GE: Managing depression in medical outpatients. N Engl J Med 2000;343:1942. Used with permission.

tic level. If minimal or no benefit occurs by 4–6 weeks and side effects are tolerable, the dose should be increased. The full effect may not be seen for 8–12 weeks in elderly patients. If a therapeutic dose has been reached and maintained for 6 weeks and the patient has not adequately responded, one should consider switching to a different agent or augmenting with an additional agent. Although serum drug levels are not useful for SSRIs, levels of TCAs can be measured to assess adherence.

c. Side effects—Side effects differ depending on the type of antidepressant (Table 14–4). Most side effects lessen within 1–4 weeks from the start of therapy, but weight gain and sexual dysfunction may last longer. For the SSRIs, the most common side effects include nausea and sexual dysfunction. Sexual dysfunction may respond to treatment with sildenafil (Viagra), but switching antidepressant mediation or lowering the dose of SSRI and augmenting with an additional agent may be necessary. The TCAs have more anticholinergic properties and may lead to dry mouth, orthostasis, and urinary retention.

d. Cautions & interactions—

(1) Cardiovascular disease—TCAs can be associated with orthostatic hypotension and cardiac conduction abnormalities, leading to arrhythmias. Before initiation of therapy, providers should obtain an electrocardiogram and proceed with caution if conduction delays such as first-degree atrioventricular block or bundle branch block are present.

(2) Hypertension—Venlafaxine may increase diastolic blood pressure.

(3) Hepatic disease—Most antidepressants are hepatically cleared and should be used with caution in patients with liver disease. Nefazodone in particular should not be used in patients with liver disease or elevated transaminases because it has been associated with an increased risk of hepatic failure and interacts with other hepatically cleared medications, including simvastatin and lovastatin.

(4) Cognitive impairment—TCAs and certain SSRIs such as paroxetine have stronger anticholinergic effects and should be avoided in patients with cognitive impairment to avoid increasing confusion.

(5) Seizure disorders—Bupropion lowers seizure thresholds.

(6) Suicidal ideation—TCAs are lethal in overdose and should be avoided in actively suicidal patients. SSRIs are relatively safe in overdose.

2. Psychostimulants—Psychostimulants such as dextroamphetamine (5–10 mg/day) or methylphenidate (2.5–5 mg/day) are sometimes indicated as either a primary or an adjuvant treatment for depression with predominant vegetative symptoms. At the end of life, patients may not have time to wait 4–6 weeks for the benefits of antidepressant medication, and psychostimulants can be effective within hours. In the setting of depression after an acute medical illness, psychostimulants offer a fast means to enhance recovery and participation in rehabilitation. Typical side effects include insomnia and agitation, but these may be lessened by taking the medication early in the day in divided doses (morning and noon). Another common side effect is tachycardia.

3. Herbal remedies—Many herbal remedies claim to be effective in treating depression, but further evidence is still needed to determine whether these "dietary supplements" (eg, *Hypericum perforatum* [St. John's wort]) have a role in the treatment of depression. *H perforatum* should not be used in conjunction with SSRIs because the combination may lead to serotonergic syndrome, which is characterized by changes in mental status, tremor, gastrointestinal upset, headache, myalgia, and restlessness. It may lower the concentration of certain drugs, such as warfarin, digoxin, theophylline, cyclosporine, and HIV-1 protease inhibitors. Other common herbal remedies such as kavakava and valerian root have not been proven effective for treating depression. Herbal remedies should not be substituted for proven depression therapies.

C. PSYCHOTHERAPY

Cognitive–behavioral therapy (CBT), problem-solving therapy (PST), and interpersonal psychotherapy (IPT) are effective treatments for major depression either alone or in combination with pharmacotherapy. CBT focuses on identifying negative thoughts and behaviors that contribute to depression and replacing them with positive thoughts and rewarding activities. PST teaches patients techniques to identify routine problems, generate multiple solutions, and implement the best strategy. IPT focuses on recognizing and attempting to resolve personal stressors and relationship conflicts that lead to depressive symptoms.

Typically, these therapies should be continued once or twice weekly for 6–16 sessions. In patients with severe depression, combination therapy with psychotherapy and pharmacotherapy is superior to either treatment alone. Psychoanalytic and psychodynamic therapies have not proved effective for treatment of major depression.

D. ELECTROCONVULSIVE THERAPY

Electroconvulsive therapy (ECT) is an effective treatment for geriatric depression. Response rates for refractory depression are quite high at 73% for the young-old (60–74 years) and 67% for the old-old (> 75 years). Typical side effects include confusion and anterograde memory impairment, which may persist for 6 mo. ECT may be first-line therapy for severely melancholic patients, for those at high risk for suicide, and for med-

Table 14–4. Frequency of side effects associated with antidepressant medications.[a]

Medication	Sedation	Agitation	Anticholinergic effects[b]	Postural hypotension	Gastrointestinal upset	Sexual dysfunction	Weight gain	Weight loss
Selective serotonin reuptake inhibitors								
Citalopram	0	0	0	0	++	++	0	+
Ecitalopram	+	0	0	0	++	++	0	0
Fluoxetine	0	++	0	0	++	+++	0	+
Paroxetine	++	0	+	0	++	+++	0	+
Sertraline	+	+	0	0	++	+++	0	+
Tricyclics–secondary								
Desipramine	++	0	++	++	+	+	+	0
Nortriptyline	+++	0	++	++	+	+	+	0
Bicyclics								
Venlafaxine[c]	+	+	+	0	+++	++	0	+
Serotonin antagonists: mirtazapine	+++	0	++	+	0	0	++	0
Norepinephrine-dopamine reuptake inhibitors: bupropion	+	++	+	0	++	0	+	++
Serotonin antagonist and reuptake inhibitors								
Nefazodone	++	0	+	+	+	0	+	+
Trazadone	++++	0	+	++	+	0	+	+

[a]Frequency of side effects: 0, none; +, minimal; ++, low; +++, moderate; ++++, high.
[b]Including dry mouth, dry eyes, blurred vision, constipation, urinary retention, tachycardia, and confusion.
[c]May cause dose-related elevation in diastolic blood pressure; monitoring of blood pressure is recommended.

Adapted with NEJM permission from Whooley MA, Simon GE, "Managing Depression in Medical Outpatients," NEJM 2000;343(26):1942–1950.

ically ill patients whose hepatic, renal, or cardiac diseases preclude the use of other antidepressants.

E. PSYCHIATRIC THERAPY

Psychiatric consultation is recommended for those patients with a history of mania or psychosis, for those who have not responded to a trial of 1 or 2 medicines, and for those who require combination therapy or ECT. Immediate psychiatric evaluation is required for any patients who, after probing, admit to having active plans to harm themselves. Risk factors for suicide in elderly patients with major depression include older age; male gender; marital status of single, divorced, or separated and without children; personal or family history of a suicide attempt; drug or alcohol abuse; severe anxiety or stress; physical illness; and a specific suicide plan with access to firearms or other lethal means (eg, stockpiled medications). If medications and weapons are present and cannot be removed from the patient's home, then consider adding "weapon at home" to the patient's problem list to highlight potential suicide risk.

F. FOLLOW-UP

1. Pharmacotherapy—Elderly patients should be monitored closely during the initial 3 mo of treatment. Many medical outpatients who receive a prescription for an antidepressant terminate treatment during the first month, when side effects may be at a maximum and before therapeutic effects are evident. Elderly patients should be monitored closely in the first 1–2 weeks of therapy to assess side effects and encourage continued therapy. They should have a minimum of 3 visits (in person or by telephone) during the first 12 weeks of antidepressant treatment.

Elderly patients must be informed that antidepressants usually take 4–6 weeks, but may take 8 weeks or longer, to have a full therapeutic effect and that only about 50% of patients respond to the first antidepressant prescribed. Patients who have not responded after an adequate trial of medication or who have had intolerable side effects may switch either to another medication within the same class (different SSRI) or to a different class of medications. When switching among SSRIs or between TCAs and SSRIs, no wash-out period is required (with the exception of switching from fluoxetine, because of its long half-life). However, abrupt cessation of shorter acting antidepressants (eg, citalopram, paroxetine, sertraline, or venlafaxine) may result in a discontinuation syndrome with tinnitus, vertigo, or paresthesias. Referral for psychiatric consultation is recommended if a patient fails to respond to 2 different medication trials.

Once remission has been achieved, antidepressants should be continued for at least 6 mo to reduce the risk of relapse. Patients who are at high risk of relapse (2 or more episodes of depression in the past or major depression lasting more than 2 years) should be continued on therapy for 2 years or possibly indefinitely. Many recommend lifelong therapy, even if it is the patient's first episode of major depression and especially if depression is severe and related to life changes that are not expected to improve. Follow-up visits should be arranged at 3- to 6-mo intervals. If symptoms return, the medications should be adjusted or changed or the patient referred for psychiatric consultation.

If the patient and physician agree to a trial discontinuation of therapy, medications should be tapered over a 2- to 3-mo period, with at least monthly follow-up by telephone or in person. If symptoms return, the patient should be restarted on medications for at least 3–6 mo.

When patients fail to respond to adequate trials of 2 medications for major depression, a diagnosis of treatment-resistant depression is considered. One must review the case and consider that the original diagnosis may be inaccurate. What first appeared as depressive symptoms may be a manifestation of underlying anxiety or cognitive impairment that is not being adequately treated. One must then verify that the patient actually received the medication that was prescribed. A simple investigation may reveal that the patient never filled the prescription or was never given medication by caregivers. Finally, one must ensure that the patient had adequate trials of medications (6–8 weeks) and that this trial was performed at a therapeutic dose.

Any patient who has had an adequate trial of 2 different medications without acceptable response should be referred to a psychiatrist for augmentation therapy. Lithium may be used in low doses in the elderly with careful monitoring of side effects. Small doses of liothyronine (T_3) can be used safely in euthyroid patients. In addition, combinations of 2 antidepressant medications may be synergistic, with low doses of 1 antidepressant enhancing response to an antidepressant of another class.

2. Structured psychotherapy—Patients who have been referred to psychotherapy must still be monitored closely by their primary care clinicians because patients tend to discontinue therapy even more frequently than antidepressant treatments. The benefits of psychotherapy are generally evident by 6–8 weeks. The addition of pharmacotherapy should be considered for patients who have not fully responded to psychotherapy alone by 12 weeks. A combination of psychotherapy and pharmacotherapy may be more effective for moderate depression than either treatment alone.

Prognosis

Depression is often a chronic or relapsing and remitting disease. Greater severity of depression, persistence of symptoms, and a higher number of prior episodes are the best predictors of recurrence. The lifetime risk of suicide in patients with major depression is 7% for men and 1% for women.

American Psychiatric Association: Diagnostic and Statistical Manual of Mental Disorders, 4th ed. American Psychiatric Association, 1994.

Hirschfeld RM et al: The National Depressive and Manic-Depressive Association Consensus Statement on the Undertreatment of Depression. JAMA 1997;277:333. [PMID: 9002497]

Sable JA et al: Late-Life Depression: How to identify its symptoms and provide effective treatment. Geriatrics 2002;57:18. [PMID: 11851203]

Whooley MA et al: Management depression in medical outpatients. N Engl J Med 2000;343:1942. [PMID: 11136266]

Wilson K et al: Antidepressants versus placebo for the depressed elderly (Cochrane Review). In The Cochrane Library (series 1). Update Software, 2003. [PMID: 114055969]

SUICIDE

Many depressed elders contemplate suicide. Primary care providers must recognize the risk factors for suicide in patients with major depression: older age; male gender; being single, divorced, or separated and without children; personal or family history of a suicide attempt; drug or alcohol abuse; severe anxiety or stress; physical illness; and a specific suicide plan with access to firearms or other lethal means. Providers should ask patients whether they ever think of hurting themselves or taking their life. If the patient responds positively, then physicians should ask whether they have a plan and, if so, what it is. Asking patients about stockpiled medications or weapons in their home is also critical in assessing the suicide risk. If medications and weapons are present and cannot be removed from the patient's home, then consider adding "weapon at home" to the problem list to highlight potential suicide risk. Actively suicidal patients with intent and plan require emergent psychiatric evaluation either through emergency departments or local psychiatric crisis units.

BIPOLAR DISORDER

ESSENTIALS OF DIAGNOSIS

- *History of manic episode: grandiosity, decreased need for sleep, pressured speech, racing thoughts, distractibility, increased activity, excessive spending, hypersexuality.*
- *May be associated with psychosis.*

- *Depressive episodes may alternate with mania.*
- *Mania may present for the first time in elderly patients, usually in those with a history of depressive episodes.*

General Considerations

Bipolar disorder is a less common diagnosis in the elderly, with an overall low prevalence of < 1% in community-dwelling elders but a 10% rate in some nursing home populations. Many patients with bipolar disease require special considerations as they age because of comorbid conditions and diminished ability to tolerate psychiatric medications. Late-onset mania is often secondary to underlying medical conditions and is frequently associated with neurological abnormalities such as cerebrovascular accident and cognitive impairment. Elderly patients with bipolar disorder have an increased 10-year mortality rate compared with those who have depression alone (70% vs. 30%).

Differential Diagnosis

DSM-IV criteria for bipolar disorder include those for major depressive episode (see Table 14–1) and for manic episode, which is defined as a distinct period of abnormally and persistently elevated, expansive, or irritable mood lasting at least 1 week and with ≥ 3 of the following symptoms: inflated self-esteem or grandiosity, decreased need for sleep, pressured speech, racing thoughts, distractibility, increase in goal-directed activity or psychomotor agitation, excessive involvement in pleasurable activities that have a high potential for painful consequences. The presence of mania is key to the differentiation between depressive disorder and bipolar disorder.

A variety of conditions may mimic a manic episode. Patients with dementia, particularly frontotemporal dementia, may be disinhibited and hypersexual. Brain tumors, cerebrovascular accidents, and partial-complex seizures may also lead to bizarre, disinhibited behaviors. Elderly patients who are prone to delirium can have waxing and waning levels of consciousness with some periods of hyperarousal. In addition, some medications may have unexpected effects in older patients. Glucocorticoids, thyroxine, and methylphenidate may lead to acute mania. Even sedative medications (eg, benzodiazepines) may have a paradoxical effect in the elderly and lead to agitation. As in younger populations, substance intoxication or withdrawal from cocaine, alcohol, or amphetamines and endocrine disorders such as hyperthyroidism or pheochromocytoma can lead to symptoms consistent with mania.

Treatment

Mood stabilizers have been the hallmark of treatment for bipolar disease. Valproic acid and carbamazepine are generally favored over lithium in the elderly because of lithium's side effect profile and narrow toxic–therapeutic window (Table 14–5). Antipsychotic medication can be used when psychotic features are present. In general, the newer antipsychotic agents such as olanzapine and risperidone are better tolerated by the elderly than the older neuroleptics with their extrapyramidal side effects and high risk of tardive dyskinesia, especially in women (Table 14–6). Olanzapine is approved as monotherapy for acute mania, although it does not have prophylactic effects against future manic episodes. Antidepressants are often used as an adjunct to mood stabilizers for patients with depression but should not be used alone because of the risk of transforming a depressive episode into a manic episode.

ANXIETY & STRESS DISORDERS
Panic Disorder

ESSENTIALS OF DIAGNOSIS

- Sudden, recurrent, unexpected panic attacks, characterized by palpitations, dizziness, sensation of dyspnea or choking.
- Attacks may include trembling, chest pain or discomfort, nausea, diaphoresis, paresthesias, and depersonalization.
- Sense of doom, fear of death.
- Persistent worry about future attacks.
- Can be accompanied by a fear of being in places where attack might occur (agoraphobia).

General Considerations

The lifetime prevalence rate of panic disorder is 1.5–2%, increasing to 4% in the primary care setting. The rate among community-dwelling elders is < 1%. Depression is also present in 50–65% of patients with panic disorder; the suicide rate for these patients is 20% higher than that for depressed patients without panic disorder. Panic disorder may be associated with agoraphobia, which can be particularly disabling in the elderly.

Differential Diagnosis

A panic attack is defined as a discrete period of intense fear or discomfort with 4 or more of the following symptoms: palpitations, sweating, trembling or shaking, shortness of breath, choking sensation, chest pain or discomfort, nausea or abdominal distress, dizziness or unsteadiness, derealization or depersonalization, fear of losing control, and fear of dying. *DSM-IV* criteria include recurrent or unexpected panic attacks, with at least 1 of the attacks having been followed by ≥ 1 mo of at least 1 of the following: persistent concern about having additional attacks, worry about the implication of the attack or its consequences, or a significant change in behavior related to the attacks.

Because the likelihood of physical disease is much higher than in younger populations, panic disorder is more difficult to distinguish from other life-threatening events in elderly patients. Acute coronary syndromes, cardiac arrhythmias, acute bronchospasm, and pulmonary embolism may lead to symptoms consistent with panic attacks. Endocrine disorders, particularly hyperthyroidism and pheochromocytoma, can mimic panic disorder. In acutely hospitalized patients, alcohol, caffeine, and tobacco withdrawal may present as agitation, worry, and other physical symptoms. Abrupt discontinuation of a short-acting antidepressant, anxiolytic, or narcotic medication may also trigger panic symptoms. Older patients who suffer from panic disor-

Table 14–5. Mood stabilizers.

Generic name	Trade name	Initial dose†	Target dose†	Comments
Lithium	Lithobid, Eskalith	300 mg qd or bid	600–1200 mg/day in divided doses bid or tid	Monitor drug levels, renal function, thyroid function; diuretics and ACE inhibitors increase levels; avoid dehydration and many NSAIDS because of toxicity
Carbamazepine	Tegretol	200 mg qd or bid	400–1000 mg/day	Monitor blood count, liver function tests, drug levels
Valproic acid	Depakote	250 mg qd or bid	500–1500 mg/day	Monitor blood count, liver function tests, drug levels

ACE, angiotensin-converting enzyme; NSAIDs, nonsteroidal anti-inflammatory drugs.

Table 14–6. Commonly used antipsychotics.

Generic name	Trade name	Initial dose (mg)	Target dosage[a] (mg/day)	Available routes of administration
Older agents				
D2 Antagonists-high potency[b]				
Haloperidol	Haldol	0.5	0.5–1	PO, IV, IM, depot
Newer agents:				
Serotonin Dopamine Receptor Antagonists				
Risperidone	Risperdal	0.5	1–1.5	PO
Olanzapine	Zyprexa	2.5	2.5–5	PO
Quetiapine	Seroquel	25	50–200	PO

[a]Target dose is the usually effective dose for organic psychosis or agitation in the elderly. Patients with formal thought disorder may require higher doses in consultation with a psychiatrist.
[b]Typical antipsychotics carry an increased risk relative to atypical antipsychotics of extrapyramidal side effects, including akathisia, bradykinesia, rigidity, and tardive dyskinesia.

der often have comorbid psychiatric diagnoses such as posttraumatic stress disorder (PTSD), generalized anxiety disorder, and depression.

Treatment

CBT has been proven effective for the treatment of panic disorder. Patients often go into a complete remission after as few as 12 weekly sessions. CBT is particularly helpful in preventing relapse and treating agoraphobia. Antidepressants, particularly SSRIs and TCAs, are helpful. Benzodiazepines may also be used as a brief adjunctive therapy while awaiting the clinical response to antidepressants or CBT. Whenever possible, long-term therapy with benzodiazepines should be avoided because of the potential risk of falls, cognitive impairment, and dependence.

Perhaps the most important aspect of treatment is education for the patient and family. Understanding the symptoms of panic disorder and developing ways of coping are essential for effective management of the disease.

Social & Specific Phobias

ESSENTIALS OF DIAGNOSIS

- *A phobia is an irrational fear leading to intentional avoidance of a specific feared object, event, or situation.*
- *Exposure to this phobic object may result in symptoms similar to those of a panic attack.*
- *Patient is aware that his or her fear is irrational.*

General Considerations

The prevalence of phobias is 5–6% in the elderly. Phobias present with features similar to panic disorder but are triggered by a specific event. Late-onset phobias are often associated with a recent life event such as a fall or injury. Social phobias affect 3% of the elderly and can lead to increasing isolation. Simple phobias are thought to be more common than social phobias, affecting 5–12% of the general population.

Differential Diagnosis

Social phobia (also known as social anxiety disorder) is defined by *DSM-IV* criteria as a marked and persistent fear of social situations. Exposure to these situations provoke anxiety and may lead to a panic attack. The patient realizes that the fear is excessive and either avoids the situation or endures it with great anxiety. The avoidance or anxiety associated with the situation interferes with the patient's normal routine, occupation, or relationships. Specific phobia is a fear of certain objects or situations with acknowledgment that the fear is unreasonable. Specific phobias may also impair a patient's ability to function normally.

In the elderly, new phobic symptoms may represent delusions associated with dementia or delirium. Patients with dementia or delirium are not typically aware of the irrational nature of their delusions in contrast to patients with phobia. Less common causes of phobia include brain tumors or cerebrovascular accidents. The psychiatric differential diagnosis of phobia includes depression, schizophrenia, and schizoid and avoidant personality disorders. Social phobia and alcohol dependence often coexist; therefore, probing for alcohol use is an important part of the assessment. Although both phobic disorders and panic disorder may present with panic attacks, patients with phobias do not experience recurrent unexpected attacks; rather, their anxiety symptoms are always associated with a specific object or situation.

Treatment

The first-line therapy for specific phobias is behavioral therapy. Techniques may include relaxation therapy, cognitive restructuring, and systematic exposure to the feared object or situation. Use of antidepressants, particularly SSRIs, may be beneficial for generalized social phobia. Beta-adrenergic antagonists such as propranolol may also be effective treatments when administered before a foreseeable feared event or situation. Benzodiazepine use may be necessary but in general should be used with caution because of adverse effects on balance and cognition. Most patients are able to adapt or overcome their phobias and can lead relatively normal lives; if not, they should be referred for evaluation by a mental health specialist.

Generalized Anxiety Disorder

ESSENTIALS OF DIAGNOSIS

- *Unrealistic or excessive worry about 2 or more life circumstances.*
- *Worry is recurrent and difficult to control.*
- *Physiological symptoms of restlessness, fatigue, irritability, muscle tension, and sleep disturbance.*

General Considerations

Anxiety symptoms are often a normal reaction to the surrounding environment. Anxiety disorders tend to begin in early adulthood and continue throughout a patient's lifetime with periods of relapses and remissions. The lifetime prevalence of generalized anxiety disorder is 5%; estimates in elders range from 2–7%. Anxiety may increase in the elderly as a result of isolation, loss of independence, illness, disability, and bereavement.

Differential Diagnosis

The diagnosis of generalized anxiety disorder is characterized by the following according to *DSM-IV* criteria:

- Excessive anxiety and worry about 2 or more life circumstances occurring more days than not for at least 6 mo.

- Worry is difficult to control.
- Anxiety and worry are associated with at least 3 of the following: restlessness, easy fatigability, difficulty with concentration, irritability, muscle tension, sleep disturbance.

Diagnosing generalized anxiety in elders can be complicated because many underlying illnesses may have similar symptoms. The differential diagnosis for generalized anxiety disorder includes the physical illnesses discussed previously for panic disorder. In addition, chronic medication or substance use and subsequent withdrawal may lead to anxiety symptoms. Caffeine, nicotine, and alcohol are common culprits. Elderly patients are much more sensitive to commonly used over-the-counter medications such as pseudoephedrine, which may cause restlessness, anxiety, and confusion. Up to 54% of patients who suffer from generalized anxiety disorder have comorbid depression. Obsessive–compulsive disorder, somatoform disorder, and personality disorders may also present with symptoms of anxiety. Psychiatric consultation should be initiated if the diagnosis is in question.

Treatment

CBT is one of the most effective treatments for generalized anxiety disorder. Relaxation techniques and biofeedback may also alleviate symptoms. Several antidepressants (paroxetine, extended-release venlafaxine) also have significant anxiolytic properties and may be effective for both anxiety and depression. When depression and anxiety occur together, one should treat the depression first; doing so may improve the symptoms of both disorders. Anxiolytic medications such as buspirone (5–30 mg twice daily) may be effective. Benzodiazepines should be used with caution in the elderly because they can cause a paradoxical effect and may also lead to falls and cognitive impairment.

Posttraumatic Stress Disorder

ESSENTIALS OF DIAGNOSIS

- *History of exposure to a traumatic event.*
- *Intrusive thoughts, nightmares, and flashbacks.*
- *Avoidance of thoughts, feelings, or situations associated with the trauma.*
- *Isolation, detachment from others, emotional numbness.*
- *Symptoms of arousal such as sleep disturbance, irritability, and hypervigilance.*

- Frequently associated with depression and substance abuse.

General Considerations

PTSD is associated with a lifetime prevalence of 1.2% in women and 0.5% in men. Symptoms of PTSD may persist into older age. In addition, symptoms can remain hidden until an older age when patients have new experiences (deaths, medical illness, disability) that trigger memories of former events or lose the capacity to compensate for lifelong symptoms because of cognitive impairment or other medical illness. However, some studies have shown that increased age may actually protect against the development of PTSD. Other protective factors include marriage, social support, and higher socioeconomic status.

Differential Diagnosis

Per *DSM-IV* criteria, the patient has been exposed to a traumatic event in which he or she experienced or witnessed an event outside the range of usual human experience. Symptoms may be grouped into 3 categories and may persist for > 1 mo.

1. Persistent reexperience of the traumatic event by ≥ 1 of the following: recurrent and intrusive recollections, dreams, acting or feeling as if the traumatic event were recurring (reliving experience, hallucinations, illusions, and dissociative flashbacks).
2. Avoidant symptoms with ≥ 3 of the following: avoiding thoughts, feelings, activities, places, or people associated with the trauma; inability to remember important aspects of the trauma; decreased interest in activities; feeling of detachment from others; restricted range of affect or sense of foreshortened future
3. Arousal symptoms indicated by ≥ 2 of the following: difficulty falling or staying asleep, irritability or outbursts of anger, difficulty concentrating, hypervigilance, or an exaggerated startle response.

Other anxiety disorders can present with symptoms of hyperarousal similar to those in patients with PTSD. Major depressive disorder and adjustment disorders can also present with numbing or avoidant symptoms. During a period of bereavement, patients can have visions or dreams about the deceased. Other psychotic disorders may be confused with PTSD, but patients with PTSD may also experience psychotic-like symptoms during severe episodes. Substance use or withdrawal

may contribute to symptoms. Organic brain syndrome resulting from prior head injury may be associated with symptoms similar to those of PTSD; the presence of visual hallucinations is particularly suggestive of an organic cause. Patients with delirium may also appear hyperaroused or be prone to illusions. There is a high comorbidity of depression and alcohol abuse among patients with PTSD.

Treatment

Antidepressants, particularly SSRIs and TCAs, are indicated for treatment of PTSD (see Table 14–3). Both individual and group CBTs are also effective in the treatments and may be used alone or in combination with pharmacological therapy. Antiadrenergic agents such as clonidine may be helpful for symptoms of increased arousal, although one must consider related side effects such as orthostasis. Benzodiazepines can often worsen symptoms of PTSD and should be avoided. Antipsychotic medications are occasionally necessary for the treatment of associated psychotic symptoms (see Table 14–5).

SCHIZOPHRENIA & PSYCHOTIC DISORDERS

 ESSENTIALS OF DIAGNOSIS

- Loss of ego boundaries and gross impairment in reality testing.
- Prominent delusions or auditory or visual hallucinations.
- Flat or inappropriate affect
- Disorganized speech, thought processes, or behavior.

General Considerations

Psychotic symptoms may be due to a long-standing psychotic illness that has persisted into older age or may present for the first time in later life in association with underlying medical conditions, especially dementia. Estimates for schizophrenia in the elderly population range from 0.1–0.5%. The prevalence of other psychotic syndromes such as paranoid ideation is higher, estimated at 4–6% in the elderly population, and is frequently associated with dementia. Patients with Alzheimer's disease have a particularly high incidence of psychosis; 50% manifest psychotic symptoms within 3 years of diagnosis.

Differential Diagnosis

The diagnostic criteria for schizophrenia include ≥ 2 of the following characteristic symptoms present for at least 1 mo: delusions, hallucinations, disorganized speech, grossly disorganized or catatonic behavior, or negative symptoms such as flattened affect. These symptoms must also be associated with social or occupational dysfunction. Patients commonly will not volunteer psychotic symptoms unless specifically asked by their provider after a trusting relationship has been established. If psychosis is suspected, it is important to ask patients and family members specifically about auditory and visual hallucinations, delusions, ideas of reference, and paranoid ideation. Visual hallucinations are associated more strongly with underlying organic cause.

Especially in the elderly, new psychotic symptoms carry a vast and complicated differential. New-onset psychotic symptoms can be attributed to medications, changes in environment, organic causes, including dementia, or a combination of these factors. Because psychosis may be the presenting sign of dementia, any elderly patient with new-onset psychosis should have a thorough cognitive screen. Prominent visual hallucinations are one of the hallmarks of Lewy body dementia. Patients with Alzheimer's disease frequently have fixed delusions regarding people stealing their possessions or marital infidelity. The dementia associated with Parkinson's disease may include negative symptoms of schizophrenia, such as flat affect.

Other central nervous system diseases such as brain tumors, partial seizures, multiple sclerosis, or cerebral systemic lupus erythematosus can also cause psychotic symptoms. Patients with major depression or bipolar disorder may experience psychotic features. Infections, endocrinopathies (thyroid, diabetes, adrenal), and nutritional deficiencies (vitamin B_{12}, thiamine) may lead to psychosis. Finally, elderly patients can be especially sensitive to medications that trigger psychotic symptoms such as steroids or levodopa. Because of the large differential diagnosis, collateral information regarding the patient's baseline mental status, psychiatric history, and onset of symptoms is critical in the evaluation of psychotic symptoms.

Treatment

A. PHARMACOTHERAPY

Antipsychotic agents such as risperidone, olanzapine, quetiapine, and clozapine are the mainstays of treatment for psychotic symptoms (see Table 14–6). Ziprasidone has been approved by the Federal Drug Administration, but data in the elderly are not yet available. Because of their lower incidence of extrapyramidal side effects, these agents are much better tolerated than the older antipsychotic agents, such as haloperidol and trifluoperazine (Stelazine). However, haldoperidol remains the treatment of choice in hospitalized patients requiring intravenous medications for acute psychosis or agitation, because none of the newer agents is available in intravenous form. Unlike older neuroleptics, which mainly treat positive symptoms (eg, delusions, hallucinations), the newer agents effectively manage both positive and negative psychotic symptoms (eg, flat affect, social withdrawal). The main side effects of newer agents are sedation and dizziness. Patients may experience akathisia and parkinsonism (eg, stiffness and rigidity) and, with longer term use, tardive dyskinesias, although the risk of such side effects is lower than with high-potency traditional antipsychotic drugs. Risperidone has been associated with a slightly increased incidence of strokes in patients with dementia. Unlike other newer agents, ziprasidone does not appear to cause weight gain and is useful in the treatment of obese patients. However, it is associated with QT prolongation and thus should be avoided in patients with underlying conduction disease and QT prolongation at baseline. Clozapine is often the treatment of choice for patients with severe resistant psychosis and those with disabling tardive dyskinesias. Clozapine, however, carries a 1–2% risk of agranulocytosis and, therefore, requires weekly blood monitoring. In addition, both clozapine and olanzapine have been associated with glucose dysregulation and thus should be used with caution in patients with diabetes mellitus. Dosages of antipsychotics used in elderly patients with dementia or acute delirium tend to be lower than those required for management of other psychotic disorders and may be only necessary for short periods of time (see Table 14–6).

To decrease inappropriate use of psychotropic medications and improve the quality of care in long-term care facilities, the Health Care Finance Administration's 1987 Omnibus Reconciliation Act outlined indications and prescribing guidelines for psychoactive medications used in the treatment of psychotic disorders and agitated behaviors associated with organic brain disorders. This act requires documentation of response in terms of specific target symptoms and careful monitoring of side effects. To avoid long-term side effects such as tardive dyskinesia, OBRA also recommends trial dose reductions of neuroleptics unless clinically contraindicated because of severity of symptoms.

B. BEHAVIORAL THERAPY

Behavioral therapy may be effective for the management of psychosis and after the acute episode has resolved. Providing a stable living environment is critical to the successful treatment of psychosis. Medical compliance is difficult without close supervision by a family or staff member. Adult day facilities provide structured programs for patients and give critical respite to caregivers, thus allowing patients to remain in the community longer than they would otherwise be able to without nursing home care.

Dada F et al: Generalized anxiety disorder in the elderly. Psychiatr Clin North Am 2001;24:155. [PMID: 11225505]

Howard R et al: Late-onset schizophrenia and very-late-onset schizophrenia-like psychosis: An international consensus. Am J Psychiatry 2000;157:172. [PMID: 10671383]

Lang AJ, Stein MB: Anxiety disorders: How to recognize and treat the medical symptoms of emotional illness. Geriatrics 2001;56:24. [PMID: 11373949]

Targum SD, Abbott JL: Psychoses in the elderly: A spectrum of disorders. J Clin Psychiatry 1999;60(suppl 8):4. [PMID: 10335666]

Weintraub D, Ruskin PE: PTSD in the elderly: A review. Harv Rev Psychiatry 1999;7:144. [PMID: 10483933]

Young RC: Bipolar mood disorders in the elderly. Psychiatr Clin North Am 1997;20:121. [PMID: 9139286]

RELEVANT WORLD WIDE WEB SITES

Agency for Healthcare Research and Quality "AHCPR supported guidelines" for Diagnosis and Treatment of Depression in Primary Care: http://text.nlm.nih.gov

American Association for Geriatric Psychiatry: www.aagpgpa.org

American Medical Association: www.ama-assn.org/ama/pub/category/3457.html

Depression Awareness, Recognition, and Treatment (DART) program of the National Institute of Mental Health: www.nimh.nih.gov/publicat/index.cfm

National Center for PTSD: http://www.ncptsd.org

National Depressive and Manic-Depressive Association Depressive Association: www.ndmda.org

National Foundation for Depressive Illnesses: www.depression.org/

National Mental Health Association (Campaign on Clinical Depression): www.nmha.org/ccd

Sleep Disorders

Diana V. Jao, MD, & Cathy A. Alessi, MD

General Considerations

More than 50% of community-dwelling older persons and > 65% of long-term care facility residents experience sleeping difficulties. Fifty percent of community-dwelling older persons use over-the-counter or prescribed sleeping medications.

Two sleep states have been defined: nonrapid eye movement (NREM) sleep and rapid eye movement (REM) sleep. NREM sleep consists of 4 stages. Stages 1 and 2 are considered light sleep; stage 1 is a transition period between wakefulness and sleep. Deep, restorative sleep occurs in stages 3 and 4. A normal night of sleep usually begins with NREM sleep; the first REM period occurs after 80 min or longer. NREM and REM then alternate throughout the night, with longer REM sleep periods as the night progresses.

Changes in both sleep structure (stages of sleep) and sleep pattern (amount and timing of sleep) occur with normal aging. Stage 1 and stage 2 sleep increases or remains unchanged with aging, whereas stage 3 and stage 4 sleep characteristically decreases. Changes in REM sleep with aging are controversial. Alterations in sleep pattern include decreased sleep efficiency (time asleep divided by time in bed), normal to decreased total sleep time, increased sleep latency (time to fall asleep), earlier bedtime and earlier morning awakening, more arousals during the night, and more daytime napping. The significance of these changes is unknown but may result in sleep complaints.

Differential Diagnosis

Patients may not report sleep complaints unless specifically asked by their health care provider, and presenting symptoms overlap significantly among common sleep disorders. One suggested algorithm for screening for sleep complaints, and an approach to diagnosis and treatment is shown in Figure 15–1.

INSOMNIA

ESSENTIALS OF DIAGNOSIS

- *Complaints of poor sleep quality.*
- *Daytime symptoms of fatigue, irritability, or problems with concentration.*
- *Diagnosis is made clinically.*

General Considerations

A. SYMPTOMS & SIGNS

Insomnia is often associated with daytime symptoms such as fatigue, irritability, and problems with concentration. Four common types of complaints related to insomnia include difficulty falling asleep, midsleep awakening, early morning awakening, and nonrestorative sleep.

Insomnia can be further classified based on the duration of symptoms. Transient (or acute) insomnia persists for no more than 1 week, and short-term (or subacute) insomnia lasts from 1 week to 3 mo. Both are generally considered an adjustment sleep disorder (ie, associated with an identifiable stressor). A longer duration of symptoms is usually regarded as chronic insomnia.

B. PATIENT HISTORY

A detailed history is essential in determining the cause of insomnia. Key factors include recent stressors and symptoms of depression, anxiety, or other psychiatric disorders.

C. SPECIAL TESTS

Instruments that can be helpful in the evaluation of insomnia include sleep questionnaires, at-home sleep

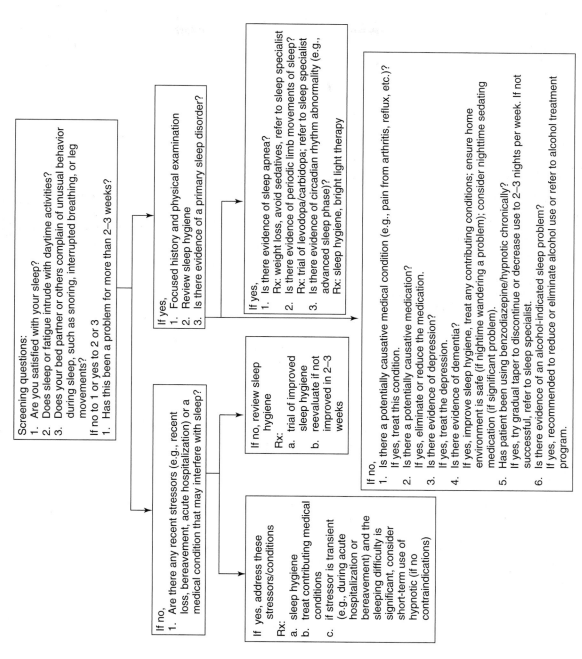

Screening questions:
1. Are you satisfied with your sleep?
2. Does sleep or fatigue intrude with daytime activities?
3. Does your bed partner or others complain of unusual behavior during sleep, such as snoring, interrupted breathing, or leg movements?

If no to 1 or yes to 2 or 3
1. Has this been a problem for more than 2–3 weeks?

If no,
1. Are there any recent stressors (e.g., recent loss, bereavement, acute hospitalization) or a medical condition that may interfere with sleep?

If yes, address these stressors/conditions
Rx:
a. sleep hygiene
b. treat contributing medical conditions
c. if stressor is transient (e.g., during acute hospitalization or bereavement) and the sleeping difficulty is significant, consider short-term use of hypnotic (if no contraindications)

If no, review sleep hygiene
Rx:
a. trial of improved sleep hygiene
b. reevaluate if not improved in 2–3 weeks

If yes,
1. Focused history and physical examination
2. Review sleep hygiene
3. Is there evidence of a primary sleep disorder?

If yes,
1. Is there evidence of sleep apnea?
   Rx: weight loss, avoid sedatives, refer to sleep specialist
2. Is there evidence of periodic limb movements of sleep?
   Rx: trial of levodopa/carbidopa; refer to sleep specialist
3. Is there evidence of circadian rhythm abnormality (e.g., advanced sleep phase)?
   Rx: sleep hygiene, bright light therapy

If no,
1. Is there a potentially causative medical condition (e.g., pain from arthritis, reflux, etc.)?
   If yes, treat this condition.
2. Is there a potentially causative medication?
   If yes, eliminate or reduce the medication.
3. Is there evidence of depression?
   If yes, treat the depression.
4. Is there evidence of dementia?
   If yes, improve sleep hygiene, treat any contributing conditions; ensure home environment is safe (if nighttime wandering a problem); consider nighttime sedating medication (if significant problem).
5. Has patient been using benzodiazepine/hypnotic chronically?
   If yes, try gradual taper to discontinue or decrease use to 2–3 nights per week. If not successful, refer to sleep specialist.
6. Is there evidence of an alcohol-indicated sleep problem?
   If yes, recommended to reduce or eliminate alcohol use or refer to alcohol treatment program.

Figure 15–1. Algorithm for screening for sleep complaints and an approach to diagnosis and treatment.

logs, symptom checklists, psychological screening tests, and interview of bed partners.

Polysomnography is not indicated for the routine evaluation of transient or chronic insomnia. Other sleep diagnostic studies are available, such as portable sleep studies, wrist activity monitors, and static charge sensitive beds, but insufficient evidence exists to make specific recommendations about their usefulness in primary care.

Differential Diagnosis

The causes of insomnia are commonly psychiatric/psychological problems, symptoms related to underlying medical illnesses, effects of medications, or problems in the sleep–wake cycle. In fact, multiple factors may contribute to insomnia in the older patient. Excessive stress, depression, anxiety, and bereavement most characteristically result in early morning awakening, increased sleep latency, and more nighttime wakefulness.

Many medical conditions can interfere with sleep, including neuropathic pain, rheumatological conditions, malignancy pain syndromes, dyspnea resulting from cardiac or pulmonary illness, gastroesophageal reflux disease, and nighttime urination.

Medications reportedly account for 10–15% of cases of insomnia. Common offending agents include corticosteroids, respiratory medications (eg, pseudoephedrine, β_2-agonists, theophylline), cardiovascular medications (eg, furosemide and quinidine), and antidepressants (eg, buproprion, fluoxetine, paroxetine, sertraline, and venlafaxine). Some antidepressants can induce somnolence or insomnia, depending on the dose (eg, desipramine, nortriptyline, and imipramine). Many other agents can disrupt sleep, such as cimetidine, phenytoin, caffeine, and nicotine. Caffeine is an ingredient in many nonprescription medications, sodas, candies, and teas, and many people are unaware that they are ingesting caffeine-containing products. Nighttime alcohol use can interfere with sleep because of effects leading to a lighter and shorter duration of sleep along with decreased REM sleep. Withdrawal from sedative–hypnotic agents also can lead to worsening insomnia.

Treatment

A. Nonpharmacological

1. Sleep hygiene—Patients with sleeping difficulty should routinely be educated on the concepts of good sleep hygiene (Table 15–1). Potential benefits include improvement in sleep pattern and a decrease in the use of sleeping medications. Sleep hygiene education seeks to reduce insomnia through modification of lifestyle and environmental factors. Measures to improve sleep hygiene should be recommended in patients with sleep-

Table 15–1. Examples of measures to improve sleep hygiene.

1. Regular morning rising time.
2. Avoid daytime napping or limit to < 1 h in the morning or early afternoon.
3. Exercise during the day but not in the evening and before bedtime.
4. Avoid caffeine, nicotine, and alcohol in the evening.
5. Avoid excessive fluid intake at night to reduce nighttime urination.
6. Avoid large meals before bedtime, but a light snack may promote sleep.
7. Follow a nighttime routine of preparation for bedtime and wear comfortable bedclothes.
8. Ensure a comfortable nighttime environment, minimizing noise and light and keeping room temperature comfortable.

ing difficulties, but specific measures may not be effective in all patients. It can be extremely helpful for the patient to keep a sleep log to record specific sleep hygiene measures used and their effectiveness.

2. Behavioral therapy—Behavioral therapy has been equally effective in patients who experience difficulty falling asleep, midsleep arousals, and early morning awakenings. Stimulus control therapy teaches patients to recondition maladaptive sleep-related behaviors. Sleep restriction therapy seeks to improve sleep efficiency by causing modest sleep deprivation (ie, limiting time in bed) and then gradually increasing time in bed as sleep efficiency improves. Cognitive interventions include instructing patients to help change their misunderstandings regarding sleep.

Relaxation techniques educate patients in recognizing and relieving tension and anxiety. However, relaxation techniques may be somewhat less effective in the older population than the other behavioral techniques mentioned.

Behavioral therapy appears to be as effective as medications for short-term insomnia. Chronic insomnia is best managed with behavioral interventions because of the greater likelihood of long-term effectiveness and lower risk of side effects.

3. Bright light therapy—Bright light therapy (exposure to sunlight or commercially available light boxes) has also been used to improve sleep and circadian rhythm problems in older people. This therapy appears promising, and some evidence for its efficacy has been demonstrated. Bright light does have potential side effects including eye strain and headache, in addition to photosensitizing effects for patients on medications such as amiodarone and hydrochlorthiazide.

B. PHARMACOLOGICAL

1. Prescription medications—When considering whether to prescribe a sleeping medication, one should consider the duration of symptoms, type of symptoms (eg, problem with sleep onset vs. awakening during the night), agent characteristics, and cost.

Benzodiazepines and related drugs are commonly prescribed for sleep (Table 15–2). Long-acting benzodiazepines (eg, flurazepam) should not be used in older patients because of the risk of daytime carryover (sedation), falls, and fractures. Short- and intermediate-acting benzodiazepines can be used in older people; however, caution is warranted because of the risk of tolerance to the hypnotic effects of the medication and the potential for rebound insomnia on withdrawal. These agents may also result in an increased risk of falls, and their half-life can be longer in older people.

Nonbenzodiazepine hypnotics (eg, zolpidem and zaleplon) seem to have a better action profile, with fewer side effects, including less tolerance and less rebound insomnia on withdrawal, compared with benzodiazepines. Zolpidem (with a serum half-life of approximately 2.5 h) can be used for patients who have difficulty falling asleep. Zaleplon (with a serum half-life of 1 h) may be used to treat midsleep awakening if the patient has ≥ 4 h of additional sleep time before awakening. There is also reportedly no daytime carryover with this medication. However, caution is warranted in using even the newer sleeping medications for the management of chronic insomnia in the elderly.

Antidepressants with sedating side effects are also commonly used as sleeping medications. Sedating antidepressants are commonly prescribed at night for depressed patients who also report insomnia. Alternatively, nonsedating antidepressants taken during the daytime are sometimes prescribed for these depressed individuals, with the addition of a low dose of a sedating antidepressant (eg, 25–50 mg trazodone) at night for sleeping difficulty. These agents appear to have fewer problems with habituation compared with benzodiazepines, but response to this treatment is variable. The antidepressant amitriptyline is sedating but should not be used in older patients because of its strong anticholinergic side effects.

2: Nonprescription medications—Over-the-counter sleeping aids often contain a sedating antihistamine (eg, diphenhydramine) alone or in combination with an analgesic. Diphenhydramine and similar compounds are generally not recommended for older people because of potent anticholinergic effects and the development of tolerance to sedating effects over time. A bedtime dose of an analgesic alone (eg, acetaminophen) may be a safe and helpful alternative in some older people. Some people use alcohol at bedtime as a "nightcap" to help them sleep. Although alcohol does cause some initial drowsiness, it can interfere with sleep later in the night and may actually worsen the insomnia symptoms.

Melatonin has also been used to promote sleep. In general, there is a decrease in melatonin levels with age and in individuals with Alzheimer's disease. Melatonin therapy appears to be effective in older insomniacs with demonstrated melatonin deficiency. However, melatonin measurements are not routinely available, and its use in insomniacs without melatonin deficiency is controversial. In addition, melatonin formulations are unregulated.

Chesson A et al: Practice parameters for the evaluation of insomnia. Sleep 2000;23:237. [PMID 10737341]

Morin CM et al: Behavioral and pharmacological therapies for late-life insomnia: A randomized controlled trial. JAMA 1999; 281:991. [PMID 10086433]

Table 15–2. Examples of commonly used prescription sleeping medications in older people.

Generic name (trade names)	Class	Usual dose range in older people	Half-life
Lorazepam (Ativan)	Intermediate-acting benzodiazepine	0.25–2 mg	8–12 h
Temazepam (Restoril)	Intermediate-acting benzodiazepine	15–30 mg	8–10 h (up to 30 h in older people)
Estazolam (ProSom)	Intermediate-acting benzodiazepine	0.5–2.0 mg	12–18 h
Zolpidem (Ambien)	Nonbenzodiazepine, imidazopyridine (short acting)	5–10 mg	1.5–4.5 h (10 h in cirrhosis)
Zaleplon (Sonata)	Nonbenzodiazepine, pyrazolopyrimidine (short acting)	5–10 mg	1 h
Trazodone (Desyrel)	Sedating antidepressant	25–150 mg	2–4 h

Morin CM et al: Nonpharmacological treatment of late-life insomnia. J Psychosom Res 1999;46:103. [PMID 10098820]

Sateia MJ et al: Evaluation of chronic insomnia. Sleep 2000;23: 243. [PMID 10737342]

EXCESSIVE DAYTIME SLEEPINESS

Problems with excessive daytime sleepiness may suggest a serious underlying sleep disorder. This excessive sleepiness is not simply the fatigue or tiredness that can occur with a variety of disorders. Excessive daytime sleepiness implies an irresistible desire to sleep and an inability to stay awake, even when it is quite abnormal to fall asleep. The 2 common conditions that are capable of inducing excessive daytime sleepiness in older people are sleep apnea and periodic limb movements disorder (PLMD). Restless legs syndrome (RLS), although related to PLMD, does not commonly present as excessive daytime sleepiness.

SLEEP APNEA

 ESSENTIALS OF DIAGNOSIS

- *Snoring, choking, and altered breathing during the night.*
- *Daytime sleepiness.*
- *Morning headache and cardiovascular complications may be present.*
- *Polysomnography is used to confirm the diagnosis.*

General Considerations

Sleep apnea is the cessation (or marked decrease) of airflow, which disrupts sleep. In obstructive sleep apnea (OSA), apnea is associated with the collapse of oropharyngeal structures, with continued ventilatory effort in the rib cage and abdomen.

Clinical Findings

A. SYMPTOMS & SIGNS

Increased body mass index is the most important predictor of sleep apnea, although not all patients with sleep apnea are obese. Other risk factors include male gender and older age; prevalence rates of up to 40% are reported in people aged 65 and older. There is some evidence for a higher prevalence among individuals with dementia.

Excessive daytime sleepiness is the most common complaint in OSA. In addition, many patients complain of morning headache. The bed partner can be very helpful in reporting the typical symptoms of loud snoring, apnea, choking, and gasping sounds.

The clinical consequences of sleep apnea appear to relate to sleep fragmentation, hypoxia, and hypercapnia. Sleep apnea is associated with cardiovascular disease and increased morbidity and mortality rates. Other adverse consequences include cognitive impairment and a higher rate of motor vehicle accidents.

B. SCREENING METHODS

Several different screening methods for sleep apnea have been suggested. The "I SNORED" (*I*nsomnia, *S*noring, *N*ot breathing/*N*octurnal choking, *O*besity [BMI > 29], *R*estorative sleep, *E*xcessive daytime hypersomnolence, and *D*rugs) test seems to have only modest predictive value in sleep laboratory studies (in which there is a high prevalence of sleep-disordered breathing). Its usefulness in a general medical population needs additional testing.

The gold standard for diagnosing OSA is nocturnal polysomnography. Based on the sleep study, an apnea–hypopnea index is calculated as the number of apnea and hypopnea events per hour of sleep.

Referral to a sleep specialist (in particular for polysomnography) is indicated in the evaluation of suspected sleep apnea. Some experts also recommend polysomnography when the initial diagnosis is uncertain or when the treatment is unsuccessful.

Treatment

The severity of associated symptoms is considered in making treatment decisions because all treatments are associated with some consequences. Nonsurgical approaches include weight loss, avoidance of alcohol and sedative use, and avoidance of the supine sleeping position. Oral–dental devices that reposition the jaw or tongue are also available. Continuous positive airway pressure (CPAP) is quite effective. Some patients may find CPAP uncomfortable, but a variety of CPAP devices are available to meet patients' needs. For those who fail or are unable to tolerate CPAP, surgical revision can be considered. Surgical procedures offer mixed results, varying from ~30% with laser-assisted uvuloplasty to ~90% for mandibular-maxillary advancement.

PERIODIC LIMB MOVEMENT DISORDER & RESTLESS LEGS SYNDROME

General Considerations

The reported prevalence of periodic limb movements during sleep ranges from 20–60% among older adults.

PLMD can present as insomnia or excessive daytime sleepiness. Frequent sleep interruptions as a result of PLMD can cause nonrestorative sleep, daytime sleepiness, and fatigue.

Reported prevalence of RLS ranges from 2–15%. RLS generally causes insomnia, nighttime restlessness, and discomfort but can also lead to excessive daytime sleepiness when severe.

RLS and periodic limb movements often coexist; the latter are present in 80% of patients with RLS. The prevalence of these 2 disorders increases with age. The cause of neither condition is known, but increased age, positive family history, pregnancy, uremia, and low iron stores have been suggested as risk factors.

Clinical Findings

A. Symptoms & Signs

PLMD is characterized by recurring episodes of stereotypic rhythmic movements during sleep, generally involving the legs. The movements occur as often as every 20–40 s throughout the night.

RLS is characterized by an uncomfortable, irresistible urge to move the legs, usually associated with paresthesias and motor restlessness. The upper extremities are less commonly involved. There is usually a worsening of symptoms at rest and relief with motor activity. The symptoms are generally most pronounced in the evening or at night, occurring before the onset of sleep or occasionally with awakenings during the night. Patients may have difficulty falling asleep.

B. Special Tests

Polysomnography is used for the evaluation of PLMD.

Differential Diagnosis

The diagnosis of PLMD is reserved for individuals with periodic limb movements during sleep plus a sleep disturbance that is not explained by the presence of another disorder.

The diagnosis of RLS is made clinically based on the patient's symptoms, but PLMD cannot be adequately evaluated by history alone and requires polysomnographic confirmation.

Treatment

The treatment of PLMD depends on the severity of symptoms and their impact on the patient's general well-being.

RLS may improve with leg stretching and other maneuvers. Pharmacotherapy should be considered for RLS when these maneuvers are ineffective or when symptoms are severe.

Choice of medication for these disorders should depend on evidence of effectiveness and comorbid conditions. Dopaminergic agents are the best studied agents for both RLS and PLMD and are considered by many as the treatment of choice in older patients. Treatment near bedtime with either carbidopa-levodopa (½ to full tablet of $^{25}/_{100}$-mg tablets, or higher) or dopamine agonists (eg, pramipexole 0.125 mg, ropinirole 0.25-mg dose or higher) may be effective for both RLS and PLMD. Other dopaminergic agents are also likely effective. Oxycodone and propoxyphene have proven effective for both RLS and PLMD, but the risk of side effects with these agents limits their usefulness in the older patient. Clonazepam is effective for the treatment of PLMD and possibly RLS, but there is concern about risks of side effects with chronic use in older people. Other treatments to consider that have demonstrated some efficacy for RLS include gabapentin or iron supplementation (if ferritin level is low)

NARCOLEPSY

General Considerations

Narcolepsy is a disorder of recurrent, uncontrollable, brief episodes of sleep, which are often associated with hypnagogic or hypnopomic hallucinations, cataplexy, and sleep paralysis. This disorder rarely presents for the first time in old age.

Clinical Findings

A. Symptoms & Signs

The tetrad of symptoms for narcolepsy consists of excessive daytime sleepiness, cataplexy, sleep paralysis, and hypnagogic hallucinations.

B. Special Tests

Polysomnography typically reveals a shortened sleep latency (ie, time to fall asleep), sleep-onset REM (ie, REM sleep present soon after sleep onset), increased stage 1 sleep, and decreased sleep efficiency with increased number of arousals and awakenings. A structured daytime sleep study (the Multiple Sleep Latency Test) is also usually performed to determine the extent of daytime sleepiness and to identify sleep episodes with early onset of REM (ie, sleep-onset REM period).

Differential Diagnosis

Narcolepsy can be complicated by other sleep disorders Sleep apnea, periodic limb movements, and REM sleep behavior disorder can complicate narcolepsy.

Treatment

Treatment consists of both nonpharmacological and pharmacological interventions. Nonpharmacological interventions involve maximizing nighttime sleep, supplemented by scheduled daytime naps, and avoiding emotional situations that precipitate attacks. However, patients usually require pharmacological treatment with stimulants such as methylphenidate or the nonstimulant agent modafinil and anticataplexy agents such as tricyclic antidepressants (eg, protriptyline, clomipramine) or selective serotonin reuptake inhibitors (eg, fluoxetine, venlafaxine, paroxetine).

Chesson AL Jr et al: Practice parameters for the treatment of restless legs syndrome and periodic limb movement disorder. Sleep 1999;22:961. [PMID 10566915]

Douglas NJ: "Why am I sleepy?" Sorting the somnolent. Am J Respir Crit Care Med 2001;163:1310. [PMID: 11371393]

Hening W et al: The treatment of restless legs syndrome and periodic limb movement disorder. Sleep 1999;22:970.[PMID 10566916]

Namen AM et al: I SNORED: An acronym of sleep disordered breathing symptoms. Am J Respir Crit Care Med 2001;163:A387. [No PMID available]

CIRCADIAN RHYTHM DISORDERS

General Considerations

The cause of a circadian rhythm sleep disorder may be obvious and transient, as in time zone change (jet lag) syndrome, or more prolonged. Correlations have been made between changes in circadian rhythms and advancing age.

Clinical Findings

A. SYMPTOMS & SIGNS

Commonly, older people experience an advanced sleep phase, which leads to a pattern of an early bedtime and early morning awakening. The alteration in circadian rhythm can be marked in people who are bed bound. When the internal clock is completely desynchronized, the sleep–wake cycles become irregular, with sleep occurring during the day and wakefulness at night or alternating periods of sleep and wakefulness throughout the 24-h period.

B. SPECIAL TESTS

Polysomnography may be indicated when a persistent circadian rhythm disorder is suspected.

Treatment

Bright light exposure (eg, at ≥2500 lux) in the evening or late afternoon has been recommended as a treatment for an advanced sleep phase. Melatonin has been used to prevent and treat zone change syndrome and appears to have some efficacy in doses of 0.5–5 mg taken close to the target bedtime of the destination.

REM SLEEP BEHAVIOR DISORDER

 ESSENTIALS OF DIAGNOSIS

- Acting out dreams with movements and behaviors.
- May present with injury in patient or bed partner.
- Often associated with other neurological disorders, such as dementia and Parkinson's disease.
- Diagnosis is made by polysomnography.

General Considerations

REM sleep behavior disorder (RBD) is an REM parasomnia. Although rare in the general population, it can present in late life and occurs more commonly in men than women.

Clinical Findings

A. SYMPTOMS & SIGNS

The normal muscle atonia present during REM sleep is lost. Patients act out their lively dreams with forceful movements and behaviors during sleep. They usually present for medical care as a result of injury to themselves or their bed partners, ranging from ecchymoses to fractures. RBD has been associated with multiple central nervous system disorders, including dementia, Parkinson's disease, and progressive supranuclear palsy. RBD may precede the typical symptoms of these conditions by as many as 10 years. In addition, medications used to treat these disorders, such as cholinergic agents for Alzheimer's disease, seligiline for Parkinson's disease, and some antidepressants, have been associated with RBD.

B. SPECIAL TESTS

Polysomnography is used to confirm the diagnosis and to rule out other conditions, such as sleep apnea.

Treatment

RBD has been successfully treated with removal of the offending agent or administration of clonazepam, which has been shown to effectively suppress the abnormal sleep behaviors in up to 90% of cases. The usual starting dose of clonazepam is 0.5 mg at bedtime, increasing to 1 mg as needed. Tolerance to the therapeutic effects of clonazepam for RBD does not appear to develop over time. However, the diagnosis of RBD must be made polysomnographically before instituting chronic treatment, particularly in older patients.

SLEEP PROBLEMS IN SPECIAL POPULATIONS

Sleep Pattern in Dementia

Most research on sleep problems with dementia has focused on Alzheimer's disease. Compared with older people without dementia, those with dementia have more sleep disruption and arousals during the night along with more stage 1 and less stage 3 and stage 4 sleep. Lower sleep efficiency is also noted. Sundowning, a worsening of confusion or problematic behaviors at night, is sometimes classified as a sleep problem and is present in 12–20% of patients with dementia.

Polysomnography does not appear to be particularly effective in the diagnosis of sleep complaints related to dementia and other psychiatric disorders.

Sleep Disturbance in Nursing Home Residents

The common pattern of sleep disturbance among nursing home residents involves frequent nighttime arousals. Many factors seem to affect quality of sleep, including multiple physical illnesses and medications that can interfere with sleep, debility and inactivity, increased prevalence of primary sleep disorders, minimal sunlight exposure, and environmental factors, including frequent nighttime noise and light and disruptive nighttime nursing care activities.

Alessi CA, Schnelle JF: Approach to sleep disorders in the nursing home setting. Sleep Med Rev 2000;4:45. [No PMID available]

 EVIDENCE-BASED POINTS

- The American Academy of Sleep Medicine (AASM) Standards of Practice Committee recommends drug treatment only for individuals who meet diagnostic criteria for RLS/PLMD and have secondary insomnia or excessive sleepiness. Dopaminergic agents are the best studied and most successful agents for treatment of RLS and PLMD.
- The AASM Standards of Practice Committee recommends that providers screen for a history of sleep difficulty, focusing on common sleep disorders. Testing (such as polysomnography) should not be routinely used to screen or diagnose patients with sleep complaints, unless there are symptoms of a specific sleep disorder such as sleep apnea, periodic limb movements, narcolepsy, or violent behaviors during sleep.

RELEVANT WORLD WIDE WEB SITES

American Academy of Sleep Medicine: www.aasmnet.org

National Institutes of Health National Center on Sleep Disorders Research: www.nhlbi.nih.gov/sleep

Visual & Hearing Impairment   16

Timothy Lewis, MD, & Gregg Warshaw, MD

■ VISUAL IMPAIRMENT

General Considerations

Visual impairment, defined as best corrected visual acuity worse than 20/40 and better than 20/200 in the better seeing eye, increases rapidly with age, especially after age 75. Visual impairment often limits functional independence among older adults and correlates with physical disability, falls, social isolation, and depression. Blindness carries a range of definitions, from no vision at all to best corrected visual acuity < 20/200 in the better seeing eye.

The predominant age-related eye diseases causing visual impairment and blindness include age-related macular degeneration, cataract, diabetic retinopathy, and glaucoma. Whites most often have impairment or blindness from age-related macular degeneration, whereas blacks have higher rates of impairment and blindness from cataract, glaucoma, and diabetic retinopathy. Uncorrected refractive error is another prevalent cause of visual impairment that affects all age groups. Nearsightedness (myopia) is generally less frequent with age, whereas farsightedness (hyperopia) generally increases with age. About 33% of older individuals with acuity worse than 20/40 improve to 20/40 or better with correction of refractive error.

Clinical Findings

A. SYMPTOMS & SIGNS

Age-related eye changes include functional alterations in accommodation, acuity, refractive power, visual fields, contrast sensitivity, corneal sensation, dark adaptation, and tear production as well multiple structural changes (Table 16–1). Presbyopia, the progressive loss of lens accommodation for near vision, usually becomes apparent by 45 years of age. Individuals with presbyopia find it increasingly difficult to focus on near objects that appear blurred without use of convex lens.

B. SPECIAL TESTS

Visual acuity should be measured in each eye separately using a standard Snellen chart at 20 feet and a hand-held chart for checking near vision. The testing room should be adequately lighted, and glasses should be clean and properly aligned to optimize testing conditions. Evaluation should include inspection of the optic disk for cupping, color, and sharpness of margins. Evidence of arteriolar narrowing, hemorrhages, and exudates should also be noted during the retinal examination. Examination of the macula for pigmentary abnormalities suggestive of macular degeneration is also recommended. The nonophthalmologist's eye examination should also include inspection of the lids for entropion, ectropion, and blepharitis as well as penlight examination for corneal clarity, conjunctival redness, eyelash crusting, and pupillary reaction. Additionally, pupillary testing with the swinging flashlight test is recommended to rule out an afferent pupillary defect.

CATARACTS

ESSENTIALS OF DIAGNOSIS

- *A lens opacity that can be observed through a well-dilated pupil with an ophthalmoscope or slit lamp.*
- *Symptoms may include blurred vision, increased glare, multiple images, alterations in color, and streaking of lights at night.*
- *The 3 main types of cataract are nuclear, cortical, and posterior subcapsular.*

General Considerations

Cataracts are usually age related and are the leading cause of blindness in the world. Cataracts affect whites more frequently than other races, especially with increasing age. Severe contrast sensitivity impairment resulting from cataract disease increases at-fault automobile crash risk, even when affecting only 1 eye.

Pathogenesis

The pathogenesis of cataract formation is unknown, but its risk factors include advancing age, excessive exposure

Table 16–1. Age-related eye changes.

Functional
  Presbyopia
  Decreased refractive power
  Decreased dark adaptation
  Decreased contrast sensitivity
  Visual field constriction
  Decreased tear production, resulting in dry eyes
  Increased difficulty with upward gaze, convergence

Structural
  Lens enlargement, resulting in narrowing of the anterior
    chamber angle
  Decreased lens translucency resulting in decreased retinal
    illumination
  Increased lens stiffness and decreased curvature
  Rod cell loss
  Liquefaction of vitreous gel
  Loss of eyelid tone, resulting in entropion or ectropion
  Rising intraocular pressure

to sunlight, and smoking. Cataracts may also arise in the setting of eye trauma, toxic substance exposure, steroid medications, or systemic diseases such as diabetes.

Prevention

High-dose supplementation with antioxidant vitamins does not prevent the development or progression of age-related cataracts. The use of sunglasses and hats to block ultraviolet light (UV-B) and smoking cessation are recommended for cataract prevention. Most traumatic cataracts are preventable through the use of protective safety goggles.

Clinical Findings

A. SYMPTOMS & SIGNS

Symptoms include glare-related vision loss, difficulty with contrast sensitivity, and reduction of visual acuity. Color perception may be altered because of yellowish discoloration of the lens. A cataract produces characteristic alterations in the red reflex. A cortical cataract usually appears as peripheral dark opacities, some of which are commonly oriented radially against the red reflex. A posterior subcapsular cataract typically appears as a central area of irregular darkening of the red reflex. A dense nuclear sclerotic cataract appears as a dull gold reflection of light from the lens when the dilated pupil is viewed with a flashlight.

B. SCREENING TEST

The best method to identify older persons with clinically significant cataract is to obtain a history and per-

form a routine ophthalmological examination, including a visual acuity check. Individuals with abnormal visual acuity that does not correct with refraction need referral to an ophthalmologist for further evaluation. It is not beneficial to screen asymptomatic persons for cataracts because their detection at a preimpairment stage does not confer a more favorable prognosis.

Differential Diagnosis

The differential diagnosis of age-related cataracts includes other disorders that reduce vision and are associated with an altered red reflex. Principal among these is blood in the vitreous. Traumatic cataract is usually associated with a well-documented history of severe ocular injury, frequently an open globe injury. Intraocular diseases such as chronic uveitis, glaucoma, and retinal detachment are also associated with cataract development.

Complications

Glaucoma and lens-induced uveitis are unusual complications of cataract. Lens-induced uveitis requires extraction of the lens. Cataracts are associated with visual hallucinations in persons with Alzheimer's disease, although the role of cataract treatment as an adjunct to antipsychotic therapy in persons with dementia is unknown.

Treatment

A. EVOLUTION OF TECHNIQUES

Most individuals are acceptable candidates for cataract surgery, provided the intervention appears likely to restore vision to a satisfactory level. Acceptable candidates must be able to lie supine for 30 min or more and be free of unstable, life-threatening medical disorders. With current methods of clear cornea incision and topical anesthesia, even patients undergoing anticoagulation with coumadin are generally considered reasonable candidates. Cataract surgery is usually done in the outpatient setting and can be performed with minimal systemic medications.

Phacoemulsification (ultrasonic emulsification of the nucleus) is currently the procedure of choice for all routine cataract surgery. Visual rehabilitation takes about 1–3 weeks after phacoemulsification compared with 2–4 mo required for extracapsular cataract extraction. More than 90% of patients achieve a postoperative visual acuity of 20/40 or better.

B. INDICATIONS FOR SURGERY

Surgery is indicated if improved vision is considered attainable and would lead to improved functioning.

Surgery is unnecessary if the patient has sufficient vision to perform all important activities. When cataract surgery is indicated, visual acuity is usually 20/50 or worse. However, cataract surgery is sometimes indicated in the setting of lesser visual acuity loss when certain lens-induced diseases are present (eg, certain types of glaucoma or uveitis). Surgery may also be indicated if there is concomitant ocular disease (eg, diabetic retinopathy) that requires clear media to permit access to the retina for diagnosis or treatment.

Some patients may not benefit from cataract surgery because of preexisting cognitive problems. The decision whether to perform cataract surgery in patients with dementia should be guided by the expected impact on the individual's function and quality of life. If the demented patient is no longer reading or watching television because of cognitive impairment, improved vision is likely unnecessary. One should also consider whether cataract surgery would lessen disorientation, ambulatory fall risk, or troublesome visual hallucinations.

C. PREOPERATIVE CARE

Preoperative care should include a history and physical examination to assess the patient's perioperative medical needs. The recognition of unstable life-threatening medical conditions and factors that would preclude supine positioning for ≥ 30 min (ie, severe kyphoscoliosis or decompensated congestive heart failure) is critical. Routine preoperative tests (eg, 12-lead electrocardiogram, complete cell count, electrolytes, urea nitrogen, and creatinine) are generally unnecessary before cataract surgery and do not appear to reduce perioperative morbidity and mortality.

D. POSTOPERATIVE CARE

Prompt recognition of complications that may occur after cataract surgery is essential. The incidence of endophthalmitis is about ≤ 0.2% and may present with eye pain, conjunctival injection, or vision loss. Retinal detachment, occurring in ~0.1% of surgeries, may be heralded by photopsia (reported as sparks or flashes) and floaters. Both complications require immediate consultation with an eye surgeon. Opacification of the posterior lens capsule is a less serious complication that is easily treated with laser capsulotomy.

Prognosis

Age-related cataracts usually progress slowly over a period of years, and patients should be offered reassurance that they may never require surgery.

Age-Related Eye Disease Study Research Group: A randomized, placebo-controlled, clinical trial of high-dose supplementation with vitamins C and E and beta carotene for age-related cataract and vision loss: AREDS report no. 9. Arch Ophthalmol 2001;119:1439. [PMID: 11594943] (A lack of a protective effect of antioxidant vitamins on prevention of cataracts was demonstrated.)

Owsley C et al: Visual risk factors for crash involvement in older drivers with cataract. Arch Ophthalmol 2001;119:881. [PMID: 11405840] (Analysis of elevated crash risk among older drivers with cataract.)

Schein OD et al: The value of routine preoperative medical testing before cataract surgery. N Engl J Med 2000;342:168. [PMID: 10639542] (Routine medical testing before cataract surgery did not measurably increase safety.)

AGE-RELATED MACULAR DEGENERATION

 ESSENTIALS OF DIAGNOSIS

- *Characterized by degeneration of the macular retina, leading to symptoms of central vision loss or distortion.*
- *Often the first sign of the disease is the appearance of drusen, or yellow-white deposits apparent under the retina during the dilated eye exam.*

General Considerations

Age-related macular degeneration (AMD) damages central vision and is the leading cause of irreversible blindness in older adults. The cause is unknown, and the prevalence of AMD and its associated blindness more than triples by decade after age 70. The Age-Related Eye Disease Study Research Group confirmed other associations besides age, including race (usually white), gender (slight female predominance), family history, and history of smoking and hypertension. The disease is classified into 2 groups: atrophic (nonexudative/"dry") and neovascular (exudative/"wet"). The more severe neovascular form is responsible for ~90% of the legal blindness cases attributable to AMD.

Prevention

Smoking cessation and adequate hypertension control are recommended preventive measures for AMD. Supplementation with zinc plus antioxidants (vitamin C, vitamin E, and beta carotene) may provide a limited delay in the progression of AMD and in vision loss among patients with newly diagnosed AMD. Patients with well-established AMD featuring geographic atrophy or hemorrhagic-exudative lesions do not appear to benefit from such therapy. The risk of visual acuity loss in some persons with the neovascular form of AMD is reduced by laser photocoagulation and photodynamic therapy.

Clinical Findings

A. Symptoms & Signs

AMD results in the inability to read, drive, identify faces, or perceive details because of the loss of central macular vision. Individuals with AMD may be able to see seemingly small objects in their peripheral vision, even though they possess extensive central visual field loss. Patients can be reassured that AMD does not usually lead to total blindness because peripheral vision is usually spared. Eye involvement is usually bilateral but is frequently asymmetric. Symptoms include impaired color vision, darkened or empty areas in the visual fields (scotomas), and distortion of straight lines.

B. Funduscopic Findings

The primary retinal findings in AMD are yellow globular spots of proteinaceous material (drusen) that appear under the macular retina during dilated eye exam. As the disease progresses, chorioretinal atrophy occurs. In the neovascular form of the disease, abnormal vessels proliferate and leak fluid or blood. Fluorescence angiography may reveal the neovascular network responsible for the bleeding or exudation and provide information essential for treatment recommendations and prognostication.

Complications

Visual distortion and profound loss of central vision are the main complications of AMD. Patients should be instructed to obtain prompt ophthalmological evaluation when any visual changes occur. Patients with drusen are often instructed to look daily at an Amsler grid. This grid features a central dot on which the patient focuses separately with each eye. In the normal eye, no grid distortion appears. Perceived distortion or absence of grid lines (scotoma) may indicate fluid leakage beneath the macular retina from a choroidal neovascular membrane.

Treatment

There is no effective therapy for most patients with AMD. However, selected patients with neovascular AMD may benefit from focal photocoagulation or photodynamic therapy. Laser surgery is the main treatment

for neovascular AMD but is feasible only when the neovascular lesions are located a safe distance away from the center of the macula. The laser destroys the portion of the retina overlying the targeted vessels, leaving a permanent scotoma. The goal of laser photocoagulation therapy is to stabilize vision, although a significant proportion of patients who undergo laser therapy experience recurrent neovascularization. Patients with central vision loss affecting both eyes may benefit from referral for low-vision rehabilitation.

Prognosis

Most patients with macular drusen never experience significant central vision loss. Although regular ophthalmic examinations are generally recommended, there is no evidence that such practice is any better in terms of visual outcomes than that of having patients return promptly if they notice new visual symptoms. The natural course of neovascular AMD is toward permanent loss of central vision over a variable time period.

EVIDENCE-BASED POINTS

- The risk of visual acuity loss in small, highly selected subgroups of persons with newly detected neovascular AMD with an exudative-hemorrhagic macular lesion appears to be reduced by laser photocoagulation and photodynamic therapy.
- Prompt ophthalmic evaluation is necessary to assess the need for laser therapy whenever a patient with AMD experiences sudden vision loss.
- Hypertension and smoking are currently the only known modifiable risk factors for AMD development.

Age-Related Eye Disease Study Research Group: A randomized, placebo-controlled, clinical trial of high-dose supplementation with vitamins C and E, beta carotene, and zinc for age-related macular degeneration and vision loss: AREDS report no. 8. Arch Ophthalmol 2001;119:1417. [PMID: 11594942] (Recommends supplement of antioxidants plus zinc for select population of patients with AMD.)

Age-Related Eye Disease Study Research Group: Risk factors associated with age-related macular degeneration. A case-control study in the age-related eye disease study: Age-related eye disease study report number 3. Ophthalmology 2000;107:2224. [PMID: 11097601] (Reviews risk factors for AMD and suggests avoidance of smoking and control of hypertension to reduce risk for AMD.)

DIABETIC RETINOPATHY

ESSENTIALS OF DIAGNOSIS

- *Dilating the pupils is important when screening for the presence of diabetic retinopathy.*
- *Nonproliferative diabetic retinopathy is characterized by microaneurysms, intraretinal hemorrhages, hard exudates, macular edema, and cotton wool spots (retinal infarcts).*
- *Proliferative diabetic retinopathy is typified by neovascularization of the optic disk and retina, preretinal and vitreous hemorrhages, and development of fibrotic vitreoretinal bands, which lead to retinal wrinkling and tractional retinal detachment.*

General Considerations

Diabetic retinopathy is the third leading cause of adult blindness. The longer an individual has diabetes, the greater is the risk for diabetic retinopathy. Generally, patients who experience diabetic retinopathy have had diabetes for ≥ 20 years. Background diabetic retinopathy (BDR), also called nonproliferative diabetic retinopathy, is the initial stage. It involves loss of pericytes, capillary dilatation and associated microaneurysms, and capillary leakage, causing exudate and macular edema. The later stage, proliferative diabetic retinopathy (PDR), involves neovascularization accompanied by preretinal hemorrhage and contraction of the fibrovascular tissue.

Pathogenesis

Diabetic retinopathy is a progressive microangiopathy with characteristic small vessel damage and occlusion. The cause of the disease is not known, but it appears to involve hyperpermeability of involved vessels. In PDR, progressive retinal ischemia stimulates the formation of delicate new vessels that leak serum proteins.

Prevention

A. GLYCEMIC & BLOOD PRESSURE CONTROL

It has been proven that better glycemic control improved retinopathy outcomes in type 1 diabetics. In addition, the incidence of diabetic retinopathy among type 2 diabetics is strongly associated with glycemic and blood pressure control. Intensive insulin therapy in type 2 diabetics may reduce the relative risk of progressive retinopathy and result in a cost savings because of its beneficial effects on diabetic complications.

B. SCREENING & LASER PHOTOCOAGULATION

Detection and appropriate laser photocoagulation treatment of PDR have the potential to reduce visual loss in elderly patients with diabetes. Often-cited guidelines for diabetes care prescribe annual funduscopic examinations to screen for PDR and macular edema. However, the optimal screening interval for patients at low risk for diabetic eye complications has not been adequately determined. Patients with poor glycemic control (ie, hemoglobin $A_{1C} > 10.0\%$) are at the highest risk for diabetic retinopathy and benefit the most from aggressive annual screening. In lower risk patients (ie, those with good glycemic control, older age, and no retinopathy at baseline exam), simulation studies suggest that annual retinal screening produces little benefit that cannot be achieved with screening every 2–3 years.

Clinical Findings

A. SYMPTOMS & SIGNS

Symptoms of diabetic retinopathy include a decrease in visual acuity, contrast sensitivity, dark adaptation, and blue-yellow color perception. Visual field testing may show scotomas corresponding to areas of retinal edema and nonperfusion.

B. SPECIAL EXAMINATIONS

Diabetic retinopathy demonstrates significant variability over time; therefore, special retinal cameras are used to document details of the fundus for future comparisons. Fluorescein angiography assists in the evaluation of all forms of diabetic retinopathy and guides planning of laser treatment.

Differential Diagnosis

The differential diagnosis of diabetic retinopathy is quite extensive, including hypertensive retinopathy, branch and retinal vein occlusions, various inflammatory and autoimmune retinopathies, and even some toxicities to systemic medications. Hypertensive retinopathy is the main consideration. Accelerated hypertension can cause extensive retinopathy with hemorrhages and cotton wool spots similar to those seen in diabetic retinopathy.

Complications

A. VITREOUS HEMORRHAGE

In PDR fragile new blood vessels proliferate onto the posterior surface of the vitreous. When the vitreous starts to contract away from the retina, these blood vessels can bleed, causing massive vitreous hemorrhage, which may lead to sudden vision loss.

B. MACULAR EDEMA

This complication severely compromises visual acuity. It can occur at any level of background retinopathy or PDR. The macular retina becomes thickened (edematous), and hard exudates accumulate in the retina.

Treatment

Treatments for diabetic retinopathy vary depending on whether the patient has BDR, PDR, or both. BDR associated with macular edema in the presence of apparent or threatened visual impairment is currently treated with focal laser photocoagulation to intraretinal leak sites identified by fluorescein angiography. This treatment offers improved visual acuity in many cases. Once diagnosed with non-PDR, patients should be examined by an ophthalmologist for proliferative changes every 3–6 mo.

Moderate to severe PDR with mild to moderate vitreous hemorrhage, but without extensive vitreoretinal fibrosis or tractional retinal detachment, is currently treated by peripheral panretinal photocoagulation. This treatment induces regression of neovascularization of the optic disk and retina, which reduces the risk of severe vision loss. However, there is no compelling evidence that such treatment is beneficial in patients with mild PDR. Profound PDR with extensive vitreoretinal fibrosis, tractional retinal detachment, or dense recurring vitreous hemorrhage usually requires a surgical procedure known as posterior vitrectomy. In this procedure, intravitreal blood and vitreoretinal fibrous membranes are removed surgically.

Some patients have both BDR with clinically significant macular edema and moderate to severe PDR. Current evidence indicates that the BDR should be addressed initially and that treatment of the PDR should follow. This seems to provide a better visual outcome than treating both components simultaneously or performing panretinal photocoagulation first and focal laser treatment for macular edema second.

Prognosis

Most persons with type 1 diabetes eventually experience diabetic retinopathy. In the UKPDS trial of type 2 diabetic patients, the incidence of retinopathy after 6 years in patients with no retinopathy at baseline was about 1 in 5. In the same study, nearly 33% of patients with retinopathy at baseline experienced progressively greater retinopathy over 6 years.

EVIDENCE-BASED POINTS

- *Good glycemic control and aggressive treatment of hypertension in patients with diabetes help minimize the development and progression of diabetic retinopathy.*
- *The risk of developing severe visual loss from PDR and macular edema can be reduced significantly by the use of laser photocoagulation.*
- *It is cost-effective to perform periodic screening retinal exams in all patients with diabetes, and annual examinations are recommended, especially in those at increased risk for diabetic ocular disease (ie, hemoglobin $A_{1C} > 10\%$).*

Stratton IM et al: UKPDS 50: Risk factors for incidence and progression of retinopathy in type II diabetes over 6 years from diagnosis. Diabetologia 2001;44:156. [PMID: 11270671] (Provides data emphasizing the need for good glycemic and blood pressure control to minimize diabetic retinopathy.)

United Kingdom Prospective Diabetes Study Group: Tight blood pressure control and risk of macrovascular and microvascular complications in type 2 diabetes: UKPDS 38. BMJ 1998;12;317:703. [PMID: 9732337] (Tight blood pressure control minimizes microvascular complications in type 2 diabetes.)

Vijan S et al: Cost-utility analysis of screening intervals for diabetic retinopathy in patients with type 2 diabetes mellitus. JAMA 2000;283:889. [PMID: 10685713] (Analysis of the cost-utility of annual vs. less frequent screening intervals for diabetic retinopathy.)

Wake N et al: Cost-effectiveness of intensive insulin therapy for type 2 diabetes: A 10-year follow-up of the Kumamoto study. Diabetes Res Clin Pract 2000;48:201. [PMID: 10802159] (Prospective cost-effectiveness analysis of intensive insulin therapy regarding diabetic microvascular complications.)

GLAUCOMA

ESSENTIALS OF DIAGNOSIS

- *Diagnosis is based on optic disk examination, intraocular pressure, and visual field measurement.*
- *Diagnosis is made on the basis of routine periodic ophthalmoscopy and tonometry.*

General Considerations

Glaucoma is a group of diseases traditionally defined by a triad of signs, including at least 2 of the following: elevated intraocular pressure (IOP), optic disk cupping, and visual field loss. Secondary and congenital forms of glaucoma exist; however, primary glaucomas (open angle and closed angle) are the more prevalent forms in older populations. Primary open-angle glaucoma (POAG) is a chronic disease that accounts for > 90% of all cases, whereas primary closed-angle glaucoma accounts for < 10%.

The prevalence of POAG is greatest in black and Hispanic populations. Individuals with a positive family history of glaucoma have an estimated 3-fold increased risk.

Prevention

Vision loss resulting from glaucoma cannot be reversed, but its progression can be prevented by early diagnosis and treatment. Periodic glaucoma screening is critical for high-risk groups such as blacks, Hispanics, and those with a family history of glaucoma. The American Academy of Ophthalmology recommends periodic eye examinations to identify patients at risk for glaucoma. Current guidelines recommend screening every 2–4 years for patients aged 40–64 years and every 1–2 years for those ≥ 65 years.

Clinical Findings

A. Symptoms & Signs

The loss of vision is unnoticeable until a significant amount of nerve damage has occurred. In POAG symptoms may be subtle, consisting of blurred vision, halos around lights, and impaired dark adaptation. Classically, vision loss starts in the nasal field (temporal retina). In contrast, patients with acute primary closed-angle glaucoma may have blurred vision, severe headache, nausea, vomiting, corneal edema, and a mid-dilated pupil.

B. Special Examinations

1. Tonometry—Elevated IOP alone is neither sufficient nor necessary as a diagnostic criterion for glaucoma. In the normal eye, IOP ranges from 10–21 mm Hg. POAG can exist in individuals who have a normal IOP during 1 or more measurements. A patient identified as having isolated intraocular hypertension does not necessarily have POAG; however, such a patient should be monitored for POAG periodically.

2. Optic disk assessment & gonioscopy—Glaucomatous optic atrophy leads to enlargement of the optic disk cup and associated disk pallor. Optic disk cupping is also associated with nasal displacement of the retinal vessels on the disk. Asymmetry of the optic disks in size and shape, or a cup–disk ratio > 0.5 in the setting of elevated IOP is highly suggestive of glaucomatous atrophy.

Gonioscopy measures the anatomic configuration of the anterior chamber angle and determines whether the eye has an open angle or a closed angle.

3. Visual field examination—Periodic visual field examination is essential to the diagnosis and follow-up of glaucoma. The field loss pattern, progression, and correlation with optic disk changes aid in monitoring disease progression.

Differential Diagnosis

Acute primary angle closure glaucoma must be differentiated from other disorders that cause acute painful unilateral visual loss. Relevant conditions include inflammation of the iris, the ciliary body, and the anterior uveal tract, all of which cause mildly decreased vision, which is often associated with photophobia. All are diagnosed clinically with a slit-lamp examination. Acute conjunctivitis is also a diagnostic possibility, but, unlike closed-angle glaucoma, it manifests little or no pain and no vision loss.

Complications

If uncontrolled, glaucoma usually results in progressive visual loss. The rate and extent of visual loss depend greatly on the type of glaucoma and individual characteristics of the patient. In chronic POAG there appears to be 2 distinct groups of patients: (1) those who seem not to lose vision progressively or who lose vision slowly and to a limited extent over long periods of time if untreated or inadequately treated and (2) those who seem to worsen progressively even if appropriate treatment is provided in a timely manner.

Treatment

Treatments for glaucoma focus on lowering IOP. Several modern analyses have demonstrated the importance of IOP control in the reduction of visual field deterioration in open-angle glaucoma. The treatment goal is to stabilize visual field loss and optic nerve damage. Both medical and surgical therapies help to achieve this goal.

A. Medical Therapy

The majority of topically applied glaucoma medicines lower IOP through a reduction in aqueous production or resistance to outflow. Topically applied β-adrenergic antagonists have been a mainstay in the initial treatment of chronic POAG. The other major drug classes include α-adrenergic agonists, muscarinic agonists (ie, pilocarpine), and carbonic anhydrase inhibitors (topical or oral). In recent years, several new ocular hypotensive medications have become available, including prostaglandin analogs, carbonic anhydrase inhibitors, and combination drugs.

All the medications used to treat glaucoma can have clinically important local and systemic adverse effects in elderly patients (Table 16–2). It is, therefore, prudent to include ophthalmic medications in the routine medication review for all older adults. Nasolacrimal occlusion, a technique aimed at reducing the risk of adverse systemic effects from topical eye medications, is difficult for older patients possessing limited dexterity.

B. Surgical Therapy

Surgery may be used to lower IOP in patients refractory to medical therapy. The most common surgical procedure for this purpose is laser trabeculoplasty. Additional measures may be necessary, including continued topical medications or filtering operations such as iridectomy or trabeculectomy.

Prognosis

Without treatment open-angle glaucoma may progress insidiously to complete blindness. Patients with medically controlled IOP that is achieved before the occurrence of extensive glaucomatous damage have a good prognosis.

Kwon YH et al: Rate of visual field loss and long-term visual outcome in primary open-angle glaucoma. Am J Ophthalmol 2001;132:47. [PMID: 11438053] (Lower IOP proved to be associated with slower visual field decline.)

Weih LM et al: Prevalence and predictors of open-angle glaucoma: Results from the visual impairment project. Ophthalmology

Table 16–2. Topical ophthalmic agents used for glaucoma.

Class	Drugs	Usual dosage[a]	Adverse effects
Beta-adrenergic antagonists	Betaxolol (Betoptic)	0.5%, 1 drop twice daily	Bronchospasm, congestive heart failure, bradycardia, depression, impotence
	Levobunolol (Betagan)	0.5%, 1 drop once or twice daily	
	Timolol (Timoptic, Betimol)[b]	0.25% and 0.5% solution, 1 drop once or twice daily	
Sympathomimetics	Dipivefrin (various)	0.1%, 1 drop twice daily	Tachyarrhythmias, increased blood pressure, anxiety, headache, tremor, eye discomfort, papillary dilatation, allergic conjunctivitis
	Epinephrine (various)	0.25–2.0%, 1–2 drops once or twice daily	
Cholinergic miotics	Carbachol (various)	0.01–3.0%, 1–2 drops up to 3 times per day	Miosis, eye or brow pain, blurred vision, myopia, bronchospasm, pulmonary edema
	Pilocarpine (various)	1–10%, 1 drop three to four times daily	
Carbonic anhydrase inhibitors	Brinzolamide (Azopt)	1%, 1 drop three times daily	Stinging, blurred vision, blepharitis, bitter taste, alopecia, dry mouth
	Dorzolamide (Trusopt)	2%, 1 drop three times daily	
Prostaglandin analogs	Bimatoprost (Lumigan)	0.03%, 1 drop once daily	Increased iris pigmentation, conjunctival hyperemia, ocular irritation, infection (upper respiratory tract infections), headache, abnormal liver function tests, and hirsutism
	Latanoprost (Xalaten)	0.005%, 1 drop once or twice daily in the evening	
	Travoprost (Travatan)	0.004%, 1 drop once daily	
	Unoprostone isopropyl (Rescula)	0.15%, 1 drop twice daily	

[a]Concentration and dosage of medications must be adjusted to the response of the patient.
[b]Verapamil should be used with extreme caution in patients taking ophthalmic timolol because of the potential for additive effects on prolonging atrioventricular conduction, and causing hypotension and left ventricular failure.
From American Society of Health-System Pharmacists: Drug Information. American Society of Health-System Pharmacists, 2002. Used with permission.

2001;108:1966. [PMID: 11713063] (Strongest risk factor for glaucoma was a positive family history, after adjusting for age.)

OCULAR VASCULAR DISEASES

Vascular diseases such as retinal vascular occlusions and anterior ischemic optic neuropathy associated with temporal arteritis increase in frequency and severity in old age. These disorders can lead to catastrophic vision loss. Patients with giant cell (temporal) arteritis usually have systemic symptoms and signs. Occult giant cell arteritis initially presents with visual symptoms and ocular signs without any systemic symptoms or signs. Giant cell arteritis should be suspected in a patient with visual loss and clinical findings of arteritic anterior ischemic optic neuropathy, central retinal artery occlusion, or posterior ischemic optic neuropathy. Urgent corticosteroid administration is begun, followed by a diagnostic evaluation. The evaluation should include measurement of the sedimentation rate and C-reactive protein and biopsy of the temporal artery.

LOW-VISION REHABILITATION

Interventions for low vision can improve the outlook for many visually impaired older adults and reduce their sense of isolation. A low-vision evaluation by a professional is recommended. Numerous agencies serving the visually impaired (private or state supported) and organizations such as the American Academy of Ophthalmology, American Optometric Association, National Eye Institute, and Lighthouse International offer additional resources.

Low-vision aids and rehabilitation strategies are designed to enhance quality of life for the low-vision patient. Optical devices such as stand magnifiers, high-powered spectacles, hand magnifiers, and closed-circuit magnification systems enhance visual acuity by enlarging the retinal image. Nonoptical devices include large-print reading material, "talking books," and writing guides. The U.S. Library of Congress administers a free library program of braille and audio materials circulated to eligible borrowers by postage-free mail and publishes a directory of publishers and distributors of large-type books and periodicals. Reading devices such as the Kurzweil machine are available in some public institutions such as libraries. This machine reads typed print out loud in a synthesized voice to permit increased independence for visually impaired persons. In some cities, closed-circuit radio reading services offer daily newspapers, magazines, and books. Rehabilitation programs exist that provide mobility training and training for activities of daily living tailored to the visually impaired.

Sometimes the simple act of making patients aware of low-vision services opens opportunities that ultimately improve quality of life.

RELEVANT WORLD WIDE WEB SITES

American Academy of Ophthalmology: www.aao.org/news/eyenet (Provides informational pamphlets and resource list.)

Macular Degeneration International: www.maculardegeneration .org (Scientifically reviewed web site offering information and support for patients with AMD and their families; it includes information on low-vision aids.)

Lighthouse International: www.lighthouse.org (Features services such as a catalog of nonoptical devices and a guidebook for visually impaired older adults.)

National Eye Institute: www.nei.nih.gov (Lists helpful resources and provides information to low-vision individuals and their families and includes information on outreach programs aimed at health care professionals to increase awareness of low-vision issues and resources.)

National Eye Institute: Vision Problems in the U.S.—Prevalence of Adult Vision Impairment and Age-Related Eye Diseases in America: www.nei.nih.gov/eyedata (Detailed report on U.S. prevalence data regarding the 4 main eye diseases.)

■ HEARING IMPAIRMENT

General Considerations

More than 33% of individuals ≥ 65 years have hearing loss. The incidence of hearing loss is estimated to double per decade, beginning with 16% at 60 years of age and proceeding to 32% at 70 years and 64% at 80 years. When matched for age, males tend to have worse hearing than females.

A. THE AGING AUDITORY SYSTEM & PRESBYCUSIS

The most common pattern of hearing loss in older adults is presbycusis, a bilateral high-frequency sensorineural hearing loss that occurs with advancing age. Pure-tone threshold sensitivity diminishes with aging. Hearing declines gradually in the majority (97%) of the population; those older than 55 years lose hearing at a rate of 9 dB/decade. Hearing loss is also compounded by complex central auditory disability. This phenomenon appears at a mean age of 60 years but has great individual variation in its progression thereafter.

B. SPEECH DISCRIMINATION

Speech discrimination is also reduced with aging. Older persons generally have more difficulty understanding speech when there is any element of speech degradation or unfavorable signal-to-noise ratio, such as degraded pronunciation or transmission, rapid speech, or speech heard against a backdrop of other conversations. Speech recognition with simultaneous sentence competition begins to deteriorate slowly starting in the fourth decade of life, a decline that accelerates after the seventh decade.

Prevention

Patients should be screened for a history of excessive noise exposure and educated about the importance of noise avoidance and the use of hearing protective devices. Noise-induced hearing loss is permanent but largely preventable. It begins at the higher frequencies (3000–6000 Hz) and develops gradually as a consequence of cumulative exposure to excessive sound levels. Patients should be warned about work or recreational activities that generate excessive noise exposure such as lawn mowing (90 dB), stereo headphone use (100 dB), or firearm use (140–170 dB). Hearing loss can develop after chronic exposures equal to an average decibel level of 85 dB or higher for an 8-h period.

Hearing loss secondary to ototoxic drugs can be minimized by careful attention to proper drug dosing, patient risk profiles, and early recognition of ototoxicity. Common classes of ototoxic drugs are listed in Table 16–3. Sensorineural hearing loss associated with aminoglycosides or chemotherapeutic agents is permanent.

Clinical Findings

A. SYMPTOMS & SIGNS

Hearing loss is often heralded by its functional consequences, including diminished speech understanding, social isolation, mood alteration, and apparent decline in cognitive performance. The clinical signs and symptoms may occur insidiously. Therefore, identification of hearing impairment sometimes requires direct questioning under challenging listening conditions. The patient should be asked about difficulty hearing speech in large groups, soft voices, or telephone conversations. Collateral history from a spouse or other individuals familiar with the patient's hearing performance may be useful. Some patients deny hearing difficulty, fearing stigmatization associated with wearing a hearing aid. If symptoms are not acknowledged, diagnosis and treatment of hearing loss may be delayed until the impairment is well advanced.

B. SCREENING TESTS

No single screening procedure is ideal. Screening tests such as the whispered voice, the finger rub, and the tuning fork test have been studied with relatively few patients and examiners, and inadequate data exist regarding interobserver reliability and observer repeatability.

The Hearing Handicap Inventory for the Elderly–Screening Version (HHIE-S; Table 16–4) is a reliable and valid self-assessment inventory for identifying disabling hearing impairment among elderly patients in the ambulatory setting. The HHIE-S was found to have a

Table 16–3. Ototoxic medications.

Antibiotics
Aminoglycosides
Erythromycin
Tetracycline
Vancomycin
Antimalarials
Chloroquinine[a]
Quinine[a]
Antineoplastics
Cisplatin
Bleomycin
5-Fluorouracil
Nitrogen mustard
Salicylates
Aspirin[a]
Diuretics
Loop diuretics[a]

[a]Hearing loss and tinnitus are reversible with these agents.

Table 16–4. The hearing handicap inventory for the elderly–screening.

Does a hearing problem cause you to feel embarrassed when you meet new people?
Does a hearing problem cause you to feel frustrated when talking to a member of your family?
Do you have difficult hearing when someone speaks in a whisper?
Do you feel handicapped by a hearing problem?
Does a hearing problem cause you difficulty when visiting friends, relatives, or neighbors?
Does a hearing problem cause you to attend religious services less often than you would like?
Does a hearing problem cause you to have arguments with family members?
Does a hearing problem cause you difficulty when listening to television or radio?
Do you feel that any difficulty with your hearing limits/hampers your personal or social life?
Does a hearing problem cause you difficulty when in a restaurant with relatives or friends?

Answers are scored as yes (4), sometimes (2), and no (0). Total point range, 0–40; 0–8, no self-perceived handicap; 10–22, mild to moderate handicap; 24–40, significant handicap. Adapted with permission from Ventry IM, Weinstein BE: Identification of elderly people with hearing problems. ASHA 1983;25:37. Used with permission.

sensitivity of 76% and a specificity of 71% for scores of > 8 compared with the gold standard of pure-tone audiometry. The HHIE-S is easy to use in general practice, and the resulting interventions reduce hearing handicap. Self-assessment inventories appear to have an advantage over pure-tone audiometry in identifying patients who are willing to accept further evaluation and treatment.

A more reliable, practical, and accurate screening method uses a portable audiometer housed within an otoscope or connected to earphones. The audiometer presents pure tones at 500, 1000, 2000, and 4000 Hz. Using a 40-dB definition of hearing impairment as the gold standard, one such device (Audioscope; Welch Allyn, Inc.) has a sensitivity ranging from 87–96% and a specificity ranging from 70–90%.

C. Physical Examination

An important focus of the routine otological examination is the identification of reversible causes of conductive hearing loss. These include otitis externa, cerumen impaction, foreign objects obstructing the external auditory canal, and osteoma. Assessment of the integrity and mobility of the tympanic membrane is also indicated. Tuning fork tests such as the Rinne and the Weber tests allow differentiation of conductive and sensorineural hearing loss.

D. Audiological Evaluation

If office-based screening suggests hearing impairment, the patient should be referred to an audiologist for formal evaluation. An audiologist will perform an audiogram to answer the following 3 questions:

1. Is a sensorineural, conductive, or mixed hearing loss present?
2. Is the loss unilateral or bilateral?
3. At what frequencies (testing for octave frequencies of 250–8000 Hz) does the loss occur?

The vertical axis of the audiogram shows hearing level (HL) measured in decibels ranging from very soft 10 dB to a very loud 110 dB. The 0-dB pure-tone HL represents the average hearing sensitivity threshold for young adults. The horizontal axis specifies the frequencies of the presented pure tones. The most critical frequencies for speech reception and understanding are 500, 1000, 2000, and 3000 Hz.

The audiogram measures hearing levels for air conduction and bone conduction of pure tones at the specified frequencies in each ear separately. Air conduction testing measures the function of the entire auditory system from the ear canal through the middle ear to the cochlea and its afferent neural pathways to the brain. Therefore, loss in air conduction can be due to a disorder anywhere in the auditory system. To better locate

the anatomic site of the hearing disorder, pure-tone bone conduction is also performed. Sound transmitted via bone conduction bypasses the outer ear and middle ear. When hearing loss is identified by air conduction and bone conduction, a sensorineural hearing loss is present (Figure 16–1). When air conduction results suggest hearing loss but bone conduction results are normal, a conductive hearing loss is present.

A complete audiological assessment also measures speech sensitivity and speech discrimination. Assessment of the speech reception threshold (SRT) involves presenting 2-syllable words to 1 ear at a time and measuring the softest level at which 50% of the words can be identified. The SRT should be within 10 dB of the pure-tone average (PTA) thresholds of 500, 1000, and 2000 Hz and thus serves to verify the reliability of the pure-tone threshold levels. Speech discrimination is evaluated by presenting a list of monosyllabic words to each ear at a comfortable loudness (typically 40 dB above the PTA) and recording the percentage of correct responses. On a scale ranging from 0–100%, speech discrimination scores of 90–100% are considered normal. Better speech discrimination scores correlate with better prognosis for hearing aid success.

Pure-tone air conduction, bone conduction, SRT, and speech discrimination assessment constitute the es-

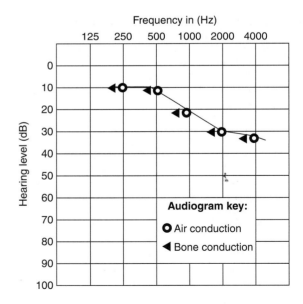

Figure 16–1. Audiogram illustrating sensorineural hearing loss. This pattern is typical of age-related hearing loss; the hearing level is normal for low frequencies but impaired for higher frequencies to a similar degree for air and bone conduction.

sential audiological testing for patients with hearing loss. Audiological procedures such as brainstem auditory evoked potentials, electrocochleography, and acoustic reflex testing are available for more specialized site-of-lesion testing. These specialized tests may be used when evaluating asymmetric sensorineural hearing loss, a suspected eighth nerve lesion, or a central auditory disorder.

Cochlear and eighth nerve lesions can be distinguished by immitance-based evaluation of the stapedius reflex. Brainstem auditory evoked potentials are used in the diagnosis of acoustic tumors. Referral to an otolaryngologist is recommended when a patient has a hearing impairment that is inconsistent with presbycusis, experiences acute or unilateral hearing loss, or has a speech discrimination impairment that is disproportionate to the degree of hearing loss.

Differential Diagnosis

Presbycusis is the predominant cause for hearing loss among older individuals. The other causes fall into 3 categories: sensorineural, conductive, and mixed loss. Mixed loss refers to a combination of conductive and sensorineural hearing loss. A variety of diseases cause hearing loss of each type (Table 16–5). Disorders of the outer ear and middle ear cause conductive hearing loss by disrupting the process of sound transmission via the external canal, tympanic membrane, and ossicular chain. Disorders of the inner ear cause sensorineural hearing loss by damaging the cochlea, eighth cranial nerve, or internal auditory canal.

A. OUTER EAR CAUSES

1. Infection—Infection of the external auditory canal (EAC) causes conductive hearing loss when there is resultant blockage of the external auditory canal. Typically, such blockage occurs as a result of inflammation and edema of the canal. Otitis externa causes ear pain and canal edema.

2. Tumors—Certain tumors can cause occlusion of the EAC, leading to conductive hearing loss. Canal tumors such as squamous carcinoma can be mistaken for otitis externa; the diagnosis is provided by biopsy.

A. MIDDLE EAR CAUSES

1. Infection—Otitis media, although more common in children, also causes conductive hearing loss in adults. The fluid that accumulates in the middle ear interferes with normal tympanic membrane vibration during sound transmission.

2. Tumors—Tumors of the middle ear (eg, squamous cell carcinoma) are rare compared with benign growths such as cholesteatoma. Management is surgical.

Table 16–5. Causes of hearing loss.

Conductive
Outer ear causes
External otitis
Trauma
Cerumen
Psoriasis
Osteoma
Exostosis
Squamous cell carcinoma
Middle ear causes
Otitis media
Tympanic membrane perforation
Cholesteatoma
Otosclerosis
Glomus tumors
Temporal bone trauma
Paget's disease
Sensorineural
Inner ear causes
Presbycusis
Noise exposure
Ménière's disease
Ototoxic drugs
Meningitis
Viral cochleitis
Barotrauma
Acoustic neuroma
Meningioma
Multiple sclerosis
Vascular Disease

3. Cholesteatoma—Symptoms such as hearing loss and recurrent ear drainage should prompt investigation for a cholesteatoma. By definition, a cholesteatoma is a growth of desquamated stratified squamous epithelium that originates on the surface of the eardrum and often becomes cystic as it grows within the middle ear. Its formation is associated with tympanic membrane trauma or abnormal retraction resulting from impaired eustachian tube function. Cholesteatoma can cause erosion of the ossicular chain and mastoid; subsequent complications include hearing loss, brain abscess, vertigo, and facial nerve paralysis. Management requires referral to an otolaryngologist for surgical treatment.

4. Otosclerosis—Otosclerosis refers to bony overgrowth affecting the footplate of the stapes, leading to its fixation and subsequent conductive hearing loss. Treatment involves either hearing amplification or stapedectomy. Systemic bone diseases such as Paget's disease and immunological diseases such as rheumatoid arthritis can also lead to conductive hearing loss.

5. Tympanic membrane perforation—A perforation of the tympanic membrane arises commonly from trauma or infection. The degree of conductive hearing loss depends on the location and size of the perforation. An audiogram is needed to measure hearing function. An inspection of the tympanic membrane is useful to identify skin that has become trapped on the undersurface of the tympanic membrane and could result in cholesteatoma formation.

6. Vascular—Benign paragangliomas such as glomus tympanicum or jugulare tumors arising in the middle ear can cause conductive hearing loss. On pneumoscopy, they often appear as a red, blanchable mass behind the tympanic membrane. In addition to hearing loss, they can cause bone erosion and damage to cranial nerves 7–12.

C. Inner Ear Causes

1. Presbycusis—Presbycusis is the most common type of hearing loss among the aged. Hearing loss that deviates from its characteristic pattern (bilateral, symmetric, high-frequency hearing loss) should prompt further otological evaluation.

2. Noise—Noise is the second most common cause of sensorineural hearing loss after presbycusis. Noise-induced hearing loss characteristically features a notched pattern of sensory threshold shift on the audiogram.

3. Infection—Both viral cochleitis and bacterial meningitis are causes of sensorineural hearing loss. Infection can cause profound hearing loss by destroying the cochlear inner hair cells, which are unable to regenerate in mammals. Treatment is sometimes possible with a cochlear implant. Viral cochleitis usually presents as sudden sensorineural hearing loss. Other causes of sudden hearing loss that should be considered include vascular ischemic events, acoustic neuroma, Ménière's disease, multiple sclerosis, and perilymph fistulas.

4. Ménière's disease—Ménière's disease causes hearing loss that is almost always low frequency and is typically episodic with periods of vertigo, hearing loss, tinnitus, and aural fullness. The associated hearing loss may become permanent over time and involve other frequencies.

5. Trauma—Trauma in the form of blunt head injury or barotrauma can cause inner ear as well as middle ear damage, leading to hearing loss. Transverse temporal bone fractures cause a fracture through the inner ear and result in a dead ear.

6. Tumors—Tumors of the inner ear are usually benign. Acoustic neuroma, the most common benign tumor in this region, originates from the eighth cranial nerve. Patients with an acoustic neuroma are most commonly either asymptomatic or complain of unilateral sensorineural hearing loss, although they can also have other symptoms such as unilateral tinnitus, dizziness, or headaches. Other tumors causing sensorineural hearing loss include meningioma and lipoma.

7. Endocrine & systemic—Metabolic abnormalities can cause sensorineural hearing loss. Diabetes, with its attendant small vessel disease, can cause cochlear ischemia. Other causes include hyperthyroidism and hypothyroidism and systemic illnesses such as syphilis.

8. Iatrogenic—The potential ototoxicity of medications assumes greater importance in older patients who receive a disproportionately high percentage of all prescription drugs. The aminoglycosides are the best known ototoxic drugs. Tobramycin and amikacin are more cochleotoxic, whereas gentamicin and streptomycin are more vestibulotoxic. Hearing levels should be monitored whenever ototoxic medications are administered.

9. Neurogenic—Stroke, transient ischemic attacks, multiple sclerosis, and Arnold-Chiari malformations are neurogenic causes of sensorineural hearing loss.

Complications

The complications of hearing impairment affect functional, emotional, social, and cognitive domains. Predisposed to social isolation and communication difficulties, individuals with hearing loss may experience depression or other mood disorders. A hearing-impaired individual can be mistaken to have dementia.

Treatment

Successful rehabilitation of elderly patients with hearing loss is a complex process performed by clinical audiologists. A holistic approach to this process involves consideration of patients' status in at least 4 domains: communication (auditory and audiovisual speech reception, hearing disability, and conversational fluency), physical (manual dexterity, general health, and visual status), psychological (attitude, depression, mental status, and motivation), and social (physical and social environments). The most important strategy for rehabilitation of hearing loss among the elderly is the hearing aid. Additional approaches include education in speech reading, auditory training, and use of assistive listening devices.

A. Hearing Aids

1. Efficacy—Hearing aids significantly improve the quality of life (eg, increase in social and emotional function and communication function and decrease in depression) of patients with sensorineural hearing loss.

Patients should be advised that acclimatization to hearing aids, and their full benefits, typically occurs after ≥ 1 mo.

2. Candidacy & audiology referral—The amount of hearing loss is less crucial than patient awareness and acceptance of hearing loss, communication difficulties, and motivation to try amplification. Patients with hearing loss not amenable to medical or surgical treatment (ie, presbycusis) should be referred to a clinical audiologist. The audiologist should recommend a type of hearing aid or aids based on the patient's hearing needs and goals, provide training in the use of amplification and other selected rehabilitative approaches, review the advantages and limitations of hearing aids, and provide supportive follow-up.

3. Selection & fitting—Selection and fitting procedures for hearing aids have become increasingly complex with the development of "high-tech" hearing aid features, including miniaturized styles, programmability, multimicrophone technology, and digital signal processing capabilities. With symmetric hearing loss, binaural hearing aid fitting provides the most benefit. Hearing aids come in several basic types, but all are designed to increase the intensity of sound and deliver it to the ear with maximal fidelity. Body hearing aids, now somewhat outdated, are the largest in size. They were traditionally used by persons with severe-profound hearing loss or those who lacked the dexterity to manipulate smaller hearing aids. Behind-the-ear (BTE) hearing aids have a case that fits behind the ear and conduct sound through a tube to an ear mold in the ear canal. Modern BTE hearing aids have greater amplification than the traditional body hearing aids.

In-the-ear (ITE) hearing aids are self-contained, fitting into the external ear, and are preferred by many patients because of their cosmetic appeal and ease of insertion and adjustment. In-the-canal hearing aids fit entirely into the outer portion of the ear canal and are even less visible. They provide sound amplification similar to most BTE and ITE hearing aids. However, they pose a problem for patients with dexterity problems because their tiny size hampers insertion and adjustment. Completely-in-the-canal hearing aids are the smallest and most expensive aids and fit entirely within the ear canal. They are suitable for patients with mild to moderate hearing impairment, good manual dexterity, and an ear canal free of adverse medical conditions.

Semi-implantable hearing aids were introduced in the late 1990s. These devices may eventually offer a reliable option for hearing-impaired patients who cannot wear an occlusive ear mold (eg, because of severe external otitis). A prototype model has a transducer that is attached directly to the ossicular chain and linked by telemetry to an externally worn audioprocessor.

Hearing aids also differ in their internal features and electronic circuitry and are classified as nonprogrammable, programmable analog, or digital. Terms used in the discussion of hearing aids, including circuitry options, are summarized in Table 16–6. Programmable hearing aids with a directional microphone have been found to be the most effective. However, the cost-effectiveness of hearing aids with advanced electronic features needs to be determined.

4. Cost—Audiology evaluations are covered by Medicare, but hearing aids are not. In many states, Medicaid will pay for hearing aids. The cost of hearing aids ranges from about $500–$3000. Digital hearing aids cost 2–3 times that of high-quality conventional analog aids. Programmable digital aids may be programmed to meet individual needs and adjust automatically to changing levels of environmental sound, but a midrange model costs about $1400.

B. COCHLEAR IMPLANTS

Cochlear implants have become widely accepted as a means of hearing rehabilitation in people with advanced sensorineural hearing loss who are unable to gain effective speech recognition with hearing aids. In appropriately selected patients, cochlear implantation improves communication ability and leads to positive psychological and social benefits; furthermore, the surgery appears to be safe and well tolerated in geriatric patients. Multichannel cochlear implants have been found to improve hearing-related quality of life and compare favorably with other accepted medical interventions in terms of cost-effectiveness (~$15,000 per quality-adjusted-life-year).

C. ASSISTIVE LISTENING DEVICES

In difficult listening situations, such as noisy public places, a variety of assistive listening devices (ALDs) are available to provide further benefit to hearing-impaired individuals. ALDs usually consist of a microphone placed close to the desired sound and a means by which sound is transmitted directly to the listener. Examples of ALDs include infrared or FM radio listening systems for televisions, stereos, concerts, and church sermons.

Some additional devices currently available to aid hearing-impaired individuals include amplified telephones that are hearing-aid compatible, portable telephone amplifiers, text telephones, signaling systems that make lamps flash on and off when the telephone or doorbell rings, vibrating alarm clocks, televisions with closed captioning, and flashing smoke detectors.

D. COMMUNICATION STRATEGIES

Individuals with hearing impairment can learn techniques that improve communication effectiveness, including speech reading. Speech reading uses interpreta-

Table 16–6. Hearing aid terminology.

Option	Description
Nonprogrammable hearing aid	Offers good sound quality at a reasonable price; limited flexibility in adjustments.
Programmable analog hearing aid	Digital/analog hybrid. Sound is converted to voltage waveform; the filtering process is programmable.
Digital hearing aid	Sound is converted to digital computer code, which undergoes processing via a digital signal processor.
Telecoil	Circuitry that helps people talk on telephone by converting eletromagnetic signal from telephone to amplified sound.
Compression	Circuitry that keeps loud sounds from being overamplified while dynamically increasing the volume of soft sounds.
Channels	Refers to the number of frequency bands into which the incoming signal is divided. Programmable aids with multiple channels can reduce the intensity of a loud low-pitched sound, with minimal effect on an incoming high-frequency channel.
Memories	Aids with multiple memories have several different signal processing schemes that are stored and can be selected by the user to suit differing listening situations (ie, quiet room vs. a situation with background noise).
Remote control	Allows remote adjustment of many hearing aid functions, such as on/off, volume, memories, telecoil.
Omnidirectional microphone	Picks up sounds form all directions (the standard microphone).
Directional microphone	Incorporates noise cancellation circuitry for improved speech understanding in noisy environments.

From Klein AJ, Weber PC: Hearing aids. Med Clin North Am 1999;83:139. Used with permission.

tion of lip movements, facial expressions, body movements, and gestures to enhance understanding of speech. Speech reading is usually taught together with hearing aid orientation by audiologists. Communication with hearing-impaired elderly persons is also facilitated when the speaker's face is in full view of the listener (within 2–3 ft), background noise is reduced, and speech is delivered with adequate pauses between sentences. One should avoid shouting and attempt to speak clearly at a slightly louder than normal intensity. When repetition is necessary, it is often most effective to paraphrase the message or write key words.

EVIDENCE-BASED POINTS

- *Hearing aids significantly improve the quality of life of patients with sensorineural hearing loss. Programmable hearing aids with directional microphones outperform less expensive nonprogrammable models.*
- *Cochlear implantation is a cost-effective means of auditory rehabilitation for individuals with advanced sensorineural hearing loss that cannot be adequately treated with hearing aids.*

RELEVANT WORLD WIDE WEB SITES

National Institute on Deafness and Other Communication Disorders: www.nidcd.nih.gov/ (This site provides a wealth of information on hearing disorders and is useful for laypersons and professionals. It also includes links to > 140 hearing-related organizations.)

REFERENCES

Vision

Munoz B et al: Causes of blindness and visual impairment in a population of older Americans: The Salisbury Eye Evaluation Study. Arch Ophthalmol 2000;118:819. [PMID: 10865321] (Current epidemiology of blindness and visual impairment in the United States.)

Rodriguez J et al: Causes of blindness and visual impairment in a population-based sample of U.S. Hispanics. Ophthalmology 2002;109:737. [PMID: 11927431] (Presents important epidemiology data on visual impairment in this growing ethnic population.)

Shingleton BJ et al: Blurred vision. N Engl J Med 2000;343:556. [PMID: 10954765] (Excellent review of blurred vision for the nonophthalmologist/primary care physician.)

Hearing

Buchman CA et al: Cochlear implants in the geriatric population: Benefits outweigh risks. Ear Nose Throat J 1999;78:489. [PMID: 11318481] (Review of cochlear implants' role in hearing rehabilitation.)

Hands S: Hearing loss in over-65s: Is routine questionnaire screening worthwhile? J Laryngol Otol 2000;114:661. [PMID: 11091826] (Prospective study of a practical hearing loss screening tool.)

Jennings CR, Jones NS: Presbycusis. J Laryngol Otol 2001;115:171. [PMID: 11244520] (Review of presbycusis and epidemiology of hearing loss.)

Johnson CE et al: A holistic model for matching high-tech hearing aid features to elderly patients. Am J Audio 2000;9:112. [PMID: 11200187] (Review of methods for matching hearing aid features to older patients based on a holistic model.)

Klein AJ, Weber PC: Hearing aids. Med Clin North Am 1999;83:139. [PMID: 9927966] (Review of modern hearing aid assessment and technologies.)

Mulrow CD, Lichtenstein MJ: Screening for hearing impairment in the elderly: Rationale and strategy. J Gen Intern Med 1991;6:249. [PMID: 2066832] (Classic evidence-based review of screening tests for hearing impairment.)

Palmer CS et al: A prospective study of the cost-utility of the multi-channel cochlear implant. Arch Otolaryngol Head Neck Surg 1999;125:1221. [PMID: 10555693] (Cost-utility analysis of cochlear implantation.)

Rabinowitz PM: Noise-induced hearing loss. Am Fam Physician 2000;61:2749. [PMID: 10821155] (Review of noise-induced hearing loss for the primary care physician.)

Ventry IM, Weinstein BE: Identification of elderly people with hearing problems. ASHA 1983;25:37. [PMID: 6626295] (Original presentation of the classic screening questionnaire, The Hearing Handicap Inventory for the Elderly-Screening Version.)

Welsh LW et al: Function of a hearing aid under stressful conditions. Ann Otol Rhinol Laryngol 2000;109:929. [PMID: 11051433] (Review of the aging auditory system and comparison of auditory function of normal persons to hearing-aided patients.)

Yueh B et al: Randomized trial of amplification strategies. Arch Otolaryngol Head Neck Surg 2001;127:1197. [PMID: 11587599] (Addresses the issue of whether technologies such as programmable circuits and directional microphones are worth the added expense.)

Syncope & Dizziness

David M. Sengstock, MD, MS, & Mark A. Supiano, MD

SYNCOPE

ESSENTIALS OF DIAGNOSIS

- *Sudden but brief loss of consciousness and postural tone with rapid recovery.*
- *Cardiovascular disorders cause most syncope and presyncope in the elderly.*
- *Syncope itself is not a diagnosis but rather a symptom of an underlying disorder.*

General Considerations

The incidence of syncope increases dramatically with advancing age. The incidence of syncope per 1000 person-years increases from 6 in the sixth decade of life to 11 in the seventh decade. The incidence is 17 and 20 for men and women, respectively, in the eighth decade. Almost 50% of emergency room visits for syncope are made by persons 65 years of age or older.

Clinical Findings

The diagnostic workup should be guided by clinical information obtained from the history and physical examination. Helpful historical information, physical examination findings, and ECG findings are listed in Table 17–1.

A. SYMPTOMS & SIGNS

The pathognomonic feature of syncope is a sudden loss of consciousness and postural tone resulting from a decrease in cerebral blood flow. The loss of consciousness is brief, and recovery is rapid and spontaneous. A patient who experiences both dizziness and an episode of fainting has sustained a syncopal event.

B. PATIENT HISTORY

History should include other syncope events, the patient's general medical problems, details of activities engaged in just before the syncopal event, and any associated symptoms.

Patients with a history of falls or fall-related injury should be assessed for preceding syncope to rule out a cardiac cause. All patients should be questioned about chest pain, palpitations, and dyspnea on exertion. An assessment of cardiac risk should include a family history of sudden or unexplained death. The patient's medication list should be carefully reviewed.

Information from witnesses, if available, provides a valuable complement to clinical history supplied by the patient. Although rhythmic movements may be seen during a syncopal event, witnesses will generally describe the patient as motionless and flaccid. Post-event confusion is not commonly seen with syncope; prolonged confusion is more consistent with a seizure.

Noncardiac causes for syncope occur much less frequently in elderly individuals but can still lead to considerable morbidity from falls. To elicit noncardiac causes, the patient should be asked about any associated activity such as coughing, urination/defecation, or eating. If an emotionally stressful event occurred just before the syncope, a vasovagal cause for the syncope should be considered. Associated warm feeling, diaphoresis, or flushing as well as gastrointestinal symptoms such as nausea support this diagnosis.

Examining the history of a sudden loss of consciousness can help differentiate psychiatric from vasovagal causes. Fainting accompanying an emotionally stressful event is not true syncope because the physiological vagal reflex does not occur in this condition. In the history, an individual with a psychiatric cause for fainting reports frequent attacks. Despite frequent events, there is no physical injury from a fall. Although seizure-like activity may also occur, loss of bowel/bladder control, injury, and postevent confusion are absent.

C. CARDIAC EXAMINATION

Cardiac examination should include assessment of the patient's carotid pulse. Delayed upstroke or low volume is consistent with aortic stenosis. Palpation for a displaced point of maximal impulse and extra sounds on auscultation raise the index of suspicion for cardiomyopathy. Auscultation may provide evidence for valvular heart disease. All patients should also undergo a resting

Table 17–1. Helpful history, physical examination, & ECG findings.

Variable	Description
History	
Risk factors	Diabetes, cardiac disease, prolonged bed rest, psychiatric history
Review	Medication list
Provoking situation	Emotional stress, frequent occurrence
Temporal	Acute onset, spontaneous recovery, postictal confusion
Prior activity	Cough, urination, defecation, swallowing, meal ingestion
Prior movement	Standing, head turn
General symptoms	Warmth, nausea, flushing
Cardiac symptoms	Chest pain, palpitations, dyspnea
Physical Examination	
Pulse	Delayed upstroke, low amplitude
Cardiac	Arrhythmia, displaced PMI, murmurs, S_3
Carotid	Bruits, carotid massage[a]
Neurologic	Focal deficits
Other examinations	Orthostatic blood pressure measurements, stool occult blood testing
ECG	
Acute changes or Q waves	Acute or previous myocardial infarction
Abnormal rhythm	Tachy/bradycardia, sick sinus syndrome
Abnormal interval	QT prolongation
Abnormal conduction	Heart block, bundle branch block

[a]Performed only when recent stroke, myocardial infarction, and bruits are absent.

electrocardiogram (ECG). Further evaluation will be guided by findings on examination and ECG.

D. LABORATORY TESTING

Clinical suspicion and differential diagnosis should guide laboratory testing. Hematocrit, electrolytes, and renal function tests are useful if anemia or volume depletion is suspected. However, routine testing has been shown to be of little diagnostic value. Likewise, more advanced testing such as cardiac enzymes should be reserved for situations in which the patient history supports a cardiac cause of syncope.

E. SPECIAL TESTS

1. Electrocardiography—An ECG should be part of the initial assessment for all patients with syncope. Although ECG establishes the definitive diagnosis in a minority of cases, it is relatively inexpensive and often provides useful information on the existence of organic heart disease, which may help guide future workup. ECGs can identify acute events such as myocardial infarction, arrhythmias, and conduction abnormalities. In addition, risk stratification can be done from ECG data because those with normal ECG have a favorable prognosis.

Further investigation should be based on data provided by history, examination, and ECG findings. If clear evidence for a cause is found, further assessment of that cause should be undertaken. Clinical suspicion of cardiac disease should prompt further workup.

2. Echocardiography—An echocardiogram rarely reveals significant abnormalities in individuals with normal histories and findings on physical examination. In addition, abnormalities that are uncovered may be incidental findings, unrelated to the cause of the syncopal event. Therefore, testing is reserved for patients with a clear indication, such as those with unexplained syncope but findings suggestive of valvular abnormalities. In patients with a history suggestive of an ischemic cause, stress echocardiogram may be preferable.

3. Ambulatory monitoring—Ambulatory ECG (Holter) monitoring should be reserved for patients with a history consistent with arrhythmia, such as a sudden loss of consciousness without prodrome. ECG abnormalities suggestive of arrhythmias may also warrant ambulatory monitoring. However, even in this select group, Holter monitoring may yield equivocal information. One study has shown that symptoms occurred in conjunction with arrhythmia in only 4% of patients referred for Holter monitoring. Only in this circumstance can arrhythmia be presumed as the cause for syncope.

4. Continuous-loop event recording—Continuous-loop event recorders can be used in patients with equivocal ambulatory ECG data when suspicion of arrhythmia remains. Monitors record data continuously until the patient experiences symptoms. The patient or a witness then activates the monitor to store the rhythm in the recorder's memory. An increased number of arrhythmias can be diagnosed using this method. However, this process requires considerable patient or caregiver compliance, which may limit the applicability of continuous-loop recorders.

5. Tilt-table testing—Tilt-table testing may be indicated for patients suspected of having noncardiac (neurally mediated) syncope. Although there are many variations in protocols, most commonly a patient is placed on a backboard and passively brought to a semiupright position at varying angles. Sudden hypotension and bradycardia are considered positive responses; these positive responses are believed to occur as a result of provocation of a vagal mechanism. Testing may be augmented by the addition of isoproterenol (after excluding cardiac disease) or nitroglycerin in patients who do not exhibit responses during initial tilting. Despite numerous attempts to standardize testing procedures, variations in the maximum angle used during tilt and choice of provocative agents (isoproterenol or nitroglycerin) remain. Furthermore, the reproducibility of positive findings in a geriatric population is variable, and false-positive rates have been reported to be as high as 65%. Thus, it may be difficult to interpret tilt-table testing results in geriatric populations.

6. Electrophysiological studies—Electrophysiological (EP) studies are recommended for patients with an unknown cause of syncope and ECG abnormalities or structural heart disease. Such evaluation may also be helpful when the history is consistent with cardiac syncope but stress testing and event monitoring do not yield definitive answers. The diagnostic yield of such studies approaches 50% in patients with a known history of heart disease. EP studies carry a low risk of complications. They are considered positive if the following are found: ventricular tachycardia, prolonged sinus recovery time, marked prolongation of His-ventricular intervals, infra-Hisian block, and supraventricular tachycardia with hypotension.

7. Neurological testing—Neurological testing is generally not recommended unless specifically warranted by history or physical examination. Electroencephalography (EEG) is diagnostic in < 2% of cases and, therefore, is recommended only in cases of suspected seizure.

8. Brain imaging, carotid ultrasonography, & magnetic resonance angiography—Brain imaging studies (computed tomography scan or magnetic resonance imaging) to assess for stroke or transient ischemic attack are recommended only if there is a history of seizure or if a neurological deficit is noted on physical examination.

9. Psychiatric examination—Psychiatric examination may be considered for patients with psychiatric histories or frequent syncopal episodes that do not cause injury. A hyperventilation maneuver may be useful in the diagnosis. However, a higher prevalence of cardiovascular disease in the elderly diminishes the predictive value of such tests. In general, a psychiatric cause for syncope should be considered a diagnosis of exclusion in a geriatric population.

Differential Diagnosis

Diagnostic considerations of syncope overlap with those of dizziness. Therefore, the initial step in the eval-

uation of syncope is distinguishing it from dizziness (Table 17–2). The differential diagnosis for syncope includes both benign and life-threatening conditions (Table 17–3). The majority of syncopal episodes in elderly patients is due to cardiovascular causes.

Transient ischemia and strokes increase in frequency with age, but these conditions generally do not lead to loss of consciousness unless there is an accompanying seizure. The frequency of movement-induced syncope also increases with age. For example, orthostasis affects 6–30% of ambulatory elderly patients, and its prevalence has been documented to increase with age. A syncopal episode may be the presenting sign of the condition.

Syncope can be associated with specific movements. Orthostatic hypotension should be considered when syncope occurs after moving from a recumbent to a standing position or after a prolonged stationary stand. The most commonly accepted definition of orthostasis is a decrease of > 20 mm Hg in systolic blood pressure or 10 mm Hg in diastolic blood pressure between supine and upright positions. Blood pressure should be measured in the recumbent position and then in the standing position at 1, 3, and 5 min because a fall in blood pressure may be delayed in the geriatric population.

Both carotid hypersensitivity and subclavian steal syndrome occur after head turning. Patients may report that symptoms are associated with neck pressure, including tight collars and neckties. Carotid massage may be used to detect induced atrioventricular block or other arrhythmias. However, a history of a recent stroke, myocardial infarction, and bruits on carotid examination are contraindications to this procedure. When testing for carotid hypersensitivity, continuous cardiac monitoring is a prudent precaution.

Seizure should not be overlooked as a cause for syncope because new onset of seizures is not uncommon after age 60. History of seizure and compliance with prescribed antiseizure medication should be discussed. History of an aura before the event, loss of conscious-

Table 17–2. Differentiating syncope & dizziness

Condition	Syncope	Dizziness/presyncope
Loss of consciousness	Yes	Absent
Onset of event	Abrupt	Protracted
Falls	Yes	Possible
Precipitated by stressful event	Yes	Possible
Aura before event	Possible	Possible
Bladder/bowel incontinence	Possible	Absent
Disorientation postevent	Yes	Absent

Table 17–3. Differential diagnosis of syncope.

Cause of syncope	Cause/characteristics
Situational	Vagal activity
Cough, toileting, swallowing, postprandial vasovagal	Associated only with activity
	Warmth, nausea
Movement induced	Cerebral perfusion deficit
Orthostatic hypotension	Standing, medications
Subclavian steal	Head turn
Carotid sinus hypersensitivity	Neck pressure/head turn
Psychiatric	Various causes
Anxiety/personality disorders	Frequent, no injury, no true LOC
Seizure	Neuronal discharge
Complex-partial epilepsy	Incontinence, postictal phase
Stroke with secondary seizure	Additional focal deficits
Cardiovascular	Decreased cardiac output
Myocardial infarction, Cardiomyopathy	Organic heart disease
Sinus node/pacemaker malfunction, heart block	Bradyarrhythmia induced
Ventricular/supraventricular tachycardia, torsades	Tachyarrhythmia induced
Aortic stenosis/dissection, pulmonary embolism, tamponade	Outflow obstruction

LOC, loss of consciousness.

ness, associated loss of bowel or bladder continence, and postictal confusion should be sought. Injury caused by an associated fall is also supportive. Apart from seizure, primary neurological causes for syncope are unusual. Transient ischemic attacks and stroke may produce loss of consciousness by causing a seizure and are generally accompanied by other neurological symptoms and focal findings.

Treatment

Treatment for patients with syncope should focus on the suspected underlying cause. Individuals with a cardiac cause are at risk for sudden death. Cardiac ischemia should be treated appropriately. Treatment options for arrhythmias may include pharmacological therapies or pacemaker insertion. Patients with compromised ventricular function have been shown to benefit from automatic implantable cardioverter defibrillators.

Movement-induced causes for syncope are often difficult to treat. Patients and caregivers should be educated about fall risk and lifestyle changes directed at minimizing risks. Individuals with carotid sinus hypersensitivity should avoid exacerbating factors, including tight collars or rapid neck movement. When postprandial hypotension is a problem, patients should avoid large meals as well as physical activity after eating. Patients with orthostatic hypotension should be trained to rise from supine and seated positions slowly to allow time for compensatory mechanisms and to avoid prolonged standing. Orthostatic hypotension can be exac-

erbated both by poor oral intake and by medications. One study found antihypertensives and antidepressants to be commonly associated with postural hypotension; antianginal agents, analgesics, and central nervous system depressants were also implicated. The need for these medications should, therefore, be reviewed and, if possible, the medication discontinued. Recommendations to increase fluid and salt intake can be considered, but caution is advised because hypertension may be exacerbated. Compression stockings and isometric leg exercises may be helpful. In those with particularly symptomatic episodes, fludrocortisone acetate, a synthetic mineralocorticoid, may be considered. However, efficacy data in the treatment of orthostasis are lacking.

Vasovagal events are best treated by avoidance of the trigger, if possible. If symptoms occur during toileting, safety devices such as a bathtub safety bar and a toilet seat with armrests can be recommended. Patients referred for tilt-table testing have been shown to benefit from a simple procedure of leg crossing and muscle tensing for 30 s at the onset of symptoms. Paroxetine has been shown to improve symptoms in vasovagal syncope; however, this has not been verified in a geriatric population. Pacemaker implantation as a therapy for vasovagal syncope has received considerable support. However, confirmatory studies are not yet available. Therefore, caution is advised when referring patients for pacemaker implantation.

Individuals with syncope that remains unexplained by all investigations may have a psychiatric condition. Elderly individuals with dizziness or syncope of any cause are at risk for traumatic injury. Falls represent a source of significant morbidity and mortality for elderly patients. The risk of automobile accidents is well recognized. Hazardous activity, such as driving, should be avoided during the evaluation period. Beyond this period, the length of time patients should refrain from driving is unclear; however, the American Heart Association recommends restricting a patient's driving privileges for several months.

Prognosis

Prognosis can be assessed by classifying patients as having cardiac, noncardiac, or unknown causes for syncope. Patients with cardiac problems have a much worse prognosis than those with a noncardiac or an unexplained cause.

Because the cause of syncope is not always determined and treatment options are limited, symptoms tend to recur: 15% of patients have a recurrence of syncope in an 18-mo follow-up. Patients with vasovagal syncope and those with unexplained syncope have approximately the same recurrence rates: 17% and 15%, respectively. Only 9% of the cardiac syncope patients have a recurrent episode; therapies aimed at the cardiac cause may influence recurrence rates.

EVIDENCE-BASED POINTS FOR SYNCOPE

- *Differentiation of syncope from dizziness is essential for both prognosis and evaluation strategy.*
- *Because the prevalence of cardiac disease increases with age, cardiac causes should be considered first, and all patients should have a detailed cardiac history and examination and an ECG.*
- *Morbidity resulting from falls and accidents justifies the need for evaluation and treatment of noncardiac syncope.*
- *Syncope from all causes tends to recur.*

DIZZINESS

ESSENTIALS OF DIAGNOSIS

- *Dizziness is defined by 4 symptom categories: vertigo, dysequilibrium, presyncope, and light-headedness.*

- *A single cause for dizziness is often not found, but symptoms usually resolve.*
- *Dizziness itself is not a diagnosis but rather a symptom of an underlying disorder.*

General Considerations

Dizziness is a common symptom that increases in prevalence with age. In the majority of patients, symptoms recur for at least 1 year. Despite the frequency and disabling nature of dizziness, < 50% of those seeking medical attention report relief.

Clinical Findings

The diagnostic workup should be guided by clinical information obtained from the history and physical examination. Helpful historical information, physical examination findings, and other specialized tests are listed in Table 17–4.

A. SYMPTOMS & SIGNS

Dizziness is generally defined by 4 categories of symptoms: (1) vertigo, or perception of movement; (2) dysequilibrium, or loss of balance without an abnormal sensation of movement; (3) presyncope, or feeling of impending loss of consciousness, (4) light-headedness, or vague symptoms that do not fall into any of the former 3 categories. It is important to note that these categories are nonspecific, and a disorder can present with any or all of these symptoms.

1. Vertigo—Vertigo is often due to a disorder of the peripheral labyrinth or its central connections. It is most commonly caused by a process affecting the peripheral vestibular system. Central causes, including stroke, are much less common and are usually accompanied by other deficits. On examination, peripheral vestibular disorders typically exhibit horizontal or rotary nystagmus, which develops after several seconds and diminishes with repeated tests. In contrast, central disorders exhibit immediate-onset vertical nystagmus and no attenuation over time. A central lesion caused by occlusion of the labyrinthine branch of the anterior inferior cerebellar artery will likely involve brainstem structures, which will result in specific neurological deficits. If the posterior inferior cerebellar artery is occluded, pontine or medullary structures would likely also be involved. Absence of cranial nerve or cerebellar deficits strongly argues against stroke.

Peripheral causes of vertigo are commonly accompanied by nausea, nystagmus, and postural instability. The most common peripheral causes of vertigo are

Table 17–4. History, physical examination, & further testing.

Variable	Description
"Don't miss"	Headaches, neurological deficits, syncope, melena, carbon monoxide exposure
Classification	Vertigo, dysequilibrium, presyncope, light-headedness
Review	Medication list
Associated symptoms	Depression, nausea, fluctuating hearing
Provoking situation	Emotional stress, frequent occurrence
Provoking activity	Standing, medication ingestion, turning of head, walking
Physical Examination	
ENT examination(s)	Otitis media, sinusitis
Ocular examination(s)	Nystagmus
Neurologic examination(s)	Focal deficits, Romberg test
Other examination(s)	Orthostatic blood pressure measurement, stool occult blood testing
Special examination(s)	Dix-Hallpike maneuver, gait analysis, depression screen
Specialized testing	
Further testing to consider	ENG, Neuroimaging, Audiometry

ENT, ear, nose, throat; ENG, electronystagmography

labyrinthitis, Ménière's disease, and benign positional vertigo. Acute labyrinthitis, also termed vestibular neuronitis or viral neuritis, is the most common of these. Vertigo caused by labyrinthitis develops over a period of days and generally resolves within about 1 week. However, a sense of unsteadiness may last considerably longer (weeks to months). Ménière's disease is typically characterized by low- and high- frequency hearing loss and tinnitus. Episodes of vertigo tend to recur and the hearing loss fluctuates.

Benign positional vertigo (BPV) is suggested by complaints of dizziness with a change in head position. The Dix-Hallpike maneuver is commonly used to screen for BPV and can be positive in as many as 44% of patients. This maneuver is performed by having the patient sit on the examination table with the head turned to one side. The patient is instructed to keep the eyes open throughout the test, even when dizziness is experienced. With the assistance of the examiner, the patient quickly lies down so that the ear faces downward. The examiner then checks for nystagmus. The test is repeated with the patient's head turned in the opposite direction. Hyperextension of the neck is often suggested but may not be possible because of arthritis or kyphosis. A positive test is indicated by horizontal or rotational nystagmus and symptoms of vertigo.

2. Dysequilibrium—This implies impairment of motor control, and patients describe a feeling of unsteadiness with standing or walking without sensations of vertigo. Patients do not generally complain of difficulties when sitting or lying down. Because elderly individuals may rely on compensatory mechanisms to maintain balance, they may report that low light, uneven ground, unfamiliar environments, or any condi-

tions disrupting these mechanisms accentuate dysequilibrium. Neurological impairment affecting motor control is believed to be the cause of dysequilibrium; however, visual problems can contribute. A gait analysis will be helpful.

3. Presyncope—This implies inadequate perfusion to the brain. The causes of presyncope generally overlap with those of syncope, and evaluation should proceed as for syncope, with the initial focus on cardiovascular evaluation. Orthostasis is a frequent cause of presyncope in the elderly.

4. Light-Headedness—This is a vague term that patients use to describe a wide array of sensations. The cause of this sensation may overlap with the other 3 categories of dizziness. In addition, metabolic disturbances (anemia, hypoglycemia, hypocarbia) may present. Asking the patient to hyperventilate for 30 s may reproduce symptoms. A careful history should be taken from individuals with a history of an anxious trigger, depressive symptoms, or previous treatment for depression because all of these factors are independently associated with dizziness symptoms.

B. Patient Assessment

Risk factors for dizziness (eg, cardiovascular or cerebrovascular disease, impaired hearing, orthostasis, anxiety or depression, multiple medications) should be sought. Inquiring about movements that elicit dizziness may reveal that symptoms are produced by moving from a recumbent to an upright position, rotating the neck, or walking. Associated symptoms of tinnitus, hearing changes, and nausea may help in the differential diagnosis. Symptoms of ear discomfort, sinus pain, hearing loss, and general malaise should be sought. The patient's medications should be carefully reviewed because they may be the cause of the dizziness.

C. LABORATORY TESTING

Routine laboratory testing is not recommended because it is generally of little value. However, complete blood count, serum electrolytes, blood urea nitrogen, and creatinine may be useful if anemia or volume depletion is under consideration. If metabolic causes of dizziness are suspected, appropriate blood tests should be ordered. Because dizziness can accompany any systemic viral or bacterial infection, laboratory evaluation for the suspected infection should be completed.

D. SPECIAL TESTS

1. Audiometry tests—These will often indicate isolated high-frequency hearing loss, a common condition in elderly individuals; however, this finding is of little use in the assessment of dizziness. Referral for audiometry can be useful when a patient has vertigo associated with fluctuating or unilateral hearing loss. Audiometric confirmation of a unilateral decrease in speech discrimination should prompt additional investigation, including auditory brainstem response (ABR) to assess retrocochlear pathways. If the ABR is abnormal, magnetic resonance imaging with gadolinium should be obtained to evaluate for acoustic neuroma.

2. Electronystagmography—Electronystagmography uses electrodes to detect nystagmus during head and eye movements and caloric testing. It has been recommended for all patients with prolonged dizziness to assess for vestibular dysfunction. However, the examination is uncomfortable and reportedly has a sensitivity as low as 29% for detecting vestibular disorders.

3. Cardiovascular testing—Specialized cardiovascular testing (stress tests and ECG) has not been useful in the general evaluation of dizziness. Cardiac evaluation should be reserved for patients with syncope or presyncope. Likewise, carotid testing should generally be re-

served for patients with a history or examination consistent with transient ischemic attacks.

4. Neuroimaging—Neuroimaging is generally recommended when an acute intracranial event is considered, such as a stroke or transient ischemic attack, or when the examination is not consistent with a peripheral cause for the vertigo. Imaging may also be considered in cases of refractory dizziness. EEG is generally useful only if seizure is suspected.

Differential Diagnosis

Dizziness is a nonspecific symptom, and most causes are benign and self-limited. Because dizziness is not usually an urgent problem, time is available to complete a structured evaluation. However, several diagnoses should be considered immediately when the patient first presents with dizziness (Table 17–5). Patients with presyncope who are at high risk for cardiac events should be evaluated urgently in the same manner as those with syncope. An intracranial or neurological cause such as meningitis or intracranial hemorrhage should be considered in those with dizziness and headache, especially when there is a history of infectious exposure or trauma. Anemia or volume depletion may present with dizziness, and a history of melena should be sought. Finally, carbon monoxide poisoning often presents with vague symptoms, including dizziness, and, therefore, should not be overlooked.

Treatment

A. GENERAL

All conditions in which treatment options are clear must be addressed. Depression, polypharmacy, and dehydration should be evaluated and treated appropriately. Efforts should also be directed at maximizing compensatory mechanisms. Vision should be evaluated, and patients should be encouraged to increase nighttime lighting. A cane or walker may be suggested for

Table 17–5. Differential diagnosis of dizziness.

Symptom	Possible mechanism	Diagnostic considerations
Vertigo	Disorders of labyrinth	Benign positional vertigo, labyrinthitis, Ménière's disease
	Disorders of central connections	Stroke, acoustic neuroma, mass lesion
Dysequilibrium	Impaired motor function	Peripheral neuropathy, arthritis, cerebellar disease, muscle weakness, impaired vision, medications
Presyncope	Inadequate cerebral perfusion	Orthostasis, carotid sinus hypersensitivity, cardiovascular disease, vagal reflex, medications
Light-headedness	Multiple	Any of the above, depression, anxiety

extra stability, especially for those at risk for falls. Physical therapy may be helpful when gait instability is a problem. Patients should use caution with driving or when falling is a risk. Although driving guidelines for dizzy patients are less stringent than for syncope patients, avoidance of driving is reasonable if symptoms occur continuously or unpredictably.

B. THE EPLEY PROCEDURE

The Epley procedure has become standard therapy for benign paroxysmal positional vertigo. The procedure attempts to induce dizziness, which, presumably, promotes compensation by the central nervous system. The patient is asked to sit on a bed with the head turned at a 45° angle. A pillow is placed so that, when the patient lies backward, it will be under the shoulders. The patient then lies backward quickly and waits for 30 s. The head is then turned to the opposite side, and the patient waits another 30 s. Finally, the patient rolls the body in the direction that he or she is facing and waits 30 s more. This should be carried out 3 (or more) times daily until vertigo is resolved.

C. VESTIBULAR REHABILITATION

In patients with chronic dizziness, referral for vestibular rehabilitation should be considered. Patients are asked to perform a number of eye, head, and body movements designed to reproduce dizziness. Although data supporting effectiveness are limited, a trial is reasonable because the procedure is noninvasive.

Attempts should be made to maximize functionality. Persistent dizziness can be distressing, and patients often report impairment in lifestyle because of concerns about physical harm resulting from falling, social embarrassment, and fears that symptoms signify a potentially serious illness. Alleviation of these fears should be considered an important goal. Reassurance and instruction in exercises have been shown to relieve concerns and improve functionality.

D. PHARMACOTHERAPY

Meclizine, benzodiazepines, and diphenhydramine have been recommended for the treatment of dizziness. However, the risk of sedation and falls argues against their use in older patients. Meclizine may be helpful in acute episodes of vertigo. However, its safety and effectiveness have not been proven. Therefore, its use in chronic or nonvertiginous dizziness is not recommended.

Prognosis

Dizziness usually resolves spontaneously over weeks to months. Patients should be reassured that serious disorders (brain tumor, stroke, cardiac arrhythmia) are rare.

EVIDENCE-BASED POINTS FOR DIZZINESS

- *Several important findings must not be missed when evaluating dizziness: syncope, signs of infection, mental status changes, neurological findings, and signs of fluid loss.*
- *Although the cause of dizziness often remains uncertain, the prognosis is generally favorable.*
- *Diagnosis is generally made by history and examination; laboratory and specialized testing should be used sparingly.*
- *A multifactorial approach to treatment that addresses physical/sensory impairments, polypharmacy, anxiety/depression, and poor access to fluids/nutrition will likely provide benefit.*

REFERENCES

Syncope

Bandinelli G et al: Disease-related syncope. Analysis of a community-based hospital registry. J Intern Med 2000;247:513. [PMID: 10792567]

Crane SD: Risk stratification of patients with syncope in an accident and emergency department. Emerg Med J 2002;19:23. [PMID: 11777866]

Getchell WS et al: Epidemiology of syncope in hospitalized patients. J Gen Intern Med 1999;14:677. [PMID: 10571716]

Kapoor WN: Syncope. N Engl J Med 2000;343:1856. [PMID: 11117979]

Kapoor WN et al: Psychiatric illnesses in patients with syncope. Am J Med 1995;99:505. [PMID: 7485208]

Linzer MD et al: Diagnosing syncope: Part 1. Value of history, physical examination and electrocardiography. Clinical Efficacy Assessment Project of the American College of Physicians. Ann Intern Med 1997;126:989. [PMID: 9182479]

Linzer M et al: Diagnosing syncope: Part 2. Unexplained syncope. Clinical Efficacy Assessment Project of the American College of Physicians. Ann Intern Med 1997;127:76. [PMID: 9214258]

Maddens M: Tilt-table testing in patients with syncope: What does it really tell us? J Am Geriatr Soc 2002;50:1451. [PMID: 12165007]

Raiha I et al: Prevalence, predisposing factors, and prognostic importance of postural hypotension. Arch Intern Med 1995; 155:930. [PMID: 7726701]

Sarasin FP et al: Prospective evaluation of patients with syncope: A population-based study. Am J Med 2001;111:177. [PMID: 11530027]

Soteriades ES et al: Incidence and prognosis of syncope. N Engl J Med 2002;347:878. [PMID: 12239256]

Youde J et al: A high diagnostic rate in older patients attending an integrated syncope clinic. J Am Geriatr Soc 2000;48:783. [PMID: 10894317]

Dizziness

Drachman DA: A 69-year-old man with chronic dizziness. JAMA 1998;30:2111. [PMID: 9875880]

Hoffman RM et al: Evaluating dizziness. Am J Med 1999;107:468. [PMID: 10569302]

Hotson JR, Baloh RW: Acute vestibular syndrome. N Engl J Med 1998;339:680. [PMID: 9725927]

Johansson M et al: Randomized controlled trial of vestibular rehabilitation combined with cognitive-behavioral therapy for dizziness in older people. Otolaryngol Head Neck Surg 2001; 125:151. [PMID: 11555746]

Lawson J et al: Diagnosis of geriatric patients with severe dizziness. J Am Geriatr Soc 1999;47:12. [PMID: 9920224]

Radtke A et al: A modified Epley's procedure for self-treatment of benign paroxysmal positional vertigo. Neurology 1999;53: 1358. [PMID: 10522903]

Rubin AM, Zafar SS: The assessment and management of the dizzy patient. Otolaryngol Clin North Am 2002;35:255. [PMID: 12391617]

Sloane PD et al: Dizziness: State of the science. Ann Intern Med 2001;134:823. [PMID: 11346317]

Tilvis RS et al: Postural hypotension and dizziness in a general aged population: A four-year follow-up of the Helsinki Aging Study. J Am Geriatr Soc 1996;44:809. [PMID: 8675929]

Tinetti ME et al: Dizziness among older adults: A possible geriatric syndrome. Ann Intern Med 2000;132:337. [PMID: 10691583]

Yardley L et al: Influence of beliefs about the consequences of dizziness on handicap in people with dizziness, and the effect of therapy on beliefs. J Psychosom Res 2001;50:1. [PMID: 11259793]

Cerebrovascular Disease

Enrique C. Leira, MD, & Harold P. Adams, Jr., MD

ESSENTIALS OF DIAGNOSIS

- *Stroke presents as a neurological deficit or headache of abrupt onset.*
- *Hemorrhagic strokes can be intracerebral or subarachnoid.*
- *Urgent neuroimaging studies are essential for diagnosis.*
- *Differential diagnosis must exclude nonvascular causes.*

General Considerations

Cerebrovascular disease is the third most frequent cause of death and the leading cause of disability in the United States. Stroke primarily affects the elderly. Given that the American population is aging, it is expected that the burden of disability from cerebrovascular diseases will continue to grow considerably. In the United States the majority of strokes result from insufficient blood perfusion in the brain (ischemic stroke), whereas bleeding that destroys and compresses the brain parenchyma or subarachnoid space (intracerebral or subarachnoid hemorrhage) accounts for ~20%.

Pathogenesis

There are 4 general mechanisms of ischemic stroke: arterial diseases, cardioembolism, hematological disorders, and systemic hypoperfusion (Table 18–1). Hemorrhagic stroke results from hypertension, vascular abnormalities, arteriopathies, coagulopathies, hemorrhagic transformation infarction, and brain tumors or metastasis (Table 18–2).

Clinical Findings

A. Signs & Symptoms

A stroke presents as an acute neurological deficit or an unusually severe, sudden headache. The neurological impairments reflect the area of the brain affected. Is-

chemic strokes and intracerebral hemorrhages present in a similar manner and are thus difficult to differentiate (Figure 18–1). Subarachnoid hemorrhages, however, often present as a sudden, explosive, very severe, unusual headache without other neurological signs.

Some clinical features suggest either ischemic stroke or hemorrhagic stroke. For example, in cerebral hemorrhages, the onset of the deficit tends to be very abrupt and is associated with a severe headache. The level of consciousness (LOC) on presentation can be a useful indicator: Patients with cerebral hemorrhage tend to have a more depressed LOC compared with those with ischemic stroke (Figure 18–2). Seizures at stroke onset are more common with intracerebral hemorrhage. Prominent nausea and vomiting also point to intracranial bleeding.

The presenting focal neurological symptoms are variable. Usually, a combination of motor, sensory, visual, coordination, cognitive, and language deficits is found. These deficits correlate with the site and size of the lesion. In ischemic stroke, the lesion should follow 1 or several arterial territories. The typical clinical presentation for the major forms of stroke is detailed in Table 18–3.

Subarachnoid hemorrhages typically present with an abrupt, uncharacteristically explosive headache, often during physical exertion (Figure 18–3). Nuchal rigidity may be present and reflects meningeal irritation. Depending on the extent of the hemorrhage, LOC can vary from normal (grade I) to deep coma (grade V). Focal neurological symptoms resulting from intraparenchymal extension of the hemorrhage, mass effect produced by the aneurysm, or early arterial vasospasm may be present. The abrupt central release of catecholamines, which occurs during a subarachnoid hemorrhage, can induce acute cardiac manifestations, including syncope, chest pain, arrhythmias, electrocardiographic (ECG) ischemic changes, cardiac enzyme elevation, and even cardiac arrest. Other confounding or nonspecific symptoms such as vertigo, malaise, diffuse aches, and leg or back pain can be present, adding to the difficulty in diagnosis.

B. Special Tests

The emergent tests required in the evaluation of every patient with suspected stroke include serum glucose,

Table 18–1. Causes of acute ischemic stroke.

A. Arterial diseases (hypoperfusion or artery-artery embolism)

Arteriosclerosis
    Extracranial vessels
    Intracranial large arteries
    Intracranial small perforating vessels
Arterial dissection
Vasculitis (systemic or isolated CNS)
Connective tissue disorders
Infectious (eg, neurosyphilis)
Hereditary (eg, CADASIL)
Vasospasm (eg, cocaine abuse)

B. Cardioembolism

Arrhythmia (eg, atrial fibrillation)
Structural cardiac abnormalities
    Valvular (eg, aortic stenosis)
    Myocardial wall (eg, akinetic segment)
    Chamber (eg, left atrial thrombus)
    Right–left shunt (eg, patent foramen ovale)
    Iatrogenic (eg, Prosthetic valve)
    Aortic arch arteriosclerosis
    Septic (eg, endocarditis)
    Neoplastic (eg, atrial myxoma)
    Paraneoplastic (eg, marantic endocarditis)

C. Hematological Disorders

Antiphospholipid antibody syndrome
Protein C, protein S deficiencies, factor V Leiden, prothrombin gene mutation
Hyperviscosity syndromes
Acquired hypercoagulable state (eg, secondary to neoplasm)
Sickel cell disease
Thrombocytosis
Polycythemia

D. General hypoperfusion

Cardiac arrest/syncope
Hypotension

CNS, central nervous system; CADASIL, cerebral autosomal dominant arteriopathy and subcortical ischemic leucoencephalopathy.

Table 18–2. Causes of hemorrhagic stroke.

Hypertension
    Idiopathic
    Drug induced (eg, cocaine)
Vascular abnormalities
    Arteriovenous malformations
    Aneurysms
Arteriopathies
    Amyloid angiopathy
    Primary angiitis central nervous system
    Cocaine vasculitis
Coagulopathies
    Liver disease
    Drug induced
        Anticoagulant therapy
        Thrombolytic therapy
        Chemotherapy
Hemorrhagic transformation infarction
Brain tumors/metastasis

Differential Diagnosis

The differential diagnosis of acute ischemic stroke and intracerebral hemorrhage includes subarachnoid hemorrhage, subdural/epidural hematoma, hypoglycemia, postictal (Todd's) paralysis, migraine, brain tumor/metastasis, encephalitis (eg, herpes simplex), brain abscess, demyelinating diseases (eg, multiple sclerosis), metabolic/infective/hypoxic encephalopathy (exacerbating latent deficit), and psychogenic paralysis/malingering. Postseizure paralysis can be difficult to differentiate from a stroke, especially if the seizure was not witnessed. The issue is further complicated by the fact that some strokes present with a seizure at onset. A diffusion-weighted MRI and an EEG may be helpful in this setting.

A serum glucose determination can be used to rule out hypoglycemia, which can be clinically indistinguishable from an ischemic stroke. Neuroimaging studies are necessary to differentiate between ischemic and hemorrhagic stroke. A lumbar puncture is mandatory for diagnosis when subarachnoid hemorrhage is suspected and the CT scan of the head is normal.

It is also necessary to differentiate strokes from subdural or epidural hematomas, tumors, and brain abscesses. Certain infections, such as herpes simplex encephalitis or cerebral abscesses, can mimic ischemic stroke.

Subarachnoid hemorrhage can imitate ischemic stroke if focal findings are present. Attacks of multiple sclerosis may also present like a stroke, but usually these exacerbations are more gradual in their presentation. Psychogenic paralysis can be difficult to diagnose but

prothrombin time, partial thromboplastin time, and electrolytes; complete cell and platelet blood count; ECG; noninvasive blood pressure monitoring; pulse oximeter/arterial blood gas; chest x-ray film; and unenhanced computed tomography (CT) or magnetic resonance imaging (MRI). Additional tests required emergently in selected patients include MRI/magnetic resonance angiography, cerebral angiogram, lumbar puncture, blood cultures (eg, suspected endocarditis), echocardiogram (eg, valve malfunction), electroencephalogram (EEG), pregnancy test, and neuroimaging studies.

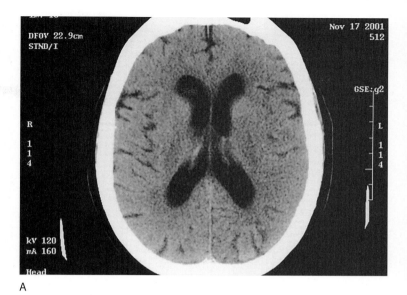

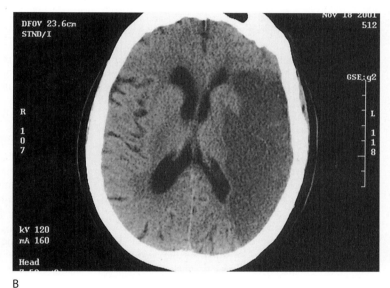

Figure 18–1. A. Computed tomography scan of a dense right hemiparesis and aphasia that started 2 h prior appears normal initially. B. Follow-up scan 24 h later shows a large infarction in the left middle artery distribution.

should be suspected in patients with unusual emotional attitudes and who present with deficits that do not follow the laws of neuroanatomy.

Complications

Early complications include extension of the infarction or hemorrhage and recurrent ischemic stroke. Hemorrhagic transformation of the infarction results from late reperfusion over a brain parenchyma with impaired vascular autoregulation. It is more commonly seen after large cardioembolic strokes and with the use of anticoagulants or thrombolytic agents. Brain edema is commonly noticeable after large infarctions. It usually reaches its maximum after 3–5 days in supratentorial lesions. However, in infratentorial strokes, brain edema can become symptomatic in the first 48 h as a result of compression of the brainstem and fourth ventricle, leading to obstructive hydrocephalus.

These complications share similar clinical manifestations: exacerbation of the previous neurological deficit, appearance of a new deficit, or a decrease in LOC.

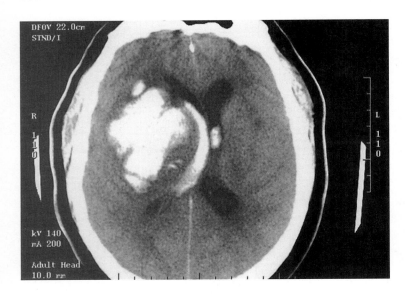

Figure 18–2. Computed tomography scan of a patient with lethargy and an abrupt left hemiparesis 1 h prior shows a large parenchymal hemorrhage that has ruptured into the lateral ventricle.

Seizures and poststroke depression are neurological complications typically seen later in the course of the stroke.

Aspiration pneumonia can occur whenever there is impaired swallowing function or decreased LOC. It usually manifests initially as a fever spike. Severe cases can lead to sepsis, respiratory failure, or acute respiratory distress syndrome. Urinary tract infection may occur, particularly in patients who require urinary catheterization. Deep venous thrombosis and pulmonary embolism often occur in immobilized patients.

Cardiac arrhythmias and myocardial infarction can follow a stroke. These events might be triggered by a central release of catecholamines. In addition, coronary artery disease and stroke share common risk factors. Falls are common in stroke patients who have gait abnormalities or who are confused or unaware of their neurological limitations. Constipation may also occur. Contractures in paralyzed limbs or pressure sores can occur as a late complication in patients who are not adequately mobilized. Early complications in stroke patients can be reduced by the implementation of the measures described in Table 18–4.

Rebleeding is a feared early complication of subarachnoid hemorrhage that justifies early identification and treatment of the aneurysm. Vasospasm typically occurs in the first week after the hemorrhage and can result in focal ischemic neurological deficits or decreased LOC. An increase in mean arterial velocities usually precedes the clinical symptoms of vasospasm. Therefore, a useful strategy in monitoring this complication is to perform repeated transcranial Doppler measurements. Communicating hydrocephalus results when blood interferes with the reabsorption of cerebrospinal fluid. It is usually manifested by a progressive deterioration in mental status. Hyponatremia and other electrolyte abnormalities can develop, leading to a worsening of the mental status and a lower seizure threshold. In addition, atelectasis, aspiration pneumonia, and gastric stress ulcers can also occur.

Treatment

A. Initial Management & Acute Ancillary Care

Table 18–5 summarizes the initial steps in the evaluation of patients with suspected stroke. The goal of any specific treatment for acute ischemic stroke is to save the area of brain tissue around the core of the infarction known as the ischemic penumbra, which is malfunctioning because of insufficient blood flow and is contributing to the total neurological deficit.

As in any other emergency, the management of acute stroke starts with assessment of the "ABC's": Airway, Breathing, Circulation. Most stroke patients do not require intubation or ventilatory support; however, those with intracerebral hemorrhage, large hemispheric infarctions, or severe brainstem lesions do. The decision to intubate is largely based on the assessment of LOC rather than respiratory parameters. Although some strokes require intubation for respiratory failure, in most instances, a decision to protect the airway is made based on the clinical likelihood of aspiration or obstruction. Acute assessment of the circulatory status includes ECG, blood pressure monitoring, and cardiac enzyme determination.

Table 18–6 summarizes the basic steps required in the general management of an acute stroke patient. Most patients with acute ischemic stroke have an ele-

Table 18-3. Symptoms of acute stroke depending on the site of the lesion.

Ischemic
  Carotid artery distribution
    Weakness (middle cerebral artery: face, arm > leg;
      anterior cerebral artery: leg > face, arm)
    Numbness (middle cerebral artery: face, arm > leg;
      anterior cerebral artery: leg > face, arm)
    Aphasia
    Dysarthria
    Hemineglect
    Visual field deficit
    Amaurosis fugax (internal carotid)
  Vertebrobasilar artery distribution
    Gait ataxia
    Dysmetria
    Dysarthria
    Dysphagia
    Nystagmus
    Vertigo
    Diplopia
    Hiccups
    Confusion
    Visual field deficits
    Weakness (including crossed findings)
    Numbness (including crossed findings)
Hemorrhagic
  Intracerebral hemorrhage
    Headache
    Lethargy/coma
    Focal symptoms similar to ischemic stroke (carotid or
      vertebrobasilar)
  Subarachnoid hemorrhage
    Severe unusual explosive headache
    Nuchal rigidity
    Lethargy/coma
    Cardiac symptoms (chest pain, syncope, arrhythmias)
    Neck, back, or leg pain
    Focal symptoms like intracerebral hemorrhage (if
      parenchymal extension, aneurysm mass effect, or
      vasospasm)

---

vated blood pressure. This elevation is usually transient and helps maintain perfusion in the ischemic penumbra. The ischemic penumbra has lost cerebral autoregulation, rendering the blood flow to that area of the brain perfusion dependent. A rapid reduction of blood pressure in a patient with moderate blood pressure elevation can result in an acute exacerbation of the neurological deficit and should be avoided. No treatment is recommended unless the mean arterial pressure is > 130 mm Hg or systolic pressure is > 220 mm Hg. Exceptions to this rule may involve cases of concomitant myocardial infarction, aortic dissection, or hypertensive end-organ damage. Another exception involves thrombolytic therapy, which requires a blood pressure < 185/110 mm Hg. If the elevated blood pressure needs to be treated, intravenous β-blocking agents are preferred because of their predictable response and minimal vasodilatory effect, a factor that could potentially worsen intracranial pressure. Labetalol should be avoided in stroke patients who are cocaine abusers. Other alternatives are sodium nitroprusside and hydralazine.

Acute stroke patients should not take food or liquid by mouth until the competency of the swallowing function is formally assessed, and intravenous fluids should be started. Peripheral intravenous access is preferred initially because central catheters constitute a relative contraindication for subsequent thrombolytic therapy. The patient should be kept flat in bed to avoid worsening of ischemia in potentially perfusion-dependent areas. Although oxygen supplementation is routinely used in the emergency setting, its usefulness is unproven.

The immediate assessment includes a rapid general and neurological exam (eg, National Institutes of Health Stroke Scale [NIHSS]) tailored to the stroke victim. The NIHSS is the standard method to evaluate stroke patients for thrombolytic therapy. The patient's NIHSS score ranges from 0 (normal) to 42, and the total score correlates with the size of the lesion and outcome at 3 mo.

B. Specific Therapies

1. Acute ischemic stroke—Acute ischemic stroke can be treated on 2 different fronts. One involves improving reperfusion, whereas the other is aimed at minimizing the neuronal damage triggered by the ischemic cascade.

Reperfusion therapy with intravenous recombinant tissue-type plasminogen activator (rt-PA) is the only approved treatment for ischemic stroke in the United States. Treatment with intravenous rt-PA increases the chances of a good outcome after an ischemic stroke if it is administered within a 3-h window. Not every case is eligible for this therapy. Patients who are candidates need to have a time of onset < 3 h, significant measurable neurological deficit, and symptoms attributed to cerebral ischemia. Table 18–7 summarizes the protocol for intravenous rt-PA treatment. Contraindications for TPA are summarized in Table 18–8.

Advanced age is not a contraindication for the use of rt-PA. However, the risk of intracerebral hemorrhage after rt-PA may increase with age. Therefore, one must use caution when administering rt-PA to elderly patients. Patients and families should be given a thorough explanation of the risks and benefits of rt-PA.

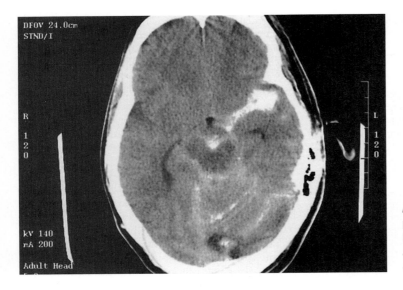

Figure 18–3. Computed tomography scan of a patient with an explosive headache and lethargy shows a subarachnoid hemorrhage that seems to originate in the left sylvian fissure.

Intra-arterial thrombolysis has the advantage of concentrating the agent at the occlusion site, which minimizes systemic bleeding. However, it is more complicated to perform because it requires the availability of emergent neurointerventional capabilities. Intra-arterial thrombolysis is an option for patients with angiographically proven major vessel occlusion and has a promising future either as an isolated therapy or in combination with intravenous thrombolysis ("bridging therapy").

Anticoagulant agents are a proven intervention in preventing recurrent cardioembolic strokes and pulmonary embolism in immobilized patients. However, they cannot be recommended to treat acute stroke in nonselected patients.

Treatment of early complications includes the use of antibiotics for aspiration pneumonia or sepsis, anticoagulants and pneumatic stocking devices, stool-bulking agents, early physical therapy, and early mobilization.

2. Hemorrhagic stroke—

a. Intracerebral hemorrhage—Intracerebral hemorrhage can be treated medically and surgically. Medical therapies include controlling arterial blood pressure, reducing intracerebral edema, preventing or treating medical complications, correcting contributing medical factors such as a bleeding diathesis, treating the specific medical cause (eg, vasculitis), and managing complications with medications such as anticonvulsants and antibiotics. Surgical interventions include ventriculostomy in patients with intraventricular extension or hydrocephalus; placement of a less invasive optic device to monitor intracranial pressure in comatose patients with poor neurological examinations; resection or embolization of an arteriovenous malformation; and evacuation of the hematoma to control increased intracranial pressure. The issue of whether hematoma evacuation is better than medical management is

Table 18–4. Measures to reduce complications after acute stroke.

Withhold feedings until swallowing function is assessed
Frequent neurological monitoring
Conservative management of blood pressure
Pneumatic compression devices or anticoagulants
   (immobilized patients)
Telemetry cardiac monitoring
Early mobilization and physical therapy
Mannitol (if evidence edema)
Antiepileptic agents (if seizures)
Antidepressant agents (if poststroke depression)

Table 18–5. Emergent evaluation of a patient with suspected stroke.

Assessment of airway, breathing, circulation
   Intubation when decreased level of consciousness
   Conservative blood pressure management
Brief history
Determination time of onset
Medications
National Institutes of Health Stroke Scale Examination
Ancillary tests
Screening for rtPA eligibility

Table 18–6. General management of patients with stroke.

Admission stroke unit/neuro-ICU
NPO/intravenous normal saline
Pneumatic leg stockings/subcutaneous anticoagulants
Blood pressure management
Ancillary tests for subtype determination
Speech/physical/occupational therapy consultations
Management of complications
Telemetry

ICU, intensive care unit; NPO, nothing by mouth.

controversial and is left to the preference of the treating physicians.

b. Subarachnoid hemorrhage—Early identification of the source of the bleeding, usually a ruptured saccular aneurysm, is critical to the treatment of subarachnoid hemorrhage. Management options include the surgical clipping of the aneurysm or intravascular embolization with metal coils. The location and shape of the aneurysm dictate which therapy is more appropriate. The patient is usually admitted to a neurointensive care unit and placed in "aneurysm precautions," which includes a quiet environment with no visitors in order to prevent rebleeding.

Complications of subarachnoid hemorrhage must be managed. Vasospasm can be treated with calcium channel antagonists (eg, nimodipine), hypervolemia-hemodilution-hypertensive therapy (triple H therapy), or cerebral angioplasty. Hydrocephalus may require frequent daily lumbar punctures for cerebrospinal fluid drainage or a lumboperitoneal shunt. Medical treatment of complications includes the correction of electrolyte abnormalities (eg, hyponatremia), antibiotics for pulmonary infections and sepsis, anticonvulsants for seizures, and mannitol infusions for cerebral edema.

Table 18–7. Protocol for use of intravenous rt-PA in acute ischemic stroke.

Total dose 0.9 mg/kg; maximum dose 90 mg
10% bolus, rest over 1 h
Avoid central, arterial catheters for 24 h
Avoid aspirin or anticoagulants for 24 h
Admit to ICU or stroke unit
Frequent blood pressure monitoring
Treat blood pressure > 185/110 mm Hg with intravenous labetalol
Neurochecks every hour

rt-PA, recombinant tissue-type plasminogen activator; ICU, intensive care unit.

Table 18–8. Contraindications for intravenous rt-PA in acute ischemic stroke.

Minor neurological deficit (NIHSS 1–2 points)
NIHSS > 22 points
Patient comatose
Deficit rapidly self-improving
Blood pressure > 185/110
Seizure at onset stroke
Abnormal CT brain (including "soft signs" of early ischemia)
Prolonged PT or PTT
Thrombocytopenia
Recent surgery, myocardial infarction, stroke, hemorrhage

rt-PA, recombinant tissue-type plasminogen activator.

C. SECONDARY PREVENTION STRATEGIES

Secondary prevention strategies in ischemic stroke should be initiated as soon as possible. The choice of strategy depends on the stroke subtype: large artery atherosclerosis (atherothrombotic), small vessel atherosclerosis (lacunar), cardioembolic, other cause, or undetermined cause. Table 18–9 lists common tests used to determine stroke subtype. Cardioembolic strokes, such as those secondary to atrial fibrillation and high-risk cardiac lesions, are better prevented by the use of oral anticoagulants. The benefit of anticoagulants for medium-risk or uncertain risk cardiac lesions, such as patent foramen ovale or atrial septal aneurysm, is not clear.

Antiplatelet agents are the first choice to prevent recurrent strokes in patients with noncardioembolic strokes. Available alternatives are aspirin, aspirin and dipyridamole, ticlopidine, and clopidogrel. Newer antiplatelet agents show a modest benefit over aspirin but

Table 18–9. Common investigations used to determine stroke subtype.

Magnetic resonance imaging
Magnetic resonance angiogram
Magnetic resonance venogram
Cerebral angiogram
Carotid duplex
Transcranial doppler
Echocardiogram (transthoracic or transesophagic)
Hematological testing
Rheumatological testing
Genetic testing
Drug screen
ESR
VDRL

ESR, erythrocyte sedimentation rate; VDRL, Venereal Disease Research Laboratories.

are more expensive or have side effects. Warfarin cannot be recommended as the first-line secondary prevention agent for patients whose strokes are not due to cardioembolism because it does not provide additional benefits compared with aspirin and has the potential for serious hemorrhagic complications. It is common practice to change the secondary prevention strategy after one agent fails, resulting in switching among different antiplatelet agents and anticoagulants after each recurrent vascular event despite the absence of supporting evidence.

A subgroup of patients with large artery arteriosclerosis may benefit from preventive surgical measures in addition to antiplatelet medical therapy. Large artery arteriosclerosis is subdivided into extracranial and intracranial disease. Patients with extracranial stenosis in the carotid artery have the option of endarterectomy. This strategy is proven for those patients with > 50% stenosis of the ipsilateral carotid artery. However, this strategy is effective only if the procedural complications (including surgery and angiogram) of death and disabling stroke can be kept at < 2%. Therefore, this approach may not be effective for high-risk medical patients or institutions without adequate experience. Age by itself is not an exclusion criterion for endarterectomy.

The technique of carotid angioplasty and stenting is an alternative to endarterectomy for patients with symptomatic carotid disease. Patients with intracranial stenosis may benefit from endovascular therapy with angioplasty and stenting.

Additional secondary prevention measures include adequate control of modifiable risk factors (in particular blood pressure), treatment of hypercholesterolemia, adequate control of diabetes, and avoidance of smoking. These measures can lower the risk of recurrent ischemic events.

Prognosis

Advanced age increases the risk of mortality after a stroke and is also a risk factor for recurrence. Disability is a more common outcome after ischemic stroke than death. The admission NIHSS score strongly predicts the outcome at 3 mo. For example, patients with an NIHSS score ranging from 0–3 have a 90% chance of a good or excellent outcome at 3 mo, whereas for those with scores ranging from 16–22 the percentage decreases to 12%.

EVIDENCE-BASED POINTS

- Intravenous rt-PA therapy is the only approved treatment available for acute ischemic stroke.

- Specialized stroke units improve outcome after an ischemic stroke.
- Aspirin and other antiplatelet drugs reduce the risk of recurrence in noncardioembolic strokes.
- Warfarin is indicated in the prevention of cardioembolic stroke (atrial fibrillation, high-risk cardiac lesions).
- Warfarin does not offer any advantage over aspirin in the prevention of noncardioembolic strokes.
- Carotid endarterectomy is a proven intervention to prevent stroke in patients with symptomatic stenosis of the carotid artery > 50%, provided that the perioperative morbidity and mortality can be kept to a minimum.
- Management of treatable risk factors is an effective measure in reducing recurrent strokes in high-risk patients.
- Anticoagulants reduce the risk of deep venous thrombosis after a cerebral infarction.
- Nimodipine is a useful agent in preventing vasospasm after a subarachnoid hemorrhage.

RELEVANT WORLD WIDE WEB SITES

American Stroke Association: www.strokeassociation.org
National Stroke Association: www.stroke.org
Stroke: stroke.ahajournals.org

REFERENCES

Adams HP Jr: Treating ischemic stroke as an emergency. Arch Neurol 1998;55:457. [PMID: 9561972]

Adams HP Jr et al: Baseline NIH Stroke Scale score strongly predicts outcome after stroke: A report of the Trial of Org 10172 in Acute Stroke Treatment (TOAST). Neurology 1999; 53:126. [PMID: 10408548]

Adams HP Jr et al: Classification of subtype of acute ischemic stroke. Definitions for use in a multicenter clinical trial. TOAST. Trial of Org 10172 in acute stroke treatment. Stroke 1993;24:35. [PMID: 7678184]

Adams HP Jr et al: Guidelines for the management of patients with acute ischemic stroke. A statement for healthcare professionals from a special writing group of the Stroke Council, American Heart Association. Circulation 1994; 90:1588. [PMID: 8087974]

Adams HP Jr et al: Guidelines for thrombolytic therapy for acute stroke: A supplement to the Guidelines for the Management of Patients With Acute Ischemic Stroke. A statement for healthcare professionals from a special writing group of the Stroke Council, American Heart Association. Stroke 1996; 27:1711. [PMID: 8784157]

Albers GW et al: Antithrombotic and thrombolytic therapy for ischemic stroke. Chest 2001;119(suppl):300S. [PMID: 11157656]

Antiplatelet Trialists' Collaboration: Collaborative overview of randomised trials of antiplatelet therapy: I. Prevention of death, myocardial infarction, and stroke by prolonged antiplatelet therapy in various categories of patients. BMJ 1994;308:81. [PMID: 8054013]

Barnett HJ et al: Benefit of carotid endarterectomy in patients with symptomatic moderate or severe stenosis. North American Symptomatic Carotid Endarterectomy Trial Collaborators. N Engl J Med 1998;339:1415. [PMID: 9811916]

Bath PM et al: Low-molecular-weight heparins and heparinoids in acute ischemic stroke: A meta-analysis of randomized controlled trials. Stroke 2000;31:1770. [PMID: 10884486]

Bath PM et al: Tinzaparin in acute ischaemic stroke (TAIST): A randomised aspirin-controlled trial. Lancet 2001;358:702. [PMID: 11551576]

Bosch J et al: Use of ramipril in preventing stroke: Double blind randomised trial. BMJ 2002;324:699. [PMID: 11909785]

Carotid and Vertebral Artery Transluminal Angioplasty Study: Endovascular versus surgical treatment in patients with carotid stenosis in the Carotid and Vertebral Artery Transluminal Angioplasty Study (CAVATAS): A randomised trial. Lancet 2001;357:1729. [PMID: 11403808]

Diener HC et al: Treatment of acute ischemic stroke with the low-molecular-weight heparin certoparin: Results of the TOPAS trial. Therapy of Patients With Acute Stroke (TOPAS) Investigators. Stroke 2001;32:22. [PMID: 11136909]

Evans A et al: Can differences in management processes explain different outcomes between stroke unit and stroke-team care? Lancet 2001;358:1586. [PMID: 11716885]

Fernandes HM et al: Surgery in intracerebral hemorrhage. The uncertainty continues. Stroke 2000;31:2511. [PMID: 11022087]

Furlan A et al: Intra-arterial prourokinase for acute ischemic stroke. The PROACT II study: A randomized controlled trial. Prolyse in acute cerebral thromboembolism. JAMA 1999;282:2003. [PMID: 10591382]

Goldstein LB: Should antihypertensive therapies be given to patients with acute ischemic stroke? Drug Saf 2000;22:13. [PMID: 10647973]

Hacke W et al: Intravenous thrombolysis with recombinant tissue plasminogen activator for acute hemispheric stroke. The European Cooperative Acute Stroke Study (ECASS). JAMA 1995;274:1017. [PMID: 7563451]

Hacke W et al: Randomised double-blind placebo-controlled trial of thrombolytic therapy with intravenous alteplase in acute ischaemic stroke (ECASS II). Lancet 1998;352:1245. [PMID: 9788453]

Hacke W et al: Thrombolysis in acute ischemic stroke: Controlled trials and clinical experience. Neurology 1999;53(suppl 4):S3. [PMID: 10532643]

Indredavik B et al: Stroke unit treatment improves long-term quality of life: A randomized controlled trial. Stroke 1998;29:895. [PMID: 9596231]

International Stroke Trial Collaborative Group: A randomised trial of aspirin, subcutaneous heparin, both, or neither among 19,435 patients with acute ischaemic stroke. Lancet 1997;349:1569. [PMID: 9174558]

Kalra L et al: Alternative strategies for stroke care: A prospective randomised controlled trial. Lancet 2000;356:894. [PMID: 11036894]

Kaste M: Thrombolysis in ischaemic stroke: Present and future: Role of combined therapy. Cerebrovasc Dis 2001;11 (suppl 1):55. [PMID: 11244201]

Larrue V et al: Risk factors for severe hemorrhagic transformation in ischemic stroke patients treated with recombinant tissue plasminogen activator: A secondary analysis of the European-Australasian Acute Stroke Study (ECASS II). Stroke 2001;32:438. [PMID: 11157179]

Le Roux PD, Winn HR: Management of the ruptured aneurysm. Neurosurg Clin North Am 1998;9:525. [PMID: 9668184]

Leira EC, Adams HP Jr: Management of acute ischemic stroke. Clin Geriatr Med 1999;15:701. [PMID: 10499931]

Lopez-Yunez et al: Protocol violations in community-based rt-PA stroke treatment are associated with symptomatic intracerebral hemorrhage. Stroke 2001;32:12. [PMID: 11136907]

Martinez-Vila E, Sieira PI: Current status and perspectives of neuroprotection in ischemic stroke treatment. Cerebrovasc Dis 2001;11(suppl 1):60. [PMID: 11240202]

Mohr JP et al: A comparison of warfarin and aspirin for the prevention of recurrent ischemic stroke. N Engl J Med 2001;345:1444. [PMID: 11794192]

National Institute of Neurological Disorders and Stroke rt-PA Stroke Study Group: Tissue plasminogen activator for acute ischemic stroke. N Engl J Med 1995;333:1581. [PMID: 7477192]

Publications Committee for the Trial of ORG 10172 in Acute Stroke Treatment (TOAST) Investigators: Low molecular weight heparinoid, ORG 10172 (danaparoid), and outcome after acute ischemic stroke: A randomized controlled trial. JAMA 1998;279:1265. [PMID: 9565006]

Sacco RL: Identifying patient populations at high risk for stroke. Neurology 1998;51(suppl 3):S27. [PMID: 98416078]

Sacco RL et al: Survival and recurrence following stroke. The Framingham Study. Stroke 1982;13:290. [PMID: 7080120]

Tong DC et al: Correlation of perfusion- and diffusion-weighted MRI with NIHSS score in acute (<6.5 hour) ischemic stroke. Neurology 1998;50:864. [PMID: 9566364]

van Gijn J, Rinkel GJ: Subarachnoid haemorrhage: Diagnosis, causes and management. Brain 2001;124(Pt 2):249. [PMID: 1157554]

Cardiac Disease

19

Michael W. Rich, MD

General Considerations

Cardiovascular diseases are the leading cause of death and major disability in both men and women in the United States, and the prevalence of cardiovascular disease increases progressively with age (Figure 19–1). Persons older than 65 account for 65% of all cardiovascular hospitalizations, and cardiovascular disease is also the most common primary diagnosis on admission to a nursing home. Older persons undergo a disproportionate number of cardiovascular procedures, and > 80% of all deaths attributable to cardiovascular disease occur in the 13% of the population older than 65. The prevalence of cardiovascular disease is similar in men and women after age 65, and women account for slightly more than 50% of all cardiovascular deaths.

The rising prevalence of cardiovascular disease with advancing age may be attributed to the cumulative effects of normal aging processes and cardiovascular risk factors.

A. Normal Aging

Normal aging is associated with extensive changes throughout the cardiovascular system that influence the epidemiology, clinical features, response to therapy, and prognosis of cardiovascular disorders in older adults. Table 19–1 summarizes the principal clinically relevant effects of normal cardiovascular aging. These changes markedly reduce cardiovascular reserve, leading to a progressive decline in peak cardiac performance, and predispose older adults to increased risk for cardiovascular complications and adverse outcomes in the presence of superimposed cardiac (eg, myocardial infarction [MI]) or noncardiac (eg, pneumonia, major surgery) conditions or procedures. Moreover, parallel age-related changes in other organ systems may further impair cardiovascular reserve or attenuate the benefit of therapeutic interventions. Finally, prevalent comorbid conditions and geriatric syndromes, polypharmacy, and an array of psychosocial, behavioral, and financial constraints may also impact presentation, compliance with prescribed treatment, and overall prognosis of older patients with cardiovascular disease.

B. Cardiovascular Risk Factors

Increasing age is the most powerful risk factor for cardiovascular disease in the United States. Other major risk factors for cardiovascular disease include hypertension, diabetes, dyslipidemia, smoking, physical inactivity, and obesity. Because the absolute number of incident cardiovascular events attributable to each of these risk factors (ie, population-attributable risk) tends to increase with age, the absolute benefit derived from treating specific risk factors is often greater in older adults. As a result, advanced age per se is rarely a contraindication to risk factor modification. In addition, because the total risk burden reflects the cumulative effects of risk factors as well as their duration and severity, and because older adults are more likely to have multiple risk factors of prolonged duration, the greatest potential benefit from aggressive risk factor modification occurs in high-risk older adults with multiple risk factors.

ACUTE MYOCARDIAL INFARCTION

 ESSENTIALS OF DIAGNOSIS

- Substernal chest discomfort lasting at least 30 min.
- ST-segment elevation or depression in 2 or more electrocardiographic leads with or without T-wave inversions or Q waves.
- Elevated levels of cardiac biomarkers, especially troponin I or T, or creatine kinase-MB.

General Considerations

Of the estimated 1.1 million recognized acute MIs occurring in the United States each year, 62% occur in persons 65 years of age or older and 37% occur in persons 75 years of age or older. In addition, case fatality rates increase markedly with age; 85% of all MI deaths occur in persons older than 65 and 60% occur in persons older than 75. Although the incidence of MI is higher in men than in women at all ages, the total number of MIs is similar in older men and women, reflecting the fact that the proportion of women in the surviv-

156

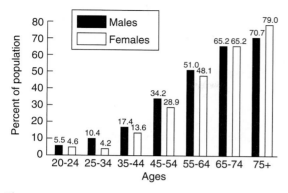

Figure 19–1. Prevalence of cardiovascular diseases in Americans.

ing population increases with age. The prevalence of silent or clinically unrecognized MI increases with age and may account for 25–30% of all MIs in the elderly. The long-term prognosis after clinically unrecognized MI is similar to that of recognized MI in older adults.

Prevention

Despite the high prevalence of coronary artery disease (CAD) and acute MI in industrialized countries, these disorders are potentially preventable through early and aggressive management of hypertension, dyslipidemia,

Table 19–1. Major effects of aging on the cardiovascular system.

Increased vascular stiffness
  Increased systolic blood pressure and pulse pressure
  Increased impedance to cardiac ejection (afterload)
Increased myocardial stiffness
  Impaired left ventricular filling
  Increased risk for heart failure with preserved left ventricular systolic function
  Increased risk for atrial fibrillation and other supraventricular arrhythmias
Diminished responsiveness to β-adrenergic stimulation
  Decreased heart rate reserve and maximum attainable heart rate
  Decreased contractile reserve
Endothelial dysfunction
  Increased risk for atherosclerosis
  Abnormal responses to physiological and pathological stimuli
Decline in sinus node function
  Increased risk for sick sinus syndrome
  Increased risk for atrial fibrillation and atrial flutter
  Impaired chronotropic responsiveness

and diabetes, combined with lifelong adherence to a pattern of behavior modification, including regular physical exercise; maintenance of desirable body weight; a diet rich in fruits, vegetables, and whole-grain products but low in cholesterol and saturated fats (including trans-saturated fats); and avoidance of tobacco products.

Aspirin, clopidogrel, β-blockers, angiotensin-converting enzyme inhibitors, and hepatic hydroxymethylglutaric coenzyme A (HMG CoA) reductase inhibitors (statins) have been shown to improve prognosis after acute MI. In addition, cardiac rehabilitation programs also reduce mortality and rehospitalizations after acute MI.

Clinical Findings

A. SYMPTOMS & SIGNS

The proportion of MI patients who have chest pain declines with age; < 50% of MI patients older than 80 complain of chest pain. Likewise, diaphoresis occurs less frequently in older patients with acute MI. Conversely, dyspnea, or acute shortness of breath, is often the presenting manifestation of acute MI in the elderly and is the most common initial symptom in persons older than 80. The prevalence of atypical symptoms, (eg, gastrointestinal disturbances, fatigue, dizziness, syncope, confusion, stroke) also increases with age, and up to 20% of patients older than 85 with acute MI have neurological complaints.

Physical findings associated with acute MI are nonspecific but may include an S_3 or S_4 gallop, new murmur of mitral regurgitation, or signs of pulmonary or systemic venous congestion, such as fine pulmonary rales or elevated jugular venous pressure. In patients with right ventricular infarction, Kussmaul's sign may be present.

B. ELECTROCARDIOGRAPHY

Classical electrocardiographic features of acute MI include ST-segment elevation of at least 1–2 mm in 2 or more contiguous leads corresponding to the anatomical distribution of the involved coronary artery (eg, leads II, III, AVF), with subsequent evolution of inverted T waves and pathological Q waves. However, the initial electrocardiogram (ECG) is often nondiagnostic in older adults because of preexisting conduction system disease (eg, left bundle branch block), presence of a ventricular pacemaker, prior MI or left ventricular (LV) hypertrophy, metabolic abnormalities or drug effects (eg, hypokalemia, digoxin), and the high prevalence of non-ST-elevation MI.

Atypical symptoms and physical findings, coupled with the high prevalence of nondiagnostic ECGs, often lead to delayed presentation and delayed recognition of acute MI. This increases the risk of complications and reduces the window of opportunity for effective intervention. Physicians should maintain a high index of suspicion for acute MI in all older patients with a wide range of unexplained cardiovascular, pulmonary, gastrointestinal, or neurological symptoms.

C. CARDIAC BIOMARKERS

Definitive diagnosis of acute MI requires documentation of an abnormal pattern of cardiac biomarkers. Troponins I and T have become the gold standard for diagnosis because of their greater sensitivity and specificity compared with the creatine kinase-MB (CK-MB) isoenzyme. Serial measures of biomarkers that exceed the normal range and exhibit a typical rise-and-fall pattern in a patient with clinical or electrocardiographic features of cardiac ischemia are diagnostic of acute MI. In the absence of recurrent ischemia, CK-MB levels peak at ~24 h after MI onset and return to normal within 48–72 h. Troponin levels usually peak at 24–72 h and may remain elevated for up to 2 weeks, especially in patients with large MIs.

Differential Diagnosis

The differential diagnosis of acute MI in the elderly includes other cardiovascular conditions as well as pulmonary, gastrointestinal, musculoskeletal, and neurological disorders. Major cardiovascular conditions that should be considered include unstable angina, aortic dissection, pericarditis, and acute pulmonary edema resulting from cardiomyopathy, valvular heart disease, or arrhythmia. Pulmonary disorders include pneumonia, pulmonary embolus, pleurisy, and pleural effusion. Gastrointestinal disorders include esophagitis or esophageal spasm, gastroesophageal reflux, peptic ulcer disease, cholelithiasis, and pancreatitis. Musculoskeletal disorders include muscular strains, costochondritis, injuries involving the cervical or thoracic spine, disorders of the shoulder joint, and chest wall trauma. Neurological conditions include stroke or transient ischemic attack, radiculopathy, and altered sensorium or delirium resulting from impaired cerebral blood flow or other causes. Psychogenic conditions, including anxiety reactions and hyperventilation syndrome, may also mimic the symptoms of acute MI.

Complications

Major complications of acute MI include heart failure (HF), hypotension, conduction disturbances (eg, bundle branch block), atrial fibrillation, myocardial rupture, and cardiogenic shock. Each of these complications is associated with worse prognosis and occurs 2–4 times more frequently in older patients. Although low-grade

ventricular arrhythmias (eg, frequent ventricular premature beats) occur more frequently in older patients, the incidence of primary ventricular fibrillation is lower.

Treatment

Table 19–2 lists the major therapeutic options for acute MI. Management of ST-elevation MI and non-ST-elevation MI differs with respect to the use of early reperfusion therapy but is otherwise similar.

A. GENERAL MEASURES

Maintenance of adequate arterial oxygenation and relief of chest discomfort are important goals. Supplemental oxygen should be provided to maintain a minimum arterial oxygen saturation of 90%. Intravenous morphine should be administered in 2- to 4-mg boluses as needed for relief of chest pain, monitoring closely for signs of respiratory depression, bradycardia, hypotension, and impaired sensorium. Sublingual nitroglycerin should be administered acutely for the treatment of ischemic chest pain or dyspnea. Patients with persistent chest pain or signs of pulmonary congestion should receive topical nitroglycerin or an intravenous nitroglycerin infusion, titrated to control symptoms while avoiding excessive blood pressure (BP) reduction (ie, systolic BP < 90 mm Hg, change in systolic BP from baseline > 20 mm Hg, or signs of hypoperfusion, such as impaired mental status). In patients with signs of right ventricular infarction

Table 19–2. Management of acute myocardial infarction.

General measures
    Oxygen to maintain arterial saturation ≥ 90%
    Morphine for pain and dyspnea
    Nitroglycerin for ischemia and heart failure
Reperfusion therapy
    Fibrinolysis
    Primary angioplasty/stenting
Antithrombotic therapy
    Aspirin
    Heparin/low-molecular-weight heparin
    Glycoprotein IIb/IIIa inhibitors
    Clopidogrel
β-blockers
Angiotensin-converting enzyme inhibitors
Other agents
    Nitrates
    Angiotensin receptor blockers
    Calcium channel blockers
    Lipid-lowering agents
    Antiarrhythmic agents
    Magnesium

(acute inferior MI with elevated jugular venous pressure, Kussmaul's sign, or ST elevation in right precordial leads), nitroglycerin may precipitate severe hypotension and should be given cautiously or avoided.

B. REPERFUSION THERAPY

Recanalization of the involved coronary artery within 6–12 h of MI onset substantially reduces mortality and morbid complications. Reperfusion can be achieved either pharmacologically, through the use of fibrinolytic agents, or mechanically, through the use of percutaneous coronary angioplasty with or without intracoronary stent implantation. In general, mechanical reperfusion is more effective than fibrinolysis. Intracranial hemorrhage occurs less frequently with mechanical reperfusion, particularly in patients older than 75, in whom the risk of intracranial bleeding is 1–2% with fibrinolytic therapy. Mechanical reperfusion has been shown to benefit patients with either ST-elevation or non-ST-elevation MI. Fibrinolytic therapy is only effective in ST-elevation MI and is contraindicated for the treatment of non-ST-elevation MI. Because of limited access to catheterization facilities, intravenous fibrinolysis is the most commonly used reperfusion strategy in the United States.

1. Fibrinolytic therapy—Currently, 5 fibrinolytic agents are approved for intravenous use for the treatment of acute MI in the United States: streptokinase, alteplase, anistreplase, reteplase, and tenecteplase (Table 19–3). Despite substantial clinical experience with these agents, the value of fibrinolytic therapy in patients older than 75 remains controversial. Use of fibrinolytic agents in this group should probably be restricted to those who fulfill criteria for fibrinolysis and who can be treated within 6 h of symptom onset (Table 19–4).

2. Percutaneous coronary angioplasty—Mechanical reperfusion (ie, percutaneous coronary intervention with or without stenting) is associated with improved outcomes in patients of all ages and may be superior to fibrinolysis in older patients. Early angiography and coronary intervention may be associated with improved short- and long-term outcomes in patients with either ST-elevation or non-ST-elevation infarctions. Consequently, mechanical reperfusion, if available, is now the preferred strategy in most older patients with documented acute MI.

C. ANTITHROMBOTIC THERAPY

1. Aspirin—Aspirin is indicated for all patients with acute coronary heart disease (CHD) regardless of age and should be continued indefinitely in all patients with documented CHD. The recommended dosage in the acute setting is 160–325 mg daily; dosages of 75–325 mg daily are suitable for long-term use.

2. Heparin—Intravenous unfractionated heparin is indicated in patients with acute MI complicated by recurrent ischemia, atrial fibrillation, or extensive damage to the anterior wall and apex of the heart. Heparin is also indicated in patients receiving a short-acting fibrinolytic agent (eg, recombinant tissue-type plasminogen activator) and those receiving a glycoprotein IIb/IIIa inhibitor. Routine use of intravenous heparin in other situations is of unproven benefit and may be associated with increased risk of bleeding complications and prolonged hospital stay.

Low-molecular-weight (LMW) heparins such as enoxaparin and dalteparin provide more stable anticoagulation than unfractionated heparin and offer the advantage of subcutaneous administration without the need to monitor activated partial thromboplastin time (aPTT). In addition, LMW heparins have been associated with improved clinical outcomes. LMW heparin therapy is indicated in all patients with non-ST-elevation MI, but the benefits in patients with ST-elevation MI are less well established.

3. Glycoprotein IIb/IIIa inhibitors—These agents are potent antiplatelet agents that block the final pathway leading to platelet aggregation; abciximab, integre-

Table 19–3. Properties of fibrinolytic agents.

Variable	Streptokinase	Alteplase	Anistreplase	Reteplase	Tenecteplase
Usual dose	1.5 MU	100 mg[a]	30 units	20 units	0.5 mg/kg
Plasma half-life (min)	20–30	4–8	90	15	20
Fibrin specificity	Low	High	Moderate	High	Very high
Reperfusion efficacy	Moderate	High	Moderate	Very high	High
Hemorrhagic stroke risk	Very low	Low	Very low	Low	Low
Major bleeding risk	Low	Low	Low	Low	Low
Allergic reactions	Yes	No	Yes	No	No
Cost	Low	High	High	High	High

[a]Weight adjusted.

Table 19–4. Criteria for fibrinolytic therapy in older adults.

Indications	Contraindications

Symptoms of acute MI within 6–12 h of onset[a]
ST elevation ≥ 1 mm in 2 or more contiguous limb leads
  or ≥ 2 mm in 2 or more contiguous precordial leads or
  left bundle branch block not known to be present previously
	Absolute
	  Previous hemorrhagic stroke at any time
	  Any stroke or cerebrovascular event within 1 year
	  Known intracranial neoplasm
	  Suspected aortic dissection or acute pericarditis
	Relative
	  Blood pressure ≥ 180/110 mm Hg on presentation,
	    not readily controlled
	  Known bleeding disorder
	  Recent major trauma or internal bleeding (within
	    2–4 weeks)
	  Noncompressible vascular puncture (eg, subclavian
	    intravenous catheter)
	  Active peptic ulcer disease

[a]Within 6 h in patients ≥ 75 years old.

lin, and tirofiban reduce the risk of recurrent ischemic events and improve clinical outcomes in patients with documented MI, particularly those undergoing percutaneous coronary revascularization. In addition, the benefits of these agents are similar in younger and older patients, although the risk of bleeding is somewhat higher in the elderly; dosage adjustment may be necessary in patients with impaired renal function. Currently, the value of glycoprotein IIb/IIIa inhibitors in older patients with acute MI who are unlikely to undergo mechanical revascularization is uncertain.

4. Clopidogrel—Clopidogrel, an oral antiplatelet agent, has been shown to reduce restenosis after percutaneous coronary stent implantation in patients with or without acute coronary events. In addition, clopidogrel added to aspirin has been shown to reduce cardiovascular mortality, nonfatal MI, and nonfatal stroke by ~20% compared with aspirin alone during long-term therapy after non-ST-elevation MI. Despite this benefit, routine long-term use of clopidogrel remains controversial because of its relatively high cost. The initial dosage is 300 mg orally followed by 75 mg/day.

D. β-BLOCKERS

Early administration of intravenous β-blockers reduces mortality, recurrent ischemic events, and both supraventricular and ventricular tachyarrhythmias in appropriately selected patients with acute MI. Intravenous β-blocker therapy should be initiated as soon as possible in all patients with suspected acute MI in the absence of contraindications (ie, heart rate < 45 bpm, systolic BP < 90–100 mm Hg, PR interval ≥ 240 ms or heart block > first degree, moderate or severe pulmonary congestion, or active bronchospasm).

Intravenous metoprolol and atenolol have been approved for treatment of acute MI. Metoprolol is administered as three 5-mg boluses at 2- to 5-min intervals followed by 25 mg orally every 6 h with further dosage increases as tolerated to reach a target dose of 200 mg daily. Atenolol is administered as two 5-mg boluses at an interval of 10 min followed by 25 mg twice daily, increasing to 50 mg twice daily as tolerated. Patients receiving intravenous β-blockers should be carefully observed for bradyarrhythmias, hypotension, dyspnea, and bronchospasm, and the dose and duration of therapy should be adjusted accordingly if these side effects occur. It is prudent to use lower dosages and a slower dose titration schedule in patients older than 75 and in older patients with multiple comorbidities or unstable hemodynamics.

E. ANGIOTENSIN-CONVERTING ENZYME INHIBITORS

ACE inhibitors are clearly beneficial in reducing mortality after acute MI in patients 65–74 years of age, but there is not clear evidence of benefit in patients older than 75. Data suggest that ACE inhibitors are particularly beneficial in patients with anterior ST-elevation MIs and in patients with MIs complicated by HF or significant LV systolic dysfunction (LV ejection fraction < 40%). Early initiation of ACE inhibitor therapy is recommended for all patients with anterior MI, active HF, or significant LV dysfunction in the absence of contraindications. In addition, wider use of ACE inhibitors in patients younger than 75 may be beneficial. Contraindications to ACE inhibitors in the setting of acute MI include systolic BP < 100 mm Hg, advanced renal insufficiency (serum creatinine ≥ 2.5–3.0 mg/dL, especially if worsening renal function is evident), hyperkalemia (serum potassium ≥ 5.5 mEq/L), and known intolerance to ACE inhibitors. ACE inhibitor therapy should be initiated with captopril 6.25 mg three times a day or enalapril 2.5 mg twice daily. The dose should be gradually increased as tolerated to a maintenance dose of captopril 50 mg 3 times a day or enalapril 10 mg twice daily. Once the maintenance dose has been achieved, changing to a once-daily agent at equivalent dosage (eg, lisinopril 20–40 mg or ramipril 10 mg) is appropriate. Throughout the initiation and titration phase of ACE inhibitor therapy, BP, serum creatinine, and serum electrolytes (especially potassium) should be carefully monitored.

F. NITRATES

Nitrate preparations are effective in controlling ischemia and in treating HF in patients with acute MI.

G. ANGIOTENSIN RECEPTOR BLOCKERS

Angiotensin receptor blockers (ARBs) appear to be somewhat less effective than ACE inhibitors for improving outcomes after acute MI. Nevertheless, for patients who are appropriate candidates for ACE inhibitor therapy but who are intolerant because of cough, ARBs may provide a suitable alternative.

H. CALCIUM CHANNEL BLOCKERS

Calcium channel blockers have not been shown to improve outcomes in patients with acute MI, and the use of short-acting dihydropyridines (eg, nifedipine) may be harmful.

I. LIPID-LOWERING AGENTS

HMG CoA reductase inhibitors (statins) decrease mortality and recurrent ischemic events after acute MI. Unless contraindicated, statin therapy should be initiated early in the course of acute MI and continued indefinitely.

J. ANTIARRHYTHMIC AGENTS

Lidocaine and amiodarone are effective in the treatment of life-threatening ventricular arrhythmias in the setting of acute MI, but routine use of these agents as prophylaxis is not recommended.

K. MAGNESIUM

Routine administration of intravenous magnesium in patients with acute MI is not efficacious.

Prognosis

Approximately 15–20% of patients with acute MI die before reaching the hospital, and this proportion likely increases with advancing age. Among patients with recognized MI, both short- and long-term mortality increases progressively with age. Total mortality within 1 year after MI is ~40% among persons older than 65. Factors associated with increased mortality include older age, anterior MI, clinical HF, impaired LV systolic function, atrial fibrillation, complex ventricular arrhythmias, poor functional status, diabetes mellitus, and lack of treatment with aspirin and β-blockers. Although short-term prognosis is more favorable in non-ST-elevation MI than in ST-elevation MI, mortality rates at 2 years are similar.

ACE Inhibitor Myocardial Infarction Collaborative Group: Indications for ACE inhibitors in the early treatment of acute myocardial infarction: systematic overview of individual data from 100,000 patients in randomized trials. Circulation 1998;97:2202. [PMID: 9631869]

Antman EM et al: Early administration of intravenous magnesium to high-risk patients with acute myocardial infarction in the Magnesium in Coronaries (MAGIC) Trial: a randomised controlled trial. Lancet 2002;360:1189. [PMID: 12401244]

Berger AK et al: Primary coronary angioplasty vs. thrombolysis for the management of acute myocardial infarction in elderly patients. JAMA 1999;282:341. [PMID: 10432031]

Braunwald E et al: ACC/AHA guidelines for the management of patients with unstable angina and non-ST-segment elevation myocardial infarction. J Am Coll Cardiol 2000;36:970. [PMID: 10987629]

Braunwald E et al: ACC/AHA guideline update for the management of patients with unstable angina and non-ST-segment elevation myocardial infarction—2002. Circulation 2002; 106:1893. [PMID: 12356647]

De Boer MJ et al: Reperfusion therapy in elderly patients with acute myocardial infarction: a randomized comparison of primary angioplasty and thrombolytic therapy. J Am Coll Cardiol 2002;39:1723. [PMID: 12039482]

Dickstein K et al: Effects of losartan and captopril on mortality and morbidity in high-risk patients after acute myocardial infarction: The OPTIMAAL randomized trial. Optimal Trial in Myocardial Infarction with Angiotensin II Antagonist Losartan. Lancet 2002;360:752. [PMID: 12241832]

Fibrinolytic Therapy Trialists' Collaborative Group: Indications for fibrinolytic therapy in suspected acute myocardial infarction: collaborative overview of early mortality and major morbidity results from all randomised trials of more than 1000 patients. Lancet 1994;343:742. [PMID: 7905143]

Fox KA et al: Interventional versus conservative treatment for patients with unstable angina or non-ST-elevation myocardial infarction. The British Heart Foundation RITA 3 randomised trial. Randomized Intervention Trial of Unstable Angina. Lancet 2002;360:743. [PMID: 12241831]

Fragmin and Fast Revascularisation During Instability in Coronary Artery Disease Investigators: Long-term low-molecular-mass heparin in unstable coronary-artery disease: FRISC II prospective randomised multicentre study. Lancet 1999;354:701. [PMID: 10475180]

Krumholz HM et al: Use and effectiveness of intravenous heparin therapy for treatment of acute myocardial infarction in the elderly. J Am Coll Cardiol 1998;31:973. [PMID: 9561996]

Pearson TA et al: AHA guidelines for primary prevention of cardiovascular disease and stroke: 2002 update: consensus panel guide to comprehensive risk reduction for adult patients without coronary or other atherosclerotic vascular diseases. Circulation 2002;106:388. [PMID: 12119259]

PRISM-PLUS Study Investigators: Inhibition of the platelet glycoprotein IIb/IIIa receptor with tirofiban in unstable angina and non-Q-wave myocardial infarction. N Engl J Med 1998; 338:1488. [PMID: 9599103]

PURSUIT Trial Investigators: Inhibition of glycoprotein IIb/IIIa with eptifibatide in patients with acute coronary syndromes. N Engl J Med 1998;339:436. [PMID: 9705684]

Ryan TJ et al: 1999 update: ACC/AHA guidelines for the management of patients with acute myocardial infarction. J Am Coll Cardiol 1999;34:890. [PMID: 10483976]

Schwartz GG et al: Effects of atorvastatin on early recurrent ischemic events in acute coronary syndromes: the MIRACL study: a randomized controlled trial. JAMA 2001;285:1711. [PMID: 11277825]

Smith SC Jr et al: AHA/ACC guidelines for preventing heart attack and death in patients with atherosclerotic cardiovascular disease: 2001 update. J Am Coll Cardiol 2001;38:1581. [PMID: 11691544]

Thiemann DR et al: Lack of benefit for intravenous thrombolysis in patients with myocardial infarction who are older than 75 years. Circulation 2000;101:2239. [PMID: 10811589]

Williams MA et al: Secondary prevention of coronary heart disease in the elderly (with emphasis on patients ≥ 75 years of age): an American Heart Association scientific statement from the Council on Clinical Cardiology Subcommittee on Exercise, Cardiac Rehabilitation, and Prevention. Circulation 2002; 105:1735. [PMID: 11940556]

Yusuf S et al: Effects of clopidogrel in addition to aspirin in patients with acute coronary syndromes without ST-segment elevation. N Engl J Med 2001;345:494. [PMID: 11519503]

UNSTABLE ANGINA

ESSENTIALS OF DIAGNOSIS

- Anginal chest discomfort of increasing severity or duration.
- ST-segment depression or T-wave inversion on the ECG.
- Absence of elevation of cardiac biomarkers.

General Considerations

Unstable angina is characterized by ischemic symptoms of increasing frequency, severity, or duration; symptoms occurring with less provocation; or symptoms of recent onset occurring with minimal exertion or at rest. Patients with unstable angina are at increased risk for progression to acute MI during short-term follow-up; therefore, aggressive treatment is warranted.

Prevention

Measures effective in the primary prevention of CAD and acute MI are also efficacious in the prevention of unstable angina.

Clinical Findings

A. SYMPTOMS & SIGNS

The symptoms and physical findings of unstable angina may be indistinguishable from those of acute MI, reflecting the similar pathogenesis of these disorders.

B. ELECTROCARDIOGRAPHY

During chest pain, the ECG usually demonstrates ST-segment depression or T-wave inversion, or both, in 1 or more contiguous leads; less commonly, ST-segment elevation may be seen. Electrocardiographic changes often resolve with resolution of chest pain, so that a nondiagnostic or even normal ECG taken when the patient is free of symptoms does not exclude unstable angina. The principal feature that distinguishes unstable angina from acute MI is the lack of elevation of cardiac biomarker proteins (troponin I, troponin T, and CK-MB).

Differential Diagnosis

The differential diagnosis of unstable angina is similar to that of acute MI.

Complications

The principal complication of unstable angina is progression to acute MI. Unstable angina may also be associated with ventricular arrhythmias, including ventricular tachycardia, ventricular fibrillation, and sudden cardiac death as well as supraventricular arrhythmias, bradyarrhythmias, and acute HF.

Treatment

The primary goals of therapy for unstable angina are to relieve symptoms and prevent progression to acute MI. Patients should be hospitalized for observation and receive prompt treatment with aspirin, nitrates, and β-blockers. In patients with persistent or severe symptoms or electrocardiographic changes, nitroglycerin should be administered intravenously. Heparin should also be administered, either intravenously (unfractionated heparin) or as subcutaneous LMW heparin. Patients with marked electrocardiographic abnormalities and those for whom percutaneous coronary revascularization is planned should also be treated with an intravenous glycoprotein IIb/IIIa inhibitor. Additional therapy for unstable angina is similar to that discussed previously for non-ST-elevation MI. In most cases, patients with severe or recurrent symptoms or electrocardiographic abnormalities should undergo cardiac catheterization and coronary angiography followed by percutaneous or surgical revascularization based on anatomical findings. Patients who respond to medical therapy and have no further symptoms should undergo a stress test to stratify risk. Patients with severe ischemia, ischemia at low cardiac workload, or ischemia in association with reduced LV systolic function should proceed to catheterization. Those with less severe ischemia or a normal stress test may be managed conservatively.

Prognosis

The natural history of unstable angina is characterized by frequent progression to MI. With current therapeutic options, the short-term prognosis is favorable, and < 10% of patients hospitalized with unstable angina experience acute MI. The majority of patients with unstable angina have severe coronary atherosclerosis and are at risk for future coronary events. Aggressive treatment of coronary risk factors and implementation of other preventive measures, including aspirin, β-blockers, and ACE inhibitors, is warranted.

Antman EM et al: Enoxaparin prevents death and cardiac ischemic events in unstable angina/non-Q-wave MI. Results of the thrombolysis in myocardial infarction (TIMI) IIB trial. Circulation 1999;100:1593. [PMID: 10517729]

Braunwald E et al: ACC/AHA guideline update for the management of patients with unstable angina and non-ST-segment elevation myocardial infarction—2002. Circulation 2002; 106:1893. [PMID: 12356647]

Goodman SG et al: Randomized trial of low molecular weight heparin (enoxaparin) versus unfractionated heparin for unstable coronary artery disease: one-year results of the ESSENCE study. Efficacy and Safety of Subcutaneous Enoxaparin in Non-Q Wave Coronary Events. J Am Coll Cardiol 2000;36:693. [PMID: 10987586]

CHRONIC CORONARY HEART DISEASE

 ESSENTIALS OF DIAGNOSIS

- Chest discomfort provoked by exertion or emotional stress and relieved by rest or nitroglycerin.
- Exercise or pharmacological stress test demonstrating myocardial ischemia.
- Angiographic evidence of significant coronary artery obstruction

General Considerations

CHD is the leading cause of death in the United States in both men and women. Although the incidence and prevalence of CHD are both higher in men than in women, the rates for women increase progressively after menopause, and the greater longevity of women compared with men results in a slight predominance of women in the total number of CHD cases. The prevalence of CHD increases progressively with age, affecting 16.1% of women and 18.6% of men older than 75.

Prevention

Primary prevention of CHD may be achieved through lifelong avoidance of tobacco products, participation in regular physical exercise, maintenance of desirable body weight, consumption of a diet rich in fruits, vegetables, and whole-grain foods, and limited consumption of foods high in saturated fats and cholesterol. Early identification and aggressive treatment of hypertension, dyslipidemia, and diabetes are essential as well.

Clinical Findings

A. SYMPTOMS & SIGNS

The most common symptom of chronic CHD is central chest discomfort, often described as pressure, tightness, or heaviness, typically brought on by physical exertion or emotional stress and relieved by rest or nitroglycerin. However, many older adults with CHD, including those with prior MI or unstable angina, manifest atypical symptoms, such as dyspnea, fatigue, weakness, dizziness, or abdominal discomfort, whereas others, particularly diabetics, are entirely asymptomatic, in part because of the high prevalence of physical inactivity at older age. Thus, despite the high prevalence of CHD in the elderly, a substantial proportion of patients do not experience typical angina pectoris, and the physician must maintain a high index of suspicion for CHD in older persons with atypical symptoms or multiple risk factors.

The physical findings of chronic CHD are nonspecific but may include an S_3 or S_4 gallop, a murmur of mitral regurgitation, a laterally displaced or dyskinetic apical impulse (especially in patients with prior MI), or signs of HF (eg, pulmonary rales, elevated jugular venous pressure, peripheral edema).

C. SPECIAL TESTS

1. Electrocardiography—The ECG may demonstrate pathological Q waves in patients with prior MI. Other ECG findings are nonspecific.

2. Stress tests—The noninvasive procedure of choice for diagnosing CHD is an exercise or pharmacological stress test, usually accompanied by echocardiographic or radionuclide imaging. These tests provide 80–90% sensitivity and specificity for diagnosing CHD, although the predictive accuracy of the test is dependent on the pretest likelihood that the patient has the disease. In general, it is preferable to perform an exercise test if the patient is capable of doing so. However, because many elderly patients are limited by arthritis, neurological conditions, or poor physical conditioning, it is often necessary to perform a pharmacological stress test in older patients (eg, dobutamine echo, adenosine sestamibi).

3. Coronary angiography—Coronary angiography remains the gold standard for determining the presence, extent, and severity of CHD as well as the suitability for percutaneous or surgical revascularization. Older patients are more likely to have multivessel disease and left main coronary artery disease.

Differential Diagnosis

The differential diagnosis of chest pain includes cardiac, vascular, gastrointestinal, pulmonary, neurological, musculoskeletal, and psychogenic causes. In patients with recent onset or progression of symptoms suggestive of ischemia, the possibility of unstable angina or acute MI must be considered.

Complications

The major complications of chronic CHD are progression to an acute coronary event (MI, unstable angina), development of HF because of the cumulative effects of myocardial injury or infarction (ischemic cardiomyopathy), and development of conduction abnormalities or arrhythmias, including ventricular tachycardia and ventricular fibrillation. Sudden cardiac death is the initial manifestation of CHD in up to 20% of cases.

Treatment

The goals of therapy for chronic CHD are to control symptoms and prevent major complications. Optimal treatment involves lifestyle modifications, attention to risk factors, pharmacological interventions, and, in selected patients, percutaneous or surgical revascularization.

A. Lifestyle Modifications

Patients with CHD, regardless of age, should be strongly advised to discontinue the use of all tobacco products. Gradual weight reduction through a program of diet and regular exercise should be encouraged in overweight patients (body mass index > 25–30 kg/m^2). Patients with CHD should eat a balanced diet rich in fruits, vegetables, and whole grains while limiting intake of saturated fats (including partially hydrogenated oils) and cholesterol. Patients should also engage in a total of at least 20–30 min of moderate intensity physical activity on most days of the week unless limited by active cardiovascular symptoms or other medical conditions. Walking, stationary cycling, and swimming are suitable exercise modalities for most older adults. When beginning an exercise program, patients should be instructed to start at a slow and comfortable pace, gradually increasing the duration of exercise over a period of weeks. The addition of flexibility and strengthening exercises is also beneficial to overall health. Patients who have suffered an MI or who have had coronary bypass surgery should be strongly encouraged to participate in a formal cardiac rehabilitation program. Such programs have been associated with reduced mortality, improved exercise tolerance and quality of life, and enhanced mood and sense of well-being.

B. Risk Factors

Smoking should be discouraged. Antihypertensive therapy should be titrated to maintain a resting BP < 140/90 mm Hg (< 130/80 mm Hg in diabetics and patients with HF or renal insufficiency). The lipid profile should be monitored and the low-density lipoprotein (LDL) cholesterol level reduced to < 100 mg/dL through dietary modifications and, if necessary, lipid-lowering agents. Diabetes should be controlled through diet and medications to achieve a hemoglobin A1C level of < 7 g/dL. Obesity and physical inactivity should be addressed through lifestyle modifications.

C. Pharmacotherapy

1. Aspirin—Long-term use of aspirin in patients with CHD markedly reduces the risk of death, MI, and stroke. The absolute benefit is greatest in high-risk patients, including those older than 65. The optimal dose of aspirin is unknown, but 75 mg once daily provides benefits equivalent to higher doses with a lower risk of side effects, including bleeding. In patients intolerant to low-dose aspirin, clopidogrel 75 mg daily is an acceptable alternative.

2. β-Blockers—β-Blockers reduce the risk of death and reinfarction after MI. β-Blockers are also highly effective antianginal agents and appear to reduce the incidence of coronary events in patients with chronic CHD. In patients without prior MI, the optimal dose of β-blockers is unknown, but a rational therapeutic goal is to gradually increase the dose until the patient has no or minimal ischemic symptoms and the resting heart rate is < 60–65 bpm. Older patients may be less tolerant of β-blockers because of the effects of aging on sinus node function and the presence of comorbidities (eg, pulmonary disease); dosages should, therefore, be adjusted accordingly.

3. Nitrates—Sublingual nitroglycerin remains the drug of choice for treatment of an acute episode of angina. As a result of drying of the oral mucosa, nitroglycerin spray may be more effective than tablets in older patients. Older patients may also be more likely to experience orthostatic hypotension with nitroglycerin; they should be advised to take the medication in a sitting or reclining position. Long-term nitrates are effective antianginal agents but have not been shown to improve clinical outcomes. In addition, tolerance to nitrates develops rapidly, requiring a daily 6- to 8-h nitrate-free interval. Several oral and transdermal nitrate preparations are available for chronic use.

4. Calcium channel blockers—Calcium channel blockers are effective antihypertensive and antianginal agents, but they have not been shown to improve clinical outcomes in patients with CHD. In addition, they may be associated with worsening HF and, with the exception of amlodipine and felodipine, should be avoided in patients with impaired LV systolic function. Verapamil and diltiazem may slow heart rate and conduction through the atrioventricular (AV) node, especially when used in combination with a β-blocker, thus increasing the risk of bradyarrhythmias and syncope in older patients with sinus node dysfunction (sick sinus syndrome) or impaired AV nodal conduction. Verapamil and, to a lesser extent, diltiazem also impair gastrointestinal motility and may lead to constipation or ileus.

5. ACE inhibitors—ACE inhibitors do not exert a direct anti-ischemic effect, but ramipril reduces mortality and major cardiovascular events in a broad range of patients with established vascular disease or diabetes. In addition, ACE inhibitors improve outcomes in patients with reduced LV systolic function with or without symptoms. Thus, initiation of an ACE inhibitor should be strongly considered in all older adults with established CHD in the absence of contraindications.

6. Angiotensin receptor blockers—ARBs have been shown to improve outcomes in patients with diabetes and in hypertensive patients with LV hypertrophy; however, the value of these agents in patients with CHD is unproven. Currently, routine use of an ARB in patients with CHD is not recommended, but they are an appropriate alternative in patients who require an ACE inhibitor but are intolerant of these agents because of cough.

7. Lipid-lowering agents—HMG CoA reductase inhibitors (statins) reduce mortality and cardiovascular morbidity in patients with CHD, and the benefits extend to patients at least up to the age of 85. Current recommendations are to initiate statin therapy to reduce the LDL cholesterol level to < 100 mg/dL in patients with established CHD or diabetes who do not respond to diet alone. As with other medications, it is advisable to start with a lower dose and titrate the drug more slowly in patients older than 75.

8. Warfarin—Warfarin is indicated in patients with CHD complicated by atrial fibrillation or LV mural thrombus with embolization. Warfarin can also be used as an alternative to aspirin in aspirin-intolerant patients. Older patients are at increased risk for bleeding complications with warfarin, especially during concomitant treatment with nonsteroidal anti-inflammatory drugs (NSAIDs).

D. REVASCULARIZATION

Percutaneous coronary revascularization and coronary artery bypass surgery are highly effective in improving symptoms and quality of life in older patients with CHD; > 50% of all revascularization procedures in the United States are now performed in patients older than 65. On the other hand, both coronary angioplasty and bypass surgery are associated with increased mortality and major complications in the very elderly, especially patients older than 80; thus, careful selection of candidates for revascularization procedures is paramount. In general, percutaneous coronary revascularization is associated with lower mortality and major morbidity (including stroke, delirium) as well as much more rapid recovery compared with coronary bypass surgery in elderly patients. However, the need for repeat revascularization procedures is higher after angioplasty, and long-term outcomes are similar. Thus, both procedures represent suitable options for older patients with severe symptomatic CHD, and the choice of procedure should be based on anatomical considerations, prevalent comorbidities, and patient preferences. Up to 50% of elderly patients undergoing coronary bypass surgery may experience a decline in cognitive function in the perioperative period. Although these cognitive deficits are transient in many patients, a significant proportion may exhibit persistent cognitive impairment during long-term follow-up.

Prognosis

The prognosis of chronic CHD is highly variable. Although some patients remain minimally symptomatic or asymptomatic for decades, others experience marked disability despite multiple therapeutic interventions. Still others succumb to the disease after suffering a large MI or fatal arrhythmia. Factors that adversely influence prognosis include older age, male gender, more severe CHD, more severe HF or LV systolic dysfunction (lower ejection fraction), more severe symptoms or functional limitations, presence of diabetes or atrial fibrillation, and presence of significant ventricular arrhythmias.

Ades PA: Cardiac rehabilitation and secondary prevention of coronary heart disease. N Engl J Med 2001;345:892. [PMID: 11565523]

American Diabetes Association: Standards of medical care for patients with diabetes mellitus. Diabetes Care 2002;25:213. [PMID: 11772918]

Dahlof B et al: Cardiovascular morbidity and mortality in the Losartan Intervention for Endpoint Reduction in Hypertension study (LIFE): a randomised trial against atenolol. Lancet 2002;359:995. [PMID: 11937178]

Dargie HJ: Effect of carvedilol on outcome after myocardial infarction in patients with left-ventricular dysfunction: the CAPRICORN randomised trial. Lancet 2001;357:1385. [PMID: 11356434]

Dickstein K et al: Effects of losartan and captopril on mortality and morbidity in high-risk patients after acute myocardial infarction: the OPTIMAAL randomised trial. Lancet 2002;360:752. [PMID: 12241832]

Expert Panel on Detection, Evaluation, and Treatment of High Blood Cholesterol in Adults: Executive summary of the third report of the National Cholesterol Education Program (NCEP) expert panel on detection, evaluation, and treatment of high blood cholesterol in adults (Adult Treatment Panel III). JAMA 2001;285:2486. [PMID: 11368702]

Heart Protection Study Collaborative Group: MRC/BHF heart protection study of cholesterol lowering with simvastatin in 20,536 high-risk individuals: a randomised placebo-controlled trial. Lancet 2002;360:7. [PMID: 12114036]

Newman MF et al: Longitudinal assessment of neurocognitive function after coronary-artery bypass surgery. N Engl J Med 2001;344:395. [PMID: 11172175]

Pearson TA et al: AHA guidelines for primary prevention of cardiovascular disease and stroke: 2002 update: consensus panel guide to comprehensive risk reduction for adult patients without coronary or other atherosclerotic vascular diseases. Circulation 2002;106:388. [PMID: 12119259]

Williams MA et al: Secondary prevention of coronary heart disease in the elderly (with emphasis on patients ≥ 75 years): an American Heart Association scientific statement from the Council on Clinical Cardiology subcommittee on exercise, cardiac rehabilitation, and prevention. Circulation 2002; 105:1735. [PMID: 11940556]

Yusuf S et al: Effects of an angiotensin-converting-enzyme inhibitor, ramipril, on cardiovascular events in high-risk patients. The Heart Outcomes Prevention Evaluation Study Investigators. N Engl J Med 2000;342:145. [PMID: 10639539]

■ VALVULAR HEART DISEASE

AORTIC STENOSIS

ESSENTIALS OF DIAGNOSIS

- *Chest pain, shortness of breath, dizziness, syncope.*
- *Harsh systolic ejection murmur at the right upper sternal border radiating to the carotid arteries.*

- *Echocardiography demonstrates a calcified aortic valve with increased systolic velocities and reduced orifice area.*

General Considerations

Aortic stenosis (AS) increases in prevalence with age and affects 15–20% of men and women older than 80. Approximately 2–3% of persons older than 75 experience AS of sufficient severity to warrant consideration for aortic valve replacement. AS is the second most common indication for major cardiac surgery in the elderly (after coronary bypass surgery).

Prevention

There are no known interventions for prevention of AS in the elderly; however, statins may slow the rate of progression.

Clinical Findings

A. Symptoms & Signs

The classic triad of symptoms associated with severe AS includes exertional angina, dizziness or syncope, and dyspnea or orthopnea. However, AS in the elderly is often occult until it reaches an advanced stage because sedentary older persons may experience few symptoms or may attribute their symptoms to another disease or to old age.

Significant AS is almost invariably associated with a ≥ grade II systolic ejection murmur that is usually harsh and best heard in the right second intercostal space with radiation to the carotid arteries. The murmur may be difficult to hear in obese patients and in those with increased chest diameter because of chronic lung disease, whereas in others it may be best heard at the apex. Murmurs that peak in late systole tend to be associated with more severe AS, but the intensity of the murmur often diminishes in patients with severe LV failure. Other physical findings include an LV heave, S_4 gallop, and reduced intensity or absence of the A_2 component of the second heart sound. Classically, the carotid upstroke is delayed in patients with severe AS, but this finding may be masked in older patients with stiff, noncompliant vessels.

B. Special Tests

1. Electrocardiography—The ECG often demonstrates LV hypertrophy, and the chest radiograph frequently reveals LV prominence.

2. Echocardiography—Echocardiography is the noninvasive procedure of choice for diagnosing AS. Typical echocardiographic features include a moderately or severely thickened and calcified valve with restricted opening. Doppler examination reveals increased mean and peak velocities across the valve, and the continuity equation permits estimation of the effective aortic valve area. A calculated aortic valve area of 1.1–1.5 cm^2 indicates mild AS, 0.8–1.1 cm^2 moderate AS, and < 0.8 cm^2 severe AS.

3. Cardiac catheterization—Because ~50% of older patients with severe AS have obstructive CAD, cardiac catheterization with coronary angiography is indicated for all patients with AS for whom aortic valve replacement is being considered. Catheterization can also provide definitive information about the severity of AS when the echocardiogram is nondiagnostic.

Differential Diagnosis

Aortic sclerosis (ie, thickening of the aortic valve cusps without valvular stenosis) occurs more frequency with age and is a marker for increased cardiovascular morbidity and mortality. The symptoms of AS may mimic many other cardiac and noncardiac diseases, including CAD, HF, arrhythmia, and chronic lung disease. Likewise, the physical findings, ECG, and chest radiograph are often nonspecific. The physician must, therefore, maintain a high index of suspicion in patients with symptoms possibly attributable to AS in association with a systolic ejection murmur. Echocardiography and cardiac catheterization are diagnostic.

Complications

The major complications of untreated severe AS include progressive HF, ischemia, syncope, and sudden death as a result of ventricular arrhythmias or asystole. Sudden death occurs predominantly in patients with severe symptomatic AS but occasionally represents the initial manifestation of the disease.

Treatment

There is no effective medical therapy for severe AS. All patients with a heart murmur resulting from AS should receive antibiotic prophylaxis for dental work and other procedures in accordance with American Heart Association (AHA) guidelines. Vasodilators, including nitrates and ACE inhibitors, should be administered with caution in patients with moderate or severe AS because of the risk of hypotension. Once symptoms develop, patients with severe AS should be referred for aortic valve replacement because the prognosis is poor in the absence of definitive therapy.

Aortic valve replacement is the procedure of choice for patients with severe symptomatic AS, and the results of valve replacement are excellent. In patients with significant CAD, coronary bypass surgery is performed concomitantly. Factors that militate against surgery include dementia, severe pulmonary disease, advanced frailty, and reluctance to undergo the procedure. In patients older than 75, most cardiac surgeons will implant a bioprosthetic valve, which has acceptable durability in this age group and obviates the need for long-term anticoagulation. Operative mortality rates for octogenarians undergoing aortic valve replacement are 4–7%; most patients report substantial improvement in symptoms and functional status after recovery.

Prognosis

Without surgery, median survival in elderly patients with severe symptomatic AS is 18–24 mo, and the prognosis is worse for patients with HF. After aortic valve replacement, survival is similar to that for persons of comparable age in the general population.

AORTIC INSUFFICIENCY

 ESSENTIALS OF DIAGNOSIS

- Dyspnea, fatigue, palpitations, chest pain.
- Decrescendo diastolic murmur in the left third and fourth intercostal spaces.
- Echocardiography demonstrates aortic insufficiency.

General Considerations

The prevalence of aortic insufficiency (AI) increases with age, but few cases are severe enough to warrant valve surgery.

Prevention

Appropriate treatment of hypertension and dyslipidemias may reduce the risk of aortic root aneurysms and dissection. Early treatment of syphilis is effective in preventing syphilitic aortitis.

Clinical Findings

A. Symptoms & Signs

Patients with acute severe AI generally have symptoms of overt HF, those with mild or moderate chronic AI are usually asymptomatic, and those with chronic severe AI report progressive exercise intolerance, shortness of breath, orthopnea, and fatigue. Palpitations and chest pain are less prominent features.

In patients with acute severe AI, the clinical picture is dominated by signs of LV failure, including shortness of breath and pulmonary congestion. A diastolic murmur of AI may be present. In patients with mild to moderate chronic AI, a short early diastolic decrescendo murmur is often the only physical finding. In those with chronic severe AI, the diastolic murmur becomes louder, occasionally reaching grade V or VI, and longer, often persisting throughout diastole with presystolic accentuation. The LV apical impulse is often diffuse and displaced laterally and inferiorly. An S_3 gallop is often present and may be palpable. BP is characterized by a widened pulse pressure and especially by a low diastolic BP. Peripheral manifestations of severe chronic AI include bounding pulses, head bobbing, Quincke's pulses (capillary pulsations), and femoral bruits with light compression of the artery.

B. SPECIAL TESTS

1. Chest radiography—In patients with acute severe AI, the chest radiograph reveals pulmonary edema, often in association with a normal cardiac silhouette. In patients with chronic severe AI, the heart size is usually markedly increased.

2. Electrocardiography—Electrocardiographic findings are nonspecific, but LV hypertrophy may be evident in patients with severe chronic AI.

3. Imaging studies—Transthoracic and transesophageal echocardiography, computed tomography, and magnetic resonance imaging are useful noninvasive techniques for evaluating AI. In most cases, transthoracic echocardiography is the initial procedure of choice. In patients with acute severe AI, a short eccentric jet of AI is often visualized, along with early closure of the mitral valve. In mild to moderate chronic AI, the AI jet is visualized but the echocardiogram may be normal otherwise. In chronic severe AI, the left ventricle is usually dilated and there is a prominent AI jet. Echocardiography may also provide valuable insight into the cause of AI, such as infective endocarditis, flail aortic valve leaflet, or aortic root aneurysm or dissection.

4. Cardiac catheterization—In most cases, cardiac catheterization is not necessary to diagnose and quantify AI. However, elderly patients who require surgery for AI should undergo coronary angiography.

Differential Diagnosis

Acute severe AI usually manifests as severe LV failure that may not respond to conventional therapy. The differential diagnosis includes other causes of acute pulmonary edema, such as acute MI, severe hypertension, and cardiac arrhythmia. Other causes of chronic HF must be considered in the differential diagnosis of severe chronic AI.

Complications

Acute severe AI is often associated with intractable HF and death without surgical intervention. The course of chronic severe AI is insidious and gradually progressive over many years, ultimately leading to severe HF.

Treatment

Acute severe AI complicated by HF requires prompt surgical intervention, usually consisting of aortic valve replacement. Medical stabilization while awaiting surgery should be directed at the underlying cause (eg, aortic dissection) and at the treatment of HF with diuretics and vasodilators. Afterload reduction with intravenous nitroprusside may result in marked clinical improvement but rarely obviates the need for surgery.

Patients with chronic AI, especially if moderate or severe, should receive antibiotic prophylaxis for dental work and other procedures. BP should be treated aggressively in accordance with current guidelines. Mild chronic AI requires no additional treatment. Patients with moderate or severe chronic AI should be treated with ACE inhibitors or other afterload-reducing agents to slow disease progression. Patients with severe chronic AI should undergo serial echocardiography at regular intervals. Criteria for aortic valve replacement include onset of HF symptoms, decline in LV ejection fraction to < 50%, or progressive LV dilatation with an end-systolic dimension > 5.5 cm by echocardiography.

For patients with acute severe AI, surgical outcomes are dependent on the severity of HF and hemodynamic compromise as well as the cause of AI. In chronic AI patients, results of surgery are excellent in those with preserved LV function and minimal symptoms but are less favorable in those with markedly dilated ventricles, significantly reduced systolic function, or severe symptoms. Bioprosthetic valves are usually implanted in elderly patients requiring aortic valve replacement for severe AI.

Prognosis

Patients with acute severe AI complicated by HF have a high mortality rate unless aortic valve replacement is performed promptly. The short- and intermediate-term prognosis for patients with mild or moderate chronic AI is favorable because the condition often remains stable for many years. Patients with severe chronic AI who are asymptomatic and have stable ventricular function have a good short- and intermediate-term prognosis. However, once symptoms of HF or significant LV dysfunction develop, the prognosis is poor unless aortic valve surgery is performed.

MITRAL STENOSIS

 ESSENTIALS OF DIAGNOSIS

- *History of rheumatic fever or prior streptococcal infection.*
- *Exertional fatigue, hemoptysis, symptoms of heart failure.*
- *Opening snap and mid-diastolic rumbling murmur.*
- *Echocardiogram demonstrating thickened mitral valve with restricted motion.*

General Considerations

Mitral stenosis (MS) is relatively rare in the elderly, with a reported prevalence of < 1% in the United States.

Prevention

Rheumatic heart disease can be prevented by prompt identification and treatment of group A β-hemolytic streptococcal infections. No interventions have been shown to prevent or slow the development of mitral valve annulus calcification.

Clinical Findings

A. Symptoms & Signs

The clinical course of MS is often insidious, and there may be an interval of several decades after an episode of acute rheumatic fever before symptoms of MS develop. Classic symptoms include exertional fatigue, a gradual decline in exercise tolerance, hemoptysis, dyspnea, and orthopnea. Not uncommonly, older patients with MS have symptoms resulting from new-onset atrial fibrillation, such as palpitations or acute HF.

Rheumatic mitral stenosis is characterized by an opening snap in early diastole followed by a mid-diastolic rumbling murmur. The murmur is low pitched, best heard at the apex or in the left lateral decubitus position, and intensified by tachycardia. There may be presystolic accentuation during sinus rhythm. Earlier

occurrence of the opening snap and longer duration of the diastolic murmur are associated with more severe stenosis. All of these features may be absent in patients with MS because of mitral annular calcification. Additional findings associated with MS may include evidence for pulmonary hypertension (right ventricular heave, augmented P_2) and evidence for biventricular failure (pulmonary rales, elevated jugular venous pressure, and peripheral edema).

B. Special Tests

1. Chest radiography—The chest radiograph may demonstrate calcification in the region of the mitral valve, evidence for left atrial or right ventricular enlargement, and increased vascular markings in the lower lung fields.

2. Electrocardiography—The ECG demonstrates left atrial enlargement or atrial fibrillation; right axis deviation and signs of right ventricular hypertrophy may also be present.

3. Echocardiography—Echocardiography is the diagnostic procedure of choice because it can reliably determine the presence of MS of either rheumatic or calcific origin, assess disease severity, estimate left atrial size, and evaluate for rheumatic or calcific involvement of other cardiac valves.

4. Coronary angiography—In elderly patients with severe MS being considered for cardiac surgery, coronary angiography is indicated to evaluate for obstructive CAD.

Differential Diagnosis

The differential diagnosis includes other cardiac and pulmonary conditions that may produce symptoms and signs of left- or right-sided HF as well as conditions that may cause atrial fibrillation or pulmonary hypertension.

Complications

Major complications of MS include chronic progressive HF and atrial fibrillation. Atrial fibrillation resulting from MS is associated with a high rate of thromboembolic events, which may approach 20% per year in those not receiving anticoagulation.

Treatment

Patients with MS should receive antibiotic prophylaxis for endocarditis in accordance with AHA guidelines. Those with atrial fibrillation should receive warfarin to maintain an international normalized ratio (INR) of 2.5–3.5 and β-blockers, diltiazem, verapamil, or digoxin, or a combination, to maintain a resting heart rate of < 80 bpm and a peak exercise heart rate of

< 115 bpm. Patients with HF should receive diuretics to relieve congestive symptoms and edema. Vasodilator therapy (eg, ACE inhibitors) has not been shown to be beneficial in the absence of LV systolic dysfunction.

Percutaneous mitral valve balloon valvotomy, open commissurotomy, and mitral valve replacement are effective treatments for severe MS in selected patients, and persons with moderate to severe symptoms unresponsive to medical management should be considered for one of these procedures. Percutaneous mitral valvotomy is the procedure of choice in patients with favorable anatomy, which includes pliable valve leaflets, absence of severe calcification, and no more than mild mitral regurgitation. Although percutaneous valvotomy has achieved excellent results in elderly patients who are suitable candidates for the procedure, most older patients are excluded because of excessive calcification of the mitral apparatus or more severe mitral regurgitation. These patients are not suitable candidates for open mitral valve commissurotomy for the same reasons; therefore, mitral valve replacement is the only option. Mitral valve replacement is associated with somewhat higher risks than aortic valve replacement, and symptomatic improvement may be less than in patients treated for aortic stenosis. In addition, patients undergoing mitral valve replacement with either a bioprosthetic or mechanical valve for MS require long-term anticoagulation with warfarin. Despite these limitations, long-term outcomes after mitral valve replacement are generally favorable.

Prognosis

MS runs a protracted course, and the 10-year survival rate in patients with minimal or no symptoms is > 80%. Once limiting symptoms develop, the prognosis is much worse, and few patients survive 10 years. In untreated patients with severe MS, 60–70% die from progressive HF, 20–30% from systemic embolization, and 10% from pulmonary embolism.

MITRAL REGURGITATION

ESSENTIALS OF DIAGNOSIS

- Exertional dyspnea or fatigue, orthopnea, peripheral edema.
- Holosystolic murmur at the apex radiating to the axilla.
- Echocardiography demonstrates mitral regurgitation.

General Considerations

Mitral regurgitation (MR) is the most common valvular disorder in the elderly, but in most cases surgical intervention is not required. Nonetheless, MR is the second most common reason for valve surgery in the elderly (after AS).

Prevention

Therapies directed at preventing the various disorders that cause acute or chronic MR may reduce the prevalence of this condition.

Clinical Findings

A. Symptoms & Signs

The clinical findings of MR are dependent on acuity and severity. Mild acute MR is usually well tolerated, but acute MR of moderate severity (eg, complicating acute MI) may be associated with dyspnea and signs of pulmonary edema. Acute severe MR (eg, from papillary muscle rupture) is almost always associated with acute pulmonary edema and respiratory failure and may result in rapid hemodynamic deterioration and death. Chronic mild or moderate MR is usually asymptomatic, and chronic severe MR is often well tolerated as long as LV function is preserved. Once LV dysfunction develops, patients with severe chronic MR typically experience symptoms and signs of left-sided HF, including exertional dyspnea, orthopnea, an S_3 gallop, and pulmonary rales. As the disease progresses, signs of right-sided HF, including elevated jugular venous pressure and peripheral edema, may ensue.

Physical findings associated with acute, severe MR, in addition to signs of HF, include a harsh early systolic murmur best heard at the apex. In patients with severe HF, the murmur may be difficult to appreciate, and the absence of a systolic murmur does not preclude acute severe MR. An S_3 gallop and signs of pulmonary hypertension may be present. Chronic MR is characterized by an apical holosystolic murmur radiating to the axilla, back, or across the precordium. In patients with mitral valve prolapse, a mid-systolic click may be heard, followed by the MR murmur. In patients with severe chronic MR, the apical impulse is usually laterally displaced, and an S_3 gallop may be present.

B. Special Tests

1. Chest radiography—In acute severe MR, the chest radiograph demonstrates pulmonary edema, but the heart size is often normal. In chronic severe MR the heart size is increased and left atrial enlargement is usually evident; pulmonary congestion may be present.

2. Electrocardiography—The ECG in acute severe MR typically shows a sinus tachycardia but is otherwise unremarkable unless the MR is due to an acute coronary ischemic event. In chronic severe MR the ECG reveals left atrial enlargement or atrial fibrillation; in advanced stages there may be evidence of right ventricular hypertrophy.

3. Echocardiography—Echocardiographic findings depend on the cause, chronicity, and severity of MR. A regurgitant MR jet is invariably present, and color Doppler techniques permit a qualitative assessment of MR severity. LV function may be hyperdynamic (eg, acute severe MR resulting from chordal rupture), normal (eg, moderate chronic MR), or impaired (eg, MR resulting from ischemic or dilated cardiomyopathy). The left atrial size is often normal in acute MR but becomes progressively dilated in severe chronic MR. The mitral valve may appear structurally normal or there may be evidence of myxomatous degeneration, rheumatic involvement, endocarditis, or a flail leaflet. For patients in whom the cause or severity of MR remains in doubt after transthoracic echocardiography, the transesophageal approach provides excellent visualization of mitral valve anatomy and function.

4. Cardiac Catheterization—Cardiac catheterization with left ventriculography is also helpful in assessing MR severity and determining LV function. However, the role of catheterization is principally limited to evaluating hemodynamics, pulmonary pressures, and coronary anatomy in patients with severe MR who are being considered for mitral valve surgery.

Differential Diagnosis

The differential diagnosis of MR includes numerous other conditions that may result in the clinical findings of left- or right-sided HF. Often, multiple such conditions coexist in elderly patients, and it may be difficult to determine the extent to which the patient's symptoms are due to MR or other causes.

Complications

Acute severe MR is almost always associated with pulmonary congestion and may be complicated by respiratory failure, hemodynamic decompensation, and death resulting from cardiogenic shock. Complications of chronic severe MR include progressive LV failure eventually leading to death, pulmonary hypertension, and atrial fibrillation.

Treatment

A. PHARMACOTHERAPY

Treatment of chronic MR should be directed at the primary cause when feasible. BP control should be opti-

mized and antibiotic prophylaxis administered before dental work and other procedures, except in patients with mild MR in the absence of structural abnormalities of the mitral valve (including mitral valve prolapse). Mild chronic MR usually requires no specific therapy, but patients with moderate or severe chronic MR should be treated with ACE inhibitors for afterload reduction. Patients intolerant to ACE inhibitors should receive ARBs or the combination of nitrates and hydralazine. Atrial fibrillation should be treated with rate-controlling agents and anticoagulation with warfarin. HF should be managed with diuretics, ACE inhibitors, β-blockers, and digoxin as appropriate.

B. SURGERY

Acute severe MR complicated by pulmonary edema or hemodynamic instability requires urgent surgical intervention. Placement of an intra-aortic balloon pump may help stabilize the patient before surgery. Other measures include diuresis, vasodilator therapy to reduce afterload as tolerated, and endotracheal intubation if needed for respiratory failure.

Surgical options for the treatment of severe MR include mitral valve repair and mitral valve replacement. Whenever feasible, mitral valve repair is preferred because it preserves the integrity of the mitral valve apparatus and obviates the need for long-term anticoagulation (unless atrial fibrillation is present). Valve surgery is indicated in patients with acute MR complicated by significant HF and in those with severe chronic MR associated with moderate or severe symptoms, ejection fraction > 30%, and LV end-systolic dimension < 5.5 cm by echocardiography.

Elderly patients with severe LV dysfunction or markedly dilated left ventricles respond poorly to surgery and should be managed medically. Results of surgery for ischemic MR also tend to be less favorable than for nonischemic MR. Other factors that influence surgical outcomes include older age, prevalent comorbidities, and symptom severity. Although mitral valve surgery in elderly patients is associated with significant morbidity and mortality, long-term outcomes are favorable, with symptomatic improvement in the majority of patients.

Prognosis

The prognosis of nonoperated acute severe MR complicated by pulmonary edema is poor; the majority of patients die within hours to days. The prognosis for mild to moderate chronic MR is good. The clinical course of severe chronic MR is highly variable, but patients should be monitored closely with serial echocardiograms because the development of significant symptoms or progressive LV dilation or dysfunction is a harbinger of poor outcome and mandates prompt consideration of surgical intervention.

Asimakopoulos G et al: Aortic valve replacement in patients 80 years of age and older: survival and cause of death based on 1100 cases: collective results from the UK Heart Valve Registry. Circulation 1997;96:3403. [PMID: 9396434]

Bellamy MF et al: Association of cholesterol levels, hydroxymethylglutaryl coenzyme-A reductase inhibitor treatment, and progression of aortic stenosis in the community. J Am Coll Cardiol 2002;40:1723. [PMID: 12446053]

Bonow RO et al: Guidelines for the management of patients with valvular heart disease: executive summary. Circulation 1998;98:1949. [PMID: 9799219]

Dajani AS et al: Prevention of bacterial endocarditis. Recommendations by the American Heart Association. JAMA 1997;277:1794. [PMID: 9178793]

Krasuski RA et al: Comparison of results of percutaneous balloon mitral commissurotomy in patients ≥ 65 years with those in patients aged < 65 years. Am J Cardiol 2001;88:994. [PMID: 11703995]

Otto CM et al: Association of aortic-valve sclerosis with cardiovascular mortality and morbidity in the elderly. N Engl J Med 1999;341:142. [PMID: 10403851]

HEART FAILURE

 ESSENTIALS OF DIAGNOSIS

- *Exertional dyspnea, fatigue, orthopnea, lower extremity swelling.*
- *Pulmonary rales, elevated jugular venous pressure, peripheral edema.*
- *Echocardiography reveals LV systolic or diastolic dysfunction.*

General Considerations

Incidence and prevalence of HF increase exponentially with age, reflecting the increasing prevalence of hypertension and CHD at older age and the marked reduction in cardiovascular reserve that accompanies normative aging. There is a 4-fold increase in the incidence of HF between ages 65 and 85. Although the incidence of HF is higher in men than in women at all ages, women comprise slightly more than half of prevalent HF cases because of the increased proportion of women among older adults.

HF is currently the most common cause of hospitalization in the Medicare age group; 77% of the nearly 1 million annual hospitalizations for HF involve persons older than 65. HF is also a major source of chronic disability in the elderly and is the most costly Medicare diagnosis-related group.

Prevention

Primary prevention of HF is feasible through aggressive treatment of the major conditions that cause HF (ie, hypertension and CHD). Antihypertensive therapy reduces the risk of incident HF by as much as 50% in older adults. The greatest benefit is seen in octogenarians with systolic hypertension. Similarly, treatment of other coronary risk factors may prevent or delay the onset of CHD, thus reducing the risk of HF.

Clinical Findings

A. Symptoms & Signs

Symptoms include exertional shortness of breath, effort intolerance, fatigue, cough, orthopnea, paroxysmal nocturnal dyspnea, and swelling of the feet and ankles. However, exertional symptoms are less prominent in the elderly in part because of reduced physical activity. Conversely, altered sensorium, irritability, lethargy, anorexia, abdominal discomfort, and gastrointestinal disturbances are more common symptoms of HF in the elderly.

Signs of HF include tachycardia, tachypnea, an S_3 or S_4 gallop, pulmonary rales, elevated jugular venous pressure, hepatojugular reflux, hepatomegaly, and dependent edema. In severe HF, the pulse pressure may be narrowed, and there may be signs of impaired tissue perfusion, such as cool skin, central or peripheral cyanosis, and diminished cognition. Depending on the cause of HF, additional findings may include marked hypertension (especially systolic hypertension), a dyskinetic apical impulse, a murmur of aortic or mitral origin, or peripheral signs of endocarditis. As with symptoms, the signs of HF in the elderly are often nonspecific or atypical.

B. Special Tests

1. Chest radiography—The chest radiograph often reveals cardiomegaly, pleural effusions, and signs of pulmonary venous congestion and alveolar edema. However, difficulties in obtaining a high-quality chest film and the presence of concomitant pulmonary disease may result in nondiagnostic radiographic findings.

2. Electrocardiography—ECG may reveal tachy- or bradyarrhythmias, LV hypertrophy, left atrial enlargement, or signs of ischemia or prior infarction. Although these findings may be helpful in determining the cause of HF, they are of limited value in establishing the diagnosis.

Although certain features are more common in patients with systolic HF (prior MI, S_3 gallop), whereas others suggest diastolic HF (marked hypertension, S_4 gallop), there is considerable overlap. Therefore, it is essential to assess LV function in all patients with a new HF diagnosis.

3. Echocardiography—In most cases, echocardiography is the preferred test for evaluating LV function. Echocardiography provides a wealth of information regarding atrial and ventricular chamber size and wall thickness, valve function, LV diastolic filling, and pericardial disorders. Alternatives to echocardiography include radionuclide angiography (MUGA) and magnetic resonance imaging.

4. Stress test—A stress test should be considered if severe CHD is suspected.

5. Cardiac catheterization—Cardiac catheterization is not recommended in the routine diagnostic evaluation of patients with HF but should be considered if there is evidence of significant CHD or valvular heart disease that may require percutaneous or surgical intervention. In patients undergoing cardiac catheterization for other reasons, LV function can be evaluated with contrast ventriculography.

Differential Diagnosis

The diagnosis of HF is usually straightforward in patients with severe symptoms and a chest radiograph demonstrating pulmonary edema but may be more difficult in patients with mild to moderate HF and atypical symptoms. Other causes of dyspnea and fatigue in older individuals include acute and chronic pulmonary disease (chronic obstructive lung disease, restrictive lung disease, pneumonia, pulmonary emboli), obstructive sleep apnea, obesity, anemia, hypothyroidism, poor physical conditioning, and depression. Lower extremity edema, in the absence of other signs of HF, may be due to venous insufficiency, renal or hepatic disease, or medications (especially calcium channel blockers). An elevated brain natriuretic peptide (BNP) level may be helpful in differentiating dyspnea of cardiac origin from that resulting from pulmonary or other causes, but the role of BNP in the diagnosis of HF in elderly patients remains to be established.

In addition to establishing a diagnosis of HF and determining cause, it is also important to identify factors that may contribute to worsening HF symptoms. Common precipitants of HF exacerbations in older adults include nonadherence to dietary restrictions or medications, myocardial ischemia or infarction, uncontrolled hypertension, arrhythmias (especially atrial fibrillation or flutter), anemia, systemic illness (eg, pneumonia, sepsis), iatrogenesis (eg, postoperative volume overload, blood transfusions), and adverse drug reactions (eg, NSAIDs).

Complications

Complications of HF include progressive symptoms and functional decline, recurrent hospital admissions as a result of acute exacerbations, supraventricular and ventricular arrhythmias, which may lead to syncope or sudden death, and, less frequently, deep vein thrombosis or mural thrombus formation with systemic embolization.

Treatment

The goals of HF therapy are to alleviate symptoms, improve functional capacity and quality of life, reduce hospitalizations, and maximize functional survival. Optimal management of the older HF patient involves identification and treatment of the underlying cause and precipitating factors, implementation of an effective pharmacotherapeutic regimen, and coordination of care through the use of a multidisciplinary team. Management of HF in the elderly is often complicated by the presence of comorbid conditions that may influence both the clinical course and treatment (Table 19–5). Thus, it is essential that HF management be individualized, with due consideration given to concomitant ill-

Table 19–5. Impact of common comorbidities in older patients with heart failure.

Condition	Impact
Renal dysfunction	Exacerbated by diuretics, ACE inhibitors
Chronic lung disease	Diagnostic uncertainty, difficulty in assessing volume status
Cognitive dysfunction	Interferes with compliance and patient assessment
Depression, social isolation	Interferes with compliance, worsens prognosis
Postural hypotension, falls	Aggravated by vasodilators, β-blockers, diuretics
Urinary incontinence	Aggravated by diuretics, ACE inhibitors (cough)
Sensory deprivation	Interferes with compliance
Nutritional disorders	Exacerbated by dietary restrictions
Polypharmacy	Increased drug interactions, decreased compliance
Frailty	Exacerbated by hospitalization, increased fall risk

ACE, angiotensin-converting enzyme.

nesses, prognosis, expectations, lifestyle, and therapeutic preferences.

A. Multidisciplinary Care

Despite major advances in HF therapy, hospital readmission rates remain high; noncompliance, social factors, and inadequate follow-up are major contributors to early readmission. A multidisciplinary approach to HF management is designed to address the medical, behavioral, psychosocial, and economic aspects of care through a coordinated delivery system that provides comprehensive patient education, fosters provider adherence to evidence-based guidelines for HF treatment, and ensures effective follow-up through telephone contacts, home health visits, and office appointments. Common features of successful interventions include a nurse coordinator, intensive patient education and promotion of self-management skills (eg, daily weights), and close follow-up (especially after hospital discharge). Multidisciplinary HF care is recommended for older patients with moderate or severe chronic HF, especially those at increased risk for adverse outcomes because of comorbidities, social isolation, depression, or a history of recurrent hospitalizations.

B. Pharmacotherapy

Current HF guidelines focus on systolic HF and acknowledge that optimal management of patients with diastolic HF is unknown. It is thus important to distinguish patients with predominantly systolic HF (LV ejection fraction < 45%) from those with predominantly diastolic HF (LV ejection fraction ≥ 45%) because pharmacotherapy of the former is largely evidence based, whereas treatment of the latter remains empiric.

C. Systolic Heart Failure

ACE inhibitors are the cornerstone of therapy for patients with impaired LV systolic function, whether symptomatic or asymptomatic, and available evidence indicates that older patients treated with ACE inhibitors experience improved quality of life, fewer symptoms and hospitalizations, and decreased mortality. ACE inhibitors approved for treatment of HF in the United States are listed in Table 19–6, along with recommended initial and maintenance dosages. Potential adverse effects of ACE inhibitors include worsening renal function, hyperkalemia, and hypotension. Therefore, close monitoring of renal function, electrolytes, and BP is warranted during initiation and titration of ACE inhibitor therapy. Cough occurs in up to 20% of patients receiving ACE inhibitors and may be severe enough to require discontinuation of therapy in 5–10% of cases, but there is no evidence that this occurs more frequently in the elderly. In patients who are unable to tolerate ACE inhibitors because of cough, ARBs are an

Table 19–6. Angiotensin-converting enzyme inhibitors for systolic heart failure.[a]

Agent	Starting dose	Target dose
Captopril	6.25 mg tid	50 mg tid
Enalapril	2.5 mg bid	10–20 mg bid
Lisinopril	2.5–5 mg qd	20–40 mg qd
Ramipril	1.25–2.5 mg qd	10 mg qd
Quinapril	10 mg bid	40 mg bid
Fosinopril	5–10 mg qd	40 mg qd

[a]Agents approved by the Food and Drug Administration for the treatment of heart failure in the United States.

acceptable alternative. However, they have not been shown to be equivalent to ACE inhibitors and should not be considered a first-line therapy for HF. The combination of hydralazine and isosorbide dinitrate is an additional option in patients unable to take ACE inhibitors or ARBs.

β-Blockers have been shown to reduce mortality and hospitalizations in patients with moderate to severe HF. These agents are recommended for all patients with stable HF in the absence of contraindications. Major contraindications to β-blockers include resting heart rate < 45 bpm, systolic BP < 90–100 mm Hg, markedly prolonged PR interval or heart block > first degree, active bronchospasm, and decompensated HF. β-Blockers approved for the treatment of HF in the United States include metoprolol and carvedilol. The starting dosage for metoprolol is 12.5 mg twice daily, and for carvedilol 3.125 mg twice daily. The dose should be increased gradually, at no less than 2-week intervals, to achieve daily dosages of 100–200 mg for metoprolol and 50 mg for carvedilol. With proper patient selection and dose titration, most HF patients tolerate β-blockers without difficulty. However, some may experience a transient increase in symptoms, and a small minority may require discontinuation of therapy because of severe side effects.

Digoxin is a mild inotropic agent that improves symptoms and reduces hospitalizations in patients with moderate HF but has no effect on total mortality. The benefits of digoxin in octogenarians are similar to those in younger patients. Digoxin is recommended in HF patients who remain symptomatic despite other therapy. The volume of distribution and renal clearance of digoxin are reduced in older patients. As a result, a digoxin dosage of 0.125 mg once daily is usually sufficient; patients with reduced renal function may require lower dosages. Serum digoxin levels of 0.5–1.1 ng/mL are therapeutic. Higher levels provide no additional benefit but increase the risk of toxicity. Routine monitoring of serum digoxin levels is not recommended, but a level should be obtained whenever toxicity is suspected. Side effects associated with digoxin include bradycardia, heart block, supraventricular and ventricular arrhythmias, gastrointestinal disturbances, and central nervous system disorders (especially visual changes). Hypokalemia, hypomagnesemia, and hypercalcemia increase the risk of digoxin toxicity, and a variety of medications, including quinidine, amiodarone, and verapamil, are associated with an increase in serum digoxin levels.

Diuretics, with the exception of spironolactone and eplerenone, have not been shown to improve clinical outcomes in HF patients, but they are nonetheless essential for relieving congestion and edema and for maintaining a euvolemic state. Some patients with mild HF may respond to a thiazide diuretic, but most will require a more potent loop diuretic, such as furosemide. Patients should be instructed to restrict dietary sodium intake to no more than 2 g/day, and the diuretic dosage should be adjusted to maintain euvolemia, as reflected by daily-recorded weights that are within 2 lb of the patient's predetermined dry weight. Patients with more severe HF or refractory volume overload may benefit from the addition of metolazone 2.5–10 mg daily. Diuretics are commonly associated with potassium and magnesium loss, and older patients are at increased risk for diuretic-induced electrolyte disturbances. Therefore, serial monitoring of electrolytes is warranted, and supplements should be prescribed as needed. Overdiuresis may also result in hypotension, fatigue, and worsening renal function.

Spironolactone has been shown to reduce mortality by up to 30% in patients with advanced HF resulting from severe LV systolic dysfunction. The dose of spironolactone is 12.5–25 mg once daily. Spironolactone is contraindicated in patients with serum creatinine > 2.5 mg/dL or serum potassium > 5.0 mEq/L,

and serum electrolytes and renal function should be assessed within 1–2 weeks after initiating therapy. Up to 10% of patients treated with spironolactone experience painful gynecomastia requiring discontinuation of therapy.

Current pharmacotherapy of systolic HF is summarized in Figure 19–2. All patients with LV systolic dysfunction should receive an ACE inhibitor, and all symptomatic patients should receive a β-blocker unless contraindicated. Diuretics should be prescribed and the dosage adjusted to maintain euvolemia. Digoxin should be added to the regimen of patients with persistent symptoms despite other therapeutic measures, and spironolactone should also be prescribed for patients with advanced HF symptoms unless contraindicated.

D. DIASTOLIC HEART FAILURE

Because the majority of older patients with diastolic HF have hypertension or CHD, primary therapy for diastolic HF entails aggressive management of these conditions. Thus, BP should be maintained at levels no higher than 130–140/80–90 mm Hg, and CHD should be controlled with medications and percutaneous or surgical revascularization if appropriate. Older patients with impaired LV diastolic filling are at increased risk of atrial fibrillation, and this arrhythmia is a common precipitant of acute HF. In such cases, restoration and maintenance of sinus rhythm is desirable. In patients with persistent or chronic atrial fibrillation, the ventricular response should be well controlled with β-blockers, calcium channel blockers (diltiazem or verapamil), or digoxin.

In patients with symptomatic diastolic HF, judicious use of diuretics is indicated to relieve congestion and correct volume overload. However, overdiuresis should be avoided because patients with diastolic HF are preload dependent, and insufficient LV preload re-

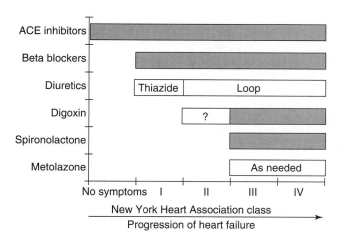

Figure 19–2. Pharmacological treatment of systolic heart failure.

duces cardiac output. Additional agents that may be helpful in improving symptoms and exercise tolerance in older patients with diastolic HF include ACE inhibitors, ARBs, β-blockers, calcium channel blockers, nitrates, and digoxin.

Prognosis

The prognosis for older patients with HF is poor, with 5-year survival rates of 20–25% in patients older than 65 and 2-year survival rates of 40–50% in those older than 85. Patients with diastolic HF have a more favorable short-term prognosis than those with systolic HF, but the long-term prognosis is similar. Other factors associated with a worse prognosis include older age, male gender, more severe symptoms, lower LV ejection fraction, ischemic cause, atrial fibrillation, diabetes, and high-grade ventricular arrhythmias. Approximately 50% of HF deaths occur suddenly as a result of ventricular fibrillation or asystole, whereas the remaining 50% are attributable to progressive HF.

A. END-OF-LIFE CARE

In light of the exceptionally poor prognosis associated with established HF (worse than for most forms of cancer), end-of-life issues should be addressed in all HF patients. Information should be provided about the clinical course and prognosis, and patients should be encouraged to express their preferences for end-of-life care and should assign durable power-of-attorney. In patients with end-stage HF and persistent severe symptoms despite optimal medical therapy, referral for hospice care should be considered.

Brophy JM et al: β-Blockers in congestive heart failure. a Bayesian meta-analysis. Ann Intern Med 2001;134:550. [PMID: 11281737]

Cohn JN et al: A randomized trial of the angiotensin-receptor blocker valsartan in chronic heart failure. N Engl J Med 2001;345:1667. [PMID: 11759645]

Flather MD et al: Long-term ACE-inhibitor therapy in patients with heart failure or left-ventricular dysfunction: a systematic overview of data from individual patients. Lancet 2000; 355:1575. [PMID: 10821360]

Gottdiener JS et al: Predictors of congestive heart failure in the elderly: the Cardiovascular Health Study. J Am Coll Cardiol 2000;35:1628. [PMID: 10807470]

Heiat A et al: Representation of the elderly, women, and minorities in heart failure clinical trials. Arch Intern Med 2002; 162:1682. [PMID: 12153370]

Hunt SA et al: ACC/AHA guidelines for the evaluation and management of chronic heart failure in the adult: executive summary. J Am Coll Cardiol 2001;38:2101. [PMID: 11738322]

Kitzman DW et al: Importance of heart failure with preserved systolic function in patients ≥ 65 years. Am J Cardiol 2001; 87:413. [PMID: 11179524]

Maisel AS et al: Rapid measurement of B-type natriuretic peptide in the emergency diagnosis of heart failure. N Engl J Med 2002;347:161. [PMID: 12124404]

McAlister FA et al: A systematic review of randomized trials of disease management programs in heart failure. Am J Med 2001; 110:378. [PMID: 11286953]

Packer M et al: Effect of carvedilol on survival in severe chronic heart failure. N Engl J Med 2001;344:1651. [PMID: 11386263]

Pitt B et al: The effect of spironolactone on morbidity and mortality in patients with severe heart failure. N Engl J Med 1999; 341:709. [PMID: 10471456]

Rathore SS et al: Association of serum digoxin concentrations and outcomes in patients with heart failure. JAMA 2003;289:871. [PMID: 12588271]

Rich MW et al: Effect of age on mortality, hospitalizations and response to digoxin in patients with heart failure: the DIG study. J Am Coll Cardiol 2001;38:806. [PMID: 11527638]

Zile MR, Brutsaert DL: New concepts in diastolic dysfunction and diastolic heart failure: part II: causal mechanisms and treatment. Circulation 2002;105:1503. [PMID: 11914262]

ARRHYTHMIAS & CONDUCTION DISTURBANCES

SICK SINUS SYNDROME

 ESSENTIALS OF DIAGNOSIS

- *Exercise intolerance, shortness of breath, fatigue, palpitations, dizziness, syncope.*
- *Sinus bradycardia, sinus pauses, paroxysmal supraventricular tachyarrhythmias accompanied by bradyarrhythmias (tachy-brady syndrome).*

General Considerations

Increasing age is associated with diffuse degenerative changes in the sinus node and atrial conduction system. The number of sinus node pacemaker cells declines with age, so that by age 75 only ~10% of the cells remain functional. In addition, conduction of the electrical impulse from the sinus node to the atrial tissues may be impaired (sinus exit block), and conduction within the atria and through the AV node is often delayed. These abnormalities in sinoatrial function, often referred to as sick sinus syndrome, predispose elderly individuals to both bradyarrhythmias (eg, inappropriate sinus bradycardia, sinus pauses, sinus arrest) and supraventricular tachyarrhythmias (atrial fibrillation, atrial flutter, atrial tachycardia). Many patients with sinoatrial dysfunction manifest both tachy- and brad-yarrhythmias, a condition referred to as tachy-brady syndrome. In the United States, sinus node dysfunction is the most common indication for permanent pace-maker implantation, accounting for approximately 50% of all pacemaker procedures.

Prevention

There are currently no known measures effective in pre-venting age-related sinoatrial dysfunction.

Clinical Findings

A. SYMPTOMS & SIGNS

Patients with sick sinus syndrome may have symptoms resulting from bradycardia, tachycardia, or both. Pa-tients with this disorder often have an asymptomatic resting sinus bradycardia, but there may be failure to increase the heart rate in response to exertion (chronotropic incompetence), resulting in exercise in-tolerance, shortness of breath, or, less commonly, angi-nal chest discomfort. Excessive sinus bradycardia may be associated with fatigue or light-headedness in addi-tion to effort intolerance. Sinus pauses more than sev-eral seconds in duration often result in severe light-headedness or syncope without premonitory symptoms. Supraventricular tachyarrhythmias may be asympto-matic or result in palpitations, dyspnea, angina, dizzi-ness, or syncope. Not uncommonly, termination of supraventricular arrhythmias is associated with pro-longed sinus pauses, resulting in dizziness or syncope.

Physical findings may include bradycardia, tachycar-dia, or an irregular rhythm. In the absence of symp-toms, BP is usually normal or elevated. Gentle carotid sinus massage may elicit an abnormal bradycardic re-sponse (sinus pause > 3 s) or reproduce the patient's symptoms of dizziness or syncope. Other physical find-ings are nonspecific.

B. SPECIAL TESTS

1. Electrocardiography—ECG often reveals sinus bradycardia with or without sinus pauses. Atrial ar-rhythmias, including atrial premature beats, atrial fibril-lation, atrial flutter, and atrial tachycardia, may also be seen. Less frequently, a slow ectopic atrial or junctional rhythm is present. When the standard 12-lead ECG is nondiagnostic in a patient with symptoms suggestive of sick sinus syndrome, 24-h ambulatory monitoring or a 30-day event recorder may be helpful.

2. Other cardiac tests—Other cardiac tests, including chest radiography, echocardiography, stress testing, and cardiac catheterization, are usually unrevealing. Rarely,

electrophysiological testing is needed to establish the di-agnosis.

Differential Diagnosis

The symptoms of sick sinus syndrome are nonspecific and may be due to a wide range of other cardiac or noncardiac causes, including CHD, HF, ventricular ar-rhythmias, aortic stenosis, pulmonary disorders (pul-monary embolus, chronic lung disease), autonomic dys-function (vagal reactions, carotid hypersensitivity syndrome, postural hypotension, postprandial hypoten-sion), hypothyroidism, hyperthyroidism, obesity, de-conditioning, pulmonary hypertension, anemia, and anxiety reactions. In addition, bradycardia and ortho-static symptoms may be due to several commonly used medications, including β-blockers (including ophthal-mological agents), diltiazem, verapamil, amiodarone and other antiarrhythmic agents, clonidine, other anti-hypertensive medications, and donepezil.

Complications

Bradyarrhythmias may be associated with falls and syn-cope, which may result in significant injury. Acute atrial fibrillation or atrial flutter with rapid ventricular response is a common precipitant of HF or acute pul-monary edema and may also be associated with non-ST-elevation MI. Patients with tachy-brady syndrome are at increased risk for thromboembolic events, includ-ing stroke. Rarely, profound bradycardia or sinus arrest may be fatal.

Treatment

Management begins with identification and treatment of other possible causes or aggravating factors. Poten-tially offending medications, such as β-blockers, should be discontinued if feasible. Electrolyte abnormalities should be corrected. Thyroid function should be as-sessed and appropriate therapy implemented if hy-pothyroidism or hyperthyroidism is detected. Addi-tional evaluation for ischemia, valve disease, pulmonary disease, or other potential causes should be undertaken on a case-by-case basis.

Patients with documented symptoms attributable to bradyarrhythmias not resulting from other treatable causes should undergo permanent pacemaker imple-mentation. Pacemaker therapy is effective in alleviating symptoms mediated by bradycardia and improves qual-ity of life in patients with effort intolerance or fatigue related to chronic bradycardia or chronotropic incom-petence. A rate-responsive dual-chamber pacing device (ie, capable of pacing both the atria and the ventricles as well as increasing the pacing rate during exercise) is preferable in patients with sinus rhythm. Such devices have been associated with improved quality of life and reduced atrial fibrillation compared with single-lead ventricular pacing.

Supraventricular tachyarrhythmias occurring in the context of tachy-brady syndrome should be managed with rate controlling agents (eg, digoxin, β-blockers, diltiazem, verapamil), anticoagulation (warfarin preferred), and antiarrhythmic agents as needed to maintain sinus rhythm. Many of the agents used to treat supraventricular tachyarrhythmias may exacerbate the associated bradyarrhythmias, necessitating pacemaker implantation.

Prognosis

Most patients with appropriately treated sick sinus syndrome are able to maintain good quality of life in the absence of other major cardiac or noncardiac conditions. The prognosis is worse in patients with tachy-brady syndrome who experience thromboembolic complications, especially stroke.

ATRIAL FIBRILLATION & ATRIAL FLUTTER

ESSENTIALS OF DIAGNOSIS

- *Palpitations, shortness of breath, chest pain, dizziness.*
- *Rapid, irregular pulse (may be regular in atrial flutter).*
- *ECG demonstrates atrial fibrillation or atrial flutter.*

General Considerations

The prevalence of atrial fibrillation increases from < 1% in persons younger than 40 to > 10% in persons older than 80. The median age of patients with atrial fibrillation is 75. Atrial fibrillation is more common in men than in women at all ages, but the proportion of women increases with age.

Prevention

Prompt identification and treatment of conditions that predispose to atrial fibrillation (eg, hyperthyroidism, electrolyte disorders) may prevent arrhythmia. Perioperative treatment of cardiac surgical patients with amio-

darone or β-blockers reduces the risk of postoperative atrial fibrillation and shortens length of hospital stay. β-Blockers also reduce the risk of postoperative atrial fibrillation in older adults undergoing major noncardiac surgery, especially chest, abdominal, or vascular procedures. Dual-chamber pacing reduces the risk of atrial fibrillation in patients with sick sinus syndrome.

Clinical Findings

A. SYMPTOMS & SIGNS

New-onset atrial fibrillation or flutter is often associated with a rapid ventricular rate, resulting in palpitations, shortness of breath, and, in some cases, chest pain, dizziness, or syncope. However, many patients are asymptomatic or minimally symptomatic, and the rhythm disturbance may be detected as an incidental finding on physical examination. Still other patients have acute pulmonary edema or a thromboembolic event, such as transient ischemic attack or stroke.

The cardinal physical finding of atrial fibrillation is an irregularly irregular rhythm. In untreated older patients, ventricular rates of 130–180 bpm are common, but rates as low as 50–70 bpm may also be seen. In atrial flutter, the rhythm is often regular, and the rate is typically either 150 bpm (2:1 block) or 75 bpm (4:1 block). However, an irregular rhythm resulting from variable AV block is also common, and it may not be possible to distinguish atrial fibrillation from atrial flutter on the basis of physical examination alone. Other physical findings are nonspecific but may include signs of HF, a mitral or aortic valvular murmur, evidence for chronic lung disease or pulmonary hypertension, or, less commonly, manifestations of hyperthyroidism.

B. SPECIAL TESTS

1. Electrocardiography—In patients with ongoing atrial fibrillation or atrial flutter, the ECG is diagnostic, revealing either an irregular rhythm without organized atrial activity (atrial fibrillation), or the classic sawtooth pattern of atrial flutter in the inferior leads (II, III, AVF). Other electrocardiographic findings may include LV hypertrophy, evidence for ischemia or prior MI, and a rightward axis suggesting pulmonary disease.

2. Chest radiography—Chest radiography may reveal cardiomegaly, left atrial enlargement, or pulmonary congestion.

3. Echocardiography—All patients with new- or recent-onset atrial fibrillation or flutter should undergo echocardiography to evaluate left atrial size, LV function, and wall thickness and to assess for the presence of valvular heart disease, pericardial disease, or pulmonary hypertension.

3. Cardiac catheterization—Cardiac catheterization is not indicated in the routine evaluation of atrial fibrillation but may be appropriate if noninvasive testing reveals severe CHD or valvular heart disease for which further intervention is contemplated.

4. Other tests—Serum electrolytes, including magnesium, should be measured, and thyroid function should be assessed, especially since atrial fibrillation may be the only clinical manifestation of hyperthyroidism in the elderly.

Differential Diagnosis

Atrial fibrillation and flutter must be distinguished from other supraventricular and ventricular tachyarrhythmias. Multifocal atrial tachycardia (MAT) is an irregularly irregular tachyarrhythmia that most commonly occurs in patients with severe chronic lung disease. The ECG demonstrates prominent P waves of varying morphology. Atrial flutter at a rate of 150 bpm may be difficult to distinguish from other supraventricular rhythms, including sinus tachycardia and paroxysmal supraventricular tachycardia (PSVT). Carotid sinus massage or intravenous adenosine 6–12 mg is often helpful in differentiating these rhythm disorders. Occasionally, wide-complex supraventricular arrhythmias may be difficult to distinguish from ventricular tachycardia. The latter condition does not respond to adenosine but may respond to lidocaine.

Complications

The most important complication of atrial fibrillation or atrial flutter is systemic embolization, which may result in stroke, MI, ischemia or infarction of abdominal viscera, or impaired circulation to the extremities. The proportion of strokes attributable to atrial fibrillation increases with age, from < 2% in persons younger than 60 to > 20% in those older than 80. Risk factors for stroke in older patients with atrial fibrillation include HF, hypertension, diabetes, and a prior thromboembolic event. The risk of embolization is lower in patients with "pure" atrial flutter, but most patients with atrial flutter also have atrial fibrillation. Other complications of atrial fibrillation and flutter include HF, non-ST-elevation MI, and syncope; these clinical events most often occur at the onset of atrial fibrillation or flutter with rapid ventricular response.

Treatment

Management of atrial fibrillation and flutter involves identification and treatment of the underlying cause and precipitating factors when feasible, controlling the ventricular rate, restoring and maintaining normal sinus rhythm, and reducing the risk of thromboembolic events.

A. RATE CONTROL

Effective control of the ventricular rate is a primary goal of therapy during both the acute and chronic phases of management. Optimal rate control is defined as a resting heart rate of 60–80 bpm and a heart rate of 90–115 bpm during moderate exercise. β-Blockers, diltiazem, verapamil, and digoxin slow conduction through the AV node, thus slowing the ventricular response rate. Although digoxin is widely used for this indication, it is less effective than other agents and is relatively ineffective in controlling the ventricular rate during exertion. In some patients with persistent symptomatic tachycardia despite aggressive pharmacological intervention, AV nodal ablation with placement of a permanent ventricular pacemaker is an effective alternative for controlling rate and reducing symptoms.

B. RHYTHM CONTROL

Restoration and maintenance of sinus rhythm offer the theoretical advantages of reducing stroke risk and avoiding the need for long-term anticoagulation. However, antiarrhythmic drugs used in the treatment of atrial fibrillation are only moderately effective and may be associated with significant side effects, including ventricular proarrhythmia. Patients with recent-onset atrial fibrillation or atrial flutter who remain significantly symptomatic despite optimal rate control, or who are poor candidates for long-term systemic anticoagulation, may benefit from cardioversion and antiarrhythmic therapy to maintain sinus rhythm.

Although patients with atrial fibrillation or flutter of < 48 h duration can safely undergo cardioversion with an acceptably low risk of thromboembolic complications, those with atrial fibrillation or flutter of longer duration should be anticoagulated with warfarin to maintain an INR of at least 2.0 for at least 3 weeks before attempting cardioversion. Alternatively, patients may undergo transesophageal echocardiography; if there is no evidence of atrial thrombus, cardioversion may be performed without delay. In either case, there is a risk of thromboembolic events for several weeks after cardioversion, and patients should be maintained on anticoagulation (INR ≥ 2.0) for a minimum of 4 weeks after cardioversion.

Cardioversion may be performed either pharmacologically or electrically. Multiple antiarrhythmic agents may restore sinus rhythm, but amiodarone is the most effective and is associated with the lowest risk of ventricular proarrhythmia. However, because of its very long half-life (1–2 mo), it may take days or even weeks of oral amiodarone loading before a therapeutic blood level is achieved. Direct current cardioversion is more effective than drug therapy in restoring sinus rhythm but is associated with a somewhat higher risk of thromboembolic complications. Once sinus rhythm has been restored, amiodarone is the most effective agent for maintaining sinus rhythm at 1 year. Sotalol, a β-blocker, is an acceptable alternative to amiodarone, but tolerability and proarrhythmia may be problematic. One-year recurrence rates are at least 30–40%; thus, long-term anticoagulation is advisable except in patients at relatively low risk for recurrence (eg, postoperative atrial fibrillation or new-onset atrial fibrillation with spontaneous reversion to sinus rhythm within 48 h), especially if a treatable cause can be identified.

C. ANTITHROMBOTIC THERAPY

Older patients with paroxysmal or chronic atrial fibrillation benefit from long-term anticoagulation with warfarin, and stroke risk is reduced by ~66%. Because increasing age is an important risk factor for thromboembolic events, older patients derive the greatest absolute benefit from warfarin therapy. Although this benefit is tempered somewhat by increased bleeding complications, including hemorrhagic stroke, current recommendations are that all older patients with nonvalvular paroxysmal or chronic atrial fibrillation receive warfarin therapy to maintain an INR of 2.0–3.0. Patients with mitral valve disease or mechanical prosthetic valves should have INRs maintained in the range of 2.5–3.5.

Patients receiving long-term warfarin treatment should be advised to avoid cauliflower, broccoli, and other dark green, leafy vegetables because these foods are high in vitamin K and antagonize the effects of warfarin. Warfarin also interacts with numerous medications, and the INR should be monitored closely after medication changes. In addition, NSAIDs markedly increase the risk of gastrointestinal bleeding in older patients taking warfarin, and these drugs should be avoided if possible.

Older patients with prior stroke, dementia, gastrointestinal bleeding, or other conditions may be at increased risk for serious hemorrhagic complications during long-term warfarin therapy. Although substantially less effective than warfarin in reducing stroke risk, with a net reduction of ~20%, aspirin in a dose of 325 mg daily may be a suitable alternative to warfarin in selected patients.

Prognosis

With proper treatment, including anticoagulation, the long-term prognosis for patients with paroxysmal or chronic atrial fibrillation or flutter is relatively good, and many patients remain essentially asymptomatic for many years, even decades. Nonetheless, persons with atrial fibrillation have reduced long-term survival compared with those with sinus rhythm, and atrial fibrillation is also associated with a worse prognosis in acute MI patients as well as in those with HF or valvular heart disease.

VENTRICULAR ARRHYTHMIAS

ESSENTIALS OF DIAGNOSIS

- *Palpitations, dizziness, syncope, shortness of breath.*
- *Wide-complex ectopic beats on the 12-lead ECG or 24-h ambulatory monitor.*

General Considerations

The prevalence of ventricular arrhythmias increases with age. In the absence of underlying cardiac disease, frequent ventricular ectopic beats are not associated with increased mortality.

Prevention

Early identification and treatment of risk factors for cardiovascular disease may reduce the risk of serious ventricular arrhythmias in older adults.

Clinical Findings

A. SYMPTOMS & SIGNS

Isolated ventricular ectopic beats (VEBs) are usually asymptomatic, but frequent VEBs may cause palpitations. Salvos of VEBs at a rapid rate (ventricular tachycardia) may result in dizziness or syncope. Occasionally, VEBs or ventricular tachycardia may trigger ventricular fibrillation.

Physical findings associated with VEBs include an intermittently irregular rhythm and cannon A waves in the jugular venous pulse. Ventricular tachycardia is associated with a rapid pulse but may or may not be associated with hypotension or signs of tissue hypoperfusion. Ventricular fibrillation is associated with absent pulse and BP. Other findings in patients with ventricular arrhythmias reflect the presence of underlying cardiovascular disease.

B. SPECIAL TESTS

1. Electrocardiography—In patients with isolated VEBs, the ECG or 24-h ambulatory monitor reveals wide-complex ectopic beats of ventricular origin (ie, not clearly preceded by a P wave). Ventricular tachycardia manifests as a wide-QRS tachycardia, which, when sustained, is usually regular. Torsades de pointes ventricular tachycardia usually occurs in the setting of marked QT-interval prolongation and has a polymorphic appearance with waxing and waning QRS amplitude. Ventricular fibrillation is a chaotic rhythm without well-defined QRS complexes.

2. Other tests—Additional evaluation in patients with significant ventricular arrhythmias is directed at assessing ventricular function and identifying potentially treatable cardiovascular disorders. An echocardiogram is indicated in most cases, and a stress test is appropriate if CHD is suspected. Cardiac catheterization is warranted in patients with CHD or valvular disorders for whom further intervention is planned. The role of electrophysiological testing for evaluation of serious ventricular arrhythmias is declining because of increasing evidence that implantable cardioverter defibrillators (ICDs) are beneficial in high-risk patients with ventricular tachycardia or resuscitated ventricular fibrillation.

Differential Diagnosis

Isolated wide-complex ectopic beats may be of supraventricular, junctional, or ventricular origin. The presence of a normal-appearing P wave preceding the ectopic beat suggests a supraventricular complex with aberrancy. Absent or retrograde P waves indicate a junctional or ventricular origin. Wide-complex tachycardias may be either supraventricular or ventricular. Patients with CHD or other major cardiac disorders are at increased risk for ventricular tachycardia. Other features that favor ventricular tachycardia include evidence for dissociation between atrial and ventricular activity, marked left- or right-axis deviation, QRS duration ≥ 160 ms, and directional QRS concordance across the precordium.

Complications

The most feared complication of ventricular arrhythmias is sudden cardiac death. Ventricular tachycardia may also be associated with syncope, HF, or angina.

Treatment

In most cases, isolated VEBs, even when frequent, require no specific therapy. In highly symptomatic patients, β-blockers are the agents of first choice. Rarely, other antiarrhythmic agents may be required to control severe symptoms, but there is no evidence that these agents reduce the risk of sudden death.

The treatment of patients with nonsustained ventricular tachycardia with or without symptoms is evolving. Patients with CHD and moderate or severe LV systolic dysfunction (ejection fraction ≤ 30%) have improved survival after implantation of an ICD. The value of ICDs in patients with nonsustained ventricular tachycardia in the absence of CHD or with CHD in the setting of preserved LV systolic function is unclear. β-Blockers reduce the risk of sudden death in patients with CHD with or without LV dysfunction and in those with nonischemic dilated cardiomyopathy. The value of other antiarrhythmic agents, including amiodarone, is unproven.

Patients with symptomatic sustained ventricular tachycardia or resuscitated sudden cardiac death outside the context of acute MI and in the absence of other treatable disorders (eg, electrolyte disturbances) should receive an ICD because these devices have been associated with substantial mortality reductions in high-risk patients. The efficacy of ICDs in preventing sudden cardiac death is similar in younger and older patients.

Prognosis

The prognosis of ventricular arrhythmias is governed by the presence, nature, and severity of underlying cardiac disease. In the absence of significant heart disease or LV systolic dysfunction, the prognosis for isolated VEBs and nonsustained ventricular tachycardia is excellent. Frequent VEBs in patients with CHD or reduced LV systolic function are a marker for increased mortality and sudden cardiac death, but there is no evidence that suppression of VEBs with antiarrhythmic drugs improves survival. Patients with nonsustained ventricular tachycardia associated with CHD and LV dysfunction, as well as those with symptomatic sustained ventricular tachycardia or resuscitated sudden cardiac death, are at high-risk for death within 1–2 years unless treated with an ICD.

Ansell J et al: Managing oral anticoagulant therapy. Chest 2001;119:22S. [PMID: 11157641]

Aronow WS et al: Prevalence and association of ventricular tachycardia and complex ventricular arrhythmias with new coronary events in older men and women with and without cardiovascular disease. J Gerontol Series A 2002;57:M178. [PMID: 11867655]

Buxton AE et al: A randomized study of the prevention of sudden death in patients with coronary artery disease. N Engl J Med 1999;341:1882. [PMID: 10601507]

Daoud EG et al: Preoperative amiodarone as prophylaxis against atrial fibrillation after heart surgery. N Engl J Med 1997; 337:1785. [PMID: 9400034]

Fuster V et al: ACC/AHA/ESC guidelines for the management of patients with atrial fibrillation: executive summary. J Am Coll Cardiol 2001;38:1231. [PMID: 11583910]

Gregoratos G et al: ACC/AHA/NASPE 2002 guideline update for implantation of cardiac pacemakers and antiarrhythmia devices: summary article. Circulation 2002;106:2145. [PMID: 12379588]

Hart RG et al: Antithrombotic therapy to prevent stroke in patients with atrial fibrillation: a meta-analysis. Ann Intern Med 1999;131:492. [PMID: 10507957]

Klein AL et al: Use of transesophageal echocardiography to guide cardioversion in patients with atrial fibrillation. N Engl J Med 2001;344:1411. [PMID: 11346805]

Lamas GA et al: Ventricular pacing or dual-chamber pacing for sinus-node dysfunction. N Engl J Med 2002;346:1854. [PMID: 12063369]

Magnano DT et al: Effect of atenolol on mortality and cardiovascular morbidity after noncardiac surgery. N Engl J Med 1996; 335:1713. [PMID: 8929262]

MERIT-HF Study Group: Effect of metoprolol CR/XL in chronic heart failure: Metoprolol CR/XL Randomised Intervention Trial in Congestive Heart Failure (MERIT-HF). Lancet 1999;353:2001. [PMID: 10376614]

Moss AJ et al: Prophylactic implantation of a defibrillator in patients with myocardial infarction and reduced ejection fraction. N Engl J Med 2002;346:877. [PMID: 11907286]

Packer M et al: Effect of carvedilol on survival in severe chronic heart failure. N Engl J Med 2001;344:1651. [PMID: 11386263]

Wyse DG et al: A comparison of rate control and rhythm control in patients with atrial fibrillation. N Engl J Med 2002; 347:1825. [PMID: 124466506]

RELEVANT WORLD WIDE WEB SITES

American College of Cardiology: www.acc.org (Features access to all guidelines published by the College as well as practice management tools)

American Heart Association: www.americanheart.org (Excellent source of materials for both practitioners and patients)

American Heart Association: www.americanheart.org/profilers (Personalized web site for care providers and patients; covers CHD, heart failure, atrial fibrillation, hypertension, and dyslipidemia)

Heart Failure Online: www.heartfailure.org (Heart failure patient education web site with modules in English and Spanish)

Heart Failure Society of America: www.abouthf.org (Heart failure patient education materials)

Heart Failure Society of America: www.hfsa.org (Informational materials for health care providers)

Society of Geriatric Cardiology: www.sgcard.org (Featuring modular slide sets on selected aspects of cardiovascular disease in older adults)

Hypertension

20

Swarna Meyyazhagan, MD, & Barbara J. Messinger-Rapport, MD, PhD

ESSENTIALS OF DIAGNOSIS

- Diastolic hypertension in the absence of major risk factors and target organ damage is defined as diastolic blood pressure ≥ 90 mm Hg.
- Systolic hypertension in the absence of major risk factors and target organ damage is defined as systolic blood pressure ≥ 140 mm Hg.
- In the presence of normal diastolic blood pressure (< 90 mm Hg), systolic hypertension is referred to as isolated systolic hypertension.

General Considerations

Hypertension in older adults is defined according to Joint National Committee on Prevention, Detection, Evaluation, and Treatment of High Blood Pressure VII (JNC VII) criteria as an elevation in systolic or diastolic blood pressure (BP). Hypertension is very common among the elderly, affecting > 50% of noninstitutionalized adults 60 years and older in the United States. It is a major risk factor for cardiovascular and cerebrovascular morbidity and mortality. Despite a slow decrease in incidence of deaths since 1965, the age-adjusted death rates from coronary disease and stroke remain high: 195.6 and 61.5 per 100,000, respectively. Coronary disease is the most common cause of death in men and women 65 years and older. Stroke is the most severely disabling condition affecting older adults.

Aging, higher body weight, smoking, reduced physical activity, and salt intake are major risk factors for hypertension. Alcohol, sleep apnea, and certain medications can also contribute to hypertension in a minority of individuals.

In the presence of normal diastolic BP (< 90), systolic hypertension is referred to as isolated systolic hypertension (ISH). Borderline systolic BP in older adults typically progresses over time into definite hypertension.

Because systolic pressure rises with age and diastolic pressure plateaus or even decreases during the sixth decade (Figure 20–1), isolated diastolic hypertension is rare in the elderly. Diastolic hypertension usually occurs in combination with systolic hypertension in older adults (diastolic–systolic hypertension).

Elevated pulse pressure (PP) is increasingly recognized as an important predictor of cerebrovascular and cardiac risk in older adults. PP increases with age in a manner parallel to the increase in systolic BP.

Differential Diagnosis

Most older hypertensives have primary or essential hypertension. Secondary hypertension refers to hypertension with an identifiable and treatable cause. Renovascular hypertension is the most common cause of treatable secondary hypertension in older persons, although it is not always surgically treatable. Less common causes in older adults include pheochromocytoma, which is rare but increases in incidence with age, Cushing's syndrome, obstructive sleep apnea, and neurological problems such as intracranial tumors.

Four common conditions in older patients are associated with or complicate the diagnosis of hypertension: "white coat," or "office," hypertension; postural, or orthostatic, hypotension, postprandial hypotension, and pseudohypertension. White coat hypertension is mild hypertension noted in the physician's office but repeatedly normal measurements at home, at work, or by ambulatory monitoring. End-organ disease, such as left ventricular hypertrophy, hypertensive retinopathy, or nephropathy, is notably absent. White coat hypertension may commonly coexist with metabolic risk factors such as hypercholesterolemia and hyperinsulinemia and may be associated with increased long-term cardiovascular mortality.

Postural hypotension is a 20-mm Hg drop in systolic BP or 10 mm Hg in diastolic BP when rising from a sitting position. Orthostatic hypotension is associated with diabetes, hypertension, low body mass index, and use of antihypertensive medications.

Postprandial hypotension is a 5–20 mm Hg drop in systolic BP after consumption of a warm meal or alcohol. The BP drop may last for 2–3 h. Postprandial hypotension can complicate identification of hypertension as well as hypertension treatment. Postprandial decreases in BP can possibly be managed through a regi-

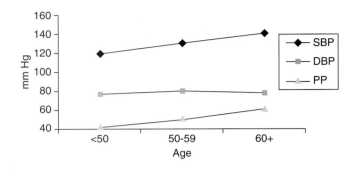

Figure 20–1. Changes in systolic blood pressure (SBP), diastolic pressure (DBP), and pulse pressure (PP) with aging. SBP and PP increase with age. DBP plateaus or peaks at approximately 55 years. Plotted using data from Framingham Heart Study.

men of small meals, limited dietary carbohydrates, and consumption of a caffeinated beverage before meals.

Pseudohypertension is a significantly higher pressure measured in the periphery (eg, brachial site) compared with a direct arterial measurement. Arterial rigidity from extensive atherosclerosis is considered to be responsible for this relatively rare phenomenon. Although it can be diagnosed by direct intra-arterial measurement, this invasive technique is usually unnecessary. The presence of Osler's sign (a palpable radial artery when BP cuff is inflated above the systolic BP) is suggestive but not diagnostic of this condition. Pseudohypertension may be suspected in those who appear resistant to an adequate drug regimen, those who become very symptomatic to a gentle pharmacological regimen, and those with very elevated BPs but no clinical evidence of end-organ disease. Incidental radiographs of the distal extremities may reveal extensive arterial calcification.

Clinical Findings

A. Symptoms & Signs

Most older hypertensives are asymptomatic. A minority may present with dizziness, palpitations, or headache. A morning headache, usually occipital, may be characteristic of stage III hypertension. End-organ damage, such as stroke, CHF, or renal failure, may be the initial presentation.

B. Patient History

A history suggesting postprandial or orthostatic hypotension may be elicited. These syndromes may reflect long-standing hypertension or the presence of associated problems that need to be considered in treating hypertension.

Patient history should be directed toward the possibility of secondary hypertension, focusing on recent weight gain, polyuria, polydipsia, muscle weakness, history of headaches, palpitations, diaphoresis, weight loss, anxiety, and sleep history (eg, daytime somnolence, loud snoring, early morning headaches).

Symptoms suspicious for target organ damage include headache, transient weakness or blindness, claudication, chest pain, and shortness of breath. Comorbid conditions such as diabetes mellitus, coronary artery disease (CAD), heart failure, chronic obstructive pulmonary disease, gout, and sexual dysfunction are important to elicit because they will impact coronary risk factor stratification and choice of initial therapy.

Medication history should include previous BP medications, current prescription drugs, over-the-counter drugs, and herbal supplements. Nonsteroidal anti-inflammatory drugs, cold medications, and some herbal supplements are particularly important because they may increase BP.

Lifestyle issues, including smoking, alcohol intake, drug use, regular exercise, and degree of physical activity, should be assessed. A dietary history targeting sodium (which can raise BP), fat intake (which can contribute to cardiovascular risk), and alcohol (which can raise BP if excessive) is important as well.

C. Physical Examination

The physical examination focuses on the confirmation of hypertension and identification of possible secondary causes. Verification of the diagnosis of hypertension can be done by measuring BP at different times using an appropriate cuff size after a comfortable rest ideally without the influence of alcohol, caffeine, or tobacco. BP is measured in both arms using standard techniques. Given the relatively high prevalence of orthostatic hypotension in older adults, standing BPs are measured as well.

D. Laboratory Tests

Complete blood count, renal and metabolic panel, lipid profile, thyroid-stimulating hormone (TSH), urinalysis, and 12-lead electrocardiogram are included in the initial evaluation.

Evidence should be sought for end-organ target disease (ie, ophthalmological vascular changes, carotid bruits, distended neck veins, third or fourth heart sound, pulmonary rales, reduced peripheral pulses). A cognitive evaluation (eg, the Mini-Mental State Examination) is also helpful in tracking longitudinal cognitive changes in the older hypertensive patient. Secondary causes, including renal bruits (renal artery stenosis); moon face, buffalo hump, and abdominal striae (Cushing's syndrome); tremor, hyperreflexia, and tachycardia (thyrotoxicosis) should be assessed.

Complications

Older persons with hypertension have higher absolute risks of cardiovascular and cerebrovascular events. They are also more likely to have other comorbid conditions that worsen these outcomes. Thus, preventing target organ damage in older adults with hypertension is vital to reducing morbidity and mortality from hypertension. Target organ damage can occur overtly, in the form of heart failure or arrhythmia, or more subtly, in the form of a neuropsychiatric deficit such as cognitive impairment. Hypertension is the major risk factor for stroke, which is the third leading cause of death and the primary cause of serious disability in adults 65 years of age and older. Approximately 66% of first strokes are attributable to hypertension; systolic hypertension is the most important risk factor. Atrial fibrillation is often a complication of hypertensive disease in older adults; 15% of strokes occur in people with atrial fibrillation.

Hypertension is also a risk factor for heart disease, including myocardial infarction, congestive heart failure (CHF), and sudden death. Diastolic dysfunction increases with age secondary to reduced vascular compliance and increased impedance to left ventricular ejection related to aging myocardium.

Other important complications include chronic renal insufficiency, end-stage renal disease, malignant hypertension, and encephalopathy. These disorders are most common with severe or poorly controlled hypertension.

Dementia, including Alzheimer's disease, may be associated with previously uncontrolled hypertension in middle-aged or older adults. The association may be particularly strong in diabetic hypertensive individuals.

American Heart Association: 2002 Heart and Stroke Statistical Update. American Heart Association, 2002.

Chobanian AV et al: The seventh report of the Joint National Committee on Prevention, Detection, Evaluation, and Treatment of High Blood Pressure: The JNC 7 report. JAMA 2003;289:2560. [PMID: 12748199]

Kannel WB: Elevated systolic blood pressure as a cardiovascular risk factor. Am J Cardiol 2000;85:251. [PMID: 10955386]

Luukinen H et al: Prognosis of diastolic and systolic orthostatic hypotension in older persons. Arch Intern Med 1999;159:273. [PMID: 99142645]

Staessen JA et al: Risks of untreated and treated isolated systolic hypertension in the elderly: Meta-analysis of outcome trials. Lancet 2000;355:865. [PMID: 10752701]

Treatment

A. HYPERTENSION

The general objective of hypertension management for both community-dwelling and nursing home patients is to reduce morbidity and mortality by early diagnosis and treatment with the least invasive methods at minimum cost. Classification of BP, stratification for cardiovascular risks, and management strategies according to JNC VII guidelines are shown in Table 20–1. Major risk factors are enumerated in Table 20–2. Treatment of hypertension in the oldest old is not clearly associated with a mortality benefit, but does appear to reduce the risk of stroke and congestive heart failure.

Little information is available to guide clinicians regarding hypertension management in nursing home residents, typically a frail, elderly group. One issue constraining hypertension treatment may be delineation of

Table 20–1. Classification of blood pressure, stratification of cardiovascular risk, & initial treatment strategies.

Class	SBP (mm Hg)		DBP (mm Hg)	Lifestyle modification	No compelling indication	With compelling indication
Normal	< 120	and	< 80	Encourage		
Prehypertension	120–139	or	80–89	Yes	No drugs	Drugs for compelling indication
Stage I	140–159	or	90–99	Yes	Thiazide first choice	Drug for compelling indication ± thiazide or other drugs
Stage II	≥ 160	or	≥ 100	Yes	Combination therapy for most, usually including thiazide; caution for orthostasis	Drug for compelling indication ± thiazide or other drugs

Adapted from Chobanian AV et al: The seventh report of the Joint National Committee on Prevention, Detection, Evaluation, and Treatment of High Blood Pressure: The JNC 7 Report. JAMA 2003;289:2560. Used with permission.

Table 20–2. Cardiovascular risk stratification in patients with hypertension.

Cardiovascular risk stratification	Target organ damage
Hypertension	Heart
Tobacco	Left ventricular hypertrophy
BMI ≥ 30	Angina or prior myocardial infarction
Physical Inactivity	Prior coronary revascularization
Dyslipidemia	Heart failure
Diabetes	Brain
Renal insufficiency	Stroke or transient ischemic attack
Age (> 55 for men, > 65 years for women)	Chronic renal disease
Family history of premature cardiovascular disease (men < 55 years, women < 65 years)	Peripheral arterial disease
	Retinopathy

Adapted from Chobanian AV et al: The seventh report of the Joint National Committee on Prevention, Detection, Evaluation, and Treatment of High Blood Pressure: The JNC 7 Report. JAMA 2003;289:2560. Used with permission.

the goals of therapy. A frail elder with multiple comorbidities may have a limited life expectancy. The potential reduction in stroke benefit from antihypertensive medication may not be realized in this case, and the side effects of the medication may be less justifiable. A higher target BP and a less aggressive approach to treatment of hypertension may be acceptable in such cases.

1. Nonpharmacological therapy—Lifestyle interventions may benefit older hypertensives and can include the following:

1. Weight reduction if overweight (5-kg threshold; 10 kg reduces BP 10–8 mm Hg). Care must be taken with older adults to maintain adequate nutrient intake should weight reduction be recommended.

2. Reduction in dietary sodium.

3. Increased consumption of fruits and vegetables and decreased consumption of dairy and animal fat (the DASH diet).

4. Limiting alcohol consumption to no more than 2 standard drinks per day for men (1 standard drink daily for women and lighter weight men). A standard drink is one 12-oz bottle of beer or wine cooler, one 5-oz glass of wine, or 1.5 oz of 80-proof distilled spirits.

5. Increasing physical activity to 30–45 min of aerobic activity 4 or more days per week. If this is not attainable, any increase in physical activity is likely to be beneficial.

6. Smoking cessation. Older adults may be less tolerant of recommended adjuvant smoking cessation therapies, such as bupropion, clonidine, and nortriptyline.

Use of nonpharmacological measures to control hypertension in the nursing home setting may be limited because residents are often limited in their activities of daily living and unable to participate in moderate exercise. Also, weight loss is a problem rather than a goal for most nursing home residents. If their diet is restricted in salt or animal and dairy fat, they may lose weight, strength, and essential nutrients.

2. Pharmacological therapy—Antihypertensive medication improves cardiovascular and cerebrovascular outcomes in older adults with BP ≥ 160/90 mm Hg. The absolute benefit of hypertension treatment tends to be greater in men, in patients aged 70 or older, in those with previous cardiovascular complications, and in the presence of wider PP. Treatment prevents stroke more effectively than coronary events, although both outcomes are improved by antihypertensive treatment.

The key to achieving maximal benefit and minimal risk in older adults is to "start low and go slow." Lower initial doses of antihypertensives minimize the risk of postural and postprandial hypotension as well as ischemic symptoms, especially in frail older adults.

Route of administration may be an issue in nursing home residents with dysphagia and those who are unwilling to take pills. A clonidine or nitroglycerin patch may be beneficial in BP management in these situations. Because orthostatic hypotension and postprandial hypotension may contribute to the risk of falling, it may be appropriate to titrate antihypertensives in the standing position. Also, BP tends to be highest before breakfast in the nursing home resident, so titration of antihypertensives later in the day may also be desirable.

Table 20–3 summarizes data on antihypertensive agents commonly used in older patients.

a. Diuretics—Thiazide and related diuretics are the preferred first-line treatment in older adults and have proved particularly effective in blacks and in salt-sensitive hypertensive patients. Diuretics have been shown

Table 20-3. Pharmacotherapy for hypertension.

Drug group	Initial dose	Typical range	Cost (30 tabs)	Indications in addition to hypertension	Side effects/comments
Diuretic					
HCTZ	6.25–12.5 mg/day	25 mg/day	$5–15	Typical first-line therapy	Hypokalemia, hypercalcemia, hyperuricemia, hyponatremia, metabolic alkalosis, increased frequency (all less likely at low doses)
Calcium channel blockers					
Dihydropyridines					
Amlodipine	2.5 mg/day	2.5–10 mg/day	$33–67	Typical first-line therapy	Flush, headache, local ankle edema (dose related)
Felodipine	2.5 mg/day	5–10 mg/day	$34–70	Typical first-line therapy	Flush, headache, local ankle edema (dose related)
Nondihydropyridines					
Verapamil	120 mg/day	120–240 mg qd–bid	$22–30	Angina, arrhythmias	Constipation, conduction block, CHF, transaminase elevation
Diltiazem (ER)	120–180 mg/day	240–480 mg/day	$30–123	Angina	Conduction block, CHF, transaminase elevation
α-Blocker					
Terazosin	1–2 mg/day	1–5 mg/day	$50	BPH, hypertension	Postural hypotension (dose related); not as beneficial as diuretic in reducing CV events
Doxazosin	1–2 mg/day	1–8 mg/day	$20–35	BPH, hypertension	Same as for terazosin
β-Blocker					
Atenolol	25 mg/day	25–50 mg/day	$5–45	CAD, systolic dysfunction	Bronchospasm, second- and third-degree heart block, fatigue, sleep disturbance; caution with diabetics, peripheral arterial disease; atenolol is renally excreted; serum levels are significantly higher in older adults and those with known renal insufficiency
Metoprolol	25 mg bid	50–100 mg bid	$15–40	CAD, systolic dysfunction	Bronchospasm, second- and third-degree heart block, fatigue, sleep disturbance; caution with diabetics, peripheral arterial disease; metoprolol is renally excreted; serum levels are significantly higher in older adults and those with known renal insufficiency

(continued)

Table 20–3. Pharmacotherapy for hypertension. (Continued)

Drug group	Initial dose	Typical range	Cost (30 tabs)	Indications in addition to hypertension	Side effects/comments
α-β Blocker					
Carvedilol	3.125 mg bid	6.25–12.5 mg bid	$55	CAD, systolic dysfunction	Bronchospasm, second- and third-degree heart block, fatigue, sleep disturbance; caution with diabetics, peripheral arterial disease; carvedilol is renally excreted; serum levels are significantly higher in older adults, and those with known renal insufficiency
Centrally acting					
Clonidine	0.1 mg bid	0.1–2 mg bid–tid	$6–30	Second- or third-line therapy or when unable to tolerate oral therapy (eg, patch)	Fatigue, dry mouth, lethargy, rebound hypertension when abruptly discontinued, fluid retention
Clonidine patch (TTS)	0.1 mg/day (TTS-1)	0.1–0.2 mg/day (TTS-1 or 2)	$42–102		
Direct vasodilators					
Hydralazine	10 mg tid or	50 mg bid–qid	$4–24	Afterload reduction in CHF	Headache, tachycardia, lupus syndrome, fluid retention
ACEIs					
Captopril	25 mg qpm 12.5 mg bid	25 mg bid–tid	$4–50	Diabetics, CHF, LV dysfunction after MI	Cough, rash, loss of taste, hyperkalemia; rarely leukopenia and angioedema
Enalapril	2.5 mg qd	5–20 mg/day	$30–100	Diabetics, CHF, LV dysfunction after MI	Cough, rash, loss of taste, hyperkalemia; rarely leukopenia and angioedema
Lisinopril	5 mg/day	10–40 mg/day	$20–50	Diabetics, CHF, LV dysfunction after MI	Cough, rash, loss of taste, hyperkalemia; rarely leukopenia and angioedema
Angiotensin-receptor blockers					
Losartan	25 mg/day	50–100 mg/day	$42–60	May be considered for diabetes, CHF if intolerant to ACEIs	Hyperkalemia, angioedema
Valsartan	80 mg/day	80–320 mg/day	$45–90	May be considered for diabetes, CHF if intolerant to ACEIs	Hyperkalemia, angioedema

HCTZ, hydrochlorothiazide; qd, every day; bid, twice daily; ER, extended release; CHF, congestive heart failure; BPH, benign prostatic hypertrophy; CV, cardiovascular; CAD, coronary artery disease; tid, 3 times daily; qpm, every night; qid, 4 times daily; LV, left ventricular; MI, myocardial infarction; ACEIs, angiotensin-converting enzyme inhibitors.

to lower cerebrovascular and cardiovascular morbidity and mortality, decrease left ventricular mass, and prevent heart failure. In low doses, thiazides have advantages of low cost and possible preservation of bone mineral density in older women. Side effects of thiazides include hypokalemia, hyponatremia, orthostatic hypotension, urinary incontinence, sexual dysfunction, and exacerbation of gout. Thiazides may be ineffective in patients with a creatinine clearance of < 30 mL/min and can be replaced by loop diuretics (eg, furosemide) when a diuretic agent is necessary.

b. Angiotensin-converting enzyme inhibitors & receptor blockers—The known renoprotective effects of angiotensin-converting enzyme (ACE) inhibitors and ACE receptor blockers (ARBs) in type 2 diabetes make ACE inhibitors and ARBs desirable first-line drugs in older diabetic hypertensives. ACE inhibitors also appear to improve vascular outcomes in high-risk patients, including diabetics and those with established vascular disease. ARBs have not been studied as extensively and are thus primarily used when there is intolerance to ACE inhibitors.

c. β-blockers—Older adults are less responsive than younger adults to β-blockers and are less likely to have BP control with β-blocker as a sole agent. In addition, compared with diuretics, β-blockers may proffer less reduction in cerebrovascular and cardiovascular events in older antihypertensive patients. However, they are warranted for the treatment of hypertensive patients with CAD for secondary prevention of myocardial infarction, for rate control with exercise in atrial fibrillation, and for reducing mortality and hospital readmission in patients with left ventricular systolic dysfunction.

d. Calcium channel blockers—Nitrendipine (not currently available in United States), a dihydropyridine calcium channel blocker (CCB) related to amlodipine and felodipine, significantly decreases the risk of cerebrovascular morbidity and mortality. Dihydropyridine CCBs available in the United States include nifedipine, amlodipine, and felodipine. However, CCBs are a heterogeneous group, and the benefits of one class of CCBs may not necessarily be extrapolated to another. Diltiazem and verapamil, 2 commonly used nondihydropyridine CCBs, have negative inotropic and chronotropic effects on left ventricular systolic function compared with amlodipine or felodipine. They may be used as adjunctive agents in patients with renal parenchymal disease and resistant hypertension but should be used with caution in systolic dysfunction.

e. α-blockers—Selective α_1-adrenergic antagonists (eg, terazosin, doxazosin) may be useful for managing hypertension in the setting of benign prostatic hypertrophy. Their major side effects are orthostatic hypotension, reflex tachycardia, and headache. The findings of slightly increased risk of stroke and cardiovascular events and a doubled risk of CHF in the doxazosin arm of the ALLHAT trial compared with chlorthalidone suggest that the α-antagonists should not be chosen as a first-line antihypertensive agent.

f. Combination drugs—JNC VII recommends that combination drug therapy be initiated for stage II hypertension (systolic BP ≥ 160 or diastolic BP ≥ 100). In the ALLHAT trial, approximately half of these high-risk older hypertensives required combination therapy. Participants on lisinopril and amlodipine were more likely to require combination therapy than those assigned chlorthalidone. This finding supports the JNC recommendation that a diuretic be a primary choice for an antihypertensive agent.

Combination drugs potentiate antihypertensive activity by acting at different sites simultaneously. Formulations that combine low doses of different classes of drugs improve BP control while minimizing the adverse effects of either drug. These drugs may in some cases be priced competitively with either of the combination agents, reducing the patient's out-of-pocket expenses as well. Lower cost, increased ease of compliance, and potential for fewer side effects make combination drugs attractive for use in older adults once the need for more than 1 agent is established.

B. DIABETES & HYPERTENSION

Type 2 diabetes is 2.5 times more likely to develop in hypertensives compared with normotensives and greatly increases cardiovascular risk. At recommended doses, there is no demonstrated increased risk of diabetes with the antihypertensive agents from the ACE inhibitors, CCB, ARB, or thiazide diuretic classes. There may be an increased risk of diabetes with β-blockers use in hypertensive individuals, but the added risk may be small compared with the benefits and the risk conferred by hypertension alone.

C. RESISTANT HYPERTENSION

Hypertension is considered resistant if BP cannot be reduced to goal with an appropriate triple-drug regimen, including a diuretic (plus ACE inhibitor, CCB, β-blocker, or ARB) and if each of the 3 drugs is at or near maximum recommended doses. With ISH in older adults, resistant hypertension is defined as the inability to lower systolic BP to < 160 mm Hg with a similar regimen.

The common causes of resistant hypertension include patient noncompliance with medications and diet, a suboptimal medication regimen, drug interaction, pseudotolerance (salt, water retention), and office hypertension. Secondary hypertension and pseudohypertension should also be considered.

When secondary causes for hypertension have been ruled out, the patient's compliance with dietary salt can be estimated by obtaining a 24-h urine collection for sodium. If the patient's hypertension remains resistant, other medications can be added to the triple therapy. Clonidine in tablet form or by transdermal patch, or another centrally acting sympatholytic agent, can be used in low doses to avoid side effects of sedation and orthostatic hypotension. Minoxidil, reserpine, and hydralazine are used cautiously because of their high rates of side effects in older patients.

ALLHAT Collaborative Research Group: Major cardiovascular events in hypertensive patients randomized to doxazosin vs chlorthalidone: The antihypertensive and lipid-lowering treatment to prevent heart attack trial (ALLHAT). JAMA 2000;283:1967. [PMID: 20248526]

Chobanian AV et al: The seventh report of the Joint National Committee on Prevention, Detection, Evaluation, and Treatment of High Blood Pressure: The JNC 7 report. JAMA 2003;289:2560. [PMID: 12748199]

Gress TW et al: Hypertension and antihypertensive therapy as risk factors for type 2 diabetes mellitus. Atherosclerosis Risk in Communities Study. N Engl J Med 2000;342:905. [PMID: 10738048]

Hansson L et al: Effect of angiotensin-converting-enzyme inhibition compared with conventional therapy on cardiovascular morbidity and mortality in hypertension: The Captopril Prevention Project (CAPPP) randomised trial. Lancet 1999; 353:611. [PMID: 10030325]

LaCroix AZ et al: Low-dose hydrochlorothiazide and preservation of bone mineral density in older adults. A randomized, double-blind, placebo-controlled trial. Ann Intern Med 2000; 133:516. [PMID: 11015164]

Messerli FH et al: Are beta-blockers efficacious as first-line therapy for hypertension in the elderly? A systematic review. JAMA 1998;279:1903. [PMID: 98296020]

Staessen JA et al: Randomised double-blind comparison of placebo and active treatment for older patients with isolated systolic hypertension. The Systolic Hypertension in Europe (Syst-Eur) Trial Investigators. Lancet 1997;350:757. [PMID: 97443133]

 EVIDENCE-BASED POINTS

- *Systolic BP and PP are more important predictors of cardiovascular risk than diastolic BP.*
- *Thiazide diuretics are effective initial therapy with significant evidence for cerebrovascular and cardiovascular event reduction.*
- *Other agents that can improve outcomes in elderly hypertensive individuals include β-blockers (especially in CAD and CHF), ACE inhibitors (in diabetic nephropathy and CHF), and dihydropyridine CCBs.*

- *α-Blockers are less effective at improving outcomes than diuretics.*
- *Effective management of hypertension may prevent disability, mortality, and cognitive decline in older adults.*

REFERENCES

ALLHAT Collaborative Research Group: Major cardiovascular events in hypertensive patients randomized to doxazosin vs chlorthalidone: The antihypertensive and lipid-lowering treatment to prevent heart attack trial (ALLHAT). JAMA 2000;283:1967. [PMID: 20248526]

Brown MJ et al: Morbidity and mortality in patients randomised to double-blind treatment with a long-acting calcium-channel blocker or diuretic in the International Nifedipine GITS study: Intervention as a goal in hypertension treatment (INSIGHT). Lancet 2000;356:366. [PMID: 10972368]

Forette F et al: Prevention of dementia in randomised double-blind placebo-controlled systolic hypertension in Europe (Syst-Eur) trial. Lancet 1998;352:1347. [PMID: 9802273]

Hansson L et al: Randomised trial of effects of calcium antagonists compared with diuretics and beta-blockers on cardiovascular morbidity and mortality in hypertension: The Nordic diltiazem (NORDIL) study. Lancet 2000;356:359. [PMID: 10972367]

Hansson L et al: Randomised trial of old and new antihypertensive drugs in elderly patients: Cardiovascular mortality and morbidity the Swedish Trial in Old Patients with Hypertension-2 study. Lancet 1999;354:1751. [PMID: 10577635]

Kjeldsen SE et al: Effects of losartan on cardiovascular morbidity and mortality in patients with isolated systolic hypertension and left ventricular hypertrophy: A losartan intervention for endpoint reduction (LIFE) substudy. JAMA 2002;288:1491.

Kostis JB et al: Prevention of heart failure by antihypertensive drug treatment in older persons with isolated systolic hypertension. JAMA 1997;278:212. [PMID: 9218667]

SHEP Cooperative Research Group: Prevention of stroke by antihypertensive drug treatment in older persons with isolated systolic hypertension. Final results of the Systolic Hypertension in the Elderly Program (SHEP). JAMA 1991;265:3255. [PMID: 2046107]

Staessen JA et al: Randomised double-blind comparison of placebo and active treatment for older patients with isolated systolic hypertension. The Systolic Hypertension in Europe (Syst-Eur) Trial Investigators. Lancet 1997;350:757. [PMID: 9297994]

RELEVANT WORLD WIDE WEB SITES

American College of Cardiology: www.acc.org

American Heart Association: www.americanheart.org

American Society of Hypertension: www.ash-us.org

Cardiosource: www.cardiosource.com

Centers for Disease Control and Prevention: www.cdc.gov/nchs/fastats/hypertens.htm

Lifeclinic: www.bloodpressure.com

National Heart, Lung, and Blood Institute: www.nhlbi.nih.gov

Peripheral Vascular & Thromboembolic Disease

Susan M. Begelman, MD, RVT

PERIPHERAL ARTERIAL DISEASE

 ESSENTIALS OF DIAGNOSIS

- Common symptoms of leg discomfort with ambulation, rest pain, nonhealing ulcers, or gangrene.
- Abnormal pulse exam in most patients.
- Evidence of systemic atherosclerosis is common.
- History of diabetes mellitus, tobacco use, hypertension, and hyperlipidemia.

General Considerations

The majority of elderly patients with peripheral arterial disease (PAD) have underlying atherosclerosis. As a result, patients with PAD have a high risk of cardiovascular and cerebrovascular morbidity and mortality. The prevalence of peripheral arterial disease rises rapidly with age. Although present in > 20% of people who are 75 or older, PAD is diagnosed by < 30% of primary care physicians.

Clinical manifestations of the disease vary. The majority of patients are asymptomatic. This may reflect the presence of limited disease or, more commonly in inactive patients, diminished capacity for ambulation that is necessary to produce intermittent claudication. PAD can also manifest as critical limb ischemia. In general, symptom severity increases with the number and length of stenotic lesions in the limb.

Risk factor modification is necessary to slow or halt progression of peripheral arterial disease and decrease the risk of cardiovascular and cerebrovascular death. Goals of therapy include cigarette smoking cessation, lowering blood pressure to < 140/90 mm Hg (< 135/85 in high-risk patients), improving glucose control with a target HbA1c < 7.0%, and lipid lowering with a target low-density lipoprotein < 100.

Good skin and foot care is essential. Many nonhealing ulcers begin with minor trauma. Therefore, patients with significant PAD should be encouraged to have a health care professional trim their toenails. Similarly, nursing home patients and individuals who have limited mobility are prone to pressure ulcers, which can become gangrenous. Regular use of devices that protect the heels can prevent unnecessary tissue or limb loss.

Clinical Findings

A. SYMPTOMS & SIGNS

Many patients are asymptomatic. Mild to moderate PAD can produce lower extremity discomfort with ambulation known as intermittent claudication. The pain is often described as an ache or "charley horse" in the calf, buttock, or thigh after a fixed distance of activity. Limb discomfort is usually relieved within minutes of activity cessation. Although some individuals will prefer to sit, most will achieve pain relief just by standing in place.

Disease progression or multiple stenotic lesions can result in rest pain (constant ischemic pain) and eventually nonhealing ulcers or gangrene. This is referred to as critical limb ischemia. Patients may have difficulty sleeping because of the constant pain and will prefer to keep the ischemic limb in a dependent position if possible. Neuropathic pain characterized by numbness and burning is seen in some patients with prolonged, severe ischemia (ischemic, monomelic neuropathy).

Skin changes are usually not present until significant PAD develops. Trophic changes, including cool, dry, shiny skin, hair loss, and thickened nails, are common but nonspecific findings. The limb can become edematous if kept dependent. Buerger's sign (also called Ratchow's sign) is the presence of rubor with limb dependency and rapid blanching with elevation. Ulcers and gangrene can develop at the tips of the toes, between 2 toes ("kissing ulcers"), and on pressure points.

A full cardiovascular examination is required to detect atherosclerosis in other arterial beds. One should record the blood pressure in both arms, the presence of carotid, aortic, and femoral artery bruits, murmurs, and the size of the abdominal aorta to exclude an aneurysm. Evidence of arrhythmias, poor cardiac output, pulmonary disease, and anemia are important to note because their presence can worsen lower extremity symptoms. Most important, a complete pulse exam includes the carotid, radial, ulnar, femoral, popliteal, dorsalis pedis, and posterior tibial pulses. They should be graded as 0 (absent), 1 (diminished), or 2 (present).

B. LABORATORY FINDINGS

Blood tests cannot be used to diagnose peripheral arterial disease, but several studies should be ordered to detect potential risk factors and comorbid diseases that may exacerbate symptoms. A complete blood count with a platelet count will reveal anemias, polycythemia, and thrombocytosis. A baseline platelet count should be drawn before exposing an individual to unfractionated heparin during the course of therapy (eg, an endovascular intervention). A fasting blood glucose level, hemoglobin A1c, urinalysis for protein and glucose, blood urea nitrogen, and creatinine can detect occult diabetes mellitus and long-standing hypertension. Renal function testing is also indicated before angiography. A fasting lipid profile should be checked. Infrequently, elderly patients will not have typical risk factors for atherosclerosis. An erythrocyte sedimentation rate to screen for vasculitis and hypercoagulable testing, including homocysteine levels, may be indicated in patients with a history of thrombosis.

C. SPECIAL TESTS

An ankle-brachial index (ABI) can easily be performed in an office setting to screen for PAD using a blood pressure cuff and a hand-held Doppler. The ABI is calculated by dividing the higher of the dorsalis pedis and posterior tibial systolic pressures for an individual leg by the higher of the two brachial pressures. An ABI < 0.9 is abnormal. Most patients with critical limb ischemia will have an ABI of < 0.4. Calcified, noncompressible arteries can be found in patients who are elderly and have diabetes mellitus, chronic renal failure, or a history of chronic steroid use. An ABI > 1.3 is unreliable. A toe-brachial index may be useful in this situation and can be performed in a vascular laboratory.

Full physiological testing includes pulse volume recordings (PVR), segmental limb pressures (SLP), and an ABI. In addition to assessing disease severity, these studies can help determine the location of disease and the likelihood that an ulcer will heal. Exercise stress testing (walking on a treadmill) increases the sensitivity of physiological testing by magnifying pressure gradients or producing them when an individual has a normal study at rest. Stress testing is contraindicated in patients with significant cardiopulmonary disease, rest pain, nonhealing ulcers, and unsteady gait requiring a cane or walker for support.

D. IMAGING STUDIES

Arterial duplex ultrasonography can be used to assess an individual's anatomy, not functional status. However, velocity gradients across stenotic lesions can be measured. An ultrasound study has the greatest clinical utility when used in conjunction with physiological testing to plan an endovascular intervention. It may be the only test available in some centers, so its limitations must be recognized. Magnetic resonance imaging can also be used to confirm the diagnosis of PAD. Like ultrasonography, it cannot directly assess functional status. In addition, this modality may not reliably differentiate between a tightly stenotic lesion and an occluded one. Except in rare circumstances, an angiogram is not necessary to diagnose PAD and should be performed only when an intervention is planned.

Differential Diagnosis

Comprehensive history and physical examinations are necessary to distinguish intermittent claudication from other causes of leg pain with ambulation, collectively known as pseudoclaudication (Table 21–1). The most common causes of pseudoclaudication are osteoarthritis of the spine causing spinal canal stenosis, osteoarthritis of the hip or knee, peripheral nerve pain, including sciatica and diabetic neuropathy, and venous claudication. The diagnosis of PAD might be delayed when older patients attribute their symptoms to arthritis or old age or when there is more than 1 cause for their leg pain.

In the absence of typical atherosclerotic risk factors, other diseases such as giant cell arteritis and remote trauma or radiation should be considered. Thrombosis of a popliteal artery aneurysm and primary vascular tumors are rare causes of intermittent claudication. Although atheroembolic disease can cause intermittent claudication, more commonly patients have rest pain, ischemic digits, and intact pedal pulses. Livedo reticularis may be present.

Treatment

In addition to risk factor modification, patients with PAD, irrespective of their symptoms and disease severity, should be prescribed an antiplatelet agent to decrease the risk of cardiovascular and cerebrovascular events. However, aspirin (81–325 mg/day) and clopidogrel (75 mg/day) have not been shown to improve peripheral arterial disease or its associated symptoms. The decision to use either antiplatelet agent alone or in combination is often determined by cost and the patient's risk of bleeding.

Table 21–1. Clinical characteristics of claudication versus pseudoclaudication.

Variable	Claudication	Pseudoclaudication
Location of discomfort	Buttock, hip, thigh, calf	Buttock, hip, thigh, calf
Type of discomfort	Ache, cramp, fatigue, weakness	Same or numbness, burning, tingling, sharp, shooting
Relationship to exercise	Yes	Variable
Time to onset after exercise	Consistent	Variable
Occurs with standing	No	Yes
Action for relief	Stand	Sit, change position
Time to relief	Seconds to minutes	Minutes to hours

A. EXERCISE REHABILITATION

A regimented walking program can significantly increase pain-free walking distance and maximal walking distance in patients with intermittent claudication. The program consists of 3–4 sessions a week, each lasting 30–60 min, during which time the individual walks on a flat surface until developing maximal pain tolerable. A rest period is then taken until the pain resolves and ambulation can be resumed. Long-term participation is required to derive and sustain the program's benefits. More improvement is often seen in a supervised exercise rehabilitation program.

B. PHARMACOTHERAPY

The 2 drugs available, pentoxifylline and cilostazol, are indicated for the reduction of symptoms from intermittent claudication but have not been shown to affect mortality. Only modest improvement in symptoms has been reported in some patients using pentoxifylline (400 mg 3 times a day with meals). A more impressive response has been demonstrated with cilostazol use (100 mg twice a day without food). Cilostazol, a phosphodiesterase inhibitor, is contraindicated in patients with congestive heart failure of any severity. β-Blockers rarely worsen symptoms and should not be withheld in most patients who require them.

C. ENDOVASCULAR INTERVENTION

Angiography is indicated when an endovascular intervention, a percutaneous angioplasty (with or without stent placement), or surgery is anticipated. The clinical indications for angiography are critical limb ischemia and lifestyle-limiting intermittent claudication. In frail patients with intermittent claudication, an assessment should first be made of the individual's ability to perform activities of daily living and quality of life. Elective angiography is warranted if the patient is limited in daily activities or the quality of life is affected by symptoms. However, for patients with critical limb ischemia aggressive intervention is required for tissue or limb salvage.

Endovascular intervention is the treatment of choice for short iliac artery stenoses. This approach is often used to fix longer iliac lesions and unilateral iliac occlusions. Single long lesions, short but heavily calcified stenoses, or multiple short stenoses in the superficial femoral and popliteal arteries (excluding the distal segment) are frequently treated with an endovascular intervention. Angioplasty is also used to improve proximal blood flow before surgery.

D. SURGERY

Individuals with PAD not amenable to an endovascular intervention should be evaluated for surgery. Every patient may not be a surgical candidate, and in the case of intermittent claudication, the decision to have surgery is elective. The length of the lesion, the arterial segment involved, the status of the inflow and distal runoff vessels, and the availability of autologous vein determine the surgical approach. In general, 5-year primary patency rates for aortoiliac reconstruction, infrainguinal bypass using autologous vein, and infrainguinal bypass using prosthetic material are > 80%, 70%, and 40% respectively.

Prognosis

Approximately 25% of patients with intermittent claudication will deteriorate; however, of those, only 20% will require an intervention. Less that 2% of all patients with PAD will ultimately require an amputation (many of these patients have diabetes mellitus or continue to smoke). However, PAD is associated with significant mortality. More than half of patients with PAD will die from coronary artery disease, nearly 20% from strokes, and an additional 10% from ruptured abdominal aortic aneurysms.

 EVIDENCE-BASED POINTS

- *An ABI should be used to screen for PAD in outpatient primary care practices.*

- *Angiography should be limited to those patients with critical limb ischemia or intermittent claudication who wish to pursue more aggressive treatment.*
- *Patients with evidence of atherosclerotic peripheral arterial disease should receive antiplatelet therapy to reduce the risk of cerebrovascular and cardiovascular morbidity and mortality.*

CHRONIC VENOUS INSUFFICIENCY

 ESSENTIALS OF DIAGNOSIS

- *Pitting edema.*
- *Skin changes, including hyperpigmentation and varicose veins.*
- *Limb pain with prolonged standing.*
- *Chronic edema resulting in ulcer formation above the medial malleolus.*

General Considerations

The venous system consists of deep veins, perforating (communicating) veins, and superficial veins (the largest of which are the saphenous veins). Chronic venous insufficiency (CVI) results when there is valvular incompetency causing reflux, obstruction preventing outflow, or both. There are primary and secondary forms of venous insufficiency. Congenital CVI is rare and usually detected during childhood. Other causes of chronic venous insufficiency should be excluded before diagnosing primary valvular incompetency.

Secondary causes of CVI are common and include multiple past pregnancies, trauma, obesity, occupations requiring prolonged standing, and leg dependency. Patients who are wheelchair bound or who have limited mobility are especially at risk for venous insufficiency. Postthrombotic syndrome resulting from direct damage of the veins or incomplete vein recanalization is a form of CVI that occurs in patients who have had a deep vein thrombosis (DVT). Vein obstruction can occur when a popliteal artery aneurysm, pelvic mass, or adenopathy compress an adjacent vein. Vein stenosis from prior instrumentation, vascular tumors, and retroperitoneal fibrosis should be considered when a cause has not been identified.

Prevention

Early institution of treatment prevents deterioration of symptoms and formation of ulcers.

Clinical Findings

A. SYMPTOMS & SIGNS

Edema usually develops slowly and initially involves only the ankle, sparing the dorsum of the foot. Typically, the skin is soft and the edema is described as "pitting." There may be minimal or no swelling early in the morning, but the edema progresses throughout the day. Constant swelling may be present in individuals who sleep in a chair or with their feet in a dependent position. Over time, the edema can progress more proximally, remain despite leg elevation, and no longer pit because of subcutaneous fibrosis.

Large varicose veins, prominent reticular veins, and multiple telangiectasias (spider veins) appear with superficial vein involvement. Incompetency at the level of the saphenofemoral junction can be detected by palpation over the area while the patient performs a Valsalva maneuver. Patients with CVI complain of pain, which is often described as a heaviness, tightness, or ache. Symptoms are more pronounced with prolonged standing and are usually relieved shortly after elevating the limb. Venous claudication, the sudden onset of "bursting" pain in the calf with ambulation, may occur in patients with significant venous obstruction.

The skin is often dry, shiny, and atrophic with a reddish, cyanotic hue when the limb is dependent. However, the limb is warm, not cool, as it is with arterial insufficiency. Eczematous dermatitis, hyperpigmentation caused by hemosiderin deposits, and ulceration, either spontaneous or resulting from minor trauma is seen in advanced stages of disease. Stasis ulcers are typically painless and often form just proximal to the medial malleolus.

B. IMAGING STUDIES

Although the diagnosis of CVI can usually be made clinically, a venous duplex ultrasonogram is helpful in identifying incompetent veins segments in both the deep and superficial systems. Ascending venography can differentiate primary from secondary disease, whereas descending venography identifies the location and competency of individual valves.

Differential Diagnosis

Not all patients with leg edema have chronic venous insufficiency. The presence of end-organ dysfunction must be excluded. History and physical examination is often sufficient to detect cirrhosis, congestive heart failure, cardiac valve disease, renal insufficiency, nephrotic syndrome, Cushing's disease, thyroid disorders, protein-losing enteropathies and other causes of malabsorption, and pulmonary hypertension.

Many medications prescribed to older patients are associated with edema formation. Common culprits include antihypertensive medications, especially the dihydropyridines, nonsteroidal anti-inflammatory drugs, steroids, and hormones (estrogen, progesterone, and testosterone). A class of oral antidiabetic drugs, the thiazolidinediones, can cause significant leg edema in a dose-dependent manner. Swelling has also been reported in patients with Parkinson's disease taking pramipexole.

Complications

Limb pain and ulceration account for the significant morbidity of this disease. Ulcer care requires frequent physician visits, and wound care products are costly. Hospitalization may be necessary for the treatment of cellulitis and ulcer débridement. Varicose veins increase the risk of DVT. Most skin changes present only a cosmetic problem.

Treatment

Because of the chronicity of this disease, lifelong treatment is required. The mainstay of therapy is a sized-to-fit compression garment. Compression stockings are graded by the degree of compression applied to the legs. Although tighter compression stockings prevent more edema and ulceration, the choice of stocking should be determined by the patient's needs and limitations. Significant compression is contraindicated in patients with moderate to severe peripheral arterial disease. Some patients will not be able to comply with therapy because of osteoarthritis in the hands or limited flexibility. If possible, use of a lightweight garment (8–15 mm Hg compression) should be encouraged. Patients should be advised to use a good moisturizer, treat tinea pedis with an antifungal agent (a common source of cellulitis in patients with CVI), avoid prolonged standing or sitting, lose weight if appropriate, and exercise. A variety of surgical techniques are available for the treatment of secondary superficial varicosities.

Prognosis

The course of severe CVI is marked by periods of ulceration. The main concerns are sepsis that develops as a result of an infected ulcer or the occurrence of a DVT with thromboembolic complications.

EVIDENCE-BASED POINTS

- Not all patients with lower extremity edema have chronic venous insufficiency.
- Sized-to-fit compression garments are the mainstay of therapy.
- The goal of treatment is to decrease morbidity from chronic limb pain and ulceration.

LYMPHEDEMA

ESSENTIALS OF DIAGNOSIS

- Unilateral limb involvement (infrequently involves both limbs).
- Nonpitting edema involving the dorsum of the foot with squaring of the toes.
- History of cellulitis, malignancy, surgery, or trauma.
- Skin changes of CVI are absent.

General Considerations

Lymphedema is a pathological condition that develops when there is malformation, dysfunction, destruction, or obstruction of the lymphatic system. There are 2 forms of this disease: primary and secondary. Primary lymphedema can present at birth (Milroy's disease), develop during the second or third decade of life (lymphedema praecox), or manifest after the fourth decade (lymphedema tarda). Some forms are familial. Secondary lymphedema accounts for the majority of cases seen in the older population. Obstruction and inflammation are the usual inciting factors. Patients who have had cellulitis, lymphangitis, pelvic or leg radiation, trauma, surgery (including lymph node dissection), and cancer (either metastatic disease or a pelvic mass) are at greatest risk for lymphedema. Filariasis and other parasitic infections should be considered in any patient who has traveled or lived in endemic areas outside the United States.

Prevention

Good foot and nail care is essential. Patients should be instructed to dry between their toes after bathing and use a topical antifungal agent if tinea pedis develops. Some individuals require chronic antibiotic therapy for recurrent cellulitis. Graduated compression stockings should be worn routinely.

Clinical Findings

A. SYMPTOMS & SIGNS

Early in the course of development patients may not recognize lymphedema; however, most have impressive unilateral lower extremity swelling. The edema initially involves the toes and extends more proximally. Typically, the toes have a squared appearance (Stemmer's sign) and the dorsum of the foot is humped. With time, the skin thickens, developing deepened creases, hyperkeratosis, and papillomatosis, and the edema becomes resistant to pitting ("woody induration"). Although the edema is characteristically painless, patients complain of general leg discomfort, heaviness, and tightness as the limb enlarges. Signs of venous insufficiency are absent.

B. IMAGING STUDIES

The diagnosis of lymphedema is suggested by history and physical examination in the absence of systemic disease. Lymphoscintigraphy is a confirmatory test that records radiolabeled tracer activity at specific time intervals, determines transit time through the lymphatics, and identifies the absence or presence and pattern of lymphatic channels and lymph node activity. Magnetic resonance imaging relies on the detection of a characteristic honeycomb pattern of edema within the epifascial plane and has the added benefit of allowing visualization of soft tissue in the limb. Computed tomography (CT) should be ordered if a pelvic malignancy is suspected.

Differential Diagnosis

Lymphedema can be difficult to distinguish from other causes of unilateral leg swelling. A venous duplex ultrasonogram is indicated if the swelling developed recently or rapidly to exclude DVT and popliteal (Baker's) cysts. Ecchymosis, especially around the ankle, is seen in patients who ruptured the medial head of the gastrocnemius muscle. Many of these patients report hearing a "pop" after stepping off a curb or walking down steps. Chronic regional pain syndrome (reflex sympathetic dystrophy) is associated with signs and symptoms of vasomotor instability, pain described as burning and aching, and a history of trauma to the limb.

Complications

Lymphedema is a disabling, chronic condition. Significant morbidity is due to a combination of the emotional, psychological, and physical aspects of this disease. Edema can limit mobility. Recurrent cellulitis and lymphangitis are common complications that can exacerbate swelling and require hospitalization for antibiotic therapy. Infrequently, patients with chronic lymphedema can develop a malignant lymphangiosarcoma heralded by the development of 1 or more flat, purple-blue skin lesions.

Treatment

The focus of treatment is on reducing and then maintaining limb size, providing emotional support, and education of patients and caregivers. In general, diuretic therapy does not have a significant impact on decreasing the amount of protein-rich fluid in the subcutaneous tissue; therefore, it is of little benefit. Leg elevation allows passive drainage but does not stimulate the lymphatics. A variety of physical therapies are now available to reduce swelling. Mechanical devices delivering sequential pressure reduce limb volume by displacing the fluid. They should be used with caution in patients with volume-dependent diseases, including congestive heart failure, valvular disease, cirrhosis, and renal insufficiency. Manual lymphatic drainage, a massage technique, stimulates lymphatic flow and decongests the limb more gradually. It is often used in combination with multilayered bandaging and exercise. Graduated compression garments are required to maintain reduced limb size. The degree of compression is determined by severity of edema, presence of peripheral arterial disease, and anticipated rate of compliance. Compliance can be difficult to achieve. Patients may have difficulty putting on tight garments. The costs of garments can be prohibitive because Medicare does not cover them. Microvascular reconstruction and debulking or excisional procedures can be performed in select cases.

EVIDENCE-BASED POINTS

- *Cellulitis is the most common secondary cause of lymphedema in the United States.*
- *Lymphoscintigraphy is the test of choice to confirm the diagnosis of lymphedema.*
- *Optimal therapy combines decongestion techniques (eg, manual lymphatic drainage), exercise, and daily use of a compression garment.*

VENOUS THROMBOEMBOLISM

ESSENTIALS OF DIAGNOSIS

- *Surgery (especially orthopedic), immobility, and malignancy are common risk factors.*
- *Typical complaints include acute limb pain and swelling for DVT; pleuritic chest pain and shortness of breath for pulmonary embolism.*
- *Physical findings are nonspecific and often absent.*
- *Noninvasive diagnostic testing includes venous duplex ultrasonography, ventilation perfusion scanning, and spiral (helical) CT.*

General Considerations

Venous thromboembolism (VTE) is a common disease with an annual incidence of approximately 1–2 per 1000 individuals. VTE has 2 clinical manifestations: DVT and pulmonary embolism (PE). The majority of symptomatic lower extremity DVT begins in the calf. Approximately 20–25% of calf vein DVT will extend into the proximal leg veins (popliteal, superficial and common femoral, iliac veins). Nearly 75% of all pulmonary emboli originate in the leg veins.

The risk of venous thromboembolism increases with advancing age independent of other factors. Several common thrombophilias have been identified, including factor V Leiden, prothrombin gene mutation 20210A, and hyperhomocysteinemia. However, hypercoagulable testing is rarely indicated in the geriatric population. These patients often have an identifiable risk factor. Myocardial infarction, stroke, congestive heart failure, nephrotic syndrome, varicose veins, inflammatory bowel disease, and obesity are independent risk factors for thrombosis. Immobility increases the risk of DVT. Likewise, hormone replacement therapy and selective estrogen receptor modulators for osteoporosis predispose women to VTE. Conditions associated with cancer treatment such as chemotherapy, surgery, radiotherapy, and central venous catheters increase VTE risk. Patients with a diagnosis of idiopathic DVT or PE should be evaluated for malignancy. The evaluation includes breast examinations, mammograms, pelvic examinations and Pap testing for women; a prostate exam and prostate-specific antigen testing for men; and a lower endoscopic examination for all individuals.

Surgery is another risk factor for VTE. The event rate after orthopedic surgery is especially high. More than 50% of patients undergoing hip and knee replacement surgery or surgery for a fractured hip will experience a DVT if prophylaxis is not given. The majority of these events involve the calf veins.

Prevention

Prophylactic measures will reduce, but not eliminate, the risk of DVT and PE and should be administered to patients at high-risk for an event. Except for minor procedures, all patients older than 60 who have surgery are considered at high risk for VTE. Likewise, prophylaxis is indicated for immobilized and hospitalized patients, especially those who have had a myocardial infarction or an ischemic stroke resulting in impaired mobility.

The type and duration of prophylaxis is determined by the clinical indication for its use and the patient's comorbidities. The goal of nonpharmacological methods is to reduce venous stasis. Graded compression elastic stockings and intermittent pneumatic compression (IPC) are best reserved for patients with a contraindication to anticoagulation or as an adjunct to pharmacotherapy. A variety of anticoagulants are available, including adjusted-dose warfarin, unfractionated heparin, low-molecular-weight heparins, and pentasaccharide (Table 21–2). The choice of drug and dose varies according to the clinical indication.

Clinical Findings

A. SYMPTOMS & SIGNS

1. DVT—Symptomatic patients typically have leg edema, pain, erythema, and warmth. Patients with concomitant involvement of the superficial venous system may have a palpable cord or dilated collateral veins. Homan's sign, calf pain with passive foot dorsiflexion, has a low sensitivity and specificity for the diagnosis of DVT.

2. PE—50% of all patients with a proximal DVT will have had an asymptomatic PE at presentation. In symptomatic patients, chest pain with inspiration, new-onset or worsening dyspnea, and palpitations are commonly reported. Lower extremity symptoms suggestive of a DVT may be present. Hemoptysis is seen infrequently. Physical findings include tachycardia, tachypnea, rales, diaphoresis, and occasionally, signs of right ventricular dysfunction.

B. LABORATORY FINDINGS

An elevated D-dimer test is seen in most patients with venous thromboembolic disease but also in the setting of recent surgery, malignancy, trauma, and active cardiopulmonary disease. Therefore, the test is most useful

Table 21–2. Dosing of anticoagulants for VTE prophylaxis and treatment.[a]

Variable	Prophylactic dose	Therapeutic dose
Unfractionated heparin	5000 U sc q8–12h	Weight-based infusion Target aPTT 50–75
Low-molecular-weight heparin		
Enoxaparin		
Abdominal surgery	40 mg sc qd	1 mg/kg sc q12h
Orthopedic surgery	30 mg sc bid	(or 1.5 mg/kg sc q12h
Medical patient	40 mg sc qd	in hospital setting)
Dalteparin		
Abdominal surgery	5000 anti-Xa U sc qd	
Orthopedic surgery	5000 anti-Xa U sc qd (hip only)	Not FDA approved
Medical patient	Not FDA approved	
Tinzaparin		
Abdominal surgery		
Orthopedic surgery	Not FDA approved	175 anti-Xa U/kg sc qd
Medical patient		
Pentasaccharide (Fondaparinux)	2.5 mg qd; approved only for DVT prophylaxis in the orthopedic patient	Not FDA approved

aPTT, activated partial thromboplastin time; FDA, Food and Drug Administration; DVT, deep vein thrombosis.
[a]Consult the package inserts for further details regarding the timing and dose of initial administration.

when performed in the outpatient setting in which these diagnoses are less likely to be present compared with the hospital setting. A normal D-dimer has a negative predictive value of 95% in patients suspected of having a DVT. The arterial blood gas can be normal or reveal a respiratory alkalosis resulting from hyperventilation in patients with PE. An elevated alveolar-arterial oxygen gradient may be detected.

C. IMAGING STUDIES

1. DVT—Duplex ultrasonography is a widely available noninvasive test. The most sensitive and specific finding is the inability to completely compress the vein and obliterate its lumen. Loss of phasicity with respiration and flow augmentation with external leg compression, the presence of intraluminal echoes, and the absence of demonstrable flow are other notable but nondiagnostic findings. Although the examination is inexpensive, it is operator dependent and less sensitive than venography in detecting calf vein thrombosis.

The gold standard study is contrast venography. The presence of an intraluminal filling defect or an abrupt cutoff is consistent with the diagnosis of a DVT. This test is more sensitive in detecting thrombosis in the calf veins, pelvic veins, and vena cava. However, it can be uncomfortable and is expensive. Occasionally, contrast-induced thrombosis occurs after venography. Venography should be used to confirm the diagnosis of DVT when the ultrasound is equivocal.

2. Pulmonary embolism—Atelectasis, pleural effusions, and parenchymal infiltrates may be present on x-ray film but are nonspecific. Classic findings such as Westermark's sign (focal oligemia), Hampton's hump (pleural-based wedge-shaped opacity), and enlargement of the pulmonary arteries are rare. Most patients will have a normal electrocardiogram or evidence of sinus tachycardia. Changes consistent with right-sided heart strain, including an $S_1Q_3T_3$ pattern (prominent S waves in lead I, a Q wave in lead III, and an inverted T wave in lead III) may be seen with large pulmonary emboli.

Ventilation–perfusion scanning, or lung scintigraphy, is performed by recording images of the lungs after intravenously injecting isotope-labeled macroaggregates of albumin and inhalation of a radioactive aerosol. Areas of "mismatch" where there is ventilation without perfusion are suggestive of a PE. The study is reported by assigning a probability of pulmonary embolism (normal, low, intermediate, or high). The diagnostic accuracy of the test improves when a pretest clinical probability is assigned. Lung scintigraphy is most helpful when interpreted as normal or high probability for PE. Otherwise, a confirmatory test may be required.

Spiral CT is more widely available than lung scintigraphy. It is inexpensive and has the advantage of detecting primary parenchymal disease. Pulmonary emboli appear as partial or complete intraluminal filling defects. Spiral CT is less sensitive in detecting peripheral emboli and must be performed with contrast; caution is necessary in patients with a decreased creatinine clearance.

Echocardiography remains an adjunctive test despite reports that it has been used to visualize thrombus. Its clinical utility in the management of PE is its ability to assess right ventricular (RV) function and estimate RV pressures. Almost half of all hemodynamically stable patients with a pulmonary embolism will have evidence of RV dysfunction. This finding is associated with an increase in mortality.

Pulmonary angiography remains the gold standard study for PE. The presence of an intraluminal filling defect or an abrupt cutoff is diagnostic. Similar to venography, it is expensive, invasive, requires contrast, and should only be used when a confirmatory test is required or an intervention is necessary.

Differential Diagnosis

Popliteal cysts and superficial thrombophlebitis can simulate a DVT with leg warmth, edema, and erythema. These diagnoses can usually be excluded using ultrasonography. A source for cellulitis is often identifiable. In general, lymphedema is painless and develops less rapidly. Chronic venous insufficiency, a potential complication of DVT, is associated with more chronic skin changes. Musculoskeletal sprains and injured muscles can be difficult to differentiate from a DVT. An acute arterial occlusion is painful and usually associated with loss of pedal pulses. Significant swelling tends to occur with limb reperfusion.

The signs and symptoms of a PE are nonspecific. They may be present with diseases involving the heart (congestive heart failure, pericarditis), lungs (asthma, pneumonia, pneumothorax), great vessels (aortic dissection), and muscles or bone (sprain, costochondritis).

Complications

Most patients who have had a DVT or PE will fully recover from the event. At least 30% of patients who have had a DVT will experience postthrombotic syndrome characterized by chronic pain and swelling in addition to other signs and symptoms of venous insufficiency. These symptoms can manifest in < 2 years. A few patients will have chronic pulmonary thromboembolism with pulmonary hypertension after a PE. The implications of this complication in the older population are unclear.

Treatment

A. ANTICOAGULATION

The mainstay of treatment is anticoagulation (see Table 21–2). Age per se is not a contraindication to anticoagulation unless the patient is actively bleeding or has a high risk for complications (eg, inability to reliably take medications because of dementia or significant fall risk). Unfractionated heparin is administered using a weight-based dosing regimen with a target activated partial thromboplastin time (aPTT) of 1.5–2.5 times the mean control value. An aPTT should be drawn before drug initiation, 6 h after starting the drug or adjusting the dose, and once daily in a hospital setting.

Low-molecular-weight (LMW) heparins are easy to administer and can facilitate outpatient therapy or early discharge from the hospital. The drugs are administered subcutaneously and do not require monitoring. LMW heparin is cleared by the kidney and should be used cautiously in patients with renal insufficiency (they are contraindicated in patients with a creatinine clearance < 30). The appropriateness of outpatient therapy must be judged for each individual patient, especially in the geriatric population. These drugs are costly and often not covered by insurance companies, including Medicare, for use on an outpatient basis.

Warfarin, the long-term anticoagulant of choice for most patients with venous thromboembolism, can be started on the same day as heparin by administering the anticipated daily dose requirement (eg, 5 mg). A 4- to 5-day overlap with heparin is necessary to ensure that all of the vitamin K-dependent factors have been adequately depleted. Patients with VTE or a known hypercoagulable state should not initially receive warfarin without simultaneous administration of another anticoagulant because of the risk of inducing a prothrombotic state by rapidly depleting protein C and S levels. The target international normalized ratio (INR) for most patients is 2.0–3.0 (higher in individuals with antiphospholipid antibody syndrome).

B. DURATION OF THERAPY

The optimal duration of therapy is not known. The decision regarding length of treatment depends on the patient's age, comorbidities, risk factors for VTE, and rate of recurrence. The duration of therapy for a patient with a reversible risk factor (eg, surgery, drugs) and a first VTE event is 3–6 mo. An idiopathic DVT or PE requires at least 6 mo of therapy. Patients with recurrent idiopathic events, some thrombophilias, and malignancy should receive long-term treatment.

C. ADJUNCTIVE THERAPIES

Inferior vena cava (IVC) filters prevent embolization of thrombi from the legs to the lungs. However, these devices do not prevent recurrent DVT or extension of preexisting thrombus. In fact, the risk of recurrent DVT is increased long term. In addition, small thrombi can pass through the device struts or around the filter via collaterals. An IVC filter should be placed in patients with a contraindication to anticoagulation (eg, bleeding, surgery), recurrent VTE events despite an elevated INR, and as an adjunct to surgical pulmonary embolectomy or thromboembolectomy. Perceived bleeding risk is important to consider in the geriatric population. For example, IVC filter placement may pose less of a risk to patients with a significant fall history.

Thrombolytic therapy is indicated in patients with a PE and hemodynamic instability. The benefits of this therapy must be weighed against the risks of bleeding. Approximately 15% of patients who are given thrombolytics will experience a significant bleed, most commonly gastrointestinal, genitourinary, or retroperitoneal. At least an additional 1–2% will have an intracranial bleed. Age over 70, recent stroke, surgery or gastrointestinal bleed, and uncontrolled hypertension are among the list of factors that increase bleeding risk. Geriatric patients with phlegmasia cerulea dolens should also be considered for thrombolytic therapy.

Prognosis

Venous thromboembolism is associated with significant morbidity and mortality. Many patients who die from PE are not diagnosed antemortem. The 3-mo mortality rate is increased by 60% in patients older than 70. Chronic thromboembolic pulmonary hypertension, a complication of pulmonary embolism, occurs infrequently. Up to 30% of patients with DVT will have postthrombotic syndrome. Sized-to-fit compression stockings decrease the risk of this complication.

EVIDENCE-BASED POINTS

- *Clinical signs and symptoms of VTE are nondiagnostic.*
- *Hypercoagulable testing in the geriatric population is rarely indicated. However, all patients with idiopathic venous thromboembolic disease should have age- and sex-specific malignancy screening.*
- *Patients in the hospital setting are at high risk for a DVT and PE. Pharmacological VTE prophylaxis should be used unless contraindicated.*
- *Although there are guidelines, the optimal duration of anticoagulant therapy is not known.*

REFERENCES

Peripheral Arterial Disease

Dawson DL et al: A comparison of cilostazol and pentoxifylline for treating intermittent claudication. Am J Med 2000;109:523. [PMID: 11063952] (An improvement in maximal and pain-free treadmill walking distance was demonstrated with cilostazol, not pentoxifylline.)

Dormandy JA, Rutherford RB: Management of peripheral arterial disease (PAD). TransAtlantic Inter-Society Consensus (TASC). J Vasc Surg 2000;31(1 Pt 2):S1. [PMID: 1066628] (A comprehensive international consensus guideline on the evaluation and treatment of intermittent claudication, acute limb ischemia, and critical limb ischemia.)

Hiatt WR: Medical treatment of peripheral arterial disease and claudication. N Engl J Med 2001;344:1608. [PMID: 11372014] (Review of risk factor modification goals, non-pharmacological therapy, and medications.)

Hirsch AT et al: Peripheral arterial disease detection, awareness, and treatment in primary care. JAMA 2001;286:1317. [PMID: 11560536] (PAD is a prevalent but underdiagnosed disease. An ABI is a useful screening tool in the outpatient setting.)

Meijer WT et al: Determinants of peripheral arterial disease in the elderly: The Rotterdam study. Arch Intern Med 2000;160:2934. [PMID: 11041900] (Identified atherosclerotic risk factors for PAD; including age of ≥ 75 years.)

Newman AB et al: Ankle-arm index as a predictor of cardiovascular disease and mortality in the cardiovascular health study. Arterioscler Thromb Vasc Biol 1999;19:538. [PMID: 10073955] (Ankle-arm index [AAI] measured in a group of patients at least 65 years old. An AAI < 0.9 was an independent risk factor for cardiovascular disease and mortality.)

Chronic Venous Insufficiency

Nicolaides AN: Investigation of chronic venous insufficiency. A consensus statement. Circulation 2000;102:e126. [PMID: 11076834] (Detailed list of diagnostic modalities for CVI.)

Ruckley CV et al: Chronic venous insufficiency: Clinical and duplex correlations. The Edinburgh Vein Study of venous disorders in the general population. J Vasc Surg 2002;36:520. [PMID: 12218976] (CVI graded by physical examination and correlated with ultrasound findings.)

Lymphedema

Badger CMA et al: A randomized, controlled, parallel-group clinical trial comparing multilayer bandaging followed by hosiery versus hosiery alone in the treatment of patients with lymphedema of the limb. Cancer 2000;88:2832. [PMID: 10870068] (Greater limb volume reduction is achieved when using multilayered bandaging in addition to a compression garment.)

Williams WH et al: Radionuclide lymphangioscintigraphy in the evaluation of peripheral lymphedema. Clin Nucl Med 2000; 25:451. [PMID: 10836695] (Describes technique. Multiple figures demonstrating various findings.)

Venous Thromboembolism

Geerts WH et al: Prevention of thromboembolism. Chest 2001; 119(suppl 1):132S. [PMID: 11157647] (American College of Chest Physicians guidelines from the sixth consensus conference on antithrombotic therapy. Exhaustive review of the literature.)

Goldhaber SZ et al: Acute pulmonary embolism: Clinical outcomes in the International Cooperative Pulmonary Embolism Registry (ICOPER). Lancet 1999;353:1386. [PMID: 10227218] (Registry of patients with pulmonary embolism showing that age older than 70 and right ventricular hypokinesis on echocardiography are predictive of an increased 3-mo mortality.)

Heit JA et al: Risk factors for deep vein thrombosis and pulmonary embolism: A population-based case-control study. Arch Intern Med 2000;160:809. [PMID: 10737280] (Hospital or nursing home confinement is among the independent risk factors for VTE.)

Hirsh J, Bates SM: Clinical trials that have influenced the treatment of venous thromboembolism: A historical perspective. Ann Intern Med 2001;134:409. [PMID: 11242501] (Good review of widely quoted studies that have influenced the standard of care for VTE treatment.)

Hyers TM et al: Antithrombotic therapy for venous thromboembolic disease. Chest 2001;119(suppl 1):176S. [PMID: 11157648] (American College of Chest Physicians guidelines from the sixth consensus conference on antithrombotic therapy.)

Kearon C et al: A comparison of 3 mo of anticoagulation with extended anticoagulation for a first episode of idiopathic venous thromboembolism. N Engl J Med 1999;340:901. [PMID: 10089183] (Trial terminated early after an increased risk of recurrent VTE was demonstrated in patients who had an idiopathic VTE and received only 3 mo of anticoagulation.)

Samama MM et al: A comparison of enoxaparin with placebo for the prevention of venous thromboembolism in acutely ill medical patients. Prophylaxis in medical patients with enoxaparin study group. N Engl J Med 1999;341:793. [PMID: 10477777] (MEDENOX study compared placebo, enoxaparin 20 mg daily, and enoxaparin 40 mg daily for VTE prophylaxis.)

Turpie AG et al: Fondaparinux vs enoxaparin for the prevention of venous thromboembolism in major orthopedic surgery: A meta-analysis of 4 randomized double-blind studies. Arch Intern Med 2002;162:1833. [PMID: 12196081] (Meta-analysis of the 4 large prospective trials using this new anticoagulant in orthopedic patients to prevent VTE.)

RELEVANT WORLD WIDE WEB SITES

HeartCenter Online: www.heartcenteronline.com/myheartdr/Articles_about_the_heart/The_Peripheral_Vascular_Center.html

Vascular Disease Foundation: www.vdf.org/PAD_Frame.htm

National Lymphedema Network: www.lymphnet.org

Circle of Hope Lymphedema Foundation, Inc.: www.lymphedemacircleofhope.org

INATE: www.inate.org

Respiratory Diseases

22

Richard W. Rissmiller, Jr, MD, & Norman E. Adair, MD

ASTHMA

ESSENTIALS OF DIAGNOSIS

- Episodic wheeze, dyspnea, cough, and chest tightness.
- Dyspnea and cough, often worse at night.
- Airflow obstruction by spirometry that is at least partially reversible.

General Considerations

Asthma is a chronic inflammatory disorder of the airways. Airway inflammation in asthma is most closely linked to allergic mechanisms. Infectious agents and air pollution may also contribute to inflammation. A genetic predisposition to asthma is recognized, primarily in the form of atopy. Elderly asthmatics may be less atopic than younger asthmatics, but elderly asthmatics are more atopic than elderly controls without asthma.

The prevalence of asthma peaks in childhood (8–10%) and declines in early adulthood. The prevalence of asthma is 6–8% past 60 years of age. Asthma can present after age 60 (late-onset asthma), but this is less common than long-standing asthma that persists into the later years of life. Asthma mortality is higher in the elderly than in younger asthmatics.

Asthma is underdiagnosed and undertreated in the elderly. Underdiagnosis stems from several factors, including attributing breathlessness to normal aging or to other disorders, primarily cardiovascular disease. In addition, the perception of bronchoconstriction is blunted in the elderly. Elderly asthmatics have less severe asthma symptoms than do younger adult asthmatics with similar degrees of airflow obstruction. Older asthmatics may have adapted to chronic obstruction or are less able to perceive airway narrowing. Thus, they may minimize symptoms and delay investigation for asthma.

Pathogenesis

Asthmatic airway inflammation, whether allergic or nonallergic, is associated with bronchial hyperreactivity. This results in airway narrowing and increased airflow resistance. Bronchial hyperreactivity can be induced by a variety of stimuli, including cold air, emotions, air pollution, and viral infections. Hyperreactive airways cause recurrent episodes of breathlessness, chest tightness, wheeze, and cough.

Long-standing airway inflammation can lead to structural changes in the airway, characterized by thickening of the airway wall and peribronchial fibrosis. Such changes can produce irreversible airway narrowing. Elderly nonsmokers with long-standing asthma have worse airflow obstruction and less reversibility after bronchodilator inhalation than elderly asthmatics whose disease is of shorter duration.

Clinical Findings

A. SYMPTOMS & SIGNS

Recurrent episodes of wheeze, breathlessness, cough, and chest tightness characterize asthma. Cough can be the only or the predominant symptom. Cough and breathlessness are commonly worse at night or in the early morning. However, if airflow obstruction becomes irreversible, as may occur with chronicity and airway remodeling, symptoms will be unremitting. This situation cannot be differentiated from chronic obstructive pulmonary disease (COPD) except when the patient has no history of tobacco exposure. Chest examination may demonstrate expiratory wheeze, diminished intensity of breath sounds, prolonged expiratory time, hyperinflation, and accessory inspiratory muscle activity. These physical signs are nonspecific and are noted in other obstructive lung diseases.

B. LABORATORY FINDINGS

Blood and sputum eosinophilia may occur in asthma but are not useful for diagnosis. The most useful laboratory investigation is spirometry, which measures the forced vital capacity (FVC) and the forced expired volume over 1 s (FEV_1). Airflow obstruction may be de-

202

fined by an FEV_1–FVC ratio of < 0.70. Airflow obstruction that is significantly reversible after inhalation of a bronchodilator is the hallmark of asthma. Significant reversibility is a 12–15% increase in FEV_1 that exceeds 200 mL in absolute volume. Spirometry is crucial for diagnosing asthma, assessing severity of airflow obstruction, and evaluating response to therapy. Additional pulmonary function testing can helpful. The diffusion capacity for carbon monoxide, a sensitive test of gas transfer, is typically normal or slightly elevated in asthma, whereas it is low in emphysema. The flow–volume loop is obtained by simultaneously measuring volume and instantaneous flow rate during forceful inspiration and expiration. Upper airway obstruction may mimic asthma and is often first suspected after identifying characteristic changes in the shape of the flow–volume loop.

C. OTHER TESTING

Diurnal measurement of peak expiratory flow over 1–2 weeks may be helpful when asthma is suspected but spirometry is normal. Peak expiratory flow is generally lowest in the morning and highest toward the midpoint of the day. Measurements should be taken before inhalation of bronchodilator medication in the morning and after treatment in the afternoon. A 20% difference between these 2 values suggests asthma.

Bronchial hyperreactivity can be assessed by demonstrating enhanced bronchial narrowing after an inhalation challenge with cold air, histamine, or, most commonly, methacholine. Bronchial hyperreactivity is not specific for asthma; it may also be seen in bronchiectasis, COPD, and allergic rhinitis without obvious asthma and after viral respiratory infections. Nevertheless, when bronchial hyperreactivity is present along with characteristic clinical findings, asthma is very likely.

Chest radiography is useful, especially with recent onset of symptoms, to rule out alternative diagnoses. Chest computed tomography (CT) may be of diagnostic value in presumed asthma that is poorly responsive to therapy or in atypical cases; central airway lesions, bronchiectasis, bronchiolar disorders, and parenchymal lung diseases may be identified.

Differential Diagnosis

Airflow obstruction and breathlessness, with or without wheeze, are features seen in asthma, COPD, vocal cord dysfunction, anatomic narrowing of the upper airway, endoluminal tumor, airway strictures, aspirated foreign bodies, bronchiectasis, and bronchiolitis and in disorders that are usually classified as interstitial lung diseases, such as sarcoidosis, lymphangioleiomyomatosis,

and Langerhan's cell histiocytosis. Chest tightness in asthma is easily confused with angina pectoris. Cough, nocturnal breathlessness, and wheeze may suggest congestive heart failure. Episodic smothering may occur with recurrent pulmonary emboli.

Some circumstances are associated with poor control or worsening asthma. Many elderly patients with asthma also have cardiovascular disease and may be receiving oral β-blocker therapy, which may exacerbate asthma. The use of a cardioselective β-blocker is less likely to precipitate bronchospasm. Aspirin and nonsteroidal anti-inflammatory drugs (NSAIDs) may produce acute bronchoconstriction in some asthmatics. Chronic sinusitis may make asthma less responsive to therapy, and aggressive medical therapy or surgical intervention may improve asthma control. Gastroesophageal reflux may also foster asthma symptoms. Antireflux therapy has been reported to improve asthma symptoms, but there is debate regarding whether airflow obstruction or medication use is improved.

Complications

Asthma causes reduced quality of life, hospitalizations, and increased health care costs. Asthma hospitalization rates are greatest in patients older than 65. Reported mortality rates from asthma are highest in the elderly.

Treatment

Drug therapy in elderly patients with asthma is the same as in younger asthmatics (Table 22–1). The goals of therapy are to prevent symptoms and exacerbations by attempting to maintain as near normal lung function as possible with minimal side effects and costs.

Avoidance of allergen exposures that induce symptoms is important. Allergen injection therapy has no proven role in older asthmatics, but referral to an allergist may be considered, especially when treatment goals are not achieved with pharmacotherapy. Data from existing studies, which involved few adults, do not indicate that multiple allergen injection immunotherapy has steroid-sparing potential and does not have a major impact on lung function.

Medications to treat asthma are separated into those that provide quick relief of symptoms and those that provide long-term control.

The quick reliever agents are the short-acting β2-agonists, typified by albuterol. Side effects are tremor, palpitations, tachycardia, and, with high doses, hypokalemia. The anticholinergic bronchodilator, ipratropium bromide, has less rapid onset but can be an acceptable bronchodilator if β2-agonists are poorly tolerated because of tremor or cardiac stimulation.

Table 22–1. Commonly used drugs for asthma.

Severity	Long-term control	Short-term control
Severe persistent	Inhaled steroids (high dose) and Long-acting β-agonist or Theophylline	Short-acting β-agonists
Moderate persistent	Inhaled steroids (low or medium dose) and Long-acting β-agonist	Short-acting β-agonists
Mild persistent	Inhaled steroids (low dose) or Cromolyn	Short-acting β-agonists
Mild intermittent	No medication needed	Short-acting β-agonists (> 22×/week may indicate need for long-term control)

Modified from National Asthma Education and Prevention Program: Expert Panel Report 2: Guidelines for the diagnosis and management of asthma. (NIH Pub No. 97–4081). National Institutes of Health, 1997.

Corticosteroids are the most potent and consistently effective long-term control medications. Inhaled corticosteroids are the principal long-term controllers. The main side effects of inhaled steroids are cough, dysphonia, and oral thrush. High-dose inhaled steroids may induce systemic effects, including rare instances of adrenal suppression, increased intraocular pressure, cataracts, and potential for increased bone loss.

Systemic corticosteroids are prescribed for short-term burst therapy to gain control of worsening symptoms but are discouraged for long-term use except in severe persistent asthma. Short-term therapy should continue until symptoms have improved or the patient achieves 80% of baseline peak expiratory flow. There is no evidence that tapering the dose prevents relapse. The side effects of systemic steroid therapy are well known: osteoporosis, aseptic necrosis of the femur, muscle weakness, immune suppression, cataracts, impaired glucose metabolism, salt retention, hypokalemia, metabolic alkalosis, bruising, and elevated intraocular pressure. If long-term systemic therapy is required, every-other-day dosing is probably preferable, and therapy to prevent osteoporosis is indicated.

Inhaled cromolyn sodium and nedocromil are long-term controllers that seem most effective in younger, atopic asthmatics. These medications are safe. However, their use in older asthmatics has been questioned.

Leukotriene receptor antagonists are long-term controllers that are taken orally once or twice daily. They are not as effective as inhaled steroids for long-term control of asthma. Leukotriene receptor antagonists are useful in aspirin-induced asthma. In persistent asthma they have marginal utility and are inferior to the combination of inhaled fluticasone-salmeterol. There are re-

ports linking leukotriene receptor antagonists with Churg-Strauss vasculitis.

Salmeterol and formoterol are long-acting β-agonists that produce bronchodilation for up to 12 h. They are useful for control of nocturnal asthma. Side effects include tachycardia, tremor, and hypokalemia. Adding a long-acting β-agonist to an inhaled steroid in moderate asthma is more effective than increasing the dose of inhaled steroid.

Sustained-release theophylline is effective in long-term control of symptoms, especially nocturnal asthma. Theophylline toxicity and relatively modest bronchodilator activity limits theophylline use in acute asthma. Serum theophylline concentrations must be monitored to maintain a relatively safe level of 10–15 μg/mL. Adverse effects at therapeutic doses include insomnia, gastric upset, increased gastroesophageal reflux, and difficulty with urination. Higher blood levels increase the likelihood of serious toxicity, including headache, nervousness, nausea, vomiting, arrhythmias, seizures, and death. Theophylline metabolism may be decreased and blood levels increased by chronic liver disease, congestive heart failure, and many medications such as macrolides, fluoroquinolones, zileuton, cimetidine, and allopurinol.

Impediments to effective control of asthma in older patients should be sought and addressed as best possible. These impediments include inadequate medication usage, which may result from cognitive impairment and poor memory, inability to use inhaler devices correctly, drug interactions, cardiovascular comorbidity, polypharmacy, and depression. In addition, the high cost of some medications can interfere with patient compliance and prevent them from reaching therapeutic goals.

Inhalation drug therapy may be administered by several methods. The pressurized metered-dose inhalers (MDIs) are the most prevalent delivery devices. Drug delivery can usually be enhanced by using a spacer attached to the MDI. A spacer acts as a holding chamber and reduces the need to precisely coordinate inhalation with actuation of the inhaler. Actuation of the MDI requires pressing on the drug canister, which can be difficult if the patient has arthritis of the hand or weakness. An attachment to the MDI is available that reduces the difficulty of actuation. Dry powder inhalers are activated by inspiration, requiring a brisk inspiratory effort but little hand–breath coordination. Nebulizers are another delivery option when MDI or dry powder inhalers are not effective.

Referral to an asthma specialist is indicated if the patient has persistent asthma symptoms or recurrent asthma exacerbations despite recommended treatment.

CHRONIC OBSTRUCTIVE PULMONARY DISEASE

ESSENTIALS OF DIAGNOSIS

- *Symptoms: dyspnea, cough, sputum production, and wheeze.*
- *Risk factors: tobacco smoke, air pollution.*
- *Spirometry: airflow obstruction that is not fully reversible.*

General Considerations

Limitation of expiratory airflow demonstrated by spirometry is the key to diagnosis. Airflow limitation is mostly due to fixed airway obstruction, which is usually progressive.

COPD is an umbrella term that refers to airflow obstruction resulting from airway and lung injury caused by inhalation of toxins and pollutants. Chronic bronchitis and emphysema are included in COPD. Chronic bronchitis is defined by symptoms of cough with sputum production for 3 mo in 2 consecutive years. Chronic bronchitis may be obstructive or nonobstructive. Airflow obstruction in chronic bronchitis is due to airway lumen compromise from thickened and inflamed bronchial walls, hypertrophy of mucus glands, smooth muscle constriction, and excess mucus. Emphysema is an anatomic lesion characterized by dilated airspaces distal to the terminal bronchiole associated with

loss of alveolar walls. Airflow obstruction in emphysema results, in part, from loss of support around airways, causing their narrowing during expiration.

The principal risk factor for COPD is tobacco smoking, which accounts for 80–90% of cases. Airflow obstruction and dyspnea typically develop after age 45. Symptomatic COPD usually occurs after 35–40 pack-years of exposure. The prevalence of COPD increases in the sixth decade, affecting equal numbers of women and men. COPD is a major cause of disability and death in most countries and contributes significantly to escalating health care costs.

Heavy exposures to occupational dusts, chemicals, and air pollution (such as biomass fuels) are additional risk factors for COPD. Low socioeconomic status, maternal smoking, subnormal lung growth, childhood respiratory illness, and airway hyperreactivity are also linked to the occurrence. The only known genetic risk factor, α1-antiprotease deficiency, is a rare cause of emphysema.

Clinical Findings

A. SYMPTOMS & SIGNS

Chronic cough with sputum production is usually the first symptom and often precedes airflow obstruction. Physical examination may be unremarkable early in the disease. Dyspnea on exertion is typically evident when the FEV_1 is reduced to 50–60% of the predicted level. Patients with predominant emphysema are notably tachypneic, display pursed-lip breathing, and tend to prefer to lean forward and support themselves using the elbows. In more advanced disease, one may observe wheezes, prolonged expiratory time, diminished breath sounds, and hyperresonance with chest percussion. Clinical signs in severe COPD include central cyanosis, ankle edema, and increased jugular venous pressure, indicating cor pulmonale and right-sided heart failure.

Exacerbations in COPD are common. An exacerbation is often caused by infection; however, in some instances, a cause cannot be identified. The symptoms of an exacerbation are worsening dyspnea (often with increased wheezing), tachypnea, and tachycardia. There may be increased cough with sputum production. The sputum may be purulent or described as tenacious and difficult to expectorate. Decreased alertness may signal hypoxemia and hypercapnia.

B. LABORATORY FINDINGS

Patients with chronic cough, sputum production, and significant exposure to risk factors should be screened with spirometry, even if they are free of dyspnea. The diagnosis of COPD is confirmed by spirometry. The FEV_1– FVC ratio is used to measure airflow obstruction. An FEV_1–FVC ratio < 70% and a postbronchodilator FEV_1 < 80% predicted indicate airflow obstruction. Additional lung function testing may include lung volumes that often display hyperinflation with increased total lung capacity and residual volume. The diffusion capacity for carbon monoxide may be reduced, and the degree of reduction correlates roughly with the severity of emphysema. Gas exchange abnormalities are more likely when FEV_1 < 40% predicted and arterial blood gas analysis is indicated. Secondary polycythemia may accompany chronic hypoxemia.

C. IMAGING STUDIES

Chest x-ray film is often unremarkable in early and moderate COPD. Advanced disease may be associated with hyperlucent lung fields, flattening of the diaphragms, increased retrosternal airspace, or thickened bronchial walls. Bullous lung disease is sometimes seen in COPD. High-resolution computed tomography (HRCT) of the chest is more sensitive than plain radiography for detecting emphysema. The routine use of computed tomography in COPD is not indicated, however. HRCT is used to examine the severity and distribution of emphysema when lung volume reduction surgery is contemplated.

It is often difficult to distinguish an exacerbation of COPD from acute pulmonary embolism (PE). Helical CT angiography can be useful when ventilation–perfusion lung scanning is not helpful.

D. SPECIAL TESTS

Screening for α_1-antitrypsin deficiency is indicated in patients who experience COPD at a young age (< 45 years) or have a strong family history of obstructive lung disease. Liver dysfunction may also be seen in this condition, especially in younger patients.

Differential Diagnosis

The differential diagnosis of obstructive lung disease includes asthma, bronchiectasis, bronchiolitis, upper airway obstruction, tracheo- or bronchomalacia, airway strictures, and endoluminal masses (tumors, amyloid, foreign bodies).

Prognosis

COPD is usually a progressive disease and a leading cause of death in older adults. The FEV_1 is a strong correlate with mortality in COPD. Age, hypoxemia, pulmonary hypertension, hypercapnia, low body weight, persistent smoking, and reduced functional capacity are additional predictors of increased mortality in COPD.

Exacerbation in COPD requiring hospitalization is associated with ~11% mortality. If the exacerbation requires intensive care, the mortality ranges from 10–50%. Mechanical ventilation for acute respiratory failure in COPD is associated with mortality ranging from 10–40%. One-year mortality after exacerbation for patients older than 65 has been reported to be > 50%.

Treatment

The goals of treatment in COPD are to prevent symptoms, prevent exacerbations, preserve lung function, and enhance quality of life.

The management of COPD is primarily symptom driven. Pharmacological therapy does not alter the progressive decline in lung function nor does it appear to affect mortality. One exception is continuous oxygen therapy in hypoxemic patients with COPD, in whom mortality is significantly improved by oxygen therapy. Smoking cessation is known to slow the rate of decline in lung function and is a key treatment goal.

The current medications used in COPD are similar to those used in asthma, but the latter usually displays a relatively large treatment effect whereas COPD does not. Bronchodilator drugs are the cornerstones of symptom control (Table 22–2).

β-Agonist bronchodilators have been the mainstays of drug therapy in COPD, and inhaled therapy is preferred. The short-acting β-agonists are primarily used as needed for symptom relief. The long-acting inhaled β-agonists are given as a scheduled dose and provide significant symptom relief in COPD, including improving exercise tolerance and possibly reducing exacerbations.

The anticholinergic bronchodilator ipratropium bromide is usually the initial drug for scheduled bron-

Table 22–2. Commonly used drugs for COPD.

Drug	Delivery/dose	Duration (h)
Short-acting β-agonist		
Albuterol	MDI 200–400 μg	4–6
	Nebulizer 2.5 mg	4–6
Long-acting β-agonist		
Salmeterol	MDI 50–100 μg	12
Formoterol	DPI 12–24 μg	12
Anticholinergic		
Ipratropium bromide	MDI 40–80 μg	6–8
	Nebulizer 500 μg	6–8
Methylxanthine		
Theophylline	Oral 300–600 mg	Varies
	Sustained release	12–24

DPI = dry powder inhaler; MDI = metered-dose inhaler.
Adapted from Pauwels RA et al: Global strategy for the diagnosis, management, and prevention of chronic obstructive pulmonary disease. NHLBI/WHO workshop summary. Am J Respir Crit Care Med 2001;163:1256. Used with permission.

chodilator therapy in COPD. There are few side effects and bronchodilation lasts 4–6 h. Compared with the β-agonist albuterol, ipratropium has similar improvement in FEV_1 but a slower onset to peak effect. Combining an anticholinergic with a β-agonist provides effective symptom control while minimizing the side effects associated with maximal doses of either single agent. A long-acting anticholinergic bronchodilator is undergoing review for use in COPD.

Theophylline has modest bronchodilator activity in COPD. Some patients prefer theophylline preparations both for convenience of oral administration and for symptom relief. Exercise performance may be improved with theophylline. Because of the narrow therapeutic window of theophylline, the need for drug level monitoring, and the potential for drug interactions, theophylline is a second-line medication in COPD.

The use of inhaled corticosteroids in COPD has been the focus of investigation. It has been shown that inhaled steroids do not improve the rate of decline in lung function. There may be an initial slight improvement in FEV_1, which may not be sustained. A reduction in the frequency of exacerbations has been noted, and symptoms may also be reduced. The current international guidelines suggest that inhaled steroids for COPD are indicated when a 4- to 6-week trial produces documented spirometric improvement and when moderate to severe COPD is associated with frequent exacerbations. Complications of therapy are uncommon, but loss of bone density has been reported. The cost–benefit ratio of inhaled steroids in COPD is unknown.

Chronic treatment with oral corticosteroids is discouraged because of the unfavorable risk–benefit ratio. No adequate trials show long-term benefits. The long-term side effects are well known.

Continuous oxygen therapy is safe and improves survival and quality of life in hypoxemic patients with COPD (Table 22–3).

Exercise training and pulmonary rehabilitation may improve shortness of breath, functional capacity, quality of life measures, and psychosocial function in COPD.

Table 22–3. Usual indications for home oxygen therapy.

1. Oxygen saturation < 88% or PaO_2 < 55 mm Hg on room air
2. Oxygen saturation < 89% or PaO_2 < 60 mm Hg on room air if there is clinical evidence of PAH, CHF, or polycythemia

These changes can be documented with rest, with activity, or during sleep with therapy appropriate for those situations. PAH, pulmonary hypertension; CHF, congestive heart failure; PaO_2, arterial oxygen tension.

Rehabilitation programs often involve multiple health care professionals with the goals of reducing symptoms and improving quality of life through exercise reconditioning, nutritional repletion, patient education, and smoking cessation. Pneumococcal vaccination and annual influenza vaccination are recommended.

Treatment algorithms in COPD involve progressive addition of medications in an effort to achieve maximum possible symptom control. A typical approach is as follows:

- Mild and intermittent symptoms: as-needed β-agonist every 2–6 h.
- Regular/daily symptoms: scheduled ipratropium bromide plus as-needed β-agonist.
- If unsatisfactory response: trial of scheduled ipratropium–β-agonist combination.
- If unsatisfactory response: addition or substitution using long-acting β-agonist.
- If unsatisfactory response: addition or substitution using slow-release theophylline.
- If unsatisfactory response: addition of inhaled steroid for 4–6 weeks, to be continued only if significant spirometric improvement is documented.
- All patients must be helped with smoking cessation.
- Hypoxemic patients should be encouraged to use continuous oxygen therapy (> 15 h/day).
- Advise pulmonary rehabilitation for persistently symptomatic patients.

Treatment of acute exacerbations involves oxygen therapy to correct hypoxemia (increasing the dose or frequency of bronchodilators), antibiotics if infection is likely, systemic corticosteroids, and avoidance of complications. Short-acting β-agonists are preferred in the acute setting, often with the addition of an anticholinergic bronchodilator. Theophylline and methylxanthines are generally avoided in the acute setting. Systemic glucocorticoids are indicated in the management of an exacerbation. This is usually given over 10–14 days, starting with a relatively high dose (40–60 mg/day). Antibiotic therapy is indicated in exacerbations when there is increased sputum volume or purulence. Common pathogens associated with exacerbations are *Streptococcus pneumoniae*, *Haemophilus influenzae*, and *Moraxella catarrhalis*.

Noninvasive intermittent positive-pressure ventilation (NIPPV) to treat respiratory failure is effective in selected patients. NIPPV reduces the need for endotracheal intubation and can shorten hospital stay. Contraindications to NIPPV include excessive secretions, impaired mentation, inability to protect the airway, and cardiovascular instability. NIPPV may also be used as a bridge between endotracheal intubation and liberation from ventilation. Currently, no evidence supports NIPPV for chronic respiratory failure resulting from COPD.

Advanced COPD, especially in the setting of comorbid conditions, should raise concern over ethical issues. It is important to address the patient's wishes regarding end-of-life care.

Lung transplantation and lung volume reduction surgery are options in highly selected patients with COPD. Optimal candidates for lung transplantation should be ≤ 65 years. Lung volume reduction surgery may be considered in selected emphysema patients up to age 75 years.

SLEEP-RELATED BREATHING DISORDERS

ESSENTIALS OF DIAGNOSIS

- *Excessive daytime sleepiness.*
- *Risk factors: obesity or anatomic narrowing of upper airway.*
- *Overnight sleep study with abnormal breathing events.*

General Considerations

Sleep-related breathing disorders (SRBDs) encompass a spectrum of respiratory events during sleep wherein ventilation deviates from the normal rhythmic tidal breathing. An apneic breathing event is defined as absence of airflow for at least 10 s. A central apnea manifests no respiratory effort, whereas an obstructive apnea is characterized by continued effort to breathe against the occluded upper airway. Hypopnea refers to reduced breathing during sleep resulting from partial occlusion of the upper airway. It is often defined as a ≥ 50% reduction in airflow for at least 10 s with an associated decline in oxygen saturation of 3%. Within the spectrum of obstructive SRBD is the upper airway resistance syndrome (UARS), in which sleep is associated with narrowing of the upper airway that is insufficient to lead to apnea or hypopnea but is capable of causing increased respiratory effort. The increased respiratory effort produces arousal from sleep, which can cause excessive daytime sleepiness. Central apnea (cessation of airflow for 10 s with absent effort to breathe) in the elderly usually takes the form of periodic breathing or Cheyne-Stokes respiration.

Obstructive sleep apnea is common in the general population, affecting ~2–4%. Epidemiological studies indicate that 20–30% of men and women older than 65 have > 5 apneic events/h of sleep. More than 50% of older adults have an apnea-hypopnea index (AHI) exceeding 5 events/h.

Obstructive sleep apnea-hypopnea syndrome (OSAHS) is defined as excessive daytime sleepiness that cannot be explained by other factors plus 2 or more additional symptoms (choking or gasping during sleep, recurrent awakenings, unrefreshing sleep, daytime fatigue, impaired concentration) and a sleep monitoring study that demonstrates ≥ 5 obstructed breathing events/h of sleep. Especially in middle age, OSAHS has been linked to increased risk for hypertension, stroke, motor vehicle accidents, neurocognitive deficits, and, possibly, death.

Many older people display an increased AHI (> 5/h) and yet seem to have relatively few OSAHS symptoms. Reasonably strong evidence links OSAHS with morbidity and excess mortality in middle age but not in old age. Despite an increased frequency of abnormal breathing events during sleep, there is less compelling evidence of associated morbidity or mortality in older patients.

Central sleep apnea is less common than obstructive sleep apnea in the general population. Advanced age is associated with an increased frequency of central apneas per hour of sleep, usually in the form of periodic breathing or Cheyne-Stokes respiration. Periodic breathing is closely associated with congestive heart failure and cerebrovascular disease. In some studies of sleep-disordered breathing in patients older than 65, 33–50% of the disordered breathing events were central apneas.

Clinical Findings

A. SYMPTOMS & SIGNS

Snoring is a prominent symptom in OSAHS. The snoring is interrupted by quiet pauses that typically terminate with an increasing struggle to breathe, followed by a loud snort reflecting arousal and opening of the collapsed upper airway. Sleep may also be characterized by body jerks and kicking as well as sleep verbalizations. Sufferers awaken feeling tired (nonrestorative sleep) and have excessive daytime sleepiness, which is the cardinal symptom. The individual may be unaware of the sleepiness. Some may have periods of microsleep during which they are unaware of surroundings but will display automatic behavior, such as driving an automobile. During wakefulness there may be cognitive dysfunction such as poor attention, forgetfulness, and irritability.

Many people with Cheyne-Stokes breathing will also complain of nonrestorative sleep and excessive daytime sleepiness.

Physical examination in OSAHS commonly reveals obesity, and there may be redundant soft tissue in the pharynx, enlarged tonsils, retrognathia, or tongue enlargement. A neck circumference > 43 cm in men or ≥ 41 cm in women increases the risk for OSAHS. The most severe cases, often with morbid obesity or concurrent COPD, will have a plethoric appearance and signs of right-sided heart failure.

B. LABORATORY FINDINGS

There are no characteristic laboratory findings. Thyroid function should be assessed if clinical findings suggest hypothyroidism. Secondary polycythemia may occur in severe cases.

C. IMAGING STUDIES

CT and magnetic resonance (MR) imaging have been used to assess upper airway size and surrounding anatomic structures but are clinically indicated in only exceptional cases. Lateral radiographs of the head and neck (cephalometry) are helpful when skeletal anomalies are present.

D. SPECIAL TESTS

A number of methods exist for monitoring breathing during sleep, ranging from overnight oximetry to technician-dependent multiple-channel recordings of electromyography, cardiac rhythm, electroencephalography, oxygen saturation, and respiratory effort and airflow (polysomnography). Polysomnography is the standard for diagnosis of SRBDs. If the criteria for OSAHS are met, a second night in the sleep laboratory is needed for a trial of continuous positive airway pressure (CPAP) to titrate the pressure until upper airway obstruction is reduced or eliminated.

Home testing and screening with overnight pulse oximetry may become acceptable tools for diagnosis. Currently, however, they are not validated to the extent that insurers will accept them as diagnostic.

Differential Diagnosis

Defining excessive daytime sleepiness is problematic with advanced age because napping becomes increasingly more frequent. Arousals from sleep and disturbed sleep are also common with age. Elders often seem to have shifted the circadian rhythm of the sleep–wake cycle forward, retiring earlier and arising earlier.

Difficulty initiating or maintaining sleep may be due to an SRBD but may also be a result of musculoskeletal discomfort, nocturia, congestive heart failure, depression, gastroesophageal reflux, and drugs or drug interactions.

Possible causes of excessive daytime sleepiness include medications, obstructive sleep apnea syndrome (and upper airway resistance syndrome), periodic limb movements in sleep (PLMSs), periodic (Cheyne-Stokes) breathing, depression, central nervous system (CNS) disease, narcolepsy, and hypothyroidism.

Medications that may cause excessive daytime sleepiness include hypnotics, antidepressants, anticonvulsants, α-agonists and α-blockers, antihistamines, and antipsychotics.

PLMSs are uncontrollable sudden, forceful, and repetitive movements, usually of the legs, that can cause arousal from light stages of sleep. Thus, similar to OSAHS, PLMSs produce poor sleep quality and lead to daytime sleepiness. This disorder is more common in the elderly. Polysomnography can determine the presence and suggest the significance of PLMSs in producing daytime sleepiness.

Complications

Obstructive sleep apnea may, in some cases, increase mortality risk. Hypertension is common in OSAHS, and the latter appears to worsen the former. Social interactions (marital and occupational) in OSAHS can be impaired by poor concentration, lagging memory, irritability, and lack of attentiveness. Motor vehicle and work accidents may be increased. When OSAHS occurs in association with COPD or marked obesity (often referred to as the overlap syndromes), abnormalities in pulmonary gas exchange are common, producing hypoxemia and hypercapnia. Pulmonary hypertension evolves and leads to right-sided heart failure.

The possible association of sleep-disordered breathing with declining cognition has been investigated in older adults. Sleep-disordered breathing is frequent in dementia, but a causal association has not been proved.

Periodic breathing (Cheyne-Stokes respiration) produces somnolence and daytime sleepiness similar to OSAHS. These patients demonstrate reduced life expectancy, presumably resulting from systolic heart dysfunction.

Treatment

Treatment options for OSAHS include general measures for sleep, CPAP provided via nose or face mask, oral appliances that enlarge the pharyngeal airway, and surgical procedures. Pharmacological therapy is not used in OSAHS but may have a role in periodic breathing or central apneas.

Sleep-related breathing events are common in the elderly, many of whom lack any symptoms. Clinical judgment is important when deciding to initiate treatment for obstructive SRBD. Symptoms, especially excessive sleepiness, in association with an abnormal number of apneic–hypopneic events or respiratory effort-related arousals are needed to consider therapy potentially worthwhile.

General measures to promote better sleep and minimize upper airway narrowing are the first consideration. Weight loss can have a substantial impact on OSAHS. Alcohol and sedating medications are to be avoided. Smoking should be eliminated. Sleeping on the side can be helpful. Nasal obstruction should be managed with antihistamines (preferably minimally sedating) and intranasal steroids. Hypothyroidism is treated with thyroid hormone.

CPAP is the principal treatment for OSAHS. Effective CPAP is associated with restoration of sleep, reduction in daytime sleepiness, and improved quality of life. Subjective improvements typically manifest within a few nights use. Hypertension may moderate, but continued antihypertensive medication will likely be needed. Compliance with CPAP is 60–70% and is improved by attention to patient education and by CPAP-induced improvement in symptoms. Complications of CPAP include nasal congestion and dryness, skin irritation from the mask, poor mask fit, noise, insufflation of the stomach, and sense of impaired breathing against the external pressure.

Several types of oral appliances are used in OSAHS, the most promising of which are mandibular advancement devices that fit over the teeth and pull the jaw forward. Snoring, sleep quality, indexes of upper airway occlusion, and symptoms have been shown to improve to varying degrees. Mandibular advancement devices are typically considered when CPAP fails or is not tolerated. These devices require at least some teeth for anchoring, which is often a problem. Acceptability of these devices in elderly patients has not been studied.

A variety of surgical procedures have been used in OSAHS. Tracheotomy is useful and reserved for life-threatening and refractory cases. Palatal surgery is useful for snoring but is inconsistently effective in OSAHS, especially the more severe cases. Tonsillectomy and adenoidectomy can be helpful in appropriate patients. Craniofacial surgery is a consideration in carefully selected older patients.

Periodic breathing/Cheyne-Stokes respiration is managed primarily by optimizing cardiac performance in those patients with congestive heart failure. Respiratory stimulants (eg, medroxyprogesterone, acetazolamide, and theophylline) have been used with variable effects and in small numbers of patients and are not currently recommended. Nocturnal oxygen by nasal cannula has been reported to reduce central apneic events and decrease nocturnal oxygen desaturation but may not improve daytime symptoms. Nasal CPAP, which carries the theoretical advantage of reducing left ventricular afterload and improving cardiac function, has shown inconsistent benefit in Cheyne-Stokes respiration.

LUNG CANCER

 ESSENTIALS OF DIAGNOSIS

- *Pathological or cytological confirmation of neoplasia.*

GENERAL CONSIDERATIONS

At least 50% of all lung cancers occur in people older than 65. Lung cancer is the most common cause of cancer mortality in the 60- to 80-year age group in both sexes. Twenty percent of all lung cancers are small cell lung carcinoma (SCLC). Adenocarcinoma is the most frequent histological subtype (30%) of non-SCLC (NSCLC), followed by squamous cell carcinoma (25%). Large cell carcinoma comprise most of the remaining NSCLCs. Only 20% of NSCLCs are resectable at diagnosis. SCLC is not surgically curable because of almost invariable dissemination at diagnosis.

The overall 5-year survival for lung cancer is 10–15%. Younger patients have a slightly better prognosis than older patients. Elimination of tobacco smoke exposure could prevent the majority of lung cancers. Chemoprevention (eg, antioxidants and retinoids) has not been shown to be useful.

Clinical Findings

A. SYMPTOMS & SIGNS

The cardinal symptoms of lung cancer are cough, dyspnea, weight loss, chest pain, and hemoptysis. Radiographs obtained for evaluation of these symptoms often are the first indication of lung cancer. At presentation, most patients with lung cancer have symptoms from either the primary tumor or metastases.

Signs of lung cancer are usually nonspecific. Localized wheeze may be produced by endobronchial tumor. Superior vena cava obstruction, supraclavicular or axillary lymphadenopathy, Horner's syndrome (unilateral exophthalmos, ptosis, miosis, and ipsilateral anhidrosis), vocal cord paralysis, and ipsilateral diaphragm paralysis are important findings that imply unresectable disease. Pleural effusion in lung cancer is usually malignant and also indicates unresectable disease. The liver may be enlarged from metastatic spread of tumor. Clubbing of the digits is occasionally seen.

Bone pain and CNS symptoms, such as headache, focal weakness, clumsiness, and uncoordination, are important to elicit, indicating the need to pursue investigation for metastatic disease with appropriate imaging studies.

Paraneoplastic syndromes are rare. They do not necessarily imply unresectability. These syndromes result from immunological epiphenomena or from hormones and cytokines produced by cancer cells.

B. LABORATORY FINDINGS

Hyponatremia resulting from syndrome of inappropriate antidiuretic hormone production is seen in both SCLC and NSCLC. Hypercalcemia is seen in squamous cell carcinoma and may be the result of osseous metastasis or hormonally mediated by tumor secretion of parathormone-related peptides or other mediators. Elevated liver enzymes should prompt imaging studies to identify hepatic metastases. Anemia and thrombocytosis may be seen in advanced lung cancer. Bone marrow involvement by tumor can produce a leukoerythroblastic picture in the peripheral blood consisting of nucleated red cell precursors and immature myeloid cells.

C. IMAGING STUDIES

Screening chest radiography for lung cancer in high-risk smokers has not been shown to improve survival and is not currently recommended by the American Cancer Society. Low-dose helical CT is a more powerful imaging method that is currently being investigated for early detection of lung cancer.

The chest radiograph is usually the first indicator that lung cancer is likely. SCLC often presents a radiographic picture with large mediastinal and hilar nodes plus a contiguous lung mass. Adenocarcinomas are typically peripheral lung masses. In comparison, squamous cell carcinomas are often centrally located masses and may be cavitary. Bronchoalveolar carcinoma, a subtype of adenocarcinoma, may display single or multiple lung masses; a nonresolving consolidative density with air bronchograms, resembling pneumonia, can be seen with bronchoalveolar cell carcinoma.

CT scanning with its enhanced resolution is helpful in further defining lung and hilar opacities, identifying mediastinal or hilar lymph node enlargement, and imaging the liver and adrenal glands.

Positron emission tomography (PET) after intravenous injection of radioactive fluorodeoxyglucose, which can differentiate normal from neoplastic cells as a result of differences in glucose metabolism, has shown value in identifying malignant lung opacities > 1 cm. PET appears more accurate than CT for identifying mediastinal lymph node metastases and can be used to direct biopsy for confirmation of nodal involvement. Whole-body PET scanning and imaging with radioisotope-labeled somatostatin analogues are promising imaging techniques for determining metastatic spread of lung cancer.

Metastases in lung cancer are commonly seen in the brain, bone, lymph nodes, liver, and adrenal glands. Any symptoms or signs referable to these areas warrant imaging studies. Surgical or needle biopsy of abnormal sites is often undertaken to confirm metastatic spread.

Treatment & Prognosis

A. NON-SMALL CELL LUNG CANCER

Surgery is the preferred treatment for completely resectable NSCLC in selected patients who are deemed suitable for thoracotomy. Surgery is potentially curative in Stage I (clinical T1N0 and T2N0) and Stage II (clinical T1N1, T2N0, and T2N1) NSCLC. Operative mortality and survival rates are acceptable in patients $\geq$ 70 years; most recent series of lung cancer surgery in the elderly indicate that age should not be a contraindication for lung cancer surgery. However, age is definitely a high-risk factor for complications and death when pneumonectomy is performed. The 30-day operative mortality for thoracotomy averages 5–8% in patients older than 70. Lobectomy is associated with mortality of ~7%. Pneumonectomy is associated with mortality of 12–15%; right pneumonectomy is least well tolerated. Some patients may be considered candidates for lesser resections or lung-sparing operations (wedge resection and segmentectomy), but cancer recurrence is higher after these lesser procedures (compared with lobectomy), and perioperative risks are not clearly reduced with lesser resections.

Operability (patient's tolerance for surgery) is assessed by history, physical examination, cardiac risk profiling, and pulmonary function testing. Unstable coronary syndromes, congestive heart failure, and myocardial infarction within 3 mo would indicate current inoperability, but effective treatment may allow subsequent reassessment. An FEV_1 < 1 L, maximal oxygen uptake < 10 mL/kg/min, and carbon monoxide diffusion test < 40% of predicted indicate inoperability.

If preoperative spirometry is normal, further pulmonary function testing is not needed. If spirometry is abnormal, full pulmonary function testing, including arterial blood gas analysis and carbon monoxide diffusion test, is advised. An FEV_1 > 1.5 L is considered sufficient to perform lobectomy and an FEV_1 > 2.0 L to perform pneumonectomy.

Poor surgical candidates with potentially resectable lung cancer (T1) can achieve 5-year survival of 20–25% with radiation therapy.

Most patients with NSCLC will have unresectable disease at presentation (75–80%). Carefully selected patients with Stage IIIA (N2) disease can benefit from extended resections; 5-year survival ranges from 20–30%. Patients with N2 disease manifested by bulky ipsilateral or subcarinal lymph node enlargement do not benefit from surgery and should be referred to radiation and medical oncology.

Stages IIIB and IV NSCLC should be referred to medical oncology. Studies have shown that patients with advanced disease who have some capacity for independent function (fair to good performance status) can benefit from chemotherapy with modest improvements in survival and better overall function and well-being compared with supportive care.

B. SMALL CELL LUNG CANCER

Combination chemotherapy is the cornerstone of treatment for SCLC. Median survival for SCLC with limited-stage disease (confined to 1 hemithorax) ranges from 15–20 mo. Median survival for extensive-stage SCLC (any extension beyond limited disease) is < 1 year.

VENOUS THROMBOEMBOLIC DISEASE

ESSENTIALS OF DIAGNOSIS

- *Advanced age is a significant risk factor for venous thromboembolic disease.*
- *A high level of suspicion and pursuit of objective testing are necessary for diagnosis.*
- *Consider pulmonary embolism when patients manifest dyspnea, tachypnea, pleuritic chest pain, tachycardia, anxiety, or hemoptysis.*
- *Pulmonary embolism is diagnosed by characteristic defects on ventilation–perfusion lung scan, helical computed tomography scan, or pulmonary angiogram.*

General Considerations

Venous thrombosis and subsequent PE (venous thromboembolic disease; VTE) are common events in hospitalized patients. Risk factors for VTE include age, prior VTE, malignancy, major surgery, hip or leg fracture, congestive heart failure, myocardial infarction, paralytic stroke, estrogen therapy (eg, prostate cancer, hormone replacement), and immobilization. Age increases the

risk for VTE in an exponential manner; the risk approximately doubles for every decade beyond age 40. Knowledge of risk factors is essential for suspecting VTE in a particular patient and for selecting appropriate prophylactic measures.

Prevention

Prophylaxis for VTE is effective and should be a key consideration in all hospitalized patients. Thromboprophylaxis should also be considered in the skilled nursing facility and other chronic care settings (Table 22–4).

Clinical Findings

A. SYMPTOMS & SIGNS

The symptoms in leg deep vein thrombosis (DVT) include swelling, increased skin temperature, and thigh or calf pain. VTE is often asymptomatic. The common symptoms in PE are dyspnea (especially if acute), pleuritic chest pain, hemoptysis, and anxiety. Syncope suggests extensive occlusion of the pulmonary vascular bed or an arrhythmia with low cardiac output. Prior cardiopulmonary disease will amplify the adverse effects and symptoms of PE. The most common signs in PE are tachypnea and tachycardia. The combination of dyspnea, pleuritic chest pain, and tachypnea are very suggestive of PE. Cyanosis may be seen in 20% of patients at presentation. Fever may be present. Hypotension is the hallmark of massive PE.

B. LABORATORY FINDINGS

Electrocardiography often shows nonspecific abnormalities in PE. Signs of acute right-sided heart strain may be seen with massive emboli. Arterial blood gas analysis often displays a reduced carbon dioxide tension (Pco_2) with respiratory alkalosis and reduced oxygen tension. However, normal values can occur and should not deter pursuit of further testing when clinical suspicion of PE exists. Absence of D-dimer in the blood measured by a validated assay argues against VTE.

C. LUNG IMAGING

The chest radiograph may be normal or have nonspecific findings in PE. Its primary utility is for excluding an alternative diagnosis such as tumor, heart failure, pneumonia, and pneumothorax. Common radiographic findings in PE are pleural effusion, segmental collapse, elevated hemidiaphragm, and focal infiltrate. A wedge-shaped lung opacity with its base toward the pleural surface (Hampton's hump) can be seen in PE. Areas of oligemia or hypovascularity of the lung (Westermark sign) are occasional findings. PE is suspected in an acutely dyspneic patient with a normal radiograph.

Table 22–4. Prevention of venous thromboembolism.

Risk group	Recommended prophylaxis
General surgery	
Low risk: minor procedure, age < 40 years, no additional risk factors	Early ambulation
Moderate risk: minor procedure, with additional risk factors; nonmajor surgery in 40–60 years, with no additional risk factors; major surgery, patients < 40 years, with no additional risk factors	LDUH, LMWH, ES, or IPC
Higher risk: nonmajor surgery in patients > 60 years or with additional risk factors; major surgery in patients > 40 years, or with additional risk factors	LDUH, LMWH, IPC device
Higher risk, with greater-than-usual risk for bleeding	Mechanical prophylaxis with IPC device
Very high risk (multiple risk factors)	LDUH or LMWH, combined with mechanical method (ES or IPC device)
Urologic surgery	
Transurethral surgery or other low-risk procedure	Prompt mobilization
Major open urological procedure	Routine prophylaxis: LDUH, ES, IPC device, or LMWH
Highest-risk group (multiple risk factors)	ES with or without IPC device plus LDUH or LMWH
Gynecologic surgery	
Brief procedure for benign disease	Prompt mobilization
Major gynecological surgery for benign disease; no additional risk factors	LDUH bid; alternatively LMWH or IPC device started just before surgery and continued several days postoperatively
Extensive surgery for malignancy	LDUH tid; for possible additional protection: LDUH plus mechanical prophylaxis with ES or IPC device
Orthopedic surgery	
Elective total hip replacement	LMWH (started 12 h before surgery, or 12–24 h after surgery; or half the usual dose 4–6 h after surgery, followed by usual high-risk dose the following day) or adjusted-dose warfarin therapy (goal INR 2.5; range, 2.0–3.0) started preoperatively or immediately postoperatively
Elective total knee replacement	LMWH or adjusted-dose warfarin (goal INR 2.5; range, 2.0–3.0)
Hip fracture surgery	LMWH or adjusted dose warfarin (goal INR 2.5, range, 2.0–3.0); possible alternative; LDUH
Medical conditions	
Acute myocardial infarction	Most patients; prophylactic or therapeutic anticoagulant therapy with SC LDUH or IV heparin
Ischemic stroke, with impaired mobility	Routine use of LDUH, LMWH, or danaparoid; if anticoagulant contraindicated: ES or IPC device
General medical patients with risk factors for VTE (cancer, bed rest, heart failure, severe lung disease)	LDUH or LMWH

ES, elastic stockings; INR, international normalized ratio; IPC, intermittent pneumatic compression device; LDUH, low-dose unfractionated heparin; LMWH, low-molecular-weight heparin.
Modified and reproduced from American College of Chest Physicians: Sixth ACCP Consensus Conference on Antithrombotic Therapy. Chest 2001;119:(1S).

Ventilation–perfusion radionuclide lung scanning has been extensively studied in the investigation of pulmonary embolus. It has advantages of being noninvasive and generally available. Ventilation–perfusion scan is rarely diagnostic and must be combined with an estimate of clinical suspicion. A high-probability scan combined with a high clinical suspicion of PE leads to a likelihood of 96%. The majority (> 80%) of the ventilation–perfusion scans for suspected PE are neither normal nor highly probable for PE (ie, a nondiagnostic study). (See Figure 22–1 for a diagnostic algorithm for acute PE.)

Pulmonary angiography (PAG) is currently the reference standard for diagnosis of PE. It is invasive, requires special equipment and expertise, and is not read-

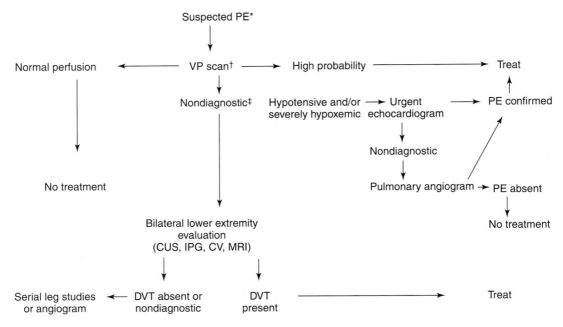

Figure 22–1. Diagnostic algorithm for acute pulmonary embolism. VP, ventilation-perfusion; CUS, compression ultrasonogram; IPG, impedance plethysmography; CV, contrast venography; MRI, magnetic resonance imaging; CT, computed tomography; MR, magnetic resonance.

ily available in most facilities. PAG is generally well tolerated in all age groups. It is most clearly indicated with hypotension or cardiovascular instability or when the ventilation–perfusion scan is indeterminate and clinical suspicion for PE is uncertain or high.

Helical (spiral) CT scanning with intravenous contrast enhancement is accurate for identifying PE in the main, lobar, and segmental pulmonary arteries. CT is not reliable for imaging emboli in subsegmental arteries (PAG has a similar limitation). Motion artifacts causing poor contrast enhancement of the vessels and other technical factors produce nondiagnostic studies in 5–10%. Helical CT scanning has the advantageous capability of potentially identifying a nonembolic cause of the patient's symptoms, which is often very useful in clinical decision making.

MR angiography is being developed as a non-contrast-requiring, noninvasive method for vascular imaging.

Echocardiography is readily available and has been used as the initial test when massive PE is suspected in a hypotensive or unstable patient.

D. VENOUS IMAGING

Proximal DVT produces the majority of PE and is itself an indication for treatment. Contrast venography is the gold standard for diagnosis of DVT but is seldom used because of the accuracy of noninvasive compression ultrasonography. Compression ultrasonography is the most common method for identifying DVT. A negative ultrasound examination cannot exclude DVT.

Compression ultrasonography is insensitive for identifying calf vein or iliac vein thrombosis, and chronic DVT will cause errors. When DVT is suspected and the initial compression ultrasonogram is negative, serial ultrasound examination every 5–7 days while withholding anticoagulation has been shown to not harm patients. Ultrasonography should not be used to screen asymptomatic high-risk patients (eg, after orthopedic surgery) for DVT because of its low sensitivity.

Pelvic vein DVT can be diagnosed with contrast venography, CT scanning, and MR imaging. MR holds considerable promise for diagnosing DVT.

Complications

PE that is promptly diagnosed and properly treated with anticoagulation results in death in < 4%. Untreated, the case-fatality rate is considerably higher. It is estimated that 50,000–200,000 people die from PE annually in the United States.

Chronic thromboembolic pulmonary hypertension is a rare complication, occurring in < 1% of PE. Surgical removal of occluding clot and fibrous tissue (pulmonary thromboendarterectomy) has been shown to help some patients with this condition.

Lower extremity DVT can produce venous valve damage and chronic venous insufficiency, causing postphlebitic syndrome characterized by swelling, pain, poor mobility, stasis dermatitis, and poorly healing ulcers.

Treatment

Unfractionated heparin has a long history as an effective treatment for VTE (Tables 22–5 and 22–6). It is

Table 22–5. Anticoagulation with unfractionated heparin.

Disease	Action
Suspected VTE	Obtain baseline APTT, prothrombin time, and CBC
	Check for contraindication to heparin therapy
	Order imaging study
	Consider giving heparin, 5000 IU pending study result
Confirmed VTE	Rebolus with heparin, 80 IU/kg; start maintenance infusion at 18 IU/kg/h
	Check APTT at 6 h to maintain a range corresponding to a therapeutic heparin level
	Check platelet count between days 3 and 5; stop heparin if platelet count falls precipitously or < 100,000/µL
	Start warfarin therapy on day 1 at 5 mg; adjust subsequent doses according to INR
	Stop heparin therapy after ≥ 4–5 days of combined therapy, when INR > 2.0
	Anticoagulate with warfarin for ≥ 3 mo (goal INR 2.5; range, 2.0–3.0)

APTT, activated partial thromboplastin time; CBC, complete blood cell count, INR, international normalized ratio.
Adapted from American College of Chest Physicians: Sixth ACCP Concensus Conference on Antithrombotic Therapy, Chest 2001; 119:(1). Used with permission.

usually administered as a continuous intravenous infusion, although intermittent subcutaneous injection is an option. Inadequate anticoagulation is associated with increased incidence of recurrent thrombosis. Weight-based dosing is advised.

Low-molecular-weight heparins (LMWHs) appear to be as effective as unfractionated heparin with the advantages of subcutaneous administration and no laboratory monitoring of activated partial thromboplastin time (APTT; Table 22–7). LMWHs appear to have a reduced risk of heparin-induced thrombocytopenia and may have a reduced risk of bleeding complications. Some studies have indicated that outpatient therapy with LMWH for selected cases of VTE is safe and effective. Complications of heparin therapy include bleeding, which correlates poorly with dose or APTT (with unfractionated heparin). Age increases the risk for bleeding complications. Another complication, heparin-induced thrombocytopenia, occurs in < 1% of patients, usually within the first 2 weeks of therapy. This syndrome may occur sooner if there has been prior exposure to heparin. Heparin-induced thrombocytopenia is associated with arterial thromboembolism and recurrent VTE; the syndrome can lead to limb loss and death. Platelet count should be checked between days 3 and 5 of therapy; if heparin is continued for a longer period the platelet count should be monitored regularly.

Warfarin is administered for 3–6 mo after an initial VTE event that is associated with a reversible or time-limited risk factor (eg, surgery or immobilization). A first-event VTE without an identifiable risk factor is treated with warfarin for ≥ 6 mo because of an expected high incidence of recurrent VTE. Ongoing risk factors such as cancer and hypercoagulability may require indefinite warfarin therapy.

Bleeding is the main complication of warfarin therapy, and the risk correlates with elevation of the international normalized ratio. Aspirin and other platelet-inhibiting drugs increase this risk. Warfarin is subject to numerous drug interactions that may either potentiate or inhibit anticoagulation. The patient's medication list should be carefully reviewed before initiating warfarin and, during maintenance therapy, the INR monitored more closely when adding or removing a drug. Another complication of coumarin drugs is skin necrosis. This uncommon condition manifests as purpuric skin lesions, which may cause extensive dermal loss, and has been associated with protein C deficiency and malignancy.

Thrombolytic agents approved for clot lysis in VTE are streptokinase, urokinase, and alteplase (recombinant tissue plasminogen activator). The principle indication for thrombolysis in VTE is hemodynamically unstable PE. Thrombolysis in PE has not improved mortality

Table 22–6. Body weight-based dosing: continuous intravenous unfractionated heparin.

APTT (s)	Dose change (IU/kg/h)	Additional action	Next APTT
< 35 (1.2 × mean normal)	+4	Rebolus 80 IU/kg	6 h
35–45	+2	Rebolus 40 IU/kg	6 h
46–70	0	—	6 h
71–90	–2	—	6 h
> 90	–3	Stop infusion 1 h	6 h

During first 24 h, repeat APTT every 6 h; thereafter once every morning unless outside therapeutic range.
APTT, activated partial thromboplastin time.
Adapted from American College of Chest Physicians: Sixth ACCP Concensus Conference on Antithrombotic Therapy, Chest 2001; 119:(1S). Used with permission.

compared with heparin anticoagulation. Severe DVT, especially when leg viability is compromised, has been treated with thrombolytic agents.

Contraindications to thrombolytic agents include previous hemorrhagic stroke, recent bleeding, intracranial neoplasm, and recent intracranial surgery. Uncontrolled severe hypertension, surgery within 10 days, recent cardiopulmonary resuscitation, and bleeding disorders are relative contraindications. The risk of in-

Table 22–7. Anticoagulation with low-molecular-weight heparin.

Disease	Action
Suspected VTE	Obtain baseline APTT, PT, CBC, platelet count
	Check for contraindication to heparin therapy
	Order imaging study
	Consider giving UFH, 5000 IU IV, or LMWH
Confirmed VTE	Give LMWH (dalteparin, enoxaparin, nadroparin, tinzaparin)
	Start warfarin therapy on day 1 at 5 mg; adjust subsequent daily dose according to INR
	Check platelet count between days 3 and 5
	Stop LMWH therapy after ≥ 4–5 days of combined therapy, when INR > 2.0
	Anticoagulate with warfarin for ≥ 3 mo (goal INR 2.5; range, 2.0–3.0)

APTT, activated partial thromboplastin time; CBC, complete blood cell count; INR, international normalized ratio of prothrombin time; UFH, unfractionated heparin; LMWH, low-molecular-weight heparin.
Adapted from American College of Chest Physicians: Sixth ACCP Concensus Conference on Antithrombotic Therapy, Chest 2001; 119:(1). Used with permission.

tracranial bleeding after thrombolysis in VTE is 1–2% and increases with age.

Interruption of the inferior vena cava with intracaval filter devices is designed to prevent recurrence of embolization to the pulmonary circulation. Indications for placement of filters are contraindication to or complication of anticoagulation, recurrent PE despite adequate anticoagulation, chronic thromboembolic pulmonary hypertension, and massive PE. Complications include recurrent venous thrombosis, chronic lower extremity edema, and filter migration.

Surgical embolectomy and catheter-directed clot extraction or clot fragmentation are potential therapeutic options in massive PE.

INTERSTITIAL LUNG DISEASE

 ESSENTIALS OF DIAGNOSIS

- *Dyspnea.*
- *Nonproductive cough.*
- *Lung crackles and clubbing on physical exam.*

General Considerations

Interstitial lung disease is a general term used to describe a large number of unrelated diffuse parenchymal pulmonary disorders. Interstitial lung diseases of known cause include those resulting from inhalation injury (inorganic dust or fumes, pneumoconioses, and organic dusts), drugs, infections, radiation, lymphangitic carcinoma, and lung disorders associated with organ transplant rejection, heart failure, and liver and renal disease.

Those of unknown cause include the idiopathic interstitial pneumonias, sarcoidosis, vasculitides, collagen vascular disorders with interstitial lung disease, heritable disorders, and Langerhan's cell histiocytosis.

Idiopathic Pulmonary Fibrosis

General Considerations

Idiopathic pulmonary fibrosis (IPF) is one of the more common idiopathic interstitial pneumonias but is nevertheless a rare condition. The prevalence of IPF increases with age, and it has its peak prevalence at or near age 70. Approximately 66% of patients with IPF are older than 65 at presentation. There is a slight male predominance. Patients usually present with exertional dyspnea and nonproductive cough. Systemic symptoms are not characteristic. Symptoms usually evolve over several months to several years, and the disease usually progressively worsens. The relatively slow evolution of dyspnea and cough may delay diagnosis. Confusion with smoking-related lung disease or heart failure can contribute to diagnostic delay. The median survival is ~3 years.

Physical examination reveals dry, bilateral inspiratory crackles, predominately at the lung bases. Clubbing of the fingers is noted in ~50% of patients. End-stage disease will display signs of pulmonary hypertension and cor pulmonale.

The working definition of IPF by international consensus is a fibrotic lung disease with a surgical lung biopsy showing usual interstitial pneumonia plus the following:

1. No known causes for interstitial lung disease.
2. Restricted lung volumes on pulmonary function testing and abnormal gas exchange.
3. Characteristic abnormalities on chest radiograph or high-resolution chest CT.

Confirmation of a diagnosis of IPF requires surgical lung biopsy. A diagnosis of IPF in the absence of a surgical biopsy is likely if all of the following major criteria and 3 of 4 minor criteria are met.

1. Major criteria
- Exclusion of known cause of interstitial lung disease.
- Lung volume restriction on pulmonary function testing.
- Bibasilar reticular opacities with minimal ground-glass attenuation on HRCT.
- Transbronchial biopsy showing no features of alternative diagnosis.
- Minor criteria
- Age > 50 years.

- Insidious onset of otherwise unexplained dyspnea.
- Duration of illness > 3 mo.
- Bibasilar inspiratory crackles of the "dry" or "Velcro" type.

Differential Diagnosis

The differential diagnosis of IPF is broad. Crackles, dyspnea, and cough are easily confused with left-sided heart failure. Collagen vascular disorders, especially systemic sclerosis and rheumatoid arthritis, and asbestosis can have features that are identical to those of IPF.

Clinical Findings

A. LABORATORY FINDINGS

Low-titer elevations in rheumatoid factor assays and antinuclear antibodies are present in up to 30% of patients, even when no underlying connective tissue disease can be identified.

Pulmonary function testing typically reveals restrictive lung disease. The vital capacity and total lung capacity will be reduced. Reduced carbon monoxide diffusing capacity and hypoxemia, initially seen with exertion and later at rest, reflect impaired gas exchange.

B. IMAGING STUDIES

Chest radiographic abnormalities in IPF include bilateral irregular nodular or reticulonodular opacities that are most visible in the lower lung and subpleural areas.

HRCT is extremely useful in evaluating ILD. The HRCT findings in IPF are relatively specific.

C. SPECIAL TESTS

Surgical lung biopsy is needed for an accurate diagnosis. Lung tissue in IPF reveals the pathological pattern of usual interstitial pneumonia. The fibrosis is patchy with interspersed normal lung. Honeycombing (cystic dilatation of distal airspaces) is common. Biopsies performed via bronchoscopy can be useful for identifying other disorders that can mimic IPF (such as sarcoidosis, infections, or cancer) but are not suitable to accurately diagnose IPF.

Prognosis

The course of IPF is variable. Occasionally, the functional and radiographic abnormalities may stabilize. However, most cases will progress and the median survival is ~3 years. Progressive respiratory failure, right-sided heart failure, coronary artery disease, pulmonary embolus, or infection may cause death. There seems to be an increased incidence of bronchogenic carcinoma in IPF. Geriatric patients with IPF, especially if they have had recent acute decline in pulmonary function or advanced fibrosis, have a poor prognosis. Indicators of longer survival include younger age at onset, female sex, and a beneficial response to corticosteroid therapy.

Treatment

There is limited evidence that any current therapy is effective. Supportive therapy with oxygen and diuretics and symptom palliation may be best for some patients. Treatment in advanced age, obesity, diabetes mellitus, severe lung impairment, advanced cardiac disease, and general debility should be carefully considered in the context of the patient's wishes for end-of-life care. If treatment is pursued, the following has been suggested:

- Prednisone 0.5 mg/kg lean body weight daily for 8 weeks, then reduced to 0.125 mg/kg daily or 0.25 mg/kg every other day; plus either
- Azathioprine starting with 25–50 mg daily and increasing by 25 mg every 2–3 weeks to the maximum dose (2–3 mg/kg lean body weight); or
- Cyclophosphamide starting with 25–50 mg/day, increasing every 1–2 weeks by 25 mg to maximum dose of 2 mg/kg lean body weight (not to exceed 150 mg daily).

Therapy should be continued, if tolerated, for at least 6 mo. If the condition worsens, treatment should be stopped. Failure of treatment is indicated by worsening symptoms, declining oxygenation, worsening opacities on radiographs or CT, or ≥ 10% decline in vital capacity or total lung capacity. If treatment fails, consultation may be undertaken to review possible alternatives. If the condition stabilizes, combination therapy should be continued. Prevention of steroid-induced osteoporosis with bisphosphonates in conjunction with calcium and vitamin D is recommended. Bone mineral density measurements at baseline and serially are advised.

Pulmonary rehabilitation may be a useful adjunct. Oxygen supplementation should be provided for patients who exhibit oxygen desaturation with exercise or at rest.

Lung transplantation is an option in IPF. However, higher posttransplant mortality with age and the limited availability of lungs for transplantation usually limit this option to patients younger than 60–65.

Other Interstitial Lung Disorders

Sarcoidosis is the most common interstitial lung disease and typically presents before age 40. Onset of sarcoidosis past age 65 is unusual.

Hypersensitivity pneumonitis (HP), also called extrinsic allergic alveolitis, has been diagnosed in all age groups. A history of exposure to an organic antigen is key to suspecting this disorder. Diagnosis requires integration of a combination of features. Management emphasizes elimination of exposure to the inciting antigen. Corticosteroids may hasten resolution in the acute or subacute presentations but is not likely to benefit chronic HP.

Drug-induced lung disease is an important cause of diffuse infiltrative lung disease and is easily overlooked. The radiographic and clinical findings in drug-induced lung diseases are varied. Presentations include acute interstitial pneumonitis, acute eosinophilic lung disease, patchy areas of organizing pneumonia (bronchiolitis obliterans organizing pneumonia, or BOOP, pattern on histology), noncardiogenic pulmonary edema, alveolar hemorrhage, and subacute and chronic lung fibrosis. A classic example of subacute lung injury and fibrosis with dyspnea and dry cough is seen in the elderly woman receiving nitrofurantoin for managing recurrent cystitis. Another classic drug-induced diffuse lung disorder in the elderly is salicylate intoxication with pulmonary edema.

Other drugs with recognized associations with 1 or more of these patterns of diffuse lung disease include NSAIDs, phenytoin, amiodarone, hydrochlorothiazide, hydralazine, propylthiouracil, busulfan, bleomycin, methotrexate, penicillamine, gold, and ergot compounds.

REFERENCES

Asthma

Chan ED, Welsh CH: Geriatric respiratory medicine. Chest 1998;114:1704. (A broad review of respiratory disorders in the elderly, including asthma.)

National Asthma Education and Prevention Program: Expert Panel Report 2: Guidelines for the diagnosis and management of asthma (NIH publication no. 97-4051). Bethesda, MD: National Institutes of Health, 1997. (Basic information on diagnosis and therapy of asthma).

Weiner P et al: Characteristics of asthma in the elderly. Eur Respir J 1998;12:564. (More severe airway obstruction in elderly patients with long-standing asthma compared with those with recent-onset disease.)

Chronic Obstructive Pulmonary Disease

McEvoy CE, Niewoehner DE: Corticosteroids in chronic obstructive pulmonary disease. Clin Chest Med 2000;21:739. (Review of systemic and inhaled steroids in COPD.)

Pauwels RA et al: Global strategy for the diagnosis, management, and prevention of chronic obstructive pulmonary disease. NHLBI/WHO Global Initiative for Chronic Obstructive Lung Disease (GOLD) Workshop Summary. Am J Respir Crit Care Med 2001;163:1256. (Evidence-based review by international committee of clinical issues in COPD.)

Stoller JK: Clinical practice: acute exacerbations of chronic obstructive pulmonary disease. N Engl J Med 2002;346:988. (Concise review of management issues in COPD exacerbations.)

Sleep-Related Breathing Disorders

American Academy of Sleep Medicine: Sleep-related breathing disorders in adults: recommendations for syndrome definition and measurement techniques in clinical research. Sleep 1999;22:667.

Leung RST, Bradley TD: State of the art: sleep apnea and cardiovascular disease. Am J Respir Crit Care Med 2001; 164:2147. (Pathophysiology and epidemiology of obstructive apnea and periodic breathing in relation to cardiovascular disease.)

Lung Cancer

British Thoracic Society: Guidelines on the selection of patients with lung cancer for surgery. Thorax 2001;56:89. (Evidence-based guidelines for assessing resectability and operability in lung cancer.)

Jaklitsch MT et al: New surgical options for elderly lung cancer patients. Chest 1999;116:480S. (Brief overview of lung cancer surgery in the elderly.)

Reif MS et al: Evidence-based medicine in the treatment of non-small cell lung cancer. Clin Chest Med 2000;21:107. (Review of the studies supporting surgical and nonsurgical therapy in NSCLC.)

Venous Thromboembolic Disease

American College of Chest Physicians: Sixth ACCP Consensus Conference on Antithrombotic Therapy. Chest 2001;119:1S. (Extensive review of the evidence for antithrombotic therapy in multiple clinical settings.)

American Thoracic Society: Clinical practice guideline. The diagnostic approach to acute venous thromboembolism. 1999; 160:1043. (Review of the evidence basis and recommendations for diagnosis of acute VTE.)

Hyers TH: State of the art: venous thromboembolism. Am J Respir Crit Care Med 1999;159:1. (Review of diagnosis and treatment of PE and DVT.)

Interstitial Lung Disease

American Thoracic Society: Idiopathic pulmonary fibrosis: diagnosis and treatment. International consensus statement. Am J Respir Crit Care Med 2000;161:646.

American Thoracic Society/European Respiratory Society: International multidisciplinary consensus classification of the idiopathic interstitial pneumonias. Am J Respir Crit Care Med 2002;165:277.

Gross TJ, Hunninghake GW: Idiopathic pulmonary fibrosis. N Engl J Med 2001;114:1704. (Review of current thinking on the pathogenesis, diagnosis, and management of IPF.)

Abdominal Complaints & Gastrointestinal Disorders

23

M. Aamir Ali, MD, & Brian E. Lacy, PhD, MD

Gastrointestinal (GI) complaints are common in the elderly and range from mild self-limited episodes of acid reflux to life-threatening episodes of bowel ischemia. Some diseases, such as diverticulitis and colon cancer, are more common in the elderly, whereas other conditions, such as acid reflux disease, may present differently. Comorbid illnesses and polypharmacy may also contribute to, and modify the presentations and outcomes of, various GI disorders in the elderly. For instance, there is an increased prevalence of peptic ulcer disease in the elderly as a result of increased nonsteroidal anti-inflammatory drug (NSAID) use, which often masks ulcer-related pain. The increased use of anticoagulation therapy leads to worse outcomes in elderly patients with ulcer-related bleeding. It is important to understand GI disorders in the context of the elderly patient, realizing that common illnesses may present and progress differently than in the younger patient and thus are often diagnosed late in their course.

■ DISORDERS OF THE ESOPHAGUS

ESSENTIALS OF DIAGNOSIS

- *Gastroesophageal reflux is experienced monthly by at least 40% of elderly persons and usually requires ongoing therapy.*
- *To maximize quality of life and minimize office visits, treatment of reflux can be started with a proton pump inhibitor along with initiation of lifestyle changes.*
- *Dysphagia may be oropharyngeal (mostly caused by neurological disorders) or esophageal; the causes of esophageal dysphagia can generally be determined by history.*

- *Esophageal cancer usually presents in an advanced stage in the elderly, with symptoms of progressive dysphagia and weight loss.*

GASTROESOPHAGEAL REFLUX DISEASE

General Considerations

Gastroesophageal reflux disease (GERD) is the most common GI disorder affecting the elderly. Symptoms affect at least 40% of the elderly U.S. population on a monthly basis and approximately 7–10% on a daily basis. Persistent symptoms can dramatically affect quality of daily life. Once symptoms develop, at least 50% of patients will have persistent symptoms or require ongoing medical therapy. Persistent, untreated, or undertreated symptoms may lead to complications of acid reflux disease, including esophagitis, peptic strictures, esophageal ulcers with bleeding, and Barrett's esophagus. These complications are more likely to occur in the elderly.

Clinical Findings

A. SYMPTOMS & SIGNS

The diagnosis of GERD can be readily made if patients complain of typical symptoms of pyrosis (substernal burning with radiation to the mouth and throat) and sour regurgitation, and if these symptoms improve with treatment. Many elderly patients with GERD have reduced symptoms because of decreased visceral sensation or the use of medications that may blunt or reduce sensation. Quite commonly, however, patients have atypical symptoms, such as a chronic cough, difficult-to-control asthma, laryngitis, or recurrent chest pain.

B. DIAGNOSTIC STUDIES

Upper endoscopy (esophagogastroduodenoscopy; EGD) should be performed in all patients with persistent symptoms of reflux despite medical therapy, patients with a history of acid reflux longer than 5 years, and those with possible complications from acid reflux. EGD is safe to perform, even in the very elderly. Unlike a barium swallow or upper GI series, EGD directly visualizes the esophagus and stomach and allows the endoscopist to perform biopsies. Patients thought to have extraintestinal manifestations of GERD should undergo ambulatory evaluation with a 24-h pH probe. Esophageal manometry is not routinely of benefit in the evaluation of patients with GERD, unless antireflux surgery is being considered.

Treatment

Many physicians advocate a step-up approach to the treatment of GERD (Table 23–1). Lifestyle modifications are suggested first. If symptoms resolve, no further treatment is required. If symptoms fail to improve, then a histamine-type 2 receptor antagonist (H$_2$RA) should be used either once or twice daily. Cimetidine is generally not recommended because of potential drug interactions and a higher incidence of adverse side effects compared with other H$_2$RAs. Persistent symptoms, or incomplete resolution of symptoms with H$_2$RA, war-

rant treatment with a proton pump inhibitor (PPI) and evaluation with upper endoscopy.

An alternative approach to the treatment of GERD is to use step-in therapy. Patients with chronic symptoms of GERD, evidence of esophagitis on EGD, or extraesophageal manifestations of GERD are prescribed lifestyle modifications and started on a PPI at the first visit. This approach leads to fewer office visits, a reduction in procedures, improved patient satisfaction, and reduced overall costs. Antireflux surgery is rarely a viable option for the elderly given the presence of comorbid conditions, increased risks of surgery, and recent data showing that ~50% of patients who undergo antireflux surgery still require the routine use of acid suppressants years later. There are no data on the utility or safety of endoscopic therapies for GERD in the elderly; thus, these procedures cannot be recommended.

ODYNOPHAGIA

Odynophagia, or painful swallowing, is an uncommon complaint in the elderly, accounting for < 5% of all visits to a gastroenterologist. Common causes are listed in Table 23–2. Precipitating factors include diminished esophageal peristalsis, erosive esophagitis, presence of

Table 23–1. Treatment of gastroesophageal reflux disease: A step-up approach.

1. **Lifestyle modifications**
   Eat smaller meals.
   Do not eat 3–4 h before going to bed.
   Minimize fats, alcohol, caffeine, and nicotine, especially at night.
   Sleep with head of bed elevated 6 in.
2. **Over-the-counter agents**
   Mylanta, Maalox, Gaviscon, Tums, Rolaids
   H$_2$RAs (Pepcid AC, Axid AR, Zantac-75)
3. **H$_2$RAs**
   Cimetidine (Tagamet; not routinely recommended because of increased incidence of side effects)
   Famotidine (Pepcid; 20 mg qd or bid)
   Nizatidine (Axid; 150 mg qd or bid)
   Ranitidine (Zantac; 150 mg qd or bid)
4. **Proton pump inhibitors**
   Esomeprazole (Nexium; 20–40 mg qd)
   Lansoprazole (Prevacid; 15–30 mg qd)
   Omeprazole (Prilosec; 20 mg qd)
   Pantoprazole (Protonix; 40 mg qd)
   Rabeprazole (Aciphex; 20 mg qd)
5. **Surgery**
   Nissen fundoplication

H$_2$RAs, histamine$_2$ receptor antagonists.

Table 23–2. Causes of odynophagia.

1. **Medications**
   Tetracycline
   Quinidine
   Doxycycline
   Alendronate
   Iron
   NSAIDs
   ASA
   Vitamin C
   Potassium chloride
2. **Infections**
   Viral (HSV, CMV, HIV, VZV)
   Bacterial (*Mycobacteria*)
   Fungal (*Candida, Asperigillus*)
3. **Acid reflux disease**
4. **Miscellaneous**
   Ischemia
   Chemotherapy
   Radiation
   Crohn's disease
   Sarcoid

NSAIDs, nonsteroidal anti-inflammatory drugs; ASA, acetylsalicylic acid; HSV, herpes simplex virus; CMV, cytomegalovirus; V2V, varicella zoster virus.

an esophageal stricture, poor fluid intake while taking pills, or taking multiple pills at once. Evaluation should begin with an EGD to permit direct inspection of the esophagus and allow biopsies, if necessary. Treatment begins with removing the offending medication (if applicable) and treating the underlying disorder, such as acid reflux disease. Patients should take pills one at a time, with adequate amounts of water, to ensure that each pill is adequately cleared from the esophagus. Fungal infections of the esophagus may be treated with either nystatin swish-and-swallow or fluconazole. Viral infections should be treated with acyclovir or famciclovir.

DYSPHAGIA

General Considerations

Dysphagia, or difficulty swallowing, is a common complaint in the elderly. Dysphagia is classified as oropharyngeal (transfer) or esophageal (transit). Oropharyngeal dysphagia refers to impaired movement of liquids or solids from the oral cavity to the upper esophagus. Painful or diseased teeth, xerostomia, poorly fitting dentures, and mandibular destruction are common causes of transfer dysphagia. Neuromuscular disorders affecting the tongue, soft palate, oropharynx, and upper esophageal sphincter may produce disturbances in normal oroesophageal movement. Neurological causes of oropharyngeal dysphagia predominate and include cerebrovascular disease, Parkinson's disease, multiple sclerosis, Alzheimer's disease, and upper motor neuron

diseases. Muscular disorders such as myasthenia gravis, polymyositis, and amyloidosis may also produce dysphagia. Finally, patients with a history of surgery or radiation to the oral cavity or neck are at risk for transfer dysphagia.

Clinical Findings

A. SYMPTOMS & SIGNS

Patients with oropharyngeal dysphagia typically cough, gag, choke, or aspirate their food during the initiation of a swallow. Those with transit dysphagia often complain of solid foods or liquids "sticking," "catching," or "hanging up" in their esophagus, and they may point to their substernal area. Using a series of questions and the algorithm outlined in Figure 23–1, the cause of esophageal (transit) dysphagia can be identified in nearly 90% of cases. Dysphagia to solids usually reflects an underlying mechanical obstruction, whereas dysphagia to both liquids and solids reflects an underlying neuromuscular disorder. Patients should be questioned to ensure they do not have either odynophagia or globus (a persistent sensation of fullness in the throat that usually improves with eating), because the evaluation and treatment of these 2 conditions is different. The physician should look for evidence of anemia and unintentional weight loss, either of which could indicate a serious disorder. The nature of the dysphagia (solids or both solids and liquids) and the temporal nature of the swallowing disorder (intermittent or progressive in nature) should be determined. Finally, asso-

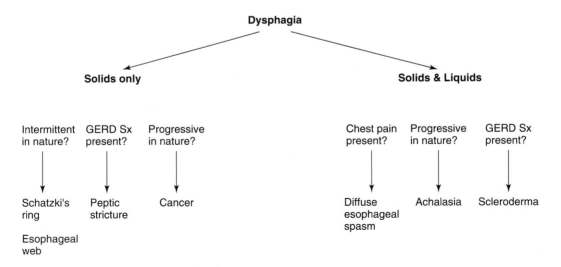

Figure 23–1. Evaluation of dysphagia.

ciated symptoms of chest pain or acid reflux should be elicited.

B. DIAGNOSTIC STUDIES

In the elderly a barium swallow is often ordered as the initial test to evaluate dysphagia. Patients should be evaluated by a speech language pathologist who can coordinate a swallowing study (modified barium swallow or videofluoroscopy) using thin, thick, and solid food materials. Upper endoscopy as the initial test has the advantage of directly inspecting the mucosa, taking biopsies if necessary, and dilating the esophagus, if a stricture or mass is present. If upper endoscopy is normal and complaints of dysphagia persist, then esophageal manometry should be performed. This is a safe and readily performed procedure that can accurately identify neuromuscular disorders that cause dysphagia.

Treatment

Treatment is directed toward the underlying disorder in addition to ensuring adequate nutrition and preventing aspiration. Patients are taught which consistency of foods can be safely swallowed, proper swallowing techniques, and how to modify their posture to improve their swallowing. Medical therapy is not effective. If aspiration occurs or the nutritional status of the patient suffers, a feeding jejunostomy or gastrostomy should be considered.

MOTILITY DISORDERS

General Considerations

Disorders of esophageal motility occur in the elderly, although age alone does not lead to a decrease in esophageal peristalsis. Presenting symptoms are usually dysphagia, chest pain, or persistent acid reflux disease. Achalasia is the most well-recognized motility disorder of the esophagus. Its prevalence increases with age; 7–12 in 100,000 elderly patients are affected. Treatment options include pneumatic dilatation, botulinum toxin injection of the lower esophageal sphincter, and surgery. Medical therapy (eg, nitrates, calcium channel blockers) is rarely effective. Surgery is an option, although it should be approached cautiously. Pneumatic dilatation produces significant relief of symptoms in many patients but is associated with a 3–10% risk of perforation. For many elderly patients, initial treatment of achalasia is best approached using botulinum toxin injection. It is safe and effective and provides symptom relief in the majority of patients for up to 9–12 mo. A second injection is often required. Side effects are un-

common and include transient chest or abdominal pain, rash, or low-grade fever.

Other common motility disorders that can occur in the elderly population include diffuse esophageal spasm, nutcracker esophagus, hypertensive lower esophageal sphincter, and ineffective esophageal motility. These conditions are diagnosed by esophageal manometry.

CANCER

General Considerations

Esophageal cancer is one of the most lethal types of cancer known; 5-year survival is ~5%. Both types of esophageal cancer, squamous cell and adenocarcinoma, are found predominantly in patients older than 60. Risk factors for squamous cell carcinoma include ethnicity (4–5 times more common in blacks than in whites), tobacco and alcohol use, previous radiation to the head or neck, achalasia, and chronic esophagitis. Barrett's esophagus, which develops in the setting of chronic acid reflux disease, is the major risk factor for adenocarcinoma of the esophagus.

Clinical Findings

A. SIGNS & SYMPTOMS

The presenting symptom for both types of cancer is the same: progressive dysphagia, first to solids and then to liquids. This is usually associated with weight loss and anemia. Odynophagia, cough, hoarseness, and recurrent pneumonia may also be present.

B. DIAGNOSTIC STUDIES

Although a barium swallow may reveal evidence of a mass, the diagnosis is made during upper endoscopy. Endoscopic ultrasonography has been shown to be more accurate than computed tomography (CT) for assessing tumor invasion.

Treatment

Surgery (esophagectomy) is recommended if the tumor is localized to the esophagus without metastasis (a T1 or T2 lesion). For patients who are poor surgical candidates or who have invasive disease, chemotherapy (5-fluorouracil, cisplatin, mitomycin C) and local irradiation may provide palliation or even cure in a select group of patients. Metallic stents are often deployed in the esophagus to improve dysphagia and minimize aspiration in those patients who are not surgical candidates. Endoscopic therapy using lasers may provide temporary relief of dysphagia by decreasing the tumor burden. In patients with nutritional compromise, endoscopically placed gastrostomy or jejunostomy tubes may be required.

DISORDERS OF THE STOMACH

ESSENTIALS OF DIAGNOSIS

- *Peptic ulcer disease is usually caused by NSAIDs or Helicobacter pylori.*
- *Complications of peptic ulcer disease are more common in the elderly.*
- *Dyspepsia is a common complaint in the elderly and requires endoscopy to rule out ulcer or cancer.*
- *Symptoms of gastric cancer are nonspecific, and diagnosis is often delayed.*

PEPTIC ULCER DISEASE

General Considerations

Peptic ulcer disease (PUD) refers to both gastric ulcers (GUs) and duodenal ulcers (DUs). Approximately 5 million cases of PUD will occur this year in the United States. The elderly are more likely to suffer complications of PUD, including hospitalization, need for blood transfusions, emergency surgery, and death. The 2 most common causes of PUD are NSAIDs and *H. pylori*.

More than 40% of elderly patients are prescribed NSAIDs, and up to 8% will be hospitalized because of a complication of NSAID use within the first year of initiating treatment. All NSAIDs increase the risk of PUD, although some appear to carry a lower risk of inducing an ulcer than others. A meta-analysis revealed that ibuprofen, at doses < 1200 mg/day, was the NSAID least likely to induce serious GI injury, with a relative risk of inducing PUD 2.1 times greater than for controls. In contrast, the relative risk of serious GI injury when using ketoprofen was 7 times higher than ibuprofen. Overall, 25% of chronic NSAID users will experience either a GU or a DU at some point in their lifetime. Cyclo-oxygenase-2 (COX-2) inhibitors have been shown to have less overall GI toxicity. However, no data exist regarding the complications of chronic use of COX-2 inhibitors in elderly patients. Aspirin may increase the risk of PUD by 1.5–3.9-fold above average.

Low-dose aspirin (75 mg/day) is generally safer than high-dose aspirin (> 300 mg/day).

Acute infection with *H. pylori* leads to a localized mucosal inflammatory response, reducing the normal gastroduodenal mechanisms that protect the mucosa from ulceration. *H. pylori* is thought to be responsible for nearly 70% of GUs and 80–90% of DUs not related to NSAID use.

Clinical Findings

A. SYMPTOMS & SIGNS

Patients may have hematemesis or coffee-ground emesis. Elderly patients with PUD may have epigastric pain; however, as many as 50% of patients will not have pain from either a GU or a DU, and suspicion of PUD is raised because of anemia or blood in the stools.

B. DIAGNOSTIC STUDIES

In patients suspected of having PUD, a complete blood cell count (CBC), prothrombin time, blood urea nitrogen (BUN), and creatinine should be obtained and stool checked for occult blood loss. Patients should be asked about a history of PUD; their use of aspirin, NSAIDs, and warfarin; and previous diagnostic studies (upper GI series, testing for *H. pylori*). Upper endoscopy should be performed in older patients suspected of having PUD to identify the lesion, perform a biopsy in the stomach for *H. pylori,* rule out a malignancy, and initiate endoscopic therapy for a bleeding ulcer, if necessary.

Complications

Hemorrhage and perforation are the most common complications of PUD and have been reported to occur in ~50% of patients older than 70.

Treatment

If an ulcer is found, therapy should be initiated with a PPI for at least 8 weeks to ensure healing. NSAIDs and aspirin should be stopped. If the patient is found to be *H. pylori* positive, double or triple antibiotic therapy should be started. In the case of a GU, healing should be documented 8–12 weeks later with follow-up EGD. Patients who require chronic NSAID or aspirin use should be treated concurrently with a PPI or misoprostol. Both agents are effective in reducing the risk of PUD in chronic NSAID users, although, as a group, the PPIs are generally better tolerated than misoprostol.

H. PYLORI

H. pylori is the most common infection worldwide. Approximately 50% of Americans aged 60 and older are infected, and the majority are asymptomatic. Acute *H. pylori* infection may lead to ulceration of the stomach or duodenum, whereas chronic *H. pylori* infection may lead to atrophic gastritis, gastric adenocarcinoma, or development of a mucosa-associated lymphoid tumor (MALT lymphoma). *H. pylori* is now considered a class I carcinogen by the World Health Organization. Testing for *H. pylori* should be performed in all individuals with a history of peptic ulcer disease or evidence of gastritis, duodenitis, or gastric atrophy or when an ulcer or erosion is identified during endoscopic or fluoroscopic examination. The diagnosis of *H. pylori* infection can be made from biopsies obtained during upper endoscopy or by detecting antibodies in the serum. Breath hydrogen tests are most useful in documenting eradication. Multiple treatment regimens have been shown to be effective in eradicating *H. pylori*. A twice-daily PPI for 10–14 days in conjunction with 2 different antibiotics (clarithromycin with either metronidazole or amoxicillin are the most effective) is the most common therapy. Eradication rates range from 75–95%, depending on the treatment regimen. The recurrence of PUD and complications of PUD are markedly reduced with *H. pylori* eradication.

DYSPEPSIA

General Considerations

Dyspepsia is defined as chronic or recurrent pain or discomfort in the upper abdomen, which is thought to arise in the upper GI tract. It is exceedingly common in clinical practice, affecting an estimated 20–30% of older adults.

Clinical Findings

A. SYMPTOMS & SIGNS

Patients may complain of upper abdominal pain, nausea, bloating, early satiety, or reflux symptoms. Dyspepsia traditionally has been classified as ulcer-like, reflux-like, or dysmotility-like; however, this classification has not been satisfactorily shown to improve either the evaluation or the treatment of patients with dyspepsia. However, it is important to distinguish patients with organic problems such as an ulcer from those with functional or nonulcer dyspepsia because the treatment and further evaluation are dramatically different.

Evaluation of dyspepsia begins with a thorough history and physical examination to determine whether the pain or discomfort arises in the GI tract or elsewhere (heart, lungs, musculoskeletal system). Patients should be asked about unintentional weight loss, odynophagia, dysphagia, a family history of GI tract cancer, and evidence of blood loss or jaundice.

B. DIAGNOSTIC STUDIES

Laboratory tests, including a CBC, erythrocyte sedimentation rate (ESR), liver function tests (LFTs), electrolytes, amylase, and lipase, should be performed. Patients should be evaluated by upper endoscopy to rule out an ulcer or cancer. Initial testing with upper endoscopy has been shown to improve quality of life and lead to a reduction in dyspeptic symptoms. If endoscopy is normal and symptoms persist, a right upper quadrant (RUQ) ultrasonogram should be performed. If this is normal and complaints persist, a solid-phase gastric emptying scan should be performed. In an older patient with persistent symptoms, concerns about occult malignancy should prompt a CT scan of the abdomen with both oral and intravenous contrast.

Treatment

Patients with persistent dyspeptic symptoms and a normal evaluation are categorized as having nonulcer dyspepsia (NUD). Treating this group of patients can be quite challenging. Few data support the routine use of antacids, antimuscarinic agents, or sucralfate. Routine treatment with H_2RAs has shown a slight benefit, but better results have been obtained with the use of once- or twice-daily PPIs. It is possible that some of the benefits of these trials occurred because patients with GERD were included in the dyspepsia category. Empiric treatment for suspected *H. pylori* does not improve patient outcomes. However, eradicating *H. pylori,* if present, does lead to a reduction in symptoms and an improvement in quality of life. Prokinetic agents (metoclopramide and erythromycin) are generally ineffective in treating patients with dyspepsia. Finally, the use of low-dose tricyclic antidepressants may improve symptoms of dyspepsia, although the mechanism of action in those patients who respond is unclear. There are no controlled, published studies to date on the use of selective serotonin reuptake inhibitors in the treatment of dyspepsia.

CANCER

General Considerations

Each year gastric cancer affects approximately 25,000 Americans, the vast majority of whom are older than 60. The overall 5-year survival rate is estimated at 16%. Nearly 95% of gastric cancers are adenocarcinomas. Carcinoids, sarcomas, and lymphomas make up the remaining 5%. Risk factors for gastric cancer include chronic atrophic gastritis, *H. pylori,* pernicious anemia, family history of gastric cancer, partial gastrectomy, tobacco use, and consumption of large quantities of salted or smoked foods.

Clinical Findings

A. Symptoms & Signs

Presenting symptoms of gastric cancer are usually vague, and this inevitably leads to a delay in diagnosis. Patients may complain of nausea, early satiety, epigastric fullness, weight loss, and abdominal pain. Physical examination may reveal a mass, a succussion splash from gastric outlet obstruction, or evidence of peripheral lymphadenopathy. Unfortunately, by the time symptoms are severe or physical examination findings are apparent, patients usually have widespread disease.

B. Diagnostic Studies

Gastric cancer is best detected by upper endoscopy because barium studies may miss early cancers or lesions in the antrum. CT scanning is useful to assess the depth of tumor invasion and the presence of lymphadenopathy. Both endoscopic ultrasonography and positron emission tomography scans are evolving technologies that may improve tumor staging.

Treatment

Surgical therapy offers the only cure for gastric cancer; however, the overall 5-year survival is poor (20–40%) and operative mortality high (15–25%). Endoscopic resection of large masses, laser therapy, and stent placement may provide palliation for some patients with obstructive symptoms. Chemotherapy and radiation do not provide any survival benefits.

■ DISORDERS OF THE COLON

ESSENTIALS OF DIAGNOSIS

- *Constipation is common in the elderly and requires careful assessment to rule out mechanical causes.*
- *Acute diarrhea is usually self-limited and caused by infections. Chronic diarrhea has many causes, and an extensive workup may be needed.*
- *Diverticulosis increases with age. Complications include bleeding, diverticulitis, and perforation.*
- *Inflammatory bowel disease (IBD) may present for the first time in older people.*

CONSTIPATION

General Considerations

Constipation can be defined as infrequent bowel movements (< 3/week), straining at stool, hard consistency, pain with defecation, or the need to digitally assist evacuation. Using all these definitions, the prevalence of constipation in the elderly in the community setting is estimated at 40%, nearly twice that of middle-aged patients. Forty-five percent of elderly patients take laxatives regularly. Interestingly, infrequent bowel movements (< 3/week) are not a common complaint in the elderly, occurring in < 5% of the community-based elderly. More commonly, elderly patients complain of straining at stool (25.6%), hard stools (27%), incomplete evacuation (22.7%), and the need to digitally assist evacuation (20%). Abdominal bloating and distention may occur, and patients may complain of rectal fullness, rectal pressure, back pain, left lower quadrant pain, or generalized abdominal discomfort. These symptoms increase in intensity as the frequency of bowel movements declines.

Constipation is most often divided into 3 general categories: slow transit constipation, pelvic floor dysfunction, and irritable bowel syndrome. However, there is often overlap between these groups. Up to 25% of patients with persistent constipation unresponsive to fiber therapy have apparently normal physiology, even after extensive evaluation. These patients are best categorized as having functional constipation.

Clinical Findings

A. Symptoms & Signs

Both over-the-counter and prescription medications should be reviewed in the history and questions asked about daily fluid and fiber intake as well as exercise. The clinician should look for coexisting neurological disorders (Parkinson's disease), systemic disorders (hypothyroidism), and musculoskeletal disorders (severe arthritis requiring narcotics), any of which could contribute to constipation (Table 23–3). One of the most important aspects of the evaluation should be to identify the patient with mechanical obstruction secondary to cancer, rectal prolapse, stricture, or a large polyp. Signs of these disorders may include unintentional weight loss, anemia, or evidence of GI bleeding.

B. Diagnostic Studies

Simple screening laboratory tests (CBC, thyroid-stimulating hormone [TSH], ESR, electrolytes) should be performed to look for evidence of anemia, hypothyroidism, or a systemic inflammatory disorder. Colon

Table 23–3. Common causes of constipation.

Irritable bowel syndrome
Slow colonic transit
Pelvic floor dysfunction (anismus, persistent puborectalis
  contraction)
Medication induced

Opiates	Anticholinergics
Calcium channel blockers	Antidepressants
Antipsychotics	Ganglion-blocking agents

Mechanical obstruction

Cancer	Large rectocele
Volvulus	Intussusception
Stricture	Anal fissure
Extrinsic compression	
Descending perineum syndrome	

Neurological disorders

Parkinson's disease	Spinal cord or sacral
Multiple sclerosis	root tumors
	Spinal cord injury
	Prior colon surgery

Systemic disorders

Hypothyroidism	Amyloid
Diabetes mellitus	Connective tissue
Congestive heart failure	disorders

Metabolic disorders

Hypokalemia	Uremia
Hypophosphatemia	Hypercalcemia
Hypomagnesemia	

Miscellaneous
  Poor fluid intake
  Immobility
  Cognitive impairment
  Autonomic neuropathy
  Diminished rectal sensation

cancer is more common in the elderly and often presents with constipation. Therefore, in patients with chronic constipation who fail to respond to simple remedies such as increasing fluid and fiber intake, colonoscopy should be performed to exclude a mechanical cause of constipation. The combination of flexible sigmoidoscopy and barium enema (BE) is an alternative approach, although smaller lesions may be missed by BE.

Differential Diagnosis

In the elderly patient, constipation may reflect an underlying malignancy; this is often the patient's primary concern. Other mechanical causes of constipation include rectal prolapse, rectal intussusception, recurrent sigmoid volvulus, extrinsic compression of the colon, and colonic

strictures secondary to previous episodes of diverticulitis. In addition, medications, neurological disorders, systemic diseases, metabolic disorders, poor fluid intake, and immobility can cause constipation (see Table 23–3).

Treatment

After mechanical causes of constipation have been ruled out, treatment should be initiated based on the primary complaint. Patients with straining and incomplete evacuation usually respond best to fluids, routinely scheduled bathroom time, and bulk-forming agents (Table 23–4). Patients with infrequent bowel movements typically respond best to osmotic agents or polyethylene glycol (PEG) solutions. These can be used safely in the elderly and do not generally interfere with the absorption of medications.

DIARRHEA

General Considerations

Patients with diarrhea most often complain of frequent stools (> 3/day) or loose stools. However, other patients use the term *diarrhea* to describe fecal incontinence or fecal urgency. The etiology of acute diarrhea (lasting < 2 weeks) in the elderly is similar to that of younger

Table 23–4. Treatment of constipation.

Initial management
  Increase fluid intake
  Exercise
  Bowel training regimen
  Education/reassurance

Second-line therapy
  Bulking agents
  Stool softeners
  Glycerin suppositories

Third-line therapy
  Osmotic agents (milk of magnesia, lactulose, sorbitol)
  PEG solutions
  Miscellaneous agents (misoprostol, colchicine, tegaserod)

Fourth-line therapy
  Stimulating agents (Senna, bisacodyl)

Agents to avoid
  Prokinetics (erythromycin, metoclopramide, cisapride)
  Lubricating agents (eg, mineral oil because of aspiration)
  Routine use of enemas (increased risk of rectal perforation
    in the elderly)

PEG, polyethylene glycol.

adults, with a few exceptions. Most cases of acute diarrhea are related to viral or bacterial infections, but it can also be caused by medications, medication interactions, or dietary supplements. *Clostridium difficile* colitis is more prevalent in the elderly because of more frequent hospitalizations, increased antibiotic use, and increased numbers of patients in institutional settings. Chronic diarrhea, lasting > 2 weeks, may result from fecal impaction, medications, irritable bowel syndrome, IBD, obstruction from colon cancer, malabsorption, thyrotoxicosis, or lymphoma. Lactase deficiency is common worldwide and is present in most individuals to some degree as they age, although it is less common in northern Europeans, North American Indians, and certain groups in Africa. Symptoms of bloating, abdominal distention, and loose stools usually begin in early adulthood, often worsening with age. Uncommon causes of diarrhea include Whipple's disease, jejunal diverticulosis, bowel ischemia, amyloidosis, lymphoma, and scleroderma with bacterial overgrowth.

Clinical Findings

A. Symptoms & Signs

A complete history and physical examination, including a rectal examination, may provide information on cause and direct further evaluation. Medication history may reveal a causative agent for the diarrhea, and recent antibiotic use may suggest *C. difficile*. A history of recent weight loss raises the concern for malignancy, IBD, microcytic colitis, malabsorption, or thyrotoxicosis. Fluid status should be assessed in all elderly patients with diarrhea because they are particularly susceptible to dehydration.

B. Diagnostic Studies

Stool cultures should be obtained to exclude infection in patients with acute diarrhea. *C. difficile* toxin assay should be obtained if there is a history of recent antibiotic use. Qualitative or quantitative stool fat should be checked in patients with steatorrhea. A TSH should also be checked as part of the initial workup of diarrhea.

In patients with *C. difficile* who fail sequential therapy with metronidazole first and then oral vancomycin, the presence of pseudomembranes should be confirmed by sigmoidoscopy or colonoscopy. Colonoscopy is also appropriate in patients with a history of weight loss, bloody diarrhea, and diarrhea lasting > 4 weeks (Table 23–5). If the colonoscopy appears grossly normal, biopsies should be obtained to rule out microscopic colitis.

Treatment

Treatment of diarrhea is based on the underlying cause. In those with no evidence of acute infection, loper-

Table 23–5. Indications for colonoscopy.

Screening at age 50 and every 10 years afterward (if no lesions identified)
First-degree family member with colon cancer
Personal history of colon cancer, colonic polyps, inflammatory bowel disease
Familial adenomatosis polyposis
Heme-occult positive stool on routine screening
Persistent change in bowel habits
Anemia secondary to blood loss from the gastrointestinal tract
Hematochezia
Unintentional weight loss
Peutz-Jeghers syndrome

amide (≤ 8/day) is generally effective in treating symptoms. Care must be exercised in the elderly with commonly used antimotility products, such as Lomotil, which contain atropine. In microscopic colitis, treatment is generally aimed at slowing colonic transit with the use of loperamide. Other alternatives include bismuth subsalicylate, prednisone, cholestyramine, or the 5-ASA products. Deodorized tincture of opium often improves symptoms in patients who fail to respond to other treatments.

DIVERTICULAR DISEASE

Diverticular disease is a disorder of industrialized nations. Diverticulosis is found in > 60% of those older than 70 and nearly 80% of those older than 80. Diverticula are outpouchings of the mucosa and submucosa that develop because of increased colonic luminal pressures. Diverticula are most commonly found on the left side of the colon; they are less common on the right side of the colon and are rarely, if ever, found in the cecum or rectum. The majority of patients who have diverticula are asymptomatic. A BE, colonoscopy, or CT scan performed for some other reason commonly identifies diverticula. Approximately 15–20% of older adults who have diverticulosis will have a complication, among them diverticular bleeding or diverticulitis.

Diverticular bleeding is characterized by the sudden onset of painless hematochezia, sometimes in large volume. Although most diverticula are present on the left side of the colon, 70% of diverticular bleeding occurs on the right side. If an episode occurs and the patient is hemodynamically stable, colonoscopy can be scheduled urgently as an outpatient. Eighty percent of diverticular bleeding will stop spontaneously. Patients should be hospitalized if bleeding persists, if they are hemodynamically unstable, or if blood loss compromises other organ systems. Evaluation includes colonoscopy to exclude sources of bleeding such as arteriovenous malformations (AVMs), ischemia, IBD, and cancer. If bleeding persists, a bleeding scan should be performed followed by angiography, if necessary. Surgical resection of the bleeding area may be required.

In uncomplicated diverticulitis, patients have lower abdominal pain (usually on the left), fever, and an elevated white blood cell count. On physical examination, the patient does not appear toxic, and there are no palpable abdominal masses or peritoneal signs. An abdominal radiograph should be performed to look for pneumoperitoneum. Treatment can be initiated in the outpatient setting with clear liquids for 2–3 days and oral antibiotics that should cover both anaerobes and gram-negative organisms. Metronidazole and a fluoroquinolone or third-generation cephalosporin for 2 weeks is generally well tolerated and very effective. The patient should call the office in 24 h and be seen 48–72 h after the initial evaluation. If no improvement occurs, the patient should be hospitalized and a CT scan of the abdomen performed.

Diverticulitis becomes complicated if an abscess, stricture, or fistula develops. Patients often have an elevated pulse or are hypotensive. Some elderly patients have lethargy or confusion. Abdominal examination may reveal a mass in the left lower quadrant or evidence of a draining fistula to the bladder, uterus, or skin. Peritoneal signs may be present. Patients with complicated diverticulitis require hospitalization. Patients should be given nothing by mouth and provided intravenous fluids. Blood cultures and an abdominal CT scan should be performed. Intravenous antibiotics should be initiated rapidly to cover both gram-negative organisms and anaerobes. If no improvement is seen within 48–72 h, an abdominal CT scan should be repeated.

Patients with an episode of diverticulitis have approximately a 35% chance of a second episode occurring within the next 5 years. Patients with > 2 episodes of diverticulitis in the same segment of colon should be referred to a surgeon for possible resection.

INFLAMMATORY BOWEL DISEASE

A second peak of IBD occurs in the U.S. population after age 65. Approximately 10–15% of all newly diagnosed cases of Crohn's disease and ulcerative colitis occur in this age group. Symptoms of Crohn's disease are similar to those in a younger population, although older patients with Crohn's disease may have fewer complaints of abdominal pain or cramps possibly because of reduced sensory thresholds or the concurrent use of multiple medications. Patients typically have a history of nonbloody diarrhea, unintentional weight loss, and fatigue. Evidence of anemia may be present (pallor, shortness of breath, reduced exercise tolerance).

Extraintestinal manifestations of Crohn's disease, including joint effusions, oral ulcers, painful nodular lesions on the extremities (erythema nodosum), uveitis, and back pain secondary to sacroileitis, commonly occur. Although Crohn's disease may develop anywhere from the mouth to the anus, in elderly patients it is less likely than in younger patients to involve large portions of the GI tract. The correct diagnosis is often delayed in the older patient because symptoms of Crohn's disease may mimic other diseases, including infectious diarrhea, ischemic colitis, lactose intolerance, medication-induced diarrhea, diverticulitis, celiac disease, microscopic colitis, or bacterial overgrowth.

Ulcerative colitis (UC) usually presents with tenesmus and frequent bloody bowel movements. Extraintestinal manifestations of UC are similar to those of Crohn's disease and also include dermatological manifestations such as pyoderma gangrenosum. Pyoderma ulcers typically appear as round or oval lesions on the shins and forearms. Elderly patients with UC are more likely to have limited left-sided disease or proctitis compared with younger patients, who often have pancolitis. The first attack of UC in an older patient is generally more severe and more likely to require steroids than that in a younger patient. Of elderly patients with UC, approximately 15% will eventually require surgery. The diagnosis of either UC or Crohn's is made based on a thoughtful physical examination and history supplemented by appropriate laboratory studies and colonoscopy. Treatment should be undertaken with gastroenterology consultation.

COLORECTAL CANCER
(See Chapter 30)

■ ANORECTAL DISORDERS

FECAL INCONTINENCE
General Considerations

For many older patients, fecal incontinence can lead to a decline in physical activity, loss of social contacts, and, eventually, isolation. The scope of the problem is impressive. Fecal incontinence is now the second leading cause of nursing home placement in the United States. Up to 7% of the elderly population have incontinence of solid or liquid stool at least once each week, and up to 50% of nursing home residents suffer from fecal incontinence. Most patients never report this problem to their clinician. Elderly men are more likely to suffer from incontinence than women. Patients are more likely to be incontinent of liquid, than solid, stool. Precipitating factors include prior surgery to the anorectal area (sphincterotomy for anal fissure, hemorrhoidectomy, episiotomy); difficult or prolonged childbirth with injury to the pudendal nerve; complete rectal prolapse; diabetic neuropathy; radiation injury to the anorectal area; IBD; and lumbosacral disease with resultant injury to L5-S4 nerve roots.

Clinical Findings

A. PHYSICAL EXAMINATION

Examination of the anorectal area can be performed with the patient in either a recumbent or a prone position. Perirectal erythema may be seen because of leakage of liquid stool. Local reflexes can be assessed by evaluating whether an anal wink is present. The external anal sphincter (EAS; striated muscle) should be assessed for evidence of mechanical injury, scar tissue, and strength during voluntary contraction. The internal anal sphincter (IAS; smooth muscle) provides most of the resting tone of the anal canal and should be assessed for resting tone. Examination should also include looking for evidence of fecal impaction, a rectal mass, hemorrhoids, rectocele, and the presence of rectal prolapse during straining.

B. SCOPE EXAMINATION

Flexible sigmoidoscopy or colonoscopy should be performed to look for a mechanical cause of incontinence (eg, large mass, fistula). Anorectal manometry can objectively measure the resting pressure of the anal canal (predominantly from the IAS), tone and contractile pressures of the EAS, and sensation within the anorectal area. Pudendal nerve testing may be required in some patients.

Treatment

In the absence of a surgically correctable cause, fecal incontinence can often be improved with behavioral interventions such as routine bathroom time 30–40 min after each meal to take advantage of the natural gastrocolic reflex. This allows emptying of the rectosigmoid colon and minimizes the chance of an accident occurring later. Bulk-forming agents should be used to create more firm stool and increase evacuation. Kegel exercises should be performed several times each day to strengthen the EAS. Loperamide may be used routinely in small doses to slow colonic transit and increase anal canal pressures. In patients with severe incontinence, a diverting colostomy or ileostomy may be required to improve quality of life.

FISSURES

Anal fissures may develop because of excessive straining or from the passage of rocky, hard stools. Patients typically complain of significant anal pain after defecation and report small amounts of bright red blood per rectum. Patients are often fearful of having another bowel movement because of persistent pain, and spasm of the anal sphincter can make examination of the area very difficult. Conservative therapy with sitz baths, stool softeners, and fiber products usually leads to healing of an acute anal fissure over 1–2 weeks. Topical nitroglycerin, calcium channel blockers, or botulinum toxin injection can be used to treat nonhealing or chronic fissures. Surgical therapy, using lateral internal sphincterotomy, may be necessary in some patients; however, fecal incontinence may develop in 3–30% of patients.

HEMORRHOIDS

Although commonly thought to develop as a result of straining and constipation, hemorrhoids may actually develop because of sliding of the lining of the anal canal. There are multiple nonsurgical treatments for hemorrhoids that do not prolapse (grade 1) or that prolapse and reduce spontaneously (grade 2). Bulking agents are commonly used to help minimize straining and the development of shear forces, although their efficacy has not been documented. Injection sclerotherapy, electrocoagulation, photocoagulation, cryotherapy, and laser therapy have proven beneficial. Rubber banding may lead to better healing and a lower rate of recurrence; however, it is more uncomfortable for the patient than the other procedures mentioned, is more difficult to perform, and is not recommended in immunocompromised patients because of an increased risk of sepsis. Surgery should be reserved for those patients with persistent symptoms who have failed nonoperative techniques.

■ GASTROINTESTINAL BLEEDING

ESSENTIALS OF DIAGNOSIS

- *Gastrointestinal bleeding is more common in the elderly and is associated with a worse outcome.*
- *Increased risk for gastrointestinal bleeding is seen with use of nonsteroidal anti-inflammatory drugs and warfarin and the presence of* Helicobacter pylori.

- Acute episodes of upper gastrointestinal bleeding usually present with hematemesis, melena, or an increased blood urea nitrogen–creatinine ratio.
- Chronic or slow upper gastrointestinal bleeding may present with anemia, melena, or a positive fecal occult blood test.
- Upper gastrointestinal endoscopy is required for evaluation of the cause of upper gastrointestinal bleeding and may also be useful in treatment.
- Lower gastrointestinal bleeding usually presents with hematochezia or a positive fecal occult blood test and requires colonoscopy for diagnosis.

UPPER GASTROINTESTINAL BLEEDING

General Considerations

Peptic ulcer disease accounts for > 50% of upper GI bleeding in the elderly. Esophagitis and gastritis are other common causes. Variceal bleeding, Mallory-Weiss tears, gastric cancer, vascular ectasias, AVMs, and aortoenteric fistulas are less common causes of upper GI (UGI) bleeding in the elderly (Table 23–6).

Clinical Findings

A. Symptoms & Signs

UGI bleeding may present with hematemesis (vomiting bright red blood), coffee-ground emesis, or melena. Chronic, slow UGI bleeding may present only with iron-deficiency anemia and a positive fecal occult blood test. Pain is an uncommon feature of UGI bleeding in

Table 23–6. Causes of GI bleeding in the elderly.

UGI bleeding	LGI bleeding
Gastric, duodenal or esophageal ulcer	Colonic diverticuli
Gastritis, duodenitis or esophagitis	Ischemic bowel disease
Esophageal varices	Inflammatory bowel disease
Mallory-Weiss tear	Angiodysplasia
Neoplasm	Infectious diarrhea
Telangiectasias	Radiation proctitis
Angiodysplasia	Postpolypectomy
	Hemorrhoids
	Stercoral ulcers

GI, gastrointestinal; UGI, upper GI; LGI, lower GI.

the elderly. Large-volume blood loss may result in circulatory collapse, syncope, or confusion. A careful medical history provides valuable information in identifying the source of UGI bleeding and in planning management. Any history of ulcer disease or liver disease, a list of all recent and current medications, including NSAIDs and anticoagulants, and patterns of alcohol use should be elicited. Physical examination includes orthostatic blood pressure and pulse measurement and evaluation for rebound tenderness and guarding. Orthostatic changes in pulse are more reliable indicators of hypovolemia than changes in blood pressure. Signs of chronic liver disease should be noted.

B. Diagnostic Studies

Laboratory evaluation includes a CBC and coagulation and chemistry profiles. The hematocrit at presentation may not accurately reflect the amount of blood lost because plasma and red cell volumes are reduced proportionally. It usually takes 24 h for extravascular fluid to restore vascular volume and reduce the hematocrit. Although a positive nasogastric lavage supports a UGI source of bleeding, a nonbloody aspirate is seen in 16% of patients with documented UGI bleeding. An elevated BUN–creatinine ratio (eg, > 35) also supports a UGI source of bleeding.

Treatment

Assessment of hemodynamic status followed, if necessary, by resuscitation of the unstable patient should precede any workup of UGI bleeding. Patients with ongoing acute UGI hemorrhage should be admitted to the intensive care unit. Anticoagulation should be stopped and reversal with fresh-frozen plasma initiated. After initial hemodynamic stabilization of the patient, upper endoscopy is performed to identify and treat the source of bleeding. If the history or physical examination suggests a variceal source, an octreotide infusion must be initiated and urgent endoscopy performed. Acid suppression with an intravenous or oral PPI has been shown to improve outcomes in patients with bleeding related to peptic ulcer disease. Patients infected with *H. pylori* should be treated.

Complications

The hospital course of the elderly patient with UGI bleeding is more likely to be prolonged by cardiac, neurological, or renal complications. Significant blood loss may unmask underlying coronary artery disease by increasing myocardial oxygen demand. UGI bleeding is associated with a mortality rate ranging from 6–44%.

Surgery for acute UGI bleeding is associated with mortality rates as high as 25%.

LOWER GASTROINTESTINAL BLEEDING

General Considerations

Colonic diverticuli and AVMs are the most frequent causes of lower GI (LGI) bleeding. IBD, bowel ischemia, NSAID-induced colitis, radiation colitis or proctitis, infections, cancer, recent polypectomy, and hemorrhoids should also be considered in the differential diagnosis (see Table 23–6).

Clinical Findings

A. SYMPTOMS & SIGNS

A positive fecal occult blood test may be the only indication of LGI bleeding. Acute LGI bleeding presents as hematochezia. Painless, large-volume hematochezia suggests a diverticular source. Abdominal pain coupled with hematochezia, especially in a patient with a history of vascular disease, suggests bowel ischemia. Loose bloody stools may occur in infections, IBD, and bowel ischemia.

B. DIAGNOSTIC STUDIES & TREATMENT

Although anemia is a consistent feature of chronic LGI bleeding, the hematocrit in patients with acute LGI bleeding may be normal until equilibrium with extravascular fluid is reached.

Stabilization of any existing hemodynamic instability is critical before proceeding with the workup of LGI bleeding. Because hematochezia may represent a briskly bleeding upper GI source in up to 10% of cases, upper endoscopy should be performed in patients with hematochezia and hemodynamic instability before proceeding with colonoscopy. Prompt colonoscopic identification and treatment of the source of bleeding should be attempted, although endoscopic treatment of diverticular bleeding is not very successful. Patients with significant bleeding despite attempted endoscopic treatment should undergo angiography with intra-arterial vasopressin infusion or angiographic embolic therapy. Surgery may benefit patients with recurrent bleeding or high transfusion requirements despite endoscopic or angiographic therapy.

Complications

LGI bleeding in the elderly is associated with a better clinical outcome than UGI bleeding. However, acute blood loss in the elderly may lead to myocardial or cerebral ischemia and renal failure.

OCCULT GASTROINTESTINAL BLEEDING

Iron deficiency anemia or a positive fecal occult blood test in the elderly patient may reflect chronic blood loss from cancer, AVMs, ulcers, or erosions in the GI tract. Evaluation should begin with a colonoscopy. If this is negative, upper endoscopy should be performed, followed, if necessary, by a small bowel follow-through to identify a source of bleeding in the small intestine.

GASTROINTESTINAL BLEEDING OF OBSCURE ORIGIN

Recurrent acute or chronic GI bleeding without an identifiable source after appropriate endoscopic and barium contrast studies is considered to be of obscure origin. Visualization of the small intestine identifies a source in many patients and may be achieved through push or sonde enteroscopy. Capsule enteroscopy is a promising new technique that, like sonde enteroscopy, allows visualization of the small bowel, although it lacks therapeutic capability. Patients requiring transfusion or hospitalization may benefit from radioisotope-tagged red blood cell scintigraphy or mesenteric angiography. Exploratory laparotomy with intraoperative enteroscopy should be reserved for patients with severe, persistent, or recurrent bleeding who do not have a diagnosis despite having undergone appropriate diagnostic testing.

■ GASTROINTESTINAL ISCHEMIA

ESSENTIALS OF DIAGNOSIS

- *Mesenteric ischemia is primarily a disease of the elderly, particularly those with underlying cardio-vascular disorders.*
- *Acute mesenteric ischemia presents with pain out of proportion to physical findings and may be caused by an embolus, thrombus, or low-output state.*
- *Selective superior mesenteric artery angiography is required for diagnosis and, often, for treatment.*
- *Chronic mesenteric ischemia presents with post-prandial pain (intestinal angina) and weight loss. It is seen in elderly patients with arteriosclerotic changes in the mesenteric circulation.*

- *Colonic ischemia presents with left lower quadrant pain and loose bloody stools. It is diagnosed by colonoscopy.*

ACUTE MESENTERIC ISCHEMIA

General Considerations

Emboli to the superior mesenteric artery (SMA) cause nearly 50% of acute mesenteric ischemia (AMI) cases, and this often occurs in the setting of underlying cardiac hypokinesis, arrhythmias, or atheromatous involvement of the aorta. SMA thrombosis causes 18–25% of AMI cases and usually occurs in patients with diffuse atherosclerotic disease. Nonobstructive mesenteric ischemia (NOMI) accounts for ~20% of AMI cases and is often seen in patients with underlying atherosclerosis who experience a low-flow state and in those taking vasoconstrictive agents or digitalis. The frequency of NOMI has been decreasing in recent years, presumably because of increased long-term use of vasodilating agents and the decreased use of digitalis. Mesenteric vein thrombosis (MVT) accounts for 5% of AMI cases and, in elderly patients, is associated with hypercoagulability from malignancy or recent abdominal surgery. Regardless of cause, AMI should be treated as an emergency and should be sought aggressively in at-risk patients.

Clinical Findings

A. SYMPTOMS & SIGNS

Abdominal pain is reported in nearly 80% of patients with AMI. Patients with NOMI are less likely to report pain than those with AMI from other causes. Often the abdominal pain is disproportional to the physical findings, which may be normal. However, as bowel necrosis develops, fever, nausea, vomiting, and hematochezia may arise, and physical findings of abdominal distension and rebound tenderness may occur. Mental confusion develops in 33% of elderly patients with AMI.

B. DIAGNOSTIC STUDIES

Laboratory abnormalities in patients with AMI include leukocytosis, metabolic acidosis, and hyperamylasemia. An abdominal plain film should be obtained, not to diagnose AMI but to exclude other causes of abdominal pain. CT scanning is useful only in the diagnosis of MVT. Magnetic resonance angiography detects proximal occlusions but often fails to detect more distal occlusion or NOMI. The test of choice to confirm the diagnosis of AMI is selective SMA angiography. This modality is both diagnostic and therapeutic because infusion of the vasodilator papaverine may be initiated if evidence of occlusion is noted on angiography.

Differential Diagnosis

The differential diagnosis in a patient with AMI includes peptic ulcer disease, acute pancreatitis, small bowel obstruction, gallstone disease, and diverticulitis.

Treatment

Early diagnosis is the key to improving outcomes in AMI. Surgical and gastroenterological consultations should be obtained soon after presentation. Management of AMI should be aggressive and begins by treating any precipitating conditions such as hypovolemia, congestive heart failure (CHF), or cardiac arrhythmias. Vasoconstrictors should be avoided in hypotensive patients. Angiography should be performed early if hypotension or hypovolemia are not present, and papaverine infusion should be initiated once vaso-occlusion or vasoconstriction is documented. Even in patients with signs of an acute abdomen, angiographic data are often helpful in the subsequent surgical management.

In the absence of peritoneal signs, proximal or major embolic occlusions are managed by papaverine infusion followed by embolectomy or thrombolysis. Distal or minor embolic occlusions or NOMI are managed expectantly with papaverine infusion and repeat angiography. Thrombotic occlusion in the patient without peritoneal signs can be managed expectantly if adequate collateralization with acceptable filling of the SMA is seen on angiography. Absence of collateralization with poor filling of the SMA warrants papaverine infusion followed by surgical revascularization. MVT discovered incidentally on a CT scan ordered for an unrelated indication can be observed or treated with a short course of anticoagulation. MVT in the patient without peritoneal signs should be treated with anticoagulation and close medical observation.

Intestinal infarction resulting in intestinal perforation and intra-abdominal sepsis is a frequent complication of AMI. Patients with AMI who present with an acute abdomen should be placed on broad-spectrum antibiotics and undergo emergency laparotomy with resection of necrotic bowel followed by a second-look operation within 24–48 h.

Prognosis

The average mortality rate for patients with AMI is 71%. The outcome is improved significantly if the diagnosis is made before intestinal infarction occurs.

CHRONIC MESENTERIC ISCHEMIA

General Considerations

Intestinal angina results from inability of atherosclerotic mesenteric vessels to meet the increased metabolic demands of digestion.

Clinical Findings

A. SYMPTOMS & SIGNS

Patients with chronic mesenteric ischemia (CMI) have abdominal pain that begins shortly after eating and resolves over 1–3 h. Symptoms may initially occur only with large meals, but with progression of the disease even small meals can trigger pain. Bloating, constipation, or diarrhea may accompany abdominal pain. Significant weight loss often results because patients develop a fear of eating. Nearly 50% of patients have an abdominal bruit, which is not specific to CMI. Intestinal infarction with bowel perforation and abdominal sepsis may occur.

B. DIAGNOSTIC STUDIES

It is important to exclude other causes of postprandial pain such as peptic ulcer disease, gastric outlet obstruction, and gallstone and pancreatic disease. Measurements of serum alkaline phosphatase, bilirubin, amylase, and lipase and performance of abdominal ultrasonography and EGD are indicated. If this initial evaluation is unrevealing, selective SMA angiography should be performed. Diagnosis based solely on angiography is problematic because patients with occlusion of even 3 splanchnic vessels can be asymptomatic.

Treatment

Occlusion of at least 2 of the 3 splanchnic vessels in a patient with CMI symptoms warrants revascularization. Surgical revascularization is the treatment of choice for CMI, with a success rate of > 90% of patients and recurrence in < 10%. In patients who are poor surgical candidates, percutaneous transluminal mesenteric angioplasty (PTMA), with or without stenting, is an option with initial success rates comparable to surgical revascularization. Higher recurrence rates have been reported among patients treated with PTMA.

COLONIC ISCHEMIA

General Considerations

The causes of colonic ischemia (CI) include IMA thrombus or embolus, CHF, cardiac arrhythmias, shock, vasculitis, hematological disorders, infections, medications (NSAIDs, digitalis, vasopressin, pseudoephedrine, sumatriptan, cocaine, amphetamines, gold), constipation, surgery, and trauma. No cause can be established unequivocally in most cases of CI. The extent of injury can range from mild reversible colopathy to gangrene or fulminant colitis. "A recent study demonstrated the presence of a congenital or acquired thrombophilic state in 72% of ambulatory patients presenting with colonic ischemia."

Clinical Findings

A. SYMPTOMS & SIGNS

Patients with CI usually present with crampy lower left quadrant pain and loose, bloody stools. Blood loss significant enough to lead to hemodynamic instability is atypical of CI and suggests other diagnoses. Physical examination often reveals abdominal tenderness of variable severity over the location of the affected portion of bowel. Peritoneal signs may be transiently present in reversible CI; the persistence of these signs for several hours suggests transmural infarction and mandates surgical exploration. Strictures, chronic colitis, gangrene resulting in perforation, and intra-abdominal sepsis are complications of CI.

B. DIAGNOSTIC STUDIES

Stool cultures should be obtained to exclude infectious colitis. The patient with suspected CI who does not have peritoneal signs should undergo a nonprepared colonoscopy or BE within 48 h of symptom onset. Colonoscopy offers higher sensitivity and the capability to obtain biopsy specimens. Patients with peritoneal signs should undergo urgent surgical exploration. CT scans are normal in up to 66% of patients with established CI.

Treatment

The patient with CI who does not have peritoneal signs should be treated with fluids, bowel rest, and broad-spectrum antibiotics. Underlying CHF or cardiac arrhythmias should be treated and vasoconstricting medications withdrawn. The patients should be monitored closely for fever, leukocytosis, or peritoneal signs. The persistence of peritoneal signs should prompt surgical exploration. Recurrence of CI occurs in only 5% of patients.

■ LIVER & PANCREAS

LIVER DISEASE

Hepatitis A occurs less frequently in the elderly than in the younger population, but the elderly may have a more severe course, with a higher risk of fulminant liver failure and death. Comorbidities and a decreased likelihood of liver transplantation contribute to the lower survival of older patients with fulminant disease.

Acute hepatitis B virus (HBV) infection is uncommon in the older population and often runs a mild and subclinical course. Symptoms, when present, include fever, malaise, arthralgias, myalgias, nausea, vomiting, abdominal pain, and jaundice. PEG interferon-α, used to treat chronic HBV in patients with decompensated liver disease, may cause increased side effects in the elderly.

Hepatitis C (HCV) is most commonly diagnosed after routine laboratory studies reveal elevated aminotransferase levels. Acute symptoms are rare and are similar to those seen in acute HBV. Older age at HCV infection is associated with increased rates of cirrhosis and mortality. Daily alcohol use worsens the prognosis. PEG interferon-α with ribavirin is the standard treatment for chronic HCV infection. Heart disease, a common affliction in the elderly, is a relative contraindication to ribavirin therapy. Despite concerns about increased side effects in the elderly, several small studies have demonstrated the safety and efficacy of interferon treatment in older patients.

Polypharmacy coupled with altered pharmacodynamics accounts for the increased incidence of drug-related hepatotoxicity in the elderly. NSAIDs, amiodarone, hepatic hydroxymethylglutaryl coenzyme A reductase inhibitors, and antituberculosis medications have been associated with hepatotoxicity in the elderly. LFTs should be monitored in patients receiving these medications.

Steep elevations in aminotransferase levels after a hemodynamic insult are typical of hepatic ischemia. Risk factors include acute myocardial infarction, CHF, valvular heart disease, cardiac arrhythmias, cardiomyopathy, sepsis, trauma, and burns. The magnitude of the aminotransferase elevation does not correlate with the extent of liver injury and does not predict outcome. Correction of hemodynamic instability leads to normalization of aminotransferase levels within 10 days.

Up to 40% of patients with primary biliary cirrhosis are elderly. Patients present with fatigue, pruritus, and elevated alkaline phosphatase levels. Diagnosis is suggested by the presence of antimitochondrial antibody (AMA) in the appropriate clinical setting and is confirmed by liver biopsy. Treatment with ursodeoxycholic acid improves survival and delays the need for liver transplantation.

More than 50% of patients with hepatocellular carcinoma (HCC) in the United States are elderly. Survival rates are significantly lower in patients diagnosed with HCC after the age of 65. Cirrhosis secondary to chronic HCV or HBV infection and alcoholic liver disease is the most frequent cause of HCC. Diagnosis is suggested by elevated alpha-fetoprotein (AFP) levels and imaging studies. Surgical resection in selected patients is the treatment of choice. Patients who are poor surgical candidates may be treated with transarterial chemoembolization. Patients with hepatic cirrhosis should be screened with liver ultrasonography and serum AFP levels every 6 mo for early detection of HCC. A CT scan of the abdomen is recommended every 1–2 years.

Age alone is not a contraindication for liver transplantation. Elderly recipients of liver transplants have the same rates of postoperative mortality and survival as younger recipients. Five-year survival, however, is lower among elderly recipients of liver transplantation. Carefully selected elderly patients with end-stage liver disease should be considered for liver transplantation.

BILIARY DISEASE

Age-related increases in cholesterol secretion in bile, combined with decreased bile acid secretion, leads to increased cholesterol saturation and, therefore, increased bile lithogenicity. Cholelithiasis is twice as common in women as in men. Cholelithiasis is often asymptomatic and is discovered during radiological studies of the abdomen performed for unrelated reasons. Ten to 25% of patients with asymptomatic gallstones will become symptomatic each decade. Symptomatic gallstone disease typically presents with RUQ pain, nausea, and vomiting. Diagnosis is suggested in the appropriate clinical setting by elevated alkaline phosphatase and bilirubin levels and is confirmed by ultrasonography.

Laparoscopic cholecystectomy is the treatment of choice for symptomatic cholelithiasis in the elderly; postoperative mortality and morbidity in selected elderly patients are comparable to that for younger patients. Poor surgical candidates may be treated with endoscopic retrograde cholangiopancreatography (ERCP) with sphincterotomy, extracorporeal shock wave lithotripsy, or ursodeoxycholic acid. Asymptomatic cholelithiasis should not be treated.

Common symptoms of cholecystitis are often blunted in older patients or are mistaken for other disease processes; thus, delays in diagnosis are common. An acute attack frequently follows a large fatty meal or awakens a patient from sleep. Symptoms consist of epigastric or RUQ pain, nausea, and vomiting. Fever and RUQ tenderness are present on physical examination. Elevations in serum bilirubin, alkaline phosphatase, aminotransferases, and white blood cell counts are characteristic. The diagnosis is made clinically and confirmed ultrasonographically. Gangrene and necrosis of the gallbladder are more common in the elderly population and are associated with increased morbidity and mortality. Cholangitis or chronic cholecystitis are other frequent complications.

Treatment of cholecystitis consists of stabilization with intravenous fluids, bowel rest, pain control, and broad-spectrum antibiotics followed by cholecystectomy. However, because older patients with acute cholecystitis frequently have significant comorbidities and hemodynamic or respiratory instability, emergent cholecystectomy often carries a high risk of complications and death. In such patients, immediate percutaneous cholecystostomy followed, after stabilization, with surgery alone or in combination with ERCP has been shown to result in favorable outcomes.

Gallbladder carcinoma is rare in the United States. Gallstone disease, female gender, and smoking are significant risk factors. The diagnosis is often made incidentally at surgery. The prognosis is poor.

BILIARY TRACT DISEASE

Choledocholithiasis may occur in as many as 50% of all elderly patients with gallstones. Common bile duct stones remain asymptomatic until they cause obstruction. Choledocholithiasis presents with recurrent attacks of RUQ pain, fever, and jaundice (Charcot's triad), often accompanied by nausea and vomiting. Hepatomegaly and RUQ tenderness may be noted on physical examination. Elevated serum and urine bilirubin levels, accompanied by elevations in serum alkaline phosphatase and aminotransferase levels, occur typically. Although ERCP was used frequently in the past for diagnosis, the demonstrated high sensitivity and specificity and the low risk associated with magnetic resonance cholangiopancreatography and endoscopic ultrasonography mandate the use of these modalities for diagnosis. Choledocholithiasis demonstrated on these studies warrants therapeutic ERCP.

Symptomatic common bile duct stones are treated with papillotomy and stone extraction during ERCP, followed by laparoscopic cholecystectomy in patients with an intact gallbladder. Fever, mental status changes, or leukocytosis accompanying the symptoms of choledocholithiasis suggest cholangitis. Such patients should be managed aggressively with broad-spectrum antibiotics and therapeutic ERCP.

PANCREATIC DISEASE

Acute pancreatitis occurs more frequently and runs a more severe course in the elderly compared with younger patients. Gallstones, medications, and cancer account for a higher proportion of acute pancreatitis in the elderly compared with younger patients. Alcohol is a common precipitating factor in both age groups. Typical presenting symptoms include epigastric pain radiating to the back along with nausea and vomiting. The diagnosis is made by elevations in amylase and lipase levels. Elevated alkaline phosphatase and bilirubin levels suggest gallstone pancreatitis, which can be confirmed by abdominal ultrasonography or CT. Patients with altered mental status or hemodynamic instability or those meeting 3 or more of Ranson's criteria (Table 23–7) should undergo a dynamic CT scan to rule out pancreatic necrosis. Bowel rest, intravenous hydration, and pain control are the cornerstones of therapy for mild acute pancreatitis. Patients with pancreatic necrosis should be placed on broad-spectrum antibiotics, and CT-guided aspiration of necrotic areas should be considered if symptoms do not improve after 5–7 days.

Endoscopic treatment of elderly patients with gallstone pancreatitis yields better outcomes than conservative treatment followed by elective cholecystectomy. Laparoscopic cholecystectomy with preoperative ERCP or intraoperative cholangiography can be performed with a postoperative risk profile comparable to that for younger individuals. In patients who are poor surgical candidates, ERCP with sphincterotomy decreases the risk for recurrent gallstone pancreatitis.

Polypharmacy places elderly patients at risk for drug-induced pancreatitis. Azathioprine, 6-mercaptopurine, estrogen, mesalamine, furosemide, and angiotensin-converting enzyme inhibitors are commonly implicated. Suspected medications should be stopped when pancreatitis is diagnosed. Other causes of pancre-

Table 23–7. Ranson's criteria.

On admission
1. Age > 55 years
2. WBC count > 16,000/μL
3. Serum glucose > 200 mg/dL
4. Serum LDH > 350 units/L
5. Serum AST > 250 units/L

Over the first 48 h
1. Increase in BUN exceeding 5 mg/dL
2. Arterial Po_2 < 60 mm Hg
3. Hematocrit drop > 10 percentage points
4. Serum calcium < 8 mg/dL
5. Base deficit > 4 mEq/L
6. Fluid sequestration exceeding 6L

Presence of 3 or more on admission predicts severe course with a sensitivity of 60–80%. WBC, white blood cell; LDH, lactate dehydrogenase; AST, aspartate aminotransferase; BUN, blood urea nitrogen; Po_2, partial pressure of oxygen.

atitis, such as hyperlipidemia or hypercalcemia, should be sought and treated if no other cause is found.

The diagnosis of chronic pancreatitis in elderly patients poses several difficulties. The structural changes commonly associated with chronic pancreatitis (ductal irregularity or dilation, calcification, abnormal echogenicity) are also observed in aging patients without pancreatitis. Because pancreatic function is maintained in the elderly, functional testing may help in establishing the diagnosis. Treatment consists of hydration, pain management, pancreatic enzyme replacement, and avoidance of alcohol.

Pancreatic cancer accounts for 5% of all cancer deaths in the United States. Painless jaundice, pruritus, and weight loss are common presenting symptoms. Elevated CA 19-9 levels suggest the diagnosis, which is confirmed by abdominal imaging or demonstration of extrinsic compression of the bile duct during ERCP. Pancreaticoduodenectomy is the only treatment with any demonstrated benefit and should be offered to selected elderly patients with high overall fitness and low comorbidity. The prognosis of pancreatic cancer remains grim.

GI MANAGEMENT OF MALNUTRITION (also see Chapter 39)

Patients who are unable to swallow or who cannot eat sufficiently to maintain adequate nutrition may be candidates for tube feeding. Nasogastric tubes are a short-term alternative. Gastrostomy or jejunostomy tubes are appropriate for patients requiring longer term tube feeding. Gastrostomy tubes allow bolus feeding and are preferable to jejunostomy tubes, which usually require continuous infusion. However, patients with gastric outlet obstruction or poor gastric emptying are not candidates for gastrostomy tubes and should receive jejunostomy tubes. Aspiration precautions (elevating the head of the bed, checking residuals) should be carefully observed because gastrostomy tube feeding does not prevent aspiration.

Chronic parenteral nutrition is appropriate only in carefully selected patients whose GI tract cannot be used. This includes patients with a nonfunctioning or obstructed GI tract, prolonged ileus, massive GI bleeding, severe malabsorption, persistent vomiting, high-output fistulas, severe pancreatitis or enterocolitis, peritonitis, and mesenteric ischemia. Complications of parenteral feeding include catheter-related thrombosis and sepsis.

ABDOMINAL PAIN

Obtaining a complete and accurate history may be difficult in elderly patients with abdominal pain because of cognitive impairment or sensory deficits that limit communication. At the same time, the classical presentations of many diseases are less common in the elderly. The ability to mount a febrile response and the sensation of pain are limited in older patients in part because of increased use of medications such as steroids and NSAIDs. Similarly, laboratory values may be normal in older patients despite the presence of considerable underlying disease. To prevent these factors from delaying diagnosis and treatment in elderly patients, the physician must use great skill in the medical interview, physical examination, and diagnostic testing.

Clinical History

The history should assess the chronology, character, location, and severity of the pain along with precipitating and alleviating factors. Chronology includes the onset, progression, and duration of pain. Pain of abrupt onset with rapid progression suggests a more aggressive cause. Characterization of the pain may help in diagnosis. Pain may be described as aching (appendicitis, diverticulitis, pelvic inflammatory disease), burning (GERD, perforated peptic ulcer), cramping (small bowel obstruction, biliary colic), boring (pancreatitis), excruciating (acute mesenteric ischemia), or tearing (ruptured abdominal aortic aneurysm). However, older patients may have limited pain or atypical presentations.

Location of the pain can also offer clues to the diagnosis. Epigastric pain and upper abdominal pain suggest a gastric, hepatobiliary, or pancreatic process. Mid-abdominal pain may represent an ileocecal process, whereas hypogastric pain suggests involvement of the colon or genitourinary structures. Shifting location of the pain may represent appendicitis or the development of peritonitis after visceral rupture. Subdiaphragmatic irritation is often referred to the shoulder. Because cardiac disease presents atypically in the elderly, any complaints of upper abdominal discomfort by patients with appropriate risk factors should raise the suspicion of coronary disease.

Severity of pain is a subjective parameter, and its usefulness is reduced further in elderly patients, whose experience of pain may be blunted because of diabetes or the use of anti-inflammatory medications. Severe pain in the absence of commensurate physical findings should raise the suspicion of acute mesenteric ischemia. Postprandial pain suggests gastric ulcers, mesenteric ischemia, pancreatitis, or biliary colic. Relief of pain with food may be reported by patients with duodenal ulcers.

A thorough medication history should be obtained. The use of NSAIDs, steroids, and anticoagulants should be noted. The possibility of drug-induced pancreatitis or hepatotoxicity should be considered.

Physical Examination

The differential diagnosis generated during the medical history should guide the physical examination. Absence of fever in older patients should not diminish the suspicion for infection because older patients frequently do not mount an appropriate febrile response to infectious agents. The abdomen should be examined for distension, ecchymoses, abnormal masses, enlarged organs, hernias, and abnormal peristalsis. Hyperperistalsis suggests obstruction or enteritis, whereas hypoperistalsis supports the diagnosis of peritonitis. An abdominal bruit, although neither sensitive nor specific, supports the diagnosis of mesenteric ischemia. The absence of rebound tenderness in the elderly should not exclude the possibility of peritonitis. Rectal and genital/pelvic examinations are an essential component of the evaluation.

Laboratory Data

The diagnostic hypotheses generated during the history and physical examination should guide the laboratory tests that are ordered. A urinalysis and CBC with differential should be ordered with the caveat that elderly patients may have significant underlying infection with normal white blood cell counts. Serum chemistry analysis provides information regarding fluid status. Amylase, lipase, and a liver chemistry profile are appropriate in the setting of upper abdominal pain.

DIAGNOSTIC IMAGING

Diagnostic tests should be ordered based on the findings of the history, physical examination, and laboratory evaluation. A set of supine and upright plain abdominal films is useful in identifying obstruction, radio-opaque gallstones, or a calcified pancreas. An upright chest x-ray film should be obtained to check for air under the diaphragm. Suspected hepatobiliary or pancreatic disease should be investigated by ultrasonography or CT scan. CT scanning is useful in demonstrating appendicitis, diverticulitis, bowel obstruction, retroperitoneal hemorrhage, and mesenteric lymph node enlargement as well as hepatobiliary and pancreatic disease. Patients suspected of having acute mesenteric ischemia should have prompt selective mesenteric angiography.

REFERENCES

Affronti J: Biliary disease in the elderly patient. Clin Geriatr Med 1999;15:571. [PMID: 10393742]

Befeler AS, Di Bisceglie AM: Infections of the liver: hepatitis B. Infect Dis Clin North Am 2000;14:617. [PMID: 10987113]

Brandt LJ, Boley SJ: AGA technical review on intestinal ischemia. Gastroenterology 2000;118:954. [PMID: 10784596]

Farrell JJ, Friedman LS: Gastrointestinal bleeding in the elderly. Gastroenterol Clin North Am 2001;30:377. [PMID: 11432297]

Ferrioli E et al: Aging, esophageal motility, and gastroesophageal reflux. J Am Geriatr Soc 1998;46:1534. [PMID: 9848814]

Greenwald DA et al: Ischemic bowel disease in the elderly. Gastroenterol Clin North Am 2001;30:445. [PMID: 11432300]

Griffin MR: Epidemiology of nonsteroidal anti-inflammatory drug-associated gastrointestinal injury. Am J Med 1998;104:23S. [PMID: 9572314]

Jensen GL et al: Nutrition in the elderly. Gastroenterol Clin North Am 2001;30:313. [PMID: 11432294]

Khuroo MS et al: A comparison of omeprazole and placebo for bleeding peptic ulcer. N Engl J Med 1997;336:1054. [PMID: 9091801]

Koutroubakis IE et al: Role of acquired and hereditary thrombotic risk factors in colon ischemia of ambulatory patients. Gastroenterology 2001;121:561. [PMID: 11522740]

Kumar S et al: Mesenteric venous thrombosis. N Engl J Med 2001;345:1683. [PMID: 11759648]

Lau JYW et al: Effect of intravenous omeprazole on recurrent bleeding after endoscopic treatment of peptic ulcers. N Engl J Med 2000;343:310. [PMID: 10922420]

Lauer GM, Walker BD: Hepatitis C virus infection. N Engl J Med 2001;345:41. [PMID: 11439948]

Martin SP, Ulrich CD: Pancreatic disease in the elderly. Clin Geriatr Med 1999;15:579. [PMID: 10393743]

Mertz H et al: Symptoms and physiology in severe chronic constipation. Am J Gastroenterology 1999;94:131. [PMID: 9934743]

Refai W, Seidner DL: Nutrition in the elderly. Clin Geriatr Med 1999;15:607. [PMID: 10393744]

Regev A, Schiff ER: Liver disease in the elderly. Gastroenterol Clin North Am 2001;30:547. [PMID: 11432305]

Rosen AM: Gastrointestinal bleeding in the elderly. Clin Geriatr Med 1999;15:511. [PMID: 10393739]

Ross SO, Forsmark CE: Pancreatic and biliary disorders in the elderly. Gastroenterol Clin North Am 2001;30:531. [PMID: 11432304]

Ruotolo RA, Evans SRT: Mesenteric ischemia in the elderly. Clin Geriatr Med 1999;15:527. [PMID: 10393740]

Soffer EE, Hull T: Fecal incontinence: a practical approach to evaluation and treatment. Am J Gastroenterology 2000;95:1873. [PMID: 10950029]

Stollman NH et al: Diagnosis and management of diverticular disease of the colon in adults. Am J Gastroenterology 1999;94:3110. [PMID: 10566700]

Varanasi RV et al: Liver diseases. Clin Geriatr Med 1999;15:559. [PMID: 10393741]

Urinary Incontinence

24

Catherine E. DuBeau, MD

ESSENTIALS OF DIAGNOSIS

- *Involuntary loss of urine sufficient to be a problem.*
- *Urinary incontinence is a syndrome, not a single disease, resulting from medical conditions, medications, or lower urinary tract disease. It can herald morbid diseases (eg, cancer and neurological conditions).*

General Considerations

The majority of persons remain continent into advanced old age, contradicting the myth that urinary incontinence (UI) is a normal consequence of aging. However, UI increases in prevalence with age. In older women, the prevalence of UI is 15–30% in the community, 50% among the homebound, and ≥ 50% in nursing home residents. In men, the prevalence is about one third that of women until age 85, when the ratio becomes 1:1.

Besides age, risk factors for UI in women are pregnancy and childbirth, pulmonary disease (because of associated cough), hysterectomy, obesity, other lower urinary tract (LUT) symptoms, neurological disorders (eg, delirium, stroke, Parkinson's disease, spinal cord injury), diabetes, and functional and cognitive impairment. In men, additional risk factors include the presence of other LUT symptoms and prostatectomy (risk greater with radical prostatectomy than with transurethral resection). Dementia is associated with UI, but the strongest correlate is impaired mobility, not cognition.

Complicating the recognition and treatment of UI is the failure of many health care providers to ask their patients about leakage and LUT symptoms, coupled with the fact that at least 50% of persons with UI never report it to a health care provider.

Fultz NH, Herzog AR: Epidemiology of urinary symptoms in the geriatric population. Urol Clin North Am 1996;23:1. [PMID: 8677528]

Thom D: Variation in estimates of urinary incontinence prevalence in the community: effects of differences in definition, population characteristics, and study type. J Am Geriatr Soc 1998;46:473. [PMID: 9560071]

Pathogenesis

Continence depends not only on LUT function but also on intact mobility, cognition, motivation, and manual dexterity. Even persons with a normally functioning LUT may experience UI if factors such as impaired mobility or cognitive impairment are present. Therefore, UI in most older persons is multifactorial and requires evaluation and treatment focused beyond the LUT alone.

A. CHIEF PRECIPITANTS

The chief precipitants of UI in older persons are age-associated changes in the LUT, comorbid disease, and medications.

1. Age-related LUT changes—These include increased prevalence of involuntary detrusor (bladder muscle) contractions; increased nocturnal diuresis; impaired detrusor contractility; decreased urine flow rate; urethral shortening and decreased elasticity in women; and prostate hyperplasia and hypertrophy in men. The relationship of UI to menopause and low estrogen levels is uncertain.

2. Comorbid diseases—These include neurological conditions (especially delirium, Parkinson's disease, stroke, spinal cord injury; rarely dementia alone [see prior discussion]), musculoskeletal conditions that impair mobility, disorders of volume (eg, congestive heart failure, pedal edema, polyuria), cancer (bladder and prostate), fecal incontinence and stool impaction, and depression. At least one third of older persons have multiple conditions.

3. Medications—See Table 24–1.

B. INCONTINENCE SUBTYPES

Incontinence can be divided into 4 major types:

1. Transient incontinence—This is caused by factors mainly outside the LUT (mnemonic DIAPPERS; Table 24–2).

2. Urge incontinence—This is coincident with or follows a strong, precipitant urge to void. A variation of

Table 24–1. Medications associated with incontinence.

Medication	Potential effects on continence

Anticholinergics
   Antihistamines
   Antiarrhythmics
   Antispasmodics
   Antiparkinsonian
   Antidiarrheals
	Impaired emptying, retention, delirium, fecal impaction

Loop diuretics	Polyuria, frequency, urgency
Psychotropics	
Antidepressants	Anticholinergics effects, sedation
Antipsychotics	Anticholinergic effect, sedation, immobility, rigidity
Sedative–hypnotics	Sedation, delirium, immobility
Narcotic analgesics	Urinary retention, fecal impaction, sedation, delirium
Alpha-adrenergic agonists	Outlet obstruction (men)
Antihypertensive agents	
Alpha-adrenergic blockers	Stress leakage (women)
Calcium channel blockers	Impaired detrusor contractility, retention; pedal edema causing nocturnal diuresis (pyridine agents)
ACE inhibitors	Associated cough leading to stress leakage
Alcohol	Frequency, urgency, sedation, delirium, immobility
NSAIDs	Pedal edema causing nocturnal enuresis
Thiazolidinediones	Pedal edema causing nocturnal enuresis

ACE, angiotensin-converting enzyme; NSAIDs, nonsteroidal anti-inflammatory drugs.
Adapted from DeBeau C: Geriatric review syllabus, 5th edition. American Geriatrics Society, 2002.

Table 24–2. Mnemonic for causes of transient incontinence.

Delirium: acute confusional state.
Infection: symptomatic UTI only, not asymptomatic bacteriuria; UI should have been of recent onset.
Atrophic urethritis/vaginitis.
Pharmaceuticals (see Table 24–1).
Psychological: severe depression, psychosis, behavioral disorders.
Excessive fluid output: high intake, diuretics (medications, caffeine, alcohol), peripheral edema, CHF, peripheral vascular disease, endocrine disorders (hypercalcemia, hyperglycemia, diabetes insipidus).
Restricted mobility (instrinsic and extrinsic causes, many of which are treatable).
Stool impaction (often with stool and bladder incontinence).

UTI, urinary tract infection; UI, urinary incontinence; CHF, congestive heart failure.
Adapted from Resnick NM: Geriatric incontinence. Urol Clin North Am 1996;23:55. Used with permission.

urge incontinence occurs in frail elderly persons who have detrusor hyperactivity with impaired contractility (DHIC), urge leakage with a high postvoid residual (without urethral obstruction).

3. Stress incontinence—This is coincident with maneuvers that increase intra-abdominal pressure (eg, coughing, running).

4. Overflow incontinence—This is impaired detrusor contractility, bladder outlet obstruction, or a combination of both.

In older women, symptoms of both urge and stress incontinence (mixed incontinence) are common. The term *overactive bladder* (OAB) denotes a syndrome that includes urgency, frequency, and nocturia with or without urge incontinence. In older persons, however, urgency and frequency may be caused by many factors besides the bladder. Thus, care should be taken not to attribute OAB symptoms initially to the LUT.

Ouslander JG et al: Overactive bladder: special considerations in the geriatric population. Am J Manag Care 2000;6(Suppl): S599. [PMID: 11183903]

Prevention

There are no evidenced-based approaches to UI prevention. Avoidance and treatment of risk factors and transient UI-associated factors may be helpful. Some experts recommend general strategies such as not forestalling voiding for long periods; avoiding diuretic beverages, artificial sweeteners, and high fluid intake; and controlling constipation.

Fonda D et al: Prevention of urinary incontinence in older people. Br J Urol 1998;82(Suppl 1):5. [PMID: not available]

Clinical Findings

A. Symptoms & Signs

Table 24–3 lists common UI and LUT symptoms with their utility in differential diagnosis. Note that UI is not associated with pelvic pain. Other causes (especially neoplastic) should be sought.

B. Clinical Examination

Patients need a full physical examination because of the multifactorial nature of UI in older persons. The examination should include cardiovascular, abdominal, and neurological systems as well as assessment of mobility and cognition.

In all patients, perineal innervation should be evaluated by checking resting and volitional anal sphincter tone and perineal sensation. The integrity of sacral roots S2-S4 (the level of the sacral micturition center) are evaluated by the anal wink and bulbocavernosus reflexes. The anal wink is done by lightly scratching (eg, with a tongue depressor) about 1 in. away from the anus, which should contract ("wink"); the reflex should be tested on the right and left sides of the anus. The same "wink" should be seen with the bulbocavernosus reflex, using the stimulus of a light squeeze of either the clitoris or glans penis. False-negative responses can occur if the patient is not completely relaxed. If unsure whether the anus visibly contracts, check by inserting a finger in the rectum and palpating for the reflexes. Pelvic floor prolapse in women is neither sensitive nor specific for UI but may impact treatment. Prolapse is best evaluated using the lower blade of a speculum to first support the posterior wall and then the anterior vaginal wall while the patient strains. Signs of pelvic muscle laxity are forward movement of the urethra (urethral hypermobility), prolapse of the anterior vaginal wall into the vagina, introitus, or beyond (cystocele), and prolapse of posterior vaginal wall (rectocele).

Table 24–3. Symptoms & signs of UI.

Symptom/sign	Utility
Urgency: sudden strong urge to void with or without leakage	Strongly suggestive of detrusor overactivity (involuntary contraction). Some patients may preempt leakage by pelvic muscle contraction or conscious effort to decrease urge sensation.
Stress: leakage coincident with maneuvers that increase intraabdominal pressure (eg, cough, sneeze, laugh, bending over, running)	Immediate leakage is sensitive sign for stress incontinence (ie, if absent, then one can be sure of its absence) but not specific. Leakage that occurs several seconds after stress maneuver and/or associated with strong urge likely a result of stress-induced detrusor overactivity.
Frequency (number of continent voids; abnormal is ≥ 8 voids/24 h)	Not specific; may result from increased fluid intake and diuretics (including caffeine) or increased diuresis (osmotic, cardiovascular, peripheral edema).
Nocturia: > 2 voids during usual sleeping hours	Not specific; may result from primary disorders of sleep (eg, obstructive sleep apnea, congestive failure, depression); nocturnal diuresis (eg, cardiovascular, pedal edema); or LUT dysfunction (detrusor overactivity, bladder outlet obstruction, decreased detrusor contractility; uncommon with stress UI).
Incomplete emptying: sense that bladder is still full after voiding	Not specific; may be associated with overflow UI, prostate disease, or medications that impair detrusor function. Frail elderly and those with peripheral neuropathy (especially diabetic) may have no sensation of impaired emptying.
Hesitancy: difficulty starting urine stream, often with need to strain	Not specific (same reasons as incomplete emptying).
Decreased force of urine stream	Not specific; although often assumed an indication of bladder outlet obstruction, also seen with impaired detrusor contractility.
Interruption of stream while voiding; urine flow stops abruptly then restarts when patient is trying to void completely	Sensitivity/specificity unknown, but suspicious for suprasacral spinal cord injury and multiple sclerosis.
Fecal incontinence	Coincident with UI when fecal impaction present or with sacral spinal cord injury.
Abrupt recent onset of UI	Sensitivity/specificity unknown but suspicious for cancer and neurological disease.

UI, urinary incontinence, LUT, lower urinary tract.

Bimanual exam should be done to check for pelvic masses. Rectal exam should check for masses and, in men, prostate nodules. Estimation of prostate size by digital exam is inexact, even among experienced clinicians.

C. LABORATORY FINDINGS

No specific laboratory findings are associated with UI. In general, renal function and urinalysis (for hematuria and, in diabetics, glycosuria) should be checked. If no recent data are available, one should also check for diabetes mellitus and vitamin B_{12} deficiency. UI should not be attributed to pyuria and bacteriuria unless UI is very recent in onset or associated with fever, dysuria, elevated white blood cell count, or otherwise unexplained inanition. In most cases, the patient will have asymptomatic bacteriuria that does not require treatment.

D. SPECIAL TESTS

Women with stress symptoms should have a stress test. To increase sensitivity, this is best done when the bladder is full with the patient in the standing position. After checking that her perineum is relaxed, the patient should be asked to give a single, vigorous cough. Immediate leakage indicates stress incontinence; delayed leakage (often of large volume and difficult to stop) or leakage that occurs after several coughs may be stress-induced urge UI (a triggered detrusor contraction).

A postvoiding residual (PVR) urine test is performed using either catheterization or ultrasonography. However, obtaining a PVR is often not possible or is impractical in primary care settings. A PVR is strongly suggested for the frail elderly (because of possible DHIC); women with a large cystocele, which can obstruct the urethra; patients on medications that suppress detrusor contractility; patients with neurological disease (other than dementia); those with previous pelvic surgery or radiation; patients who have failed empiric therapy; and men with urge UI who will be treated with antimuscarinic agents.

Urodynamic studies are not necessary in the initial evaluation of most older persons. Urodynamics should be considered for women with stress UI who desire surgery; men with elevated PVR who desire prostate surgery; patients with complex neurological disease (especially Parkinson's disease and spinal cord injury); and persons who have failed empiric therapy. This testing includes evaluation of urine flow rate, cystometric pressure with filling and voiding, assessment of urethral function, and a pressure-flow study to evaluate obstruction and detrusor contractility. The best quality testing is done with medium-rate fluid filling of the bladder and simultaneous measure of abdominal pressure; carbon dioxide cystometry is neither sensitive nor specific.

E. IMAGING

Few patients require special imaging. A renal ultrasonogram is often performed for men with a large PVR, especially if they have impaired renal function. There is no consensus on the definition of large PVR. In the setting of renal insufficiency, even lower volumes (eg, 100–200 mL) should prompt further evaluation.

F. TESTS IN FRAIL ELDERLY

Evaluation of UI in frail, institutionalized elders should be tailored to their overall functional and cognitive status and goals of care. At the same time, one should recognize the potential for treatment benefit in persons with reversible precipitants (see Table 24–1) and in those with intact mobility despite impaired cognition. Although the Minimum Data Set includes a resident assessment protocol for UI that is completed by nursing staff, full evaluation of UI is the responsibility of the patient's clinician. Stress testing is less feasible and sensitive in this population; it should still be considered for women who are suitable candidates for surgical repair or who have pulmonary conditions or take medications that could precipitate stress leakage. Guidelines for evaluation of UI in these settings are available from the American Medical Directors Association and the National Association for Continence.

Fantl JA et al: Urinary incontinence in adults: acute and chronic management *I* (clinical practice guideline no. 2, AHCPR Publication No. 96-0682). Public Health Service, Agency for Health Care Policy and Research, 1996.

Differential Diagnosis

UI can be the presenting symptom of serious underlying diseases. However, patient care goals will determine the extent of evaluation. Important conditions to consider are abdominal and pelvic malignancies (especially in the setting of hematuria or pelvic pain and sudden onset of UI); bladder stones (with recurrent urinary tract infections [UTIs] and pelvic pain); spinal cord injuries (when the neurological exam is abnormal beyond known comorbidity); and fistulas (with vaginal leakage of urine or stool). Urinary retention with overflow incontinence should be suspected in men with underlying prostate disease and in women with a large cystocele, prior pelvic surgery, or irradiation. Although uncommon beyond the sixth decade, women with nonmalignant pelvic pain, dysuria, and frequent small voids may have interstitial cystitis and should be referred for evaluation.

Complications

Morbidity associated with UI includes falls (and attendant fractures), skin infections, and pressure ulcers.

Most significant is its impact on many domains of quality of life, including psychological distress (decreased self-esteem, worry about coping strategies), impaired social interactions (at work, church, leisure time, and with intimate relationships), and limitations of activities.

Naughton MJ, Wyman JF: Quality of life in geriatric patients with lower urinary tract dysfunction. Am J Med Sci 1997; 314: 219. [PMID: 9332259]

Treatment

The model for UI treatment mirrors that of many chronic diseases: a stepped approach over time, starting with treatment of precipitating or aggravating factors (eg, comorbid disease, immobility, medications) followed by lifestyle changes, behavioral therapies, medications, and finally surgery. Combining treatments, especially behavioral and medications, works better than either alone. Older persons should have treatment individualized to their overall care goals, most bothersome aspect of UI, and desired outcomes. Table 24–4 presents treatments and evidence-based efficacy. Many of these methods work for several types of UI.

A. Lifestyle Changes

Modification of the volume and types of fluid intake can have a large impact on leakage and frequency. Patients should aim for a 24-h output of ~2 L (adjusted for body size), avoid diuretic drinks with caffeine (coffee, tea, colas), and—if nocturia is a problem—curtail late afternoon and evening intake.

B. Behavioral Treatments

Bladder retraining, prompted voiding, and habit training reduce urge and stress UI by keeping bladder volume low by regular voiding. Bladder retraining is performed with mobile, cognitively intact persons. In addition to timed voiding, patients are instructed to inhibit urgency by sitting or standing still, relaxing, and pelvic muscle contracting. They should continue to the bathroom when the urge has subsided. For frail patients, including those with impaired mobility prompted voiding (taking the patient to the toilet with praise reinforcement) and habit training (simply taking the patient to the toilet on a schedule) are effective. None have side effects. Prompted voiding and habit training depend on caregivers and, therefore, can have high personal and labor costs.

Pelvic muscle exercises (PME) strengthen the muscles that support the urethra and augment its closure. Often used for stress UI, PME may help with urge leakage as well. Similar to other muscle-strengthening regimens, PME are based on low repetitions of high-inten-sity contractions held as long as possible. A starting regimen could be 3 sets of 10 contractions (with adequate relaxation between each contraction) repeated 2–3 times per week. As patients progress, they increase the intensity and duration of each contraction. Keys to PME success are correct identification of the target muscles and motivation to continue the program. Biofeedback and weighted vaginal cones (held in the vagina while the patient is upright) can be added to help patients learn PME.

Electrical stimulation is an alternative for patients who have difficulty localizing or contracting muscles for PME. A tubular sensor with electrodes is placed in the vagina or rectum, and a low electrical current causes rhythmic pelvic muscle contractions.

C. Medications

Antimuscarinic agents that decrease parasympathetic activation of the detrusor are used for urge UI. The agents with well-established efficacy are oxybutynin and tolterodine. Both are available in immediate-release (IR) and extended-release (ER) formulations; doses are oxybutynin 2.5-5 mg 2–4 times daily (maximum, 20 mg/day), oxybutynin-ER 5–30 mg once daily, tolterodine 1–2 mg twice daily, and tolterodine-ER 2–4 mg once daily. ER formulations have similar efficacy but fewer side effects than IR formulations. A topical oxybutynin patch is now available as well (Oxytrol 3.9-mg patch every 3 days). Troublesome anticholinergic side effects in older persons are dry mouth (40% occurrence with IR forms, ≤ 20% with ER forms and a risk factor for caries), constipation, blurred vision, acute narrow-angle glaucoma, worsening of reflux, and confusion. Although the absolute number of patients studied are relatively small, oxybutynin-ER has better efficacy and tolterodine-ER better tolerability. Lack of response to one agent does not preclude response to the other.

Other agents used for treatment of urge incontinence are imipramine, hyocyamine, probanthine, and flavoxate; these have no established efficacy in older patients and are best avoided. The antidiuretic desmopressin is sometimes used to treat nocturia but must be used with caution in older persons because of the high risk of fluid retention, congestive failure, and hyponatremia.

Estrogen (oral and topical) previously was widely used in postmenopausal women with stress and urge UI. Oral estrogen with progesterone has been found to worsen UI; the data on topical estrogen are conflicting and scant (especially in older women). Estrogen is effective in reducing recurrent UTIs in women. Topical estrogen is available as a cream (Premarin), ring insert (Estring), and dissolving tablet (Vagifem).

Currently, there are no drugs available to treat stress incontinence. Duloxetine, a serotonin and norepineph-

Table 24–4. Evidence-based efficacy of urinary incontinence (UI) treatment.

Treatment	Target patient/condition	Efficacy (level of evidence)
Lifestyle changes, good bladder habits	All/all	True efficacy unknown yet should be universally tried. (5)
Behavioral		
Bladder retraining	W, M/urge, SUI	≥ 50% decrease in UI episodes in 75% of women; may be helpful for urge; insufficient evidence whether drug therapy better or useful as a supplement. (1)
Prompted voiding	W, M, F/urge, SUI	Mean reduction 0.8–1.8 UI episodes/day short term; no long-term data, increases self-initiated voiding. Suggestive evidence of short-term benefit from adding oxybutinin. (1)
Habit training	W, M, F/urge, SUI	≥ 25% decrease in UI episodes in 33% of pts. (1, 2) Compliance by staff problematic. (2)
PME	W, M/urge, SUI	Urge: role unclear; even with added bladder retraining, efficacy less than that for SUI. (2)
		For SUI (W): 56–95% decrease in UI episodes; effective for mixed UI; efficacy depends on program efficacy. (1) Most trials studied premenopausal women.
		Men with postprostatectomy UI: wide confidence intervals limit data; symptoms tend to improve over time, irrespective of management. (2)
PME and biofeedback	W, M, F/urge, SUI	Possible marginal improvement over PME alone. (2, 5) Significantly better than control and feasible in homebound. (1, but single study)
PME and vaginal cones	W/SUI	Data all from premenopausal women; 68–80% greatly improved-cured; better than no active treatment. No difference between cones and PME or electro-stimulation.
Electrical stimulation	W/urge and SUI	50–94% improved cure, but few studies. (2, 3)
Medications		
Antimuscarinic agents		Versus placebo: cure/improvement; change in UI episodes/24 h and voids/24 h. Associated with dry mouth. (1) Little likelihood that outcomes modified by age, sex, diagnosis, or choice of drug.
Oxybutynin	W, M/urge	15–60% decreases in UI episodes over placebo; side effects common, especially dry mouth. (1)
Oxybutynin-ER	W, M/urge	Efficacy same as immediate release, with lower prevalence of side effects. (1)
Tolterodine	W, M/urge	12–18% decrease in UI episodes over placebo; side effects 20% less than other antimuscarinic agents at maximum dose. (1)
Tolterodine-ER	W, M/urge	Efficacy same as immediate release, with lower prevalence of side effects. (1)
Oral estrogens	W/urge, SUI	Conflicting evidence; both decreases and increases UI. (1, 2)
Topical estrogen	W/urge, SUI	
Desmopressin	Nocturia	Approximate decrease in frequency of 1 episode/night; optimal dose unclear; risk fluid retention and hyponatremia especially in elderly. (3, 4)
Other agents	See text	No proven efficacy (1, 4, depending on agent).
Surgery		
Open abdominal retropubic suspension (eg, Marshall-Marchetti-Kranz procedure)	W/SUI	Scant data in older and/or frail women.
Anterior vaginal repair (anterior colporrhaphy)	W/SUI	Less effective than open suspension (year 1 failure rate 29% vs 14%; long term 41% vs 17%), with more repeat operations (23% vs 2%).
Laparoscopic colposuspension		Poorer outcomes than open colposuspension; role in practice uncertain. (1, 2)

(continued)

Table 24–4. Evidence-based efficacy of urinary incontinence (UI) treatment. (*continued*)

Treatment	Target patient/condition	Efficacy (level of evidence)
Needle suspensions		More likely to fail than open suspension (26% failed vs. 14%), with more complications (48% vs. 30%), in women with primary UI. (1, 2) May be as effective as anterior vaginal repair (36% failed vs. 39%). Limited data comparing with suburethral slings.
Suburethral sling procedures (including TVT)	W/SUI	No data comparing slings with other surgical or conservative treatment. Short term-cure rates with TVT similar to open abdominal retropubic suspension; complications 9%. (2, 4) GORE-TEX slings may have higher complications than rectus fascia slings. (2)
Artificial sphincter	W, M/intrinsic sphincter deficiency	Cure 77%, improvement-cure 80%, complication rate 20%. (2, 4)
Periurethral bulking agents	W/intrinsic sphincter deficiency	Cure 50% (range, 8–100%), improvement-cure 67%. (2)
Devices and palliative measures		
Catheters	W, M overflow	High morbidity: bacteriuria universal by 30 days (1); urethral and meatal trauma; bladder stones, pyelonephritis. Suprapubic catheters may decrease urethral injury in men. (2) Clean intermittent catheterization option for willing and able patients. (5)
Pessaries	W prolapse	Option for women who do not want surgery; fitting may be difficult. (5)
Garments, pads	All	Patients should try variety of products for best efficacy (2); high absorbency better for heavier leakage, shaped pads more likely to stay in place. (2)

Levels of evidence: 1, randomized controlled trials (RCTs); 2, cohort or low-quality RCT studies; 3, case-control studies; 4, case series; 5, expert opinion (modified from Oxford criteria, NHS Centre for Evidence Based Medicine (minerva.minervation.com/cebm). UI, urinary incontinence; W, women; M, men; F, frail; SUI, stress incontinence; ER, extended-release formulation; PME, pelvic muscle exercise; TVT, tension-free vaginal tape.

rine uptake inhibitor that may be released in the near future, has good to moderate efficacy in middle-aged women, although initial nausea may decrease compliance.

D. SURGERY

Numerous operations are used to treat stress UI. In general, these operations use a variety of approaches to resuspend the muscles, ligaments, and fascia that support the urethra and anterior vaginal wall. Data on long-term outcomes (beyond 5 years) and surgery in older–old women are scant. As with other surgical procedures, outcomes from more recent techniques (eg, tension-free vaginal tape) are based on case series or limited randomized trials of selected patients in tertiary centers and should be interpreted with caution.

E. PESSARIES

Pelvic organ prolapse, causing urethral obstruction with overflow UI or exacerbating stress UI, may respond to a pessary. Numerous models are available. Ring and Gelhorn pessaries often are easiest to fit in older women

and need to be changed only monthly. Cube pessaries require daily changing. Many older women with prolapse are difficult to fit because of a shortened vagina.

F. CATHETERS

Drainage catheters cause morbidity, resulting in universal bacteriuria by 30 days and increasing the rates of (1) infections with resistant organisms, (2) chronic pyelonephritis by 3 mo, and (3) urethral meatal damage. They should be reserved for patients with sacral or lower extremity wounds, those with chronic retention not amenable to other treatment, and those for whom palliative measures are too uncomfortable or disruptive (eg, end of life).

G. PALLIATIVE MEASURES

Absorbant garments and pads should be used only when all other methods have failed or when incontinence persists despite adequate, appropriate treatment. They are costly for patients, especially over time. Products range from penile shields for men to numerous varieties of pads and undergarments for both men and women. Patient advocacy organizations have information to help patients pick the product most appropriate for their type of leakage and lifestyle.

Abrams P et al (eds): Incontinence, 2nd edition. Second International Consultation on Incontinence. Health Publications Ltd, 2002.

The Cochrane Library: Update Software, 2002.

Prognosis

The majority of persons with UI will improve with treatment. Virtually no long-term outcomes data (> 5 years) exist. Whether UI severity increases over time is not clear. The finding of involuntary detrusor contractions in healthy continent older persons raises the possibility that detrusor overactivity may progress over time. However, other reasons for UI to worsen are failure of compensatory mechanisms (eg, urethral sphincter function in women), increasing comorbidity, and multiple medications.

EVIDENCE-BASED POINTS

- *UI is common but never normal in older patients, and all older persons routinely should be directly asked about lower tract symptoms.*

- *Evaluation should search for functional, comorbid, medication, and fluid balance factors that can precipitate and exacerbate incontinence.*
- *Behavioral therapies are effective for a wide variety of patients, especially when targeted to patients' functional and cognitive status.*
- *Combination of behavioral and drug therapy is more efficacious than either alone.*
- *Surgical treatment remains an effective option for older women with stress urinary incontinence.*

RELEVANT WORLD WIDE WEB SITES

General

International Continence Society: www.continet.org (Includes links to other continence organizations and resources.)
American Urological Association: www.auanet.org
American Foundation for Urologic Disease: www.afud.org
American Urogynecologic Association: www.augs.org
American Medical Directors Association: www.amda.com) (UI treatment in long-term care.)

Patient Advocacy

National Association for Continence: www.nafc.org
Simon Foundation for Continence: www.simonfoundation.org

Renal System, Fluid, & Electrolytes

Laurence H. Beck, MD

ACUTE RENAL FAILURE

ESSENTIALS OF DIAGNOSIS

- *Abrupt rise in blood urea nitrogen or serum creatinine.*
- *Oliguria common but not necessary.*
- *Early symptoms nonspecific or absent.*

General Considerations

Acute renal failure (ARF) is more common in the elderly than in younger individuals with similar precipitating factors. Serum creatinine rises 1.0–1.5 mg/dL/day in typical ARF. Recovery of renal function is less complete and mortality is higher in the elderly. Because glomerular filtration rate (GFR) normally falls progressively with aging, the aged kidney has less functional reserve, so that fluid and electrolyte complications occur earlier in the course of ARF. From a management standpoint, it is crucial to distinguish among prerenal, intrinsic renal, and postrenal failure.

Prevention

Avoidance of volume depletion and judicious use of potentially nephrotoxic drugs are the mainstays of prevention, particularly in acutely ill or hospitalized elderly patients.

Clinical Findings

A. SYMPTOMS & SIGNS

Symptoms of early ARF are nonspecific and usually reflect the underlying etiological condition (Table 25–1). In hypovolemic ARF, postural dizziness or hypotension is common. Conversely, signs of congestive heart failure (CHF) may predominate. Later in the course of ARF, uremic symptoms, including nausea, vomiting, clouded sensorium, and asterixis, may develop. Because of platelet dysfunction, bleeding or oozing occurs more readily at sites of trauma. Rhythm disturbances may occur if electrolyte abnormalities (especially hyperkalemia) develop. Tachypnea and abdominal pain may be the result of metabolic acidosis. Oliguria (< 500 mL urine/24 h) is common in hypotensive or septic ARF. With nephrotoxins, nonoliguric renal failure is more common.

B. LABORATORY FINDINGS

Stepwise increases in blood urea nitrogen (BUN) and serum creatinine concentration are typical. In prerenal and postrenal states, the BUN is increased disproportional to the creatinine, so that the BUN–creatinine ratio is usually > 20:1. Because of the decreased concentrating ability and sodium reabsorptive capacity of the aged kidney, urinary indexes (such as the urinary sodium concentration [U_{Na}], urinary osmolality [U_{Osm}], and fractional excretion of sodium [FE_{Na}]) are less useful in the elderly in distinguishing between a prerenal state and intrinsic renal failure.

Hyperkalemia is common, especially in the oliguric patient. If ARF lasts more than 2–3 days, metabolic acidosis, with low plasma bicarbonate concentration, is the rule. Early on, it is usually a hyperchloremic acidosis, but in later stages an anion gap metabolic acidosis ensues.

Urinalysis shows little abnormality in prerenal azotemia. In typical ATN, the sediment contains "dirty-brown" granular casts. If significant proteinuria is present in ARF, suspect acute glomerulonephritis (GN; see later discussion).

Differential Diagnosis

The most important diagnostic decision is to determine whether the ARF is prerenal, postrenal, or intrinsic renal failure. The most useful diagnostic tools are the physical examination and the renal sonogram. Physical examination should determine whether there are signs of hypovolemia (postural hypotension, tachycardia, dry mucous membranes, poor skin turgor) or heart failure, the principal causes of prerenal azotemia. If hypovolemia is present, a volume challenge with intravenous normal saline solution should be administered to look for reversal of oliguria and azotemia. If the patient is normovolemic at onset, a renal sonogram must be done to rule out urinary tract obstruction. The finding of hydronephrosis in the presence of ARF demands urgent

Table 25–1. Causes of acute renal failure.

Prerenal
  Dehydration
  Gastrointestinal fluid/electrolyte losses
  Burns
  Diuretics
  Congestive heart failure
  Renal artery stenosis (bilateral)
Postrenal
  Bladder outlet obstruction (eg, prostatic hypertrophy)
  Bilateral ureteral obstruction
    Kidney stones
    Bladder/prostate cancer
    Retroperitoneal fibrosis
  Intratubular obstruction
    Acute uric acid nephropathy
    Acute myeloma kidney
Intrinsic renal causes
  Acute glomerulonephritis
  Acute interstitial nephritis
  Acute tubular necrosis
    Hypovolemic
      Bleeding
      Dehydration
      Gastrointestinal losses
    Ischemic
      Congestive heart failure
      Myocardial infarction with shock
      Postoperative
    External nephrotoxins
      Aminoglycoside antibiotics
      Amphotericin B
      Cyclosporine
      Radiocontrast dyes
    Endogenous nephrotoxins
      Rhabdomyolysis
      Acute severe hemolysis
Reversible hemodynamic renal failure
  Nonsteroidal anti-inflammatory drugs
  Angiotensin-converting enzyme inhibitors

decompression with a Foley catheter or a nephrostomy. When these tests indicate intrinsic ARF and the urinalysis does not show significant proteinuria, ATN is the most likely diagnosis. One must then carefully review the history and medical record to determine the likely cause, of which there are many (see Table 25–1).

A. ACUTE TUBULAR NECROSIS

ATN occurs as a result of prolonged renal ischemia or exposure to nephrotoxins. Ischemia can occur with true volume depletion (bleeding, diarrhea, diuretic-induced hypovolemia) or from decreased cardiac output (CHF, myocardial infarction, sepsis). The postsurgical setting is a common milieu for ATN in the elderly as a result of intraoperative hypotension, myocardial ischemia or arrhythmia, or intraoperative fluid loss.

Nephrotoxic drugs, especially aminoglycoside antibiotics, are more likely to produce ATN in the elderly because of decreased rate of clearance, resulting in toxic levels. Other medications implicated in ARF in the elderly are angiotensin-converting enzyme (ACE) inhibitors and nonsteroidal anti-inflammatory drugs (NSAIDs). These cause functional ARF as a result of alterations in renal blood flow, especially in elderly individuals with poor underlying renal perfusion. This latter form of ARF is reversible if the drug is withdrawn.

Radioiodinated contrast-induced ATN is an important cause of ARF in the elderly. Risk factors include advanced age, diabetes mellitus, high or repeated dye loads, and preexisting renal insufficiency (with serum creatinine > 2.0 mg/dL). Volume expansion with saline solution and pretreatment with acetyl cysteine (Mucomyst) reduce the incidence of contrast-induced ATN.

B. PRERENAL AZOTEMIA

Volume depletion causes a disproportionate increase in BUN compared with creatinine (BUN–creatinine ratio > 20:1). The same is true of CHF. Correction of the hemodynamic instability will restore renal perfusion and correct the azotemia. However, if the hypovolemia or CHF is left untreated, ischemic ATN may result.

C. POSTRENAL (OBSTRUCTIVE) ACUTE RENAL FAILURE

If there is any possibility of urinary tract obstruction as a cause of ARF, a catheter should be inserted into the urinary bladder (to relieve outlet obstruction) and a renal ultrasonogram obtained to look for hydronephrosis. About 10–15% of cases of ARF in the elderly are due to obstruction. Oliguria or anuria is common, but some patients with postrenal failure have normal or increased urinary output resulting from nephrogenic diabetes insipidus caused by the elevated hydrostatic pressure from the obstruction.

Complications

A. HYPERKALEMIA

Hyperkalemia is most likely in oliguric patients who are postsurgical or have deep tissue infections, with resultant release of large amounts of intracellular potassium into the circulation.

B. VOLUME OVERLOAD

Volume overload can be prevented by meticulous attention to daily fluid intake and output, so that intake volume should not exceed the sum of urinary and gastrointestinal output (plus 500–700 mL/day insensible loss), unless hypovolemia is present.

C. Uremic Encephalopathy

Rapid accumulation of nitrogenous waste can cause mental confusion, lethargy, and coma, especially in the elderly individual with underlying central nervous system (CNS) disease. Asterixis is an early sign of impending encephalopathy and is usually an indicator for dialysis.

Prognosis

Mortality in ATN remains about 50%, as it has for decades. Risk factors for survival include younger age, a cause other than ischemia or sepsis, and nonoliguric ATN. In surviving patients, recovery of renal function may not be complete, particularly in elderly patients with underlying vascular disease. Diabetic patients with dye-induced ATN who are oliguric and whose serum creatinine rises to 5 mg/dL or higher rarely recover function and usually progress to end-stage renal disease (ESRD).

Clark B: Biology of renal aging in humans. Adv Renal Repl Ther 2000;7:11. [PMID: 10672914]

GLOMERULAR DISEASE

ESSENTIALS OF DIAGNOSIS

- *Proteinuria (by dipstick or quantitative).*
- *Microscopic hematuria or red blood cell casts.*
- *Hypertension is usual.*
- *Peripheral edema common.*

General Considerations

Glomerular disease in the elderly usually presents as a nephritic syndrome, often with progressive renal failure, or as nephrotic syndrome. The nephritic patient has an abrupt onset of hypertension, hematuria, decreased GFR, and fluid retention. The nephrotic patient usually has a more gradual onset, with development of peripheral edema and hypoalbuminemia.

Prevention

The causes of these conditions are generally unknown, except in certain systemic diseases, such as diabetic

nephropathy. Renal complications, including proteinuria, nephrotic syndrome, and renal insufficiency, can be prevented or delayed by tight control of plasma glucose and of hypertension.

Clinical Findings

A. Symptoms & Signs

In the elderly, the onset of nephritic syndrome is often heralded by a sudden increase in blood pressure, development of edema, or symptoms of CHF. Oliguria is common in the nephritic syndrome.

B. Laboratory Findings

The nephritic patient may have "smoky" urine or gross hematuria. Proteinuria is present, and the urinary sediment shows red blood cell casts. BUN and creatinine concentrations increase progressively, often in a pattern similar to ATN. In nephrotic syndrome, urinalysis shows heavy proteinuria, 24-h urinary protein excretion is > 3.5 g, and hypoalbuminemia and hypercholesterolemia are present. Urinalysis is often "bland," with few cellular elements. Fat-laden tubular cells, which produce characteristic "Maltese crosses" under polarized light microscopy, are often seen in the urinary sediment.

Differential Diagnosis

Most patients with a nephritic or nephrotic syndrome should be referred to a nephrologist for consultation and comanagement.

A. Nephritic Syndrome

Postinfectious GN is less common in elderly than in younger patients. The presentation is similar to poststreptococcal GN in younger individuals, although signs of fluid overload and CHF are more common. The most common clinicopathological diagnosis in elderly patients with a nephritic presentation is rapidly progressive GN (RPGN). Renal biopsy of such patients shows extensive epithelia crescent formation. About 50% of these patients are positive for antineutrophil cytoplasmic antibodies (ANCAs). The pattern of staining can distinguish between "pauci-immune" RPGN (perinuclear pattern: p-ANCA) or Wegener's granulomatosis (cytoplasmic pattern: c-ANCA). A smaller proportion of patients have serum antiglomerular basement membrane antibodies typical of Goodpasture's syndrome. Another cause of RPGN in the elderly is hepatitis C-associated cryoglobulinemia. These patients often have cutaneous vasculitis; serum complement is usually depressed.

B. Nephrotic Syndrome

The incidence of nephrotic syndrome does not change with aging, but the underlying diagnoses are skewed toward certain diseases. The most common diagnoses from biopsy series of elderly patients are membranous GN (35–40%), amyloidosis (10–12%), and minimal change disease (11%). Underrepresented in biopsy series is diabetic glomerulosclerosis, because this diagnosis is often presumed, without biopsy, in the patient with long-standing diabetes and clinical evidence of nephropathy. There is little to differentiate clinically between the different types of primary glomerular diseases. Unless there are serious contraindications, renal biopsy should be sought in the elderly patient with nephrotic syndrome because treatment protocols differ for the various diseases.

Complications

The principal complications in elderly patients with nephritic presentation are hemodynamic: hypertension, volume overload, and CHF. Patients with RPGN may experience uremic symptoms within weeks or months of onset. Nephrotic patients virtually always have peripheral edema, but some have anasarca, with ascites or pleural effusions. Hypercoagulability results from loss of antithrombin III and other proteins in the urine. The incidence of deep venous thrombosis and of renal vein thrombosis is markedly increased as a consequence.

Treatment

Treatment of primary glomerulopathies should be coordinated with a nephrologist. Management of the most common diagnosis, membranous GN, is controversial. Prednisone with or without chlorambucil has shown some benefit in populations other than the elderly. However, the potential complications of immunosuppressive therapy are increased in the elderly patient. There is no specific therapy for amyloidosis.

Nonspecific management is important. Hypertension should be treated aggressively to slow progression of renal insufficiency. Diuretics must be used with caution, particularly in nephrotic patients, who are susceptible to intravascular volume depletion and ARF.

Prognosis

Most elderly patients with RPGN and diabetic GN progress inexorably to ESRD. Membranous GN is characterized by occasional spontaneous remission, and immunosuppressive treatment may result in stabilization or reversal.

Madaio MP, Harrington JT: The diagnosis of glomerular diseases. Acute glomerulonephritis and the nephrotic syndrome. Arch Intern Med 2001;161:25. [PMID: 11146695]

RENOVASCULAR DISEASE

ESSENTIALS OF DIAGNOSIS

- *Refractory (or new-onset) hypertension after age 50.*
- *Progressive renal insufficiency.*
- *Decreased renal blood flow by Doppler or magnetic resonance angiography.*

General Considerations

Renovascular disease increases in prevalence with increasing age. Risk factors include a history of atherosclerosis, diabetes mellitus, tobacco use, and hypertension. Atherosclerotic narrowing of 1 or both renal arteries can present with hypertension and progressive renal insufficiency or without clinical manifestation. Clues to the diagnosis include onset of hypertension after age 50, refractory hypertension in the elderly, and progressive renal insufficiency in the presence of other signs of peripheral vascular disease. However, the mere presence of renal artery narrowing does not predict clinical disease. Autopsy studies in patients older than 70 demonstrate a prevalence of severe renovascular disease in up to 60–65%. Angiographic studies have indicated a similar incidence of ~70% in elders with hypertension and 35% in those who are normotensive.

Prevention

There is reason to believe that smoking cessation, tight control of diabetes, lowering of elevated cholesterol, and control of hypertension itself will decrease the incidence or progression of atherosclerotic renal disease.

Clinical Findings

A. SYMPTOMS & SIGNS

In renovascular hypertension (RVH), symptoms are similar to those of other forms of hypertension, ultimately resulting in CHF, atrial fibrillation, stroke, and myocardial infarction. Patients with RVH frequently are refractory to standard treatment, have abrupt onset of hypertension after age 50, and may have a unilateral abdominal bruit on the affected side. In atherosclerotic renovascular insufficiency, the symptoms and signs are no different from those of other forms of progressive renal failure.

B. LABORATORY FINDINGS

Urinalysis in renovascular disease usually shows mild proteinuria, with a "bland" urinary sediment consisting of hyaline and granular casts. In unilateral renal artery stenosis (RAS), BUN and creatinine are usually normal. However, the use of ACE inhibitors in such patients frequently leads to a reversible azotemia, often accompanied by hyperkalemia. This development should strongly suggest the diagnosis and lead to further testing.

C. IMAGING STUDIES

Abdominal ultrasonography shows unilateral or bilateral shrunken kidneys. More useful is Doppler ultrasonography, which can estimate renal blood flow on each side. This test is quite sensitive (> 90%) for detection of clinically significant RAS. Angiography is the most definitive test for diagnosing RAS but is also most risky, with possible atheroembolic or dye-induced renal injury as complications. Carbon dioxide subtraction angiography avoids these risks, as does magnetic resonance angiography.

The most effective screening test for RVH is captopril renography, in which renal perfusion is measured before and after administering the ACE inhibitor captopril. The affected kidney shows a dramatic decrease in perfusion after captopril.

Differential Diagnosis

RAS accounts for only ~5% of hypertension in the United States, so the much more likely diagnosis in most cases is essential hypertension. Increased age, sudden onset, and an abdominal bruit increase the likelihood of RAS, as does development of azotemia after use of an ACE inhibitor. There is little to distinguish ischemic nephropathy from other forms of progressive renal failure. The prevalence is uncertain.

Treatment

The optimal management of RVH is uncertain. Medical management may be effective. Correction of the stenosis, with angioplasty or surgical repair, although invasive, can occasionally cure and usually decrease the severity of the hypertension. Recent series of surgical revascularization report 50–70% improved; angioplasty outcomes are similar.

The management of ischemic nephropathy is even less clear because of the unpredictability of progression of the atherosclerotic narrowing. Treatment, therefore, should be individualized. In centers with excellent surgical or angioplasty technical skills, intervention may be considered, particularly in elders with few comorbidities.

Safian RD, Textor SC: Renal-artery stenosis. N Engl J Med 2001;344:431. [PMID: 11172181]

van Jaarsveld BC et al: The effect of balloon angioplasty on hypertension in atherosclerotic renal-artery stenosis. N Engl J Med 2000;342:1007. [PMID: 10749962]

CHRONIC RENAL FAILURE

ESSENTIALS OF DIAGNOSIS

- Bilaterally small kidneys by ultrasonography in most conditions.
- Progressive azotemia over time.
- Loss of urine concentrating ability (isosthenuria).

General Considerations

Elderly individuals make up the majority of new ESRD patients in the United States. The 1999 U.S. Renal Data System (USRDS) report indicated that, for 1997, of 79,000 new ESRD patients who began treatment, 51% were 65 years of age or older. Of the 300,000 patients receiving renal replacement therapy (RRT), 34% were age 65 or older. The most common causes of ESRD in elderly are diabetes and hypertension-induced nephrosclerosis.

Prevention

Rigorous control of blood pressure in patients with hypertension can prevent onset of chronic renal failure (CRF). Target blood pressure should be normal (< 130/85). ACE inhibitors are the antihypertensive drug of choice because of their beneficial effects on the renal glomerular pressure. A similar preventive effect has been shown in diabetic patients who maintain tight sugar control. Protein restriction has been shown in experimental animals to slow progression of renal failure. However, the effect in humans is relatively minor. For most patients with CRF, protein intake should not exceed 1 g/kg/day.

Clinical Findings

With minor exceptions, the symptoms, signs, and laboratory findings are no different in elderly patients with CRF than in younger patients.

A. SYMPTOMS & SIGNS

Most patients with progressive CRF experience nonspecific symptoms of fatigue and weakness. With worsening of renal failure, buildup of nitrogenous wastes leads to gastrointestinal symptoms (nausea, anorexia, hiccups) and later to neurological symptoms (somnolence, confusion, irritability). Itching may become severe, particularly in those with secondary hyperparathyroidism. Urinary frequency and nocturia are common because of a loss of concentrating function. Physical examination may reveal pallor (resulting from anemia), a yellowish tint to the skin, signs of pruritus, and bruising. Hypertension is usually present. Asterixis is a late neurological sign. In untreated end-stage patients, uremic "frost" on the skin, pericardial friction rub, and seizures may occur.

B. LABORATORY FINDINGS

Increased BUN and creatinine, progressive over time, is diagnostic. Because of decreased muscle mass (the site of creatinine production), an elderly patient with normal serum creatinine (≤ 1.0 mg/dL) implies a GFR that is only 50–60% of that of a young patient with the same serum creatinine. As a result, a serum creatinine of 3–4 mg/dL may represent ESRD in an octogenarian. To avoid the need for 24-h urine collection to measure creatinine clearance, one should estimate GFR, using the Cockcroft-Gault equation:

$$\text{Creatinine clearance} = [(140 - \text{Age}) \times$$
$$\text{Weight (kg)}] / [\text{serum creatinine concentration} \times 72]$$
$$(\text{for women, multiply by } 0.85 \text{ because}$$
$$\text{of smaller muscle mass}).$$

Anemia (resulting from decreased erythropoietin production) is common and is usually normochromic and normocytic. Hyperphosphatemia and hypocalcemia are common in untreated patients with CRF. Urinalysis usually shows granular casts, variable amount of protein, and isosthenuria (specific gravity 1.010–1.012).

C. IMAGING STUDIES

Renal ultrasonography shows bilaterally shrunken kidneys in most patients with CRF. Exceptions include adult polycystic kidney disease (very large kidneys with myriad cysts), amyloidosis (normal- to large-sized kidneys), and chronic obstructive uropathy (large kidneys with dilated collecting systems).

D. SPECIAL TESTS

Renal biopsy is used less frequently in elderly than in younger patients with undiagnosed renal failure because of concern about increased risks of complications. Patients with progressive renal failure in the setting of chronic hypertension or long-standing diabetes mellitus may have a presumptive diagnosis made without biopsy. However, presentation of a nephritic syndrome or nephrotic syndrome in the absence of diabetes warrants a serious consideration of renal biopsy to diagnose potentially treatable kidney disease.

Complications

Anemia, primarily resulting from decreased erythropoietin production, develops in most patients with CRF. The anemia is normochromic and normocytic, similar to other anemias of chronic disease.

Hyperkalemia rarely occurs spontaneously until late in CRF. The exception is diabetic glomerulosclerosis, caused by a condition of hyporeninemic hypoaldosteronism (often called Type IV renal tubular acidosis).

Cardiovascular complications, including hypertensive heart disease and CHF, are common in elderly patients with CRF. Pericarditis is a late complication of ESRD.

Unless serum phosphate and calcium concentrations are kept normal, most patients with CRF experience secondary hyperparathyroidism, characterized by bones showing osteitis fibrosis cystica. Many also have a component of osteomalacia caused by deficiency of 1,25-dihydroxyvitamin D, which is normally produced by the kidney.

Treatment

Management of CRF in the elderly does not differ importantly from that for younger patients. Treatment should be coordinated with a nephrologist in most cases by the time the serum creatinine concentration approaches 3 mg/dL.

A. CARDIOVASCULAR

Hypertension is common, and uncontrolled hypertension is a major contributor to progression of renal failure regardless of underlying cause. ACE inhibitors should generally be included in the drug regimen to preserve glomerular filtration. Because of associated coronary artery disease and valvular heart disease, CHF is common in the elderly CRF patient and should be aggressively treated to avoid a prerenal component contributing to the renal failure. Conversely, overdiuresis needs also to be avoided to prevent decreased perfusion to the already compromised kidney.

B. HYPERKALEMIA

This is more common in ARF than in CRF. However, certain types of renal disease are more likely to have a potassium excretory defect: interstitial kidney diseases and diabetic patients (with hyporeninemic hypoaldosteronism). Acute severe hyperkalemia is managed in the usual way: intravenous calcium, glucose and insulin, or bicarbonate infusion, with hemodialysis in extreme or refractory cases. Chronic hyperkalemia is best managed with a low-potassium diet and avoidance of ACE inhibitors, NSAIDs, and potassium-sparing diuretics (spironolactone, triamterene, amiloride).

C. Acidosis

Most patients with CRF have a defect in ammonia production (and thereby hydrogen ion excretion) when GFR falls to about 25% normal. The resultant metabolic acidosis has few symptoms but may contribute to chronic bone disease. More severe acidosis leads to anorexia, dyspnea, and abdominal pain. Patients whose serum bicarbonate concentration falls below 20 mmol/L should receive oral alkali (sodium bicarbonate or sodium citrate).

D. Anemia

For patients with hemoglobin concentration < 10 g/dL, intravenous or subcutaneous erythropoietin should be begun once or twice weekly. Oral iron supplementation should be added if the serum ferritin is below 100 µg/mL.

E. Calcium & Phosphorus Metabolism

Secondary hyperparathyroidism and hypovitaminosis D are usual concomitants of progressive renal failure and must be managed to prevent the serious consequences of metabolic bone disease (renal osteodystrophy). Dietary phosphorus restriction should begin when GFR decreases to 50% of normal. If serum phosphate concentration is elevated, intestinal phosphate binders, such as calcium carbonate or calcium acetate, should be begun. Aluminum hydroxide antacids also bind phosphate but should not be used chronically in the patient with CRF because of possible aluminum toxicity. Target serum calcium concentration should be 10 mg/dL. If hypocalcemia occurs despite phosphate control, oral vitamin D (or its active product 1,25-dihyroxyvitamin D) should be started.

F. Modification of Drug Doses in Chronic Renal Failure

In patients with CRF, it is important to modify drug doses for medications cleared primarily by the kidney. This is particularly true for drugs with serious dose-related toxicities (eg, aminoglycoside antibiotics, digoxin, amphotericin). Appropriate dose modifications can be found in published tables or the Physicians' Desk Reference.

G. Renal Replacement Therapy

Discussion and decision making about renal replacement therapy (RRT; peritoneal dialysis, hemodialysis, renal transplantation) should begin by consulting a nephrologist whenever an elderly patient without prohibitive comorbidities progresses toward ESRD. One can attempt a rough estimate of when RRT will be necessary by plotting 1/creatinine against time (usually a straight-line function) and projecting to the point where 1/creatinine reaches 0.10–0.13. The decision to initiate RRT in an elderly patient requires medical, ethical, and psychosocial considerations that are sometimes difficult to weigh. The decision is best made within a team approach, involving the primary physician, nephrologist, social worker, patient, and family.

Prognosis

Because of comorbidities (primarily cardiovascular disease), survival of elderly patients receiving hemodialysis or peritoneal dialysis is shorter than for younger ESRD patients. Although rates are improving, the most recent USRDS data indicate mortality rates that are 3 times as high for patients older than 75 compared to those patients aged 45–64 (46 deaths/100 patient years vs. 17.3).

Bennett WM et al: Drug prescribing in renal failure: dosing guidelines for adults. Am J Kidney Dis 1983;3:155. [PMID: 6356890]

Diabetes Control and Complications Research Group: Effect of intensive therapy on the development and progression of diabetic nephropathy in the Diabetes Control and Complications Trial. Kidney Int 1995;47:1703. [PMID: 7643540]

Levey AS et al: Dietary protein restriction and the progression of chronic renal disease: what have all of the results of the MDRD study shown? Modification of Diet in Renal Disease Study group. J Am Soc Nephrol 1999;10:2426. [PMID: 10541304]

McCarthy JR: A practical approach to the management of patients with chronic renal failure. Mayo Clin Proc 1999;74:269. [PMID: 10089997]

Ritz E, Orth SR: Nephropathy in patients with type 2 diabetes mellitus. N Engl J Med 1999;341:1127. [PMID: 10511612]

Stack AG, Messana JM: Renal replacement therapy in the elderly: medical ethical, and psychosocial considerations. Adv Renal Repl Ther 2000;7:52. [PMID: 10672917]

U.S. Renal Data System 1999 Annual Data Report: Executive summary. Am J Kidney Dis 1999;34:S9. [PMID: 10430999]

HYPONATREMIA

 ESSENTIALS OF DIAGNOSIS

- *Plasma sodium concentration (P_{Na}) < 130 mmol/L.*
- *Plasma chloride concentration (P_{Cl}) < 90 mmol/L.*

- *Plasma osmolality decreased (< 270 mOsm/kg) unless hyperglycemia has contributed to the hyponatremia.*

General Considerations

Hyponatremia is a common electrolyte disorder in the elderly, ranging from 7% in healthy ambulatory elders to as high as 15–20% in hospitalized individuals and those in chronic care facilities. In hospitalized patients, hyponatremia on admission is associated with a mortality of almost 10% compared with only 1% for those with a normal sodium concentration.

Pathophysiology

Sustained hyponatremia indicates an excess of total body water relative to total body solute, and it almost always indicates some impairment of free water excretion by the kidney. Hyponatremia indicates nothing about the state of total body sodium (TB_{Na}); this determination requires a clinical physical examination. Patients with hyponatremia must be classified as having increased TB_{Na} (the edema states), decreased TB_{Na} (hypovolemia), or normal TB_{Na} (euvolemia). The mechanism of hyponatremia differs in each of these states (Table 25–2).

Table 25–2. Causes of hyponatremia.

With decreased total body sodium content (hypovolemia)
Diarrhea
Prolonged vomiting
Diuretic-induced volume depletion
Burns
Adrenal (mineralocorticoid) insufficiency
With increased total body sodium content (hypervolemia)
Congestive heart failure
Cirrhosis
Nephrotic syndrome
Advanced renal failure
Protein-losing enteropathy
With normal total body sodium content (euvolemia)
Syndrome of inappropriate antidiuretic hormone secretion
Reset osmostat
Hypopituitarism, with secondary hypocortisolemia
Severe hypothyroidism
Psychogenic polydipsia

A. Increased Total Body Sodium (Edema States) With Hyponatremia

In CHF and cirrhosis, there is decreased effective intravascular volume, leading to volume-stimulated enhancement of salt and water reabsorption by the kidney. Furthermore, antidiuretic hormone (ADH) levels are increased, leading to inappropriate concentration of the urine, preventing water excretion and correction of the hyponatremia.

B. Decreased Total Body Sodium (Hypovolemia) With Hyponatremia

Examples are gastrointestinal losses (vomiting, diarrhea), bleeding, or diuretic-induced hypovolemia. As in CHF, there are volume-stimulated increases in renal salt and water reabsorption and volume-induced ADH release, causing a concentrated urine and preventing excretion of free water. The result is hyponatremia.

C. Normal Total Body Sodium (Euvolemia) Hyponatremia

Most patients with hyponatremia in this clinical category have the syndrome of inappropriate ADH secretion (SIADH) as a result of medical disease, pain syndromes, postsurgical state, or medications (Table 25–3).

Clinical Findings

A. Symptoms & Signs

Principal symptoms of hyponatremia, if any, relate to the CNS. Change of mental status, in the form of lethargy, forgetfulness, cognitive decline, stupor, and rarely coma, usually occur as the P_{Na} falls to ≤ 125 mmol/L. Rapid lowering of sodium concentration is more likely to produce symptoms than a gradual change to the same level. Few physical signs relate to the hyponatremia per se aside from demonstrable neuropsychological changes. Patients with hypervolemic hyponatremia usually have peripheral edema, ascites, or both and may have other typical signs of CHF. Hypovolemic hyponatremia is characterized by low blood pressure, often with significant postural drop; tachycardia; and dry mucous membranes.

B. Laboratory Tests

Hyponatremia ($P_{Na} < 130$ mmol/L), hypochloremia (< 90 mmol/L), and hypo-osmolality (usually < 270 mOsm/kg) are present. Plasma osmolality (P_{Osm}) can be estimated by the formula:

$$E_{osm} = \text{estimated osmolality} = 2 \times [\text{sodium concentration (mmol/L)}] + [\text{blood glucose (mg/dL)}/18] + [\text{BUN (mg/dL)}/2.8].$$

Table 25–3. Causes of SIADH.

Central nervous system disease
  CNS tumors
  Trauma
  Subdural hematoma
  Subarachnoid hemorrhage
  Encephalitis
Pulmonary disease
  Lung cancer (especially small cell)
  Tuberculosis
  Fungal infections
  Pneumonia
  Positive-pressure ventilation
Cancer
  Lung
  Pancreas
  Bowel
  Lymphoma
Acute psychosis
Aging (rare as sole explanation for SIADH)
Drugs
  Chlorpropamide
  Cyclophosphamide
  Vincristine
  Psychotropic medications, especially phenothiazines
  Antidepressants: SSRIs, tricyclics
  Carbamazepine
Other causes
  Pain
  Postoperative state
  Severe hypokalemia

CNS, central nervous system; SIADH, syndrome of inappropriate antidiuretic hormone secretion; SSRIs, selective serotonin reuptake inhibitors.

Hyperglycemia can lead to hyponatremia by osmotically attracting water out of the intracellular space, diluting the serum sodium concentration. The expected change in P_{Na} is a decrease of 1.6 mmol/L for every 100 mg/dL increase in blood glucose concentration.

Serum uric acid concentration is usually increased (> 7 mg/dL) in hypovolemic and hypervolemic hyponatremic patients. Conversely, in SIADH, serum uric acid concentration is typically reduced (< 4 mg/dL) as a result of increased uric acid renal clearance.

Treatment

Restriction of water intake (< 500 mL/day) should be instituted in all cases. If hypovolemia is present, give IV normal saline (or blood or plasma if bleeding is the cause of the hypovolemia). If an edema state is present, treat the underlying condition (CHF, cirrhosis). In most cases, sodium restriction (to < 1 g sodium/day) is appropriate. Limit the rate of correction of hyponatremia to 1–2 mmol/L/h. More rapid correction can lead to a serious CNS complication, central pontine myelinolysis (CPM). For individuals with severe neurological symptoms (seizure, coma), infuse a small volume of 3% sodium chloride solution intravenously to produce a rapid initial rise in serum sodium concentration and reverse some of the brain edema. A useful formula for calculating the effect of any sodium-containing infusate is as follows:

$$\text{Change in } P_{Na} = [\text{infusate sodium concentration} - P_{Na}] / [\text{total body water} - 1].$$

In a 70-kg patient with a starting P_{Na} of 112 mmol/L, 500 mL of 3% NaCl solution will raise the P_{Na} to 121 mmol/L. In such an emergency, the target for this initial treatment should be 120 mmol/L, at which point the guidelines just presented should be followed.

Prognosis

The outcome is determined primarily by the underlying illness rather than the hyponatremia per se, unless severe neurological complications have occurred, such as seizure, coma, or CPM.

Adrogue HJ, Madias NE: Hyponatremia. N Engl J Med 2000; 342:1581. [PMID: 10824078]

Beck LH: Fluid and electrolyte balance in the elderly. Geriatr Nephrol Urol 1999;9:11. [PMID:10435222]

HYPERNATREMIA

 ESSENTIALS OF DIAGNOSIS

- $P_{Na} > 150$ mmol/L.
- $P_{Cl} > 110$ mmol/L.
- $P_{Osm} > 300$ Osm/kg.

General Considerations

Hypernatremia is common in sick elderly patients. In nursing home patients requiring hospitalization, the prevalence of hypernatremia is 30% and is associated with a mortality rate of 42%.

Prevention

It is reasonable to administer regular feedings of water, either orally or via nasogastric administration, to frail nursing home patients or other individuals who are dependent on others for their water requirements.

Clinical Findings

A. SYMPTOMS & SIGNS

The symptoms of hypernatremia are similar to those of hyponatremia: Mental status changes predominate and are to be expected when the P_{Na} is > 155 mmol/L. The hypernatremic patient may have no subjective symptoms. Physical findings include the neuropsychological abnormalities associated with depressed mental status, often accompanied by poor skin turgor and dryness of mucous membranes.

A. LABORATORY FINDINGS

See Essentials of Diagnosis. Hypernatremic patients usually have elevated BUN and creatinine concentration, usually in a prerenal pattern (BUN–creatinine ratio > 20:1).

Treatment

Electrolyte-free water must be administered to reduce P_{Na} and plasma osmolality toward normal. Water can be given by mouth or nasogastric tube in the awake patient; more often, it should be infused intravenously (as dextrose and water solution). Hypotonic sodium solutions (eg, half-normal saline solution) can be given if there are concomitant signs of hypovolemia or if it is known that the preceding fluid losses consisted of sodium-containing hypotonic fluids (as in vomiting or diarrhea). The minimal volume of free water required to restore P_{Na} to normal can be estimated from the formula: Water deficit = total body water × (1 − [140/P_{Na}]) (total body water can be estimated as weight [in kg] × 60%).

Care must be taken not to correct the hypernatremia too rapidly, particularly if the abnormality has been developing over several days or more. Because of adaptive changes in brain electrolytes and other solutes, rapid correction of hypernatremia can lead to cerebral edema. A rule of thumb is to correct half of the deficit in the first 24 h, with the remaining correction taking place over the next 24–48 h.

Adrogue HJ: Hypernatremia. N Engl J Med 2000;342:1493. [PMID: 10816188]

Geriatric Rheumatology

26

David E. Blumenthal, MD

ESSENTIALS OF DIAGNOSIS

- Many rheumatic conditions, such as tendinitis or bursitis, are diagnosed by history and physical findings alone, and additional diagnostic tests are not useful.

- Many rheumatological tests are falsely positive in the elderly, so one must determine the pretest probability of disease by history and physical before ordering and interpreting laboratory tests.

- Radiographs and magnetic resonance images can document anatomic changes, but only a careful history and physical will determine the clinical relevance of the findings.

- Synovial fluid analysis is useful in determining the cause of a joint effusion and confirming a septic or crystal-induced arthritis.

- Older patients who are treated with chronic steroids should be aggressively screened and treated for osteoporosis.

General Considerations

A properly performed history and physical is essential to accurate rheumatological diagnosis. Many rheumatic conditions, such as tendinitis and bursitis, are diagnosed by history and physical findings alone, and additional diagnostic tests are not useful. The history and physical enables estimation of the pretest probability of disease and is crucial to the rational use of laboratory and imaging tests.

Autoantibody testing is frequently falsely positive in the elderly, and one must determine the pretest probability of disease by history and physical before ordering and interpreting laboratory tests. Twenty to 40% of elderly patients without rheumatic disease may have a positive antinuclear antibody (ANA), and rheumatoid factor (RF) can be found in approximately 15% of healthy older adults. The erythrocyte sedimentation rate (ESR) is a nonspecific marker of inflammation and can be increased in malignancies, infectious diseases, and any cause of tissue necrosis. The ESR increases with age, and the laboratory may only report the normal range for younger patients. To calculate a normal sedimentation rate for a male, divide age by 2; for a female, add 10 to the age and divide by 2.

Radiographs and magnetic resonance images (MRIs) can document anatomic changes, but only a careful history and physical will determine the clinical relevance of the findings. A radiograph of the knee may show changes of osteoarthritis (OA), but the patient's pain might be caused by nearby anserine bursitis or referred pain from the hip. Radiographs are most useful in detecting changes in bone. If 2 bones are closer than normal, loss of intervening articular or structural cartilage is assumed. MRI is ideal for imaging structures that are not well seen on radiographs and is particularly useful to search for meniscal tears in the knee, rotator cuff tears, compression of neural tissue in the spine, and early avascular necrosis.

Synovial fluid analysis is useful in determining the cause of a joint effusion and confirming a crystal-induced arthritis. Synovial fluid analysis is essential when the differential diagnosis includes septic arthritis. Classification of synovial fluid according to cellularity is summarized in Table 26–1. Synovial fluid should undergo cell count with differential, culture with Gram's stain, and crystal analysis by polarized light microscopy. Synovial fluid analysis for protein, pH, RF, ANA, or complement has no clinical value.

OSTEOARTHRITIS

ESSENTIALS OF DIAGNOSIS

- History suggests mechanical pain.
- Examination suggests loss of articular cartilage.
- Radiographs confirm loss of articular cartilage.
- Morning stiffness < 30 min duration, if present.

Table 26–1. Synovial fluid analysis.

Variable	Noninflammatory	Inflammatory	Septic	Hemarthrosis
Color	Pale yellow	Cloudy yellow	Cloudy/purulent	Bloody/red
WBC/mm^3	< 2000	2000–75,000	> 100,000	RBC >> WBC
WBC differential	< 25% PMNs	> 50% PMNs	> 80% PMNs	Variable

WBC, white blood cells; PMNs, polymorphonuclear leukocytes; RBC, red blood cell; >> indicates significantly greater than.

General Considerations

Thinning and fissuring of the articular cartilage is known as OA, osteoarthrosis, or degenerative joint disease (DJD). Autopsy evidence of OA can be found in most adults older than 65, and physical examination reveals OA of the hands in 70% of people older than 70. Joints commonly affected by primary OA include the knee, hip, distal interphalangeal joint (DIP), proximal interphalangeal joint (PIP), first metatarsophalangeal (MTP) joint, acromioclavicular joint, facet joints of the cervical spine, and facet joints of the lumbar spine.

Clinical Findings

Most patients complain of "mechanical" pain, which worsens with continued use of the joint and improves with rest. Morning stiffness is common but usually resolves in < 30 min. Morning stiffness lasting > 1 h, pain that keeps the patient from sleeping, and reports of impressive joint swelling suggest inflammatory rather than degenerative disease. OA patients report difficulties with activities of daily living as a result of pain, loss of strength, or diminished range of motion. Pain at rest is not usual but can be seen when the cartilage loss is severe.

Physical examination reveals osteophytes on the margins of the joints, particularly in the hands at the DIP joints (Heberden's nodes) and the PIP joints (Bouchard's nodes). Range of motion may be diminished, and there is often crepitus caused by friction within the joint. A joint effusion may be present, particularly in the knee, but warmth is minimal and synovial proliferation is absent. Degenerative disease of the hip can cause pain that is referred down the thigh to the knee. When a patient complains of knee or thigh pain, the examiner should also assess the ipsilateral hip.

Blood testing is generally not helpful in diagnosing OA but may be used to seek a cause of suspected secondary OA. Synovial fluid analysis reveals a synovial fluid white blood cell (WBC) count of < 2000/mm^3, indicating a noninflammatory condition. Radiographs show joint space narrowing, marginal osteophytes, subchondral sclerosis, and subchondral cysts. Weight-bearing radiographs may better demonstrate the cartilage loss in joints of the lower extremities. MRI can detect early loss of articular cartilage but is more costly than conventional radiography and is seldom needed to diagnose OA.

Differential Diagnosis

Because most elderly patients will have evidence of OA on physical examination or radiographs, there is a risk of erroneously ascribing pain to OA while missing another diagnosis. When joints atypical for OA are involved (eg, metacarpophalangeal joint, wrist, elbow, subtalar joint), other diagnoses should be considered. The classic symptoms and signs of OA in an unusual joint distribution should raise suspicion of secondary OA, causes of which are listed in Table 26–2. The differential diagnoses of pain in an extremity are listed in Table 26–3. A carefully performed history and physical are essential to localize the pain to its site of origin, supplemented by imaging as indicated.

Treatment

Acetaminophen, ≤ 1000 mg 4 times/day, is initial therapy. If the patient's symptoms are not controlled, non-steroidal anti-inflammatory drugs (NSAIDs), tramadol, narcotics, or glucosamine can be considered.

The risk of NSAID gastropathy and gastrointestinal bleeding increases with advancing age. Patients with

Table 26–2. Causes of secondary osteoarthritis.

Dysplasia, congenital or acquired	Metabolic
Trauma	Acromegaly
Osteonecrosis	Ochronosis
Infection	CPPD arthropathy
Chronic inflammation	Mucopolysaccharidoses
Hemarthroses, especially hemophilia	Neuropathy
Joint hypermobility	

CPPD, calcium pyrophosphate dihydrate.

Table 26-3. Differential diagnosis of peripheral joint OA.

Periarticular disease: tendinitis, bursitis
Ligament injury: sprain
Disease of structural cartilage: meniscal tear, tear of glenoid labrum
Disease of bone: fracture, malignancy, benign bone tumor, Paget's disease, osteomalacia
Disease of muscle: contusion, hematoma, pyomyositis, diabetic muscle infarction
Disease of skin or subcutaneous tissue: cellulitis, panniculitis, fasciitis
Neuropathic pain
Referred pain: hip to knee, diaphragm to shoulder, myocardium to shoulder
Ischemic pain: claudication, thromboembolic disease, vasculitis

prior GI bleeding, age > 65 years, high-dose NSAID treatment, and concomitant corticosteroid treatment are at higher risk. Bleeding risk can be lessened by use of a COX-2 selective NSAID (eg, celecoxib, rofecoxib, or valdecoxib) or concomitant use of a proton pump inhibitor or misoprostol, 200 µg 2-4 times/day as tolerated; the limiting toxicity is usually diarrhea. All NSAIDs potentially cause worsening renal function, fluid retention, or hepatic injury. Such adverse effects are more likely to occur in patients with preexisting diabetes mellitus, congestive heart failure, or chronic renal insufficiency. Limiting the NSAID dose to the lowest dose necessary to control symptoms will help minimize renal and gastrointestinal toxicity.

Some evidence suggests that glucosamine, 1500 mg daily, may retard the loss of articular cartilage seen in OA and provide some relief of pain. Adverse effects are rarely encountered, although diabetic patients may occasionally see increases in blood glucose. Although glucosamine generally appears to be safer than NSAIDs, it is sold as a nutritional supplement and thus is not regulated. Physicians should warn patients that such "nutraceuticals" may not contain standardized dosages and ingredients.

Some patients report anecdotal relief of symptoms with topical salicylates. Topical capsaicin has relieved OA pain and is available in 0.025% and 0.075% preparations. However, topical capsaicin can be locally irritating, and the patient must take care not to apply it to mucosal surfaces or the eyes.

Weight reduction can be beneficial for OA in the lower extremities. Exercise is often necessary to achieve weight reduction, which is difficult for patients with joint pain. Water aerobics and swimming may allow the patient to exercise with less pain. Quadriceps strengthening is beneficial for OA of the knees. A cane will help transfer weight from the affected joint and should be held in the hand opposite the painful limb. Proper footwear can absorb some of the force of each step.

The degree of inflammation in the OA joint is much less than that seen in inflammatory arthritis, and oral immunosuppressive treatment is not indicated in OA. However, individual patients can report significant improvement in joint pain after intra-articular corticosteroid injection. An empiric trial of corticosteroid injection may be attempted if oral medications do not provide satisfactory pain relief. If successful, repeat injections should not be performed more than every 4 mo.

Intra-articular injection of synthetic hyaluronan preparations has been shown to provide relief of OA knee pain for as much as 1 year, but there is still some uncertainty about whether the injections are superior to placebo. Little is known about safety and efficacy in joints other than the knee. Synvisc is injected into the knee weekly for 3 consecutive weeks. Hyalgan is injected into the knee weekly for 5 consecutive weeks. There is a risk of a reactive inflammatory arthritis after injection and a small risk of joint infection.

When there is severe loss of articular cartilage and the patient's quality of life is impaired, surgery should be considered. The primary goal of surgery is relief of pain. Total joint arthroplasty is usually selected for OA of the hip, knee, and shoulder. Arthrodesis (fusion) is usually preferred for the wrist, ankle, and first MTP joint.

 EVIDENCE-BASED POINTS

- *Gastropathy is a significant risk in elderly patients treated with NSAIDs.*
- *Gastroprotective strategies, including the use of COX-2 selective NSAIDs, reduce the risk of NSAID gastropathy, but other risks of NSAIDs remain.*

Chan FKL et al: Celecoxib versus diclofenac and omeprazole in reducing the risk of recurrent ulcer bleeding in patients with arthritis. N Engl J Med 2002;347:2104. [PMID: 12501222] (In this trial of patients with recent ulcer bleeding who were *Helicobacter pylori* negative, recurrent bleeding rates over 6 mo were 4.9% in patients who received celecoxib and 6.4% in those who received diclofenac plus omeprazole, a nonsignificant difference. Renal adverse events, including hypertension, peripheral edema, and renal failure, were common.)

Pavelka K et al: Glucosamine sulfate use and delay of progression of knee osteoarthritis: a 3-year, randomized, placebo-controlled, double-blind study. Arch Intern Med 2002;162:2113. [PMID: 12374520] (Results suggest that glucosamine is superior to placebo in treatment of OA and has a good safety profile.)

Raynauld J-P et al: Safety and efficacy of long-term intraarticular steroid injections in osteoarthritis of the knee. A randomized, double-blind, placebo-controlled trial. Arthritis Rheum 2003; 48:370. [PMID: not available] (Study found no deterioration of articular cartilage and some beneficial effects on joint pain, stiffness, and range of motion in the corticosteroid treatment group.)

DEGENERATIVE DISEASE OF THE SPINE

 ESSENTIALS OF DIAGNOSIS

- *History of mechanical pain in the neck, back, or extremities.*
- *History and examination should rule out compression of neural tissue.*
- *Radiographic evidence of degenerative change is common and may not explain the symptoms.*
- *Spine computed tomography or magnetic resonance imaging findings should be correlated with the symptoms and examination.*

General Considerations

Degenerative disease of the lumbar spine and facet joints is called spondylosis. Radiographic evidence of degenerative disease in the spine is almost universal in elderly people, and one should not necessarily conclude that spondylosis is the source of symptoms. Spondylosis commonly causes pain in the neck and low back but can also be responsible for isolated pain in an extremity, buttock pain, headache, and neurological dysfunction. Degenerative changes in the lumbar spine can lead to lumbar canal stenosis, characterized by neurogenic claudication in 1 or both legs.

Clinical Findings

A. SYMPTOMS & SIGNS

The patient often reports a history of chronic, gradually worsening neck or low back pain. However, because of the proximity of neural tissue, the patient may report a variety of neurological symptoms or neurogenic pain distant from the spine. Cervical spondylosis can cause occipital headaches; pain or numbness in the shoulder, arm, or hand; loss of dexterity; or lower extremity spasticity with gait disturbance. Lumbar spondylosis can lead to lumbar canal stenosis and neurogenic claudication, a pain in the legs or buttocks that worsens with prolonged standing and is relieved by sitting. Unlike vascular claudication, neurogenic claudication worsens while standing still. Nocturnal spine pain should raise concerns about a more ominous process, such as a malignancy. The sudden onset of severe spine pain suggests a fracture, possibly indicating osteoporosis.

B. PHYSICAL EXAMINATION

Physical examination should include the patient's height; alignment and range of motion of the cervical, thoracic, and lumbar spine; direct palpation of the spine and paraspinous tissues; and a careful neurological examination. Straight-leg raise testing for nerve root impingement is less sensitive in an older population with degenerative disk disease, and a negative test does not rule out foraminal encroachment. In fact, neurological examination may be normal even in the presence of compressed neural tissue. The abdomen should be examined for evidence of an abdominal process that might radiate to the back and to search for an abdominal aortic aneurysm. The possibility of vascular claudication is investigated by arterial examination of the lower extremities. Patients with postural exacerbation of symptoms should be positioned to produce the pain. Pain in the extremities that appears after standing or is reproduced by flexion–extension of the spine is suspicious for pain generated by neural compression. For patients with extremity pain, the examination should attempt to exclude joint or periarticular disease as the source of the pain.

Blood testing is generally not useful in confirming degenerative disease of the spine or resulting neural compression.

C. IMAGING STUDIES

Imaging usually begins with plain radiographs. Given the frequency of degenerative change in the elderly, the radiographs are mainly useful for excluding other vertebral processes such as fracture, infection, and malignancy. Flexion and extension views are useful if the patient reports symptoms that vary with posture. When compression of neural tissue is suspected, spine computed tomography (CT), CT myelogram, or spine MRI will be necessary for confirmation. In general, these studies are performed only if the physician plans to act on the findings by referring the patient for local injection or surgery. The images must be interpreted with caution; facet joint OA, disk flattening, and disk bulging are commonly found in asymptomatic elderly people and may not be the cause of the patient's complaint. One must confirm that the degree of the foraminal encroachment or canal stenosis is sufficiently severe and in the proper anatomic site to cause the current symptoms.

Electromyography (EMG) with nerve conduction testing can assist in confirming compression of neural tissue in the spine, ruling out more distal sites of compression, or detecting a more diffuse neuropathy. In patients with lower extremity claudication and an inconclusive history and physical, noninvasive vascular ultrasound evaluation can be helpful.

Differential Diagnosis

Other diseases of the spine, such as infection and malignancy, are often associated with severe, unremitting, or nocturnal pain. Fracture is often associated with acute onset and may or may not have an obvious initiating event. Abdominal or retroperitoneal processes radiating to the back should be considered when there are other associated risk factors (eg, vascular disease, alcoholism) or symptoms (vomiting, weight loss) or when pain is severe and acute in onset. Widespread myofascial tenderness in the back, neck, and extremities suggests a diagnosis of fibromyalgia. Tenderness that localizes specifically to 1 or more adjacent vertebral bodies is worrisome for fracture, infection, and malignancy.

Treatment

The recommendations for analgesic use are the same as those for OA. Gabapentin or one of the less anticholinergic tricyclic antidepressants, such as desipramine or nortryptiline, can be cautiously used when neurogenic pain is present. Amitriptyline should generally be avoided in older adults because of its high side effect profile.

Referral to a center specializing in pain management or spine disease may permit trials of epidural corticosteroid injection or facet joint injections. Transcutaneous electrical nerve stimulation units or dorsal column stimulators have been used, but their efficacy has not been demonstrated. Surgery is used to correct clinically significant instability and to relieve disabling symptoms of neural compression. Surgery is not generally indicated to relieve local pain in the back or neck. The success rates vary according to the nature of the problem, the operation performed, and the criteria used to measure success; however, there is a risk that the disabling symptoms will persist after operation, and the clinicians should be conservative, particularly when considering multilevel decompression in aged patients with comorbid conditions that might increase the surgical risk.

EVIDENCE-BASED POINTS

- *NSAIDs should be used with caution, as in OA.*
- *Nonsurgical therapies should be offered first; surgery is reserved for patients in intractable pain whose health dose not preclude operation.*

Atlas SJ et al: Surgical and nonsurgical management of lumbar spinal stenosis: four year outcomes from the Maine lumbar spine study. Spine 2000;25:556. [PMID: 10749631]

Amundsen T et al: Lumbar spinal stenosis: conservative or surgical management? A prospective 10-year study. Spine 2000;25: 1424. [PMID: not available]

(These studies support the use of conservative therapy initially, with surgery as a potentially effective option for patients refractory to conservative care.)

GOUT

ESSENTIALS OF DIAGNOSIS

- *Acute onset of monoarticular or polyarticular joint inflammation.*
- *Lower extremity predominance in early years.*
- *Presentations often atypical in older persons.*
- *Synovial fluid analysis is important to confirm diagnosis and exclude septic arthritis.*

General Considerations

Gout is caused by deposition of uric acid crystals in the synovium and other tissues. Chronic uric acid overload leads to microtophi, macrotophi, and acute attacks of synovitis. Premenopausal women rarely have gout, but its incidence in women rises after menopause. Polyarticular and upper extremity attacks are more prevalent in elderly persons.

Clinical Findings

A. SYMPTOMS & SIGNS

An acute attack of gouty arthritis usually occurs in the lower extremity, especially the first metatarsophalangeal (MTP) joint, midfoot, ankle, and knee. First attacks are usually abrupt and monarticular, with rapid appearance of joint swelling, tenderness, pain with motion, and erythema. Near the inflamed joint, there may be tendinitis, bursitis, and soft tissue edema.

Upper extremity attacks usually appear in the wrist, elbow, or small joints of the hands. Isolated bursitis, particularly of the olecranon or prepatellar bursae, can be seen. Acute attacks may be precipitated by trauma, binge alcohol drinking, medications that alter uric acid levels (eg, thiazide diuretics), surgery, or acute medical illness. The attack typically lasts for several days to a week or 2 and then resolves, even if untreated. With time, attacks become more frequent and are more likely to be polyarticular and to involve the upper extremity. In elderly people, the first attack may be polyarticular with multiple inflamed joints in all 4 extremities.

B. Physical Examination

Physical examination reveals erythema, warmth, swelling, and tenderness of the affected joint, with marked pain on range of motion of the joint. Pitting edema and tenosynovitis may be seen in the vicinity of the inflamed joint. Tophi may be found near the joints at risk, embedded in the olecranon or prepatellar bursae, or in the ears. The patient may be febrile from acute gout.

C. Laboratory Findings

Chronic hyperuricemia suggests that a person is at risk for gout but does not establish that the current symptoms are from gout. Serum uric acid levels can be normal at the time of a gout attack and are not helpful at the time of an acute attack. Sedimentation rate and C-reactive protein (CRP) may be elevated because of inflammation but do not differentiate acute gout from other causes of joint inflammation.

D. Imaging Studies

Radiographs will often show a joint effusion. Tophi can be seen as hazy shadows near the joint that may be stippled with calcification. An erosion of the bony cortex with an encircling lip of bone is very suspicious for a gouty tophus. As contrasted with other types of inflammatory arthritis, the periarticular bone density and the articular cartilage are usually well preserved.

Synovial fluid analysis should be performed whenever feasible to confirm the presence of monosodium urate crystals and to exclude septic arthritis. In acute gout, the synovial fluid is usually cloudy, with a synovial fluid WBC count in the inflammatory range (2000–75,000/ mm^3). Occasionally, the synovial fluid WBC count is > 100,000/mm^3, which is in the range normally associated with septic arthritis. Because gout and septic arthritis can coexist, it is prudent to treat with intravenous antibiotics while awaiting cultures when the synovial fluid WBC count is in the septic range. Occasionally, the fluid will contain so many suspended urate crystals that it may appear white and chalky, sometimes called "gout milk." Under polarized light microscopy, monosodium urate crystals are lance shaped, often the size of a WBC or larger, and strongly negatively birefringent. To perform polarized light microscopy on the biopsy tissue, the specimen should be preserved in 100% ethanol. When the urate crystal is parallel to the direction of polarization, it will appear yellow; when perpendicular, it will appear blue. Synovial biopsy is sometimes performed to rule out chronic infection.

Differential Diagnosis

When gout presents as an acute monarticular arthritis, pseudogout, infection, and hemarthrosis should be considered, particularly when there is no history of gout and a joint other than the MTP is involved. Gout does not usually affect the shoulders, hips, or spine, and pain in these locations should lead to consideration of another diagnosis. A polyarticular presentation may suggest calcium pyrophosphate deposition, rheumatoid arthritis (RA), or another polyarticular arthritis. Synovial fluid analysis will often be necessary to make a diagnosis.

Treatment

The acute attack can be aborted by NSAIDs, colchicine, or corticosteroids. Choice of agent will depend on patient comorbidities and risk profile.

Any NSAID can be effective if given in anti-inflammatory doses. Indomethacin is not well tolerated by older adults and is best avoided. There are few data on COX-2 selective NSAIDs or injectable NSAIDs in acute gout. The risk of NSAID gastropathy, worsening renal function, and fluid retention is significant in older adults, and corticosteroids may be preferable.

Colchicine in a dosage of 0.6 mg orally every 2 h is often recommended, but this regimen is not well tolerated by older adults because of frequent abdominal cramping and diarrhea. Colchicine, 0.6 mg orally every 4–12 h, is less effective but better tolerated. Other potential adverse effects of colchicine include bone marrow suppression, neuropathy, and myopathy, with increased risk in patients with renal insufficiency. Intravenous colchicine should not be used because of uncommon, but potentially fatal, toxicity.

Prednisone, 35 mg daily tapered to zero over 7–14 days, is generally effective and safe but can induce hyperglycemia or psychiatric symptoms. Methylprednisolone, 30 mg intravenously daily with subsequent taper, can be substituted in patients who cannot take oral medications. Intra-articular corticosteroids are ideal for attacks of monarticular in medium to large joints after septic arthritis has been ruled out. Depot methylprednisolone, 80 mg into the knee or 40 mg into the wrist, ankle, or elbow, is usually effective.

Prophylaxis of future attacks should be discussed with patients who have had acute gouty attacks because the risk of recurrence is high. Some patients who have had only 1 attack or have modifiable risk factors such as thiazide diuretic use can reasonably be monitored with watchful waiting.

Colchicine, 0.6 mg daily or twice daily, can provide protection against acute gout attacks but is generally not used as a first-line agent. Chronic NSAID use may also provide prophylaxis, with the usual cautions and contraindications.

Uric acid-lowering therapy with allopurinol or a uricosuric agent is generally preferred as a prophylactic approach over chronic colchicine or NSAID use. NSAIDs, colchicine, or prednisone should be given for a short duration when uric acid-lowering agents are begun, because initiation of therapy may precipitate an acute attack of gout.

Allopurinol inhibits xanthine oxidase, thus preventing formation of uric acid. It is equally efficacious in overproducers and underexcretors of uric acid. The initial dose is based on renal function (Table 26–4). Ideally, the dose is increased every 1–2 mo until the serum uric acid is < 6.0 mg/dL, but this may not be prudent in all older people. Potential adverse effects of allopurinol include rash, fever, cytopenias, dyspepsia, granulomatous hepatitis, and vasculitis. The potentially serious allopurinol hypersensitivity syndrome is characterized by rash, hepatitis, eosinophilia, and renal insufficiency. Allopurinol can potentiate the effect of warfarin, theophylline, and azathioprine.

Uricosurics can also be used and are less toxic than allopurinol. Most gout patients are underexcretors of urate, so uricosurics are theoretically sound treatments. However, they are not very effective in patients with a GFR < 60 mL/min or in patients with tophaceous gout. Their efficacy is also reduced by low-dose aspirin

therapy. They are contraindicated if the patient has had uric acid renal calculi, and the patient must drink fluids liberally to prevent stone formation. Thus, few elderly patients are good candidates for uricosuric therapy. It is considered in patients who have demonstrated intolerance of allopurinol and in the occasional patient with severe tophaceous gout whose impressive uric acid burden necessitates treatment with both allopurinol and a uricosuric. Treatment options include probenecid, 250 mg twice daily, or sulfinpyrazone, 50 mg twice daily, with gradual escalation of the dose until serum uric acid is < 6.0 mg/dL.

EVIDENCE-BASED POINTS

- *In gout patients on uric-acid lowering therapy, achieving sustained lowering of the serum uric acid to $\leq$ 6 mg/dL will permit better clearance of existing urate crystals and provide better protection against future gout attacks.*

Li-Yu J et al: Treatment of chronic gout. Can we determine when urate stores are depleted enough to prevent gout? J Rheumatol 2001;28:577. [PMID: 11296962] (Patients who achieved serum uric acid levels of $\leq$ 6 mg/dL for more than 12 mo had fewer attacks of gout and were more likely to have cleared their knee synovial fluid of urate crystals.)

CALCIUM PYROPHOSPHATE DIHYDRATE DEPOSITION DISEASE

ESSENTIALS OF DIAGNOSIS

- *Recognition of the varied clinical expressions.*
- *Demonstration of calcium pyrophosphate dihydrate crystals in joint fluid or on joint radiographs.*

General Considerations

The typical patient is a woman older than 60. The signs and symptoms of calcium pyrophosphate dihydrate (CPPD) disease vary with the clinical expression of the disease and include pseudogout (acute monarticular arthritis), pseudo-OA (gradual loss of articular cartilage

Table 26–4. Initial dose of allopurinol according to renal function.

Creatinine clearance (mL/min)	Allopurinol dosage
100	300 mg daily
80	250 mg daily
60	200 mg daily
40	150 mg daily
20	100 mg daily
10	100 mg every other day
0	100 mg twice weekly

without apparent joint inflammation), pseudorheumatoid (symmetric, polyarticular inflammatory arthritis), pseudoneuropathic (rapid destruction of one or several joints), and asymptomatic chondrocalcinosis.

Clinical Findings

A. SYMPTOMS & SIGNS

In pseudogout, acute attacks of monarticular arthritis typically occur in the shoulders, wrists, small joints of the hands, and the knees and appear similar to gout. The patient with pseudo-OA has symptoms and signs of OA. Underlying CPPD disease should be suspected when the involved joint is not usually involved by primary OA, if CPPD crystals are found on arthrocentesis, or if chondrocalcinosis is seen on radiographs. Pseudorheumatoid patients have morning stiffness, joint swelling, and gradual joint damage in a distribution similar to RA. Pseudoneuropathic patients report monarticular or oligoarticular joint pain and impressive joint destruction on radiographs but lack the neurological deficits needed to diagnose a neuropathic arthropathy.

B. SERUM TESTING

Hyperparathyroidism, hemochromatosis, hypothyroidism, amyloidosis, hypomagnesemia, and hypophosphatasia are risk factors for CPPD disease, but in most patients no underlying cause is found. Serum testing is not useful to confirm or rule out CPPD arthropathy.

C. IMAGING STUDIES

Radiographs may show features of OA, RA, or neuropathic arthropathy according to the type of presentation. Chondrocalcinosis is caused by deposition of calcium in the articular cartilage or fibrocartilage. Calcification of articular cartilage can be seen in any joint. Calcification of fibrocartilage is best seen in the menisci of the knee, triangular cartilage of the wrist, symphysis pubis, and intervertebral disks.

D. SPECIAL TESTS

Arthrocentesis reveals weakly birefringent blunt rods that are blue when parallel to the axis of polarization and yellow when perpendicular (the opposite of gout). Synovial fluid WBC counts can be > 100,000/mm^3 in attacks of pseudogout, as they can in gout, thus raising concerns about infection.

Differential Diagnosis

Because CPPD disease has such a wide variety of presentations, it mimics many other conditions, including gout, RA, OA, and neuropathic arthropathy. Synovial fluid analysis is indicated when CPPD disease is in the differential diagnosis.

Treatment

Acute attacks of synovitis are treated the same as acute attacks of gout. NSAIDs and daily colchicine can be used for prophylaxis. Unlike gout, there is no medication to remove crystals from the affected joints.

RHEUMATOID ARTHRITIS

ESSENTIALS OF DIAGNOSIS

- *Symmetric, polyarticular inflammatory arthritis with a characteristic pattern of joint involvement.*
- *Evidence of inflammation by history, examination, and laboratory tests.*

General Considerations

New-onset RA can be seen in older adults. Differentiating RA from the pseudorheumatoid presentation of CPPD or from polymyalgia rheumatica (PMR) can be difficult. RA is a systemic disease and can cause weight loss or fever. Potential extra-articular disease manifestations are listed in Table 26–5.

Clinical Findings

A. SYMPTOMS & SIGNS

The patient complains of inflammatory joint symptoms: The joints feel better with use and worse with rest; the joints stiffen with inactivity. Morning stiffness is a prominent complaint, and it takes at least 1 h for the joints to loosen up. The worst time of the day is generally several hours before and after awakening. The patient reports pain, stiffness, and swelling in a fairly

Table 26–5. Extra-articular manifestations of rheumatoid arthritis.

Rheumatoid nodules
Interstitial lung disease
Pleuropericarditis
Sjögren's syndrome
Scleritis/episcleritis/corneal melt
Digital infarcts
Vasculitis
Felty's syndrome
Lower extremity ulcers
Amyloidosis

symmetric pattern, potentially involving the PIP and MCP joints of the hands, wrists, elbows, shoulders, temporomandibular joints, cervical spine, hips, knees, ankles, and MTPs. The disease can occasionally be more asymmetric and oligoarticular (involving 2–4 joints) early in the course, but symptoms confined to 1–2 joints are not typical of RA. Patients with wrist synovitis may complain of numbness and tingling in a median nerve distribution caused by inflamed synovium in the carpal tunnel.

B. PHYSICAL EXAMINATION

Physical examination may show warmth, synovial thickening, joint tenderness, loss of hand grip strength, pain with joint motion, and loss of range of motion. Rheumatoid nodules, if present, can be seen just distal to the olecranon, over the extensor surfaces of the fingers and toes, overlying the Achilles tendon, and embedded in a chronically swollen olecranon bursa. In a patient with long-standing, poorly controlled synovitis, joint damage accumulates: ulnar deviation and subluxation of the fingers, volar subluxation of the wrist, loss of extension of the elbows, loss of abduction in the shoulders, valgus angulation of the knees, valgus angulation of the hindfoot, pes planus, plantar subluxation of the metatarsal heads, and atlantoaxial instability in the cervical spine.

RF is seen in ~80% of patients. The prevalence of false-positive RF is high in elderly people, and positive RF can be seen in chronic inflammatory states other than RA. Therefore, the presence of serum RF does not by itself confirm a diagnosis of RA and absence does not exclude it. Evidence of an acute-phase response (eg, elevated sedimentation rate, elevated CRP, low serum albumin) is almost always present. The complete blood count will usually show anemia of chronic disease, which is often normocytic but can be microcytic. Patients with Felty's syndrome will demonstrate neutropenia.

C. IMAGING STUDIES

Radiographs can be normal in the early stages. Periarticular osteopenia and joint effusions are seen initially, followed by joint space narrowing and periarticular erosions as the disease progresses. Radionuclide bone scans and joint MRI can also show the synovitis but are seldom needed for diagnosis.

D. SYNOVIAL BIOPSY

Synovial fluid is cloudy-yellow, with synovial fluid WBC count in the inflammatory range (2000–75,000/mm^3). Joint debris can be seen, but analysis for crystals is negative. Synovial biopsy shows chronic inflammation that is indistinguishable from other types of chronic synovium-based arthritis, such as psoriatic arthritis or reactive arthritis. Biopsy material may be available from joint or carpal tunnel surgery but is seldom needed to establish the diagnosis.

Differential Diagnosis

The differential diagnosis can be challenging in elderly people. RA may present with proximal symptoms, mimicking PMR. Conversely, PMR can sometimes present with some distal inflammatory changes. Polyarticular gout, pseudorheumatoid CPPD disease, psoriatic arthritis, systemic vasculitis, systemic lupus erythematosus (SLE), dermatomyositis, polymyositis, bacterial endocarditis, and paraneoplastic arthritis can mimic RA. Diagnosis is based on the overall clinical picture, laboratory studies, and synovial fluid analysis. When the diagnosis is in question, rheumatology consultation is warranted.

Treatment

Prednisone, 15–20 mg daily, usually provides satisfactory short-term control of symptoms and can be used as a bridge to more definitive treatment. Such doses are not safe for long-term use and should be weaned to < 10 mg daily as quickly as possible. Intra-articular injection of corticosteroids can provide relief in the injected joint, but the pattern of joint involvement is usually polyarticular, requiring systemic therapy.

NSAIDs provide some relief of pain and inflammation but do not protect against joint damage. Only a minority of patients—those with very mild disease—are candidates for NSAID monotherapy. NSAIDs can be used for analgesia in conjunction with more effective disease-modifying antirheumatic drugs (DMARDs). DMARDs are best supervised by a consulting rheumatologist. Methotrexate is the disease-modifying agent of choice for most patients with RA, dosed at 7.5–15 mg orally or subcutaneously every week. Potential adverse effects include alopecia, mucositis, diarrhea, cytopenias, increased hepatic transaminases, opportunistic infection, and pneumonitis. Folic acid, 1 mg daily, helps prevent adverse effects of methotrexate. For refractory patients or those intolerant of methotrexate, one can consider leflunomide, sulfasalazine, etanercept, intravenous infliximab, or combination therapy. Hydroxychloroquine is often used in combination with other immunosuppressives but rarely provides sufficient disease control by itself. Tumor necrosis factor (TNF) blockers, including etanercept, infliximab, and adalimumab, are potent inhibitors of rheumatoid synovitis. Infection is the main risk with these agents. Etanercept and adalimumab are given by subcutaneous injection, and infliximab is administered intravenously.

Joint replacement or fusion can provide pain relief for a severely damaged joint. Synovectomy of an individual joint can be done at the time of reconstructive surgery but contributes little to overall disease control because of the systemic nature of the disease.

EVIDENCE-BASED POINTS

- *Combinations of oral DMARDs provide better disease control than single DMARD therapy.*
- *The new TNF-blocking agents are quite expensive but generally more effective than the oral DMARDs.*
- *Aggressive treatment of RA provides relief of symptoms, prevents joint damage, and may prolong the life of a rheumatoid patient.*

Choi HK et al: Methotrexate and mortality in patients with rheumatoid arthritis: a prospective study. Lancet 2002;359:1173. [PMID: 11955534] (Treatment with methotrexate was associated with a reduction in the cardiovascular and noncardiovascular mortality in RA patients treated with methotrexate compared with RA patients who did not receive methotrexate. Similar reductions were not seen with other oral DMARDs.)

Genovese MC et al: Etanercept versus methotrexate in patients with early rheumatoid arthritis: two-year radiographic and clinical outcomes. Arthritis Rheum 2002;46:1443. [PMID: 12115173] (Patients treated with etanercept showed statistically significantly fewer radiographic erosions and better scores on the disability section of the Health Assessment Questionnaire.)

O'Dell JR et al: Treatment of rheumatoid arthritis with methotrexate and hydroxychloroquine, methotrexate and sulfasalazine, or a combination of the three medications: results of a two-year, randomized, double-blind, placebo controlled trial. Arthritis Rheum 2002;46:1164. [PMID: not available] (Provides additional evidence that the combination of methotrexate, sulfasalazine, and hydroxychloroquine is an effective and well-tolerated combination.)

POLYMYALGIA RHEUMATICA

ESSENTIALS OF DIAGNOSIS

- *Characteristic history.*
- *Prompt response to corticosteroid treatment.*
- *Blood tests usually show systemic inflammation but can be normal.*

- *The typical patient is a white woman approximately 70 years old.*
- *Polymyalgia rheumatica is uncommon in blacks.*
- *Fifteen to 20% of patients with polymyalgia rheumatica will have concomitant giant cell arteritis (temporal arteritis).*

Clinical Findings

A. SYMPTOMS & SIGNS

Patients reports morning stiffness and pain in the neck, upper back, shoulders, upper arms, low back, hips and proximal thighs, with difficulty arising from bed. The pain can be difficult to localize. Distal joints are often spared, although some patients report swelling and stiffness in the hands. Because PMR is a systemic inflammatory disease, patients may report fever, fatigue, malaise, anorexia, and weight loss. Patients with coexisting temporal arteritis may report headache, scalp tenderness, jaw claudication, and visual loss. Physical examination reveals stiffness and pain on motion of the shoulders. Occasionally, synovitis is seen in distal joints. Signs of temporal arteritis may be present.

Blood testing reveals evidence of systemic inflammation, including increased ESR, increased CRP, anemia of chronic disease, and low serum albumin. In up to 25% of cases, the laboratory testing can be normal, necessitating diagnosis on clinical grounds alone.

B. IMAGING STUDIES

Imaging is most useful in confirming alternative diagnoses, but one must be careful because the typical patient at risk for PMR is also at risk for a variety of degenerative diseases. MRI of the shoulders in PMR will often show subacromial bursitis but should not be considered a standard diagnostic study.

Treatment

Empiric treatment with prednisone, 20 mg daily, almost always gives prompt relief of PMR symptoms. Because the physical examination findings can be nonspecific and the laboratory testing can be normal, an empiric trial of prednisone can be useful in confirming suspected PMR. The prednisone trial must be interpreted with caution because many other diseases, including lymphoma and infection, may initially respond to prednisone. A rapid, complete alleviation of symptoms after prednisone treatment is evidence in favor of PMR. A complete lack of response to prednisone, 20 mg daily, essentially rules out PMR, and a partial but inadequate response should spur a search for an alternative diagnosis. Prednisone can be tapered to the lowest tolerated dose. Because many patients have risk factors for osteoporosis, most will require concomitant treatment with calcium, 1000–1500 mg daily, vitamin D, and a bisphosphonate. Relapses during prednisone taper are common, and patients will usually require corticosteroid treatment for 1–5 years. Patients who lack symptoms of temporal arteritis do not need to undergo a biopsy because the yield is low. Patients with symptoms of temporal arteritis in addition to PMR should be started on prednisone, 20–60 mg daily, and scheduled for a temporal artery biopsy within 1 week.

Differential Diagnosis

Cervical and lumbar spondylosis, lumbar canal stenosis, OA of the acromioclavicular joints and hips, and subacromial impingement with subdeltoid bursitis or rotator cuff disease are common in this age group, and the overlap of symptoms can make accurate diagnosis difficult. One must be careful in interpreting history, physical, laboratory, and imaging data to avoid errors. RA can present with proximal symptoms that may appear clinically similar to PMR.

Many of the immunosuppressives used in RA have been tried in PMR. Unfortunately, no steroid-sparing strategy has proved to be consistently effective. Immunosuppressives used in RA are often considered in patients who must reduce their dependence on corticosteroids.

GIANT CELL ARTERITIS

ESSENTIALS OF DIAGNOSIS

- New-onset headache, jaw claudication, scalp tenderness, loss of vision.
- Forty to 60% of patients will report concomitant symptoms of polymyalgia rheumatica.
- Acute-phase reactants (erythrocyte sedimentation rate, C-reactive protein) are usually elevated.
- Temporal artery biopsy is often diagnostic.

General Considerations

Giant cell arteritis (GCA) has significant overlap with PMR. As with PMR, the typical patient is a white woman of 70 years. Females outnumber males 2 to 1. PMR is uncommonly seen in blacks and is not seen in persons younger than 50. Blindness is the most feared complication, but it can usually be prevented by prompt corticosteroid treatment. Involvement of the aorta and proximal large arteries is seen in 10–15% of patients.

Clinical Findings

A. SYMPTOMS & SIGNS

The onset of symptoms can be either sudden or gradual. Patients complain of headache, often with scalp tenderness. Jaw claudication and visual loss are signs of ischemia. Amaurosis fugax is an ominous symptom and, if caused by GCA, predicts a significant risk of blindness. Patients may have symptoms of systemic inflammation, including fatigue, malaise, weight loss, and fever. The patient may also have symptoms and signs of PMR. Examination may reveal scalp tenderness; the temporal artery may be beaded, thickened, or tender. Retinal examination may reveal ischemia. Aortic and proximal large vessel involvement may manifest as aortic regurgitation, diminished brachial or radial pulses, or bruits.

Anemia of chronic disease and increased platelet counts are common. ESR and CRP are usually elevated, and the ESR may be > 100 mm/h. If clinical suspicion is high, a normal or minimally elevated ESR does not rule out the diagnosis. Autoantibody testing is usually negative.

Chest radiograph may show a thoracic aortic aneurysm. Contrast angiography is reserved for patients with potentially operable large vessel disease. MRI of the aorta and great vessels can be useful to diagnose large vessel involvement noninvasively.

Temporal artery biopsy should be performed to confirm the diagnosis, given the toxicities associated with empiric treatment. Corticosteroids are often started before harvesting of the artery, and the biopsy will still be diagnostic if obtained within 2 weeks of the initiation of treatment. Higher yields are obtained if the artery undergoing biopsy is abnormal on examination and is 3–5 cm in length. False-negative rates of a unilateral biopsy vary but are generally ~10%. The false-negative rate falls to < 5% if a negative biopsy is followed by immediate biopsy of the contralateral artery.

Differential Diagnosis

Patients with tension or vascular headache generally have more chronic symptoms. Acute headache or scalp pain may be seen in meningitis, primary or metastatic tumor, cervical spondylosis, glaucoma, herpes zoster, or adverse effects of medication.

Treatment

Patients with visual symptoms are treated with prednisone, 40–60 mg daily. Methylprednisolone, 500 mg intravenously twice daily, is sometimes used for patients believed to be at risk for imminent visual loss. High-dose corticosteroids are unlikely to restore vision once blindness has occurred. Prednisone, 20–40 mg daily, is usually sufficient for patients without visual symptoms. The dose can be increased to 40–60 mg/day if the presenting symptoms do not respond to the initial prednisone dose in 3–5 days. Loss of vision after the initiation of corticosteroid treatment is uncommon. The corticosteroid dose is tapered by 10–15% every 2 weeks until 10 mg of prednisone daily. Thereafter, the prednisone dose can be reduced by 1 mg/day every month. Potential adverse effects include weight gain, cushingoid body habitus, ocular cataracts, glucose intolerance, fluid retention, osteoporosis, proximal muscle weakness, pseudotumor cerebri, psychosis, and infection. ESR and CRP may be useful to follow disease activity; however, laboratory testing should be interpreted in the context of the history and physical, and one should not overtreat mild elevations of the sedimentation rate in asymptomatic patients. Relapses are common during prednisone taper, particularly during the first 18 mo. Most patients require at least 2 years of corticosteroid treatment. Given the risk of high-dose corticosteroids in a population that is typically elderly, white, and female, a steroid-sparing immunosuppressive with activity against GCA is sorely needed. Methotrexate as a steroid-sparing agent in GCA has had mixed results in randomized controlled trials. Given the importance of TNF in granuloma formation, anti-TNF therapies such as etanercept, infliximab, and adalimumab appear promising but not proven.

SEPTIC ARTHRITIS

ESSENTIAL OF DIAGNOSIS

- *Usually monarticular, sometimes polyarticular, intense joint inflammation.*
- *Arthrocentesis before administration of intravenous antibiotics.*

General Considerations

Joints become infected by hematogenous spread from a distant site, local spread of nearby osteomyelitis, or direct inoculation of the joint from trauma or a medical procedure. Risk factors include inflammatory arthritis such as RA, diabetes mellitus, advanced age, presence of a prosthetic joint, and weakened immune function.

Clinical Findings

A. SYMPTOMS & SIGNS

The infected joint is usually red, warm, swollen, and intensely painful with any movement. A fever is not necessarily present, especially in the elderly.

B. LABORATORY FINDINGS

The patient may have an increased WBC count in the peripheral blood and an increased ESR, but normal laboratory tests do not rule out septic arthritis. Blood cultures are positive in approximately 50% of patients.

C. IMAGING STUDIES

Radiographs show a joint effusion; with time, there is destruction of the joint demonstrated by loss of articular cartilage. Suspected septic arthritis of the sternoclavicular joint is best imaged by CT. A transthoracic or transesophageal echocardiogram is useful to search for valvular vegetations of bacterial endocarditis.

D. SPECIAL TESTS

Arthrocentesis and synovial fluid analysis is essential. The synovial fluid should be analyzed for cell count with differential, crystal analysis, Gram's stain, and culture. When the joint is infected by common gram-positive and gram-negative bacteria, the synovial fluid usually reveals a WBC count of > 100,000/mm^3 with > 80% polymorphonuclear neutrophils. Occasionally, the synovial fluid WBC count will be lower, particularly early in the course of infection, and lower WBC counts do not rule out infection if there is a reasonable clinical suspicion. Infection with opportunistic or atypical organisms such as *Mycobacteria* may be associated with synovial fluid WBC counts of 5000–50,000/mm^3. Synovial fluid culture usually reveals gram-positive organisms, particularly *Staphylococcus*. In the elderly, gram-negative infections are more likely to occur. The presence of urate or CPPD crystals does not rule out infection, and if the synovial fluid WBC count is > 100,000/mm, it is prudent to treat the patient for septic arthritis until cultures are complete.

Differential Diagnosis

Crystal-induced arthritis and hemarthrosis may be difficult to differentiate from septic arthritis. Polyarticular arthritis can be seen in gonococcus, Lyme disease, and bacterial endocarditis. Synovial fluid analysis is essential if septic arthritis is in the differential diagnosis.

Treatment

Empiric antibiotic treatment should be instituted before culture results. If the Gram's stain is positive, therapy is guided by the result. Oxacillin is recommended for initial therapy of community-acquired gram-positive infections and vancomycin for patients with indwelling venous catheters or suspected hospital-acquired infection. Gram-negative infections should be treated with a first-generation cephalosporin or an antipseudomonal penicillin with an aminoglycoside. If the Gram's stain is negative, the patient should receive coverage for clinically suspected organisms. Gram-negative infection is more common in the elderly, and antibiotic coverage should be appropriately broad. Antibiotic therapy should be tailored to the culture and sensitivity results and the clinical course. Home antibiotic therapy for 2–6 weeks is usually necessary, depending on the severity of the initial infection and the response to treatment.

Septic arthritis is an infection in a closed space akin to an abscess, and drainage is necessary to eradicate the infection. Needle aspiration every 1–2 days is sufficient for small to medium-size joints that are easily aspirated. Surgical arthrotomy is usually recommended for the hip and is indicated for any joint in which the purulent fluid is too thick to drain with a needle. Arthrotomy is also recommended if needle aspiration does not document a falling synovial fluid WBC count and conversion of joint cultures to negative. It may be necessary to remove a prosthetic joint or foreign body to achieve sterilization.

SJÖGREN'S SYNDROME

 ESSENTIALS OF DIAGNOSIS

- Dry eyes and mouth.
- Blood tests suggesting inflammatory autoimmune disease.
- Confirmatory ophthalmology examination or salivary gland biopsy.

General Considerations

Sjögren's syndrome is caused by autoimmune attack on the glands that make saliva and tears. Sjögren's syndrome can occur in isolation (primary Sjögren's) or can accompany another autoimmune disease, usually SLE, RA, or scleroderma (secondary Sjögren's). Other autoimmune phenomena may be associated, including pneumonitis and vasculitis.

Clinical Findings

A. Symptoms & Signs

The patient reports gradually worsening dryness of the eyes and mouth (keratoconjunctivitis sicca and xerosto-

mia). Loss of tears can lead to scratching and infection of the cornea. Loss of saliva can lead to accelerated dental caries and periodontal disease. There may be parotid gland enlargement and dryness of other mucosal surfaces such as the pharynx, trachea, and vagina. Patients may experience pneumonitis or vasculitis. Patients with pneumonitis report gradually worsening dyspnea and cough. Vasculitis can present as a purpuric rash with lower extremity predominance or multiple peripheral neuropathies (mononeuritis multiplex). Some patients experience a stocking-distribution sensory neuropathy, with tingling in the feet and neuropathic pain. In secondary Sjögren's syndrome, there will also be symptoms and signs of the primary connective tissue disease.

B. Laboratory Tests

ANA is positive in ~80% of patients, and additional autoantibody testing reveals anti-SSA (Ro) or anti-SSB (La) in 50–80%. RF is positive in 90% of patients and does not necessarily indicate coexisting RA. Polyclonal hyperglobulinemia and increased ESR are common.

Slit-lamp examination with rose bengal or equivalent stain can reveal the ocular consequences of chronically dry eyes. To test for ocular dryness, one can place a filter paper on the palpebral conjunctiva and measure the extent of wetness at 5 min (the Schirmer test); 5 mm of wetness or less is diagnostic of deficient tear production. Tests of salivary gland secretion are also available but less commonly used.

Biopsy of the minor salivary glands of the lip can be obtained under local anesthesia. The presence of focal lymphocytic infiltrates with overlying normal mucosa is consistent with Sjögren's syndrome.

Differential Diagnosis

Dry mucosal surfaces can be caused by aging or medications and parotid gland enlargement by infectious parotitis, lymphoma, and sarcoidosis. When other autoimmune phenomena are present, the differential diagnosis includes lupus and RA. Fibromyalgia is commonly seen in patients with primary Sjögren's; one must take care not to attribute the fibromyalgia symptoms to lupus or RA. The presence of widespread myofascial tenderness supports a diagnosis of fibromyalgia.

Treatment

Treatment is largely symptomatic. Liberal use of artificial tears with lubricating ointment overnight for the eyes and water and sugar-free beverages for the mouth often provides some relief. Proper oral hygiene practices and frequent visits to the dentist can prevent gum disease and loss of teeth.

Pilocarpine, 5 mg 4 times a day, or cevimeline, 30 mg 3 times a day, can be used to stimulate production of saliva. Secretogogues are not generally effective for dry eyes. Adverse effects can include sweating, flushing, diarrhea, bronchospasm, and increased intra-ocular pressure.

Immunosuppressants cannot save the lacrimal and salivary glands from autoimmune attack and are generally not used for that purpose. Hydroxychloroquine is sometimes used to treat Sjögren's-related arthralgia. True synovitis suggests secondary Sjögren's in the setting of RA or SLE and is treated accordingly. In primary Sjögren's, corticosteroids and other immunosuppressants are reserved for treatment of autoimmune attack on nonexocrine organs or systemic vasculitis. Patients with autoimmune attack confined to exocrine glands can still have impressive laboratory phenomena, including high ESR, anemia of chronic disease, positive ANA, and positive RF. One should not overreact to the laboratory phenomena and reserve immunosuppression for potentially reversible organ-threatening disease.

OTHER VASCULITIDES

ESSENTIALS OF DIAGNOSIS

- *Ischemia or hemorrhage in end-organs.*
- *Symptoms and laboratory evidence of systemic inflammation.*
- *Patterns of organ involvement, laboratory testing, and biopsy allow more specific diagnoses.*

General Considerations

Vasculitis is often suspected when a patient appears to have a systemic, inflammatory disease with ischemia or hemorrhage in a variety of end-organs. Certain physical examination signs, such as palpable purpura, cutaneous ulcers, or mononeuritis multiplex, are suspicious for the presence of vasculitis. Diagnosis of a particular type of vasculitis often requires a carefully performed history, physical, laboratory testing, imaging, and directed biopsy. Characteristics of the specific vasculitides are summarized in Table 26–6.

Clinical Findings

A. SYMPTOMS & SIGNS

Many patients will report nonspecific symptoms of chronic systemic inflammation, including fatigue, malaise, weight loss, and fever. The other symptoms and signs will differ according to the pattern of organ involvement. Involvement of the skin can present as palpable purpura, usually on the lower extremities and buttocks, or as well-demarcated ischemic ulcers. Peripheral nerve involvement is usually manifested as mononeuritis multiplex. Abdominal pain and bloody stool suggests gastrointestinal involvement. Lung involvement usually presents with dyspnea and cough. Brain or meningeal involvement is suggested by headache, seizures, altered consciousness, or focal neurological deficits. Myocardial involvement usually manifests as heart failure; symptoms of angina can be seen in coronary involvement by GCA but are rare in other vasculitides.

There is usually evidence of an acute-phase response, with increased ESR and CRP, anemia of chronic disease, increased platelet count, low serum albumin, and increased complement. Low serum complement can be seen in lupus and cryoglobulinemia. Peripheral blood eosinophilia is suggestive of Churg-Strauss vasculitis, but mild eosinophilia can be seen in other vasculitides. In the vasculitides listed in Table 26–6, ANA is usually negative, but RF is occasionally positive. Vasculitis associated with a strongly positive ANA raises concerns about lupus, Sjögren's syndrome, or RA. Antineutrophil cytoplasmic antibody (ANCA) screening is usually performed by immunofluorescence, followed by more specific enzyme immunoassay, and is most useful when

Table 26–6. Characteristics of selected vasculitides.

Diagnosis	Vessel size	Pattern of organ involvement	Diagnostic testing
Hypersensitivity	Postcapillary venule	Skin	Biopsy: leukocytoclasis
Microscopic polyangiitis	Small artery/arteriole	Skin, kidney, peripheral nerve, CNS, lung	p-ANCA, biopsy
Polyarteritis nodosa	Small–med artery	Skin, kidney, gut, peripheral nerve	Angiogram, biopsy
Wegener's granulomatosis	Small–med artery	Nose, sinuses, trachea, lung, eye, kidney	c-ANCA, biopsy
Churg-Strauss	Small–med artery	Skin, peripheral nerve, lung, heart, gut	Blood-tissue eosinophilia
Giant cell	Large artery	Head, aorta, upper extremities	Biopsy
Behçet's	Any, arteries and veins	Skin, CNS, eye, mouth, genitals, gut	Biopsy

CNS, central nervous system; ANCA; antineutrophil cytoplasmic antibody.

there is a clinical suspicion of Wegener's granulomatosis (WG) or microscopic polyangiitis (MPA). A c-ANCA pattern is seen with antibodies to proteinase 3 and is approximately 98% specific for WG; however, ANCA testing has low sensitivity and can be negative in WG patients with early disease or disease limited to the upper airway. A p-ANCA immunofluorescence pattern is seen with antibodies to myeloperoxidase and is suggestive of MPA, but it can also be seen in WG and nonvasculitic glomerular disease. High ANCA titers are more likely to be significant; low-titer positive results may be misleading and should be interpreted with caution. Patients with a clinical suspicion of polyarteritis nodosa (PAN) should be tested for antibodies to hepatitis B virus.

Plain radiographs may show pulmonary infiltrates, cardiac enlargement, or free abdominal air caused by a perforated viscus. Chest CT is more sensitive than radiography to reveal pulmonary involvement by vasculitis. Abdominal CT may reveal bowel wall edema or wedge-shaped renal infarcts. MRI of the brain is useful if there is evidence of central nervous system injury. Contrast angiograms of the renal and mesenteric arteries reveal stenoses, aneurysms, and poststenotic dilatation in patients with PAN. Contrast angiography is generally not used to diagnose WG, MPA, or hypersensitivity vasculitis because the inflamed vessels are usually too small to be seen on the angiogram.

Skin biopsy is usually performed if cutaneous vasculitis is suspected. In WG and MPA, kidney biopsy usually shows a pauci-immune glomerulonephritis; the renal biopsy does not usually directly confirm the presence of vasculitis but can be useful in excluding other causes of a pulmonary-renal syndrome, including SLE and Goodpasture's syndrome. Bronchoscopic lung biopsy does not usually provide enough tissue to confirm vasculitis but can be useful to rule out infection, malignancy, or sarcoidosis. Thoracoscopic-guided open lung biopsy is best when a definitive lung biopsy is desired, as in suspected WG, Churg-Strauss, or MPA. Endoscopic bowel biopsy is not generally useful in diagnosing vasculitis, but bowel removed at surgery should be carefully sectioned if vasculitis is clinically suspected. Sural nerve biopsy may reveal vasculitis of the vasa nervorum in patients with mononeuritis multiplex, but false-negative biopsies are common.

Nerve conduction studies can assist with differentiating mononeuritis multiplex from other causes of neurological symptoms in the extremities, including entrapment neuropathies, radiculopathies, or toxic/ metabolic neuropathies.

Differential Diagnosis

Conditions that can mimic vasculitis are summarized in Table 26–7.

Table 26–7. Differential diagnosis of vasculitis.

Bacterial endocarditis
Vascular infection: syphillis, mycotic aneurysm, infected vascular graft
Adverse effect of vasoconstrictor medications
Severe atherosclerosis
Cholesterol emboli
Buerger's disease (thromboangiitis obliterans)
Antiphosopholipid antibody syndrome
Thrombotic thrombocytopenic purpura
Scleroderma/CREST syndrome
Malignancy
Calciphylaxis
Hypereosinophilic syndrome
Atrophie blanche (livedoid vasculopathy)

CREST, calcinosis cutis, Raynaud's phenomenon, esophageal dysfunction, sclerodactyly, telangiectasia.

Treatment

Leukocytoclastic or hypersensitivity vasculitis confined to the skin (palpable purpura) can be treated by withdrawing the inciting antigen, if it can be identified. Cutaneous vasculitis associated with an acute viral infection will generally resolve as the patient recovers from the virus. Vasculitis that results from hypersensitivity to a medication is best treated by withdrawal of the medication. Chronic palpable purpura can be treated with colchicine, 0.6 mg once or twice daily, dapsone, or hydroxychloroquine. Systemic corticosteroids are often not indicated because the adverse effects can be more harmful than isolated cutaneous vasculitis.

Evidence of end-organ injury outside the skin necessitates treatment with prednisone, 1–1.5 mg/kg/day, with gradual taper over 6 mo. For significant threat to the lung, myocardium, nervous system, lung, or kidney, cyclophosphamide, 2–4 mg/kg/day, is given as a single morning daily dose. Potential toxicities of daily cytoxan include cytopenias, infection, hemorrhagic cystitis, alopecia, nausea, diarrhea, mucositis, and late malignancy. Patients should drink fluids liberally to protect the bladder from toxic metabolites. A CBC should be obtained every 1–2 weeks, and the cyclophosphamide dose should be lowered as necessary so that the WBC count does not fall below 3000/mm^3. Cyclophosphamide treatment is generally continued for 3 mo; patients who are doing well can then be switched to methotrexate, 12.5–15 mg/week. Azathioprine, 2 mg/kg/day, can substitute for methotrexate in patients with diminished renal function (serum creatinine > 1.8 mg/dL).

Osteoporosis & Hip Fractures

27

Manish Srivastava, MD, & Chad Deal, MD

ESSENTIALS OF DIAGNOSIS

- *In 1994, the World Health Organization established bone mineral density measurement criteria for the diagnosis of osteoporosis (Table 27–1).*
- *Osteoporosis is a systemic skeletal disease characterized by low bone mass and microarchitectural deterioration of the bone tissue, with a consequent increase in bone fragility and susceptibility to fracture.*
- *Osteoporosis is more common in women than in men, although the incidence among men is increasing.*
- *The prevalence of osteoporosis and osteoporotic fractures increases with age.*

General Considerations

According to the National Osteoporosis Foundation, in the United States in 2002, 32 million women and 12 million men older than 50 have either osteoporosis or low bone mass (defined as T ≤ 2.0 and ≤ 1.0, respectively). This number is expected to increase to 52 million by 2010. Of these, it is estimated that > 10 million people have osteoporosis, a figure that will rise to almost 12 million by 2010 and approximately 14 million by 2020 if additional measures are not taken to stem this disease. The prevalence of osteoporosis increases with age from 15% in women 50–59 years old to 70% in women 80 years old. The lifetime risk for fracture for a 50-year-old woman is 40–50%. A fracture is considered to be osteoporotic (fragility fracture) if it is due to relatively low trauma such as a fall from standing height or less, a force that in a young healthy adult would not be expected to cause a fracture. There is overwhelming evidence that the incidence of fracture in specific settings is closely linked to the prevalence of osteoporosis or low bone mass. In most populations, hip fracture incidence increases with age and typically peaks after age 85. With increasing life expectancy worldwide, the number of elderly individuals is increasing in every geo-graphic region. Because hip fracture incidence rates rise exponentially with age, this will result in increasing numbers of hip fractures. In 1990, there were an estimated 1.65 million hip fractures (1.2 million in women and 450,000 in men) worldwide, which is projected to increase to 6.3 million by the year 2050.

A. OSTEOPOROSIS IN WOMEN

Radiographic population surveys find that ~5% of 50- to 54-year-old white women have at least 1 prevalent radiographic vertebral fracture, and the proportion with a prevalent fracture rises to > 35% among women aged 80–85 years. The risk of an incident vertebral fracture on x-ray film is only about 0.5% in the next year in a 50-year-old white woman but increases to 2–3% per year by 80–85 years. Pelvic fractures and fractures of the proximal humerus and shaft–distal femur have an occurrence pattern that resembles that of hip fractures.

B. OSTEOPOROSIS IN MEN

There is growing awareness that osteoporosis in men is not rare, although its incidence is lower than in women. Thirty-three percent of all hip fractures worldwide occur in men. The risk factors for osteoporosis in men age 60 and older are low femoral neck bone mineral density (BMD), quadriceps weakness, low body weight, falls in the preceding year, and a history of fractures in the last 5 years. The Framingham Osteoporosis Study identified low baseline weight, weight loss, and cigarette smoking as risk factors for osteoporosis. In addition, low estradiol levels have been associated with vertebral fractures, whereas low testosterone level consistent with hypogonadism poses no significant increased risk for fracture. Age-related decline in testosterone level has been thought to play a role in decreased bone formation in elderly men.

Currently, there is no validated guideline for prevention or treatment of osteoporosis in men. Men with a history of fractures and those with known risk factors for low bone density should be targeted for prevention of osteoporosis and can be offered BMD measurement. However, the BMD threshold at which therapy should be started is unclear.

Lifestyle modifications, including increasing physical activity and cessation of smoking and alcohol, should be recommended to all men. Calcium and vitamin D sup-

Table 27–1. Diagnostic categories for osteoporosis in postmenopausal women based on World Health Organization Criteria.

Category	Definition by bone density
Normal	A value for BMD that is not > 1 SD below the young adult mean value.
Osteopenia	A value of BMD that lies between 1 and 2.5 SD below the young adult mean value.
Osteoporosis	A value for BMD that is > 2.5 SD below the young adult mean value.
Severe osteoporosis	A value for BMD > 2.5 SD or below the young adult mean in the presence of 1 or more fragility fractures.

BMD, bone mineral density.

plementation should be recommended for older men, although evidence is limited and conflicting.

The use of testosterone therapy in eugonadal men is controversial, and current data do not support any benefit associated with it. Testosterone replacement is appropriate only in the setting of proven hypogonadism in men with markedly low total testosterone levels. Currently, the roles of PTH, growth hormone, and raloxifene are being evaluated.

Clinical Findings

A. SIGNS & SYMPTOMS

Osteoporosis has no clinical manifestations until there is a fracture. Osteoporosis-associated fracture occurs most likely at sites of low bone mass. Vertebral spine and hip are the 2 common sites of fracture. Others include wrist, pelvic, proximal humerus, and shaft–distal femur.

1. Vertebral fracture—About 66% of vertebral fractures are asymptomatic; they are diagnosed as an incidental finding on chest or abdominal x-ray film. The most common sites for fractures are the lower thoracic area and upper lumbar spine. Osteoporotic fracture can lead to the acute onset of pain, typically occurring suddenly during routine activities, such as lifting or bending. The acute pain usually subsides in several weeks to months and is replaced by a chronic dull pain that usually resolves but can persist for a prolonged period.

Multiple vertebral fractures can lead to

- Increased thoracic kyphosis with height loss and development of "dowager's hump."
- Crowding of internal organs (patients note that their abdomens have become larger, that their clothes do not fit, or that they no longer have a waist).

- Complaints of pain in the muscles of the neck because patients must extend the neck to look forward.
- Reduction in the distance between the bottom of the rib cage and the top of the iliac crests, which may be associated with dyspnea and gastrointestinal complaints (eg, early satiety and constipation).
- Functional and physical limitation because of chronic pain, which leads to anxiety, depression, and loss of self-esteem and self-image.

2. Hip fracture—Hip fractures are relatively common in osteoporosis. The incidence increases with increasing age, affecting 15% of women and 5% of men by age 80. They are usually associated with a fall. Most hip fracture patients have difficulty standing, and the involved leg appears shorter and externally rotated. A patient with an impacted hip fracture may occasionally be able to walk. Intertrochanteric fractures are usually unstable and may be associated with substantial blood loss and hemodynamic compromise in the elderly. Hip fracture mortality is higher for men than for women, increases with age, and is greater for those with coexisting illnesses and poor prefracture functional status.

B. RISK FACTORS

Low bone density is an important risk factor for osteoporosis. Predictors of low bone mass include female sex, increased age, estrogen deficiency, white race, low body weight (< 127 lbs), family history of osteoporosis, and history of fracture. Cigarette smoking, alcohol abuse, and calcium or vitamin D deficiencies are also associated with osteoporosis. Residents of nursing homes and other long-term care facilities are at high risk for fractures. Most have low BMD and a high prevalence of other risk factors for fracture, including advanced age, poor physical function, low muscle strength, decreased cognition and high rates of dementia, poor nutrition, and multiple-drug regimen.

Although low BMD has been established as an important predictor of future fracture risks in women, other clinical risk factors have also been identified, among them historical factors, such as previous fracture, self-rated poor health, use of long-acting benzodiazepines, and sedentary lifestyle, and physical examination findings, such as inability to rise from a chair, poor visual performance, and resting tachycardia. The presence of 5 or more of these factors increased the rate of hip fracture in the highest tertile of BMD from 1.1/1000 woman-years to 9.9/1000 woman-years and in the lowest tertile of BMD to 27.1/1000 woman years.

Approximately 95% of hip fractures are caused by falls. Falls risk increases with advancing age for persons older than 65. Risk factors for falls include lack of physical activity, muscle weakness or balance problems, functional limitations, cognitive impairment or dementia, use of psychoactive medications, and environmental factors, including home hazards. Frequently, a fall is the result of an interaction between personal and environmental factors.

C. IMAGING STUDIES

Because 66% of vertebral fractures are asymptomatic, radiographs of the thoracic and lumbar spine are necessary to detect existing fractures. However, osteoporosis cannot be reliably diagnosed using x-ray films alone because a loss of up to 30% of bone mass is often not detected. Bone density measurement is needed to quantify osteoporosis.

D. BONE MINERAL DENSITY MEASUREMENT

BMD measurement can be used to establish the diagnosis of osteoporosis, estimate fracture risk, and identify candidates for intervention. It is also used to assess changes in bone mass over time in treated and untreated patients.

1. Indications—The National Osteoporosis Foundation (NOF) has recommended BMD testing for all white women age 65 and older and for postmenopausal women younger than 65 who have clinical risk factors (Table 27–2).

2. Measurement techniques—Several different methods are used to measure BMD (Table 27–3). Dual energy x-ray absorptiometry (DEXA) is the most common because it gives very precise measurements at clinically important sites with minimal radiation. It is the gold standard against which all other technologies are compared. The cost of DEXA is approximately $150–$250. Medicare covers the cost in all elderly

Table 27–2. National Osteoporosis Foundation recommendations for BMD testing.

Postmenopausal women (age 50–65) with risk factors for osteoporosis (besides menopause)
    Family history of osteoporosis
    Personal history of low trauma fracture at age > 45 years
    Current smoking
    Low body weight (< 127 lb)
Women age 65 years and older regardless of additional risk factors
Postmenopausal women with fractures
Women considering therapy for osteoporosis if BMD testing would facilitate such a decision
Women who have been on HT for prolonged periods

BMD, bone mineral density; HT, hormone replacement therapy.

women (> 65 years) for initial diagnosis and for follow-up after 23 mo.

3. Measurement sites—The routine DEXA examination should include scans of the hip and spine. BMD measurement at central sites (spine and hip) provides reproducible values at important sites of osteoporosis-associated fractures and also is more likely than measurement at peripheral sites to show a response to treatment in serial measurements. Peripheral sites can identify patients with low bone mass and predict fracture risk. However, peripheral sites are not as predictive for hip and spine fractures as site-specific measurement.

4. Bone density reports—Bone density data are reported as T scores and Z scores. T scores represent the number of standard deviations above or below young adult mean bone density values, whereas Z scores represent the standard deviations above or below age- and sex-matched control women. T scores are used by the World Health Organization (WHO) for establishing the diagnosis of osteopenia and osteoporosis (see Table 27–1). Each standard deviation change in the BMD increases fracture risk by 2–2.5 times. Patients with Z scores lower than −1.5 or −2.0 often have a secondary cause of osteoporosis.

5. Follow-up scans—Because annual losses of bone mass normally seen with aging are in the range of 1% per year, the precision error of current instruments (approximately 1–2% with DEXA) means that the usual interval between scans should be at least 2 years. Because high-dose steroid therapy can result in rapid bone loss in a shorter interval (6–12 mo), more frequent scans should be obtained in these patients.

E. LABORATORY EVALUATION

Despite the lack of definitive guidelines on the use of biochemical markers, such markers have the potential to provide independent or adjunctive information on decision making. The resorption markers are measured in the urine. However, blood measurements have become available (Table 27–4). Resorption markers must be measured in the morning on the second void urine because there is a large diurnal variation. The resorption markers are also independent risk factors for fracture. Women who have elevated markers are at increased risk of bone loss in the near future, and those with low bone mass may be candidates for pharmacological intervention.

Secondary causes of osteoporosis should be excluded in individuals with very low bone densities before rendering a diagnosis of idiopathic or primary osteoporosis. The common secondary causes are listed in Table 27–5 along with laboratory tests required to evaluate each disease. Men are more likely to have a secondary cause of osteoporosis than women. The most com-

Table 27–3. Bone mineral density measurement techniques.

Technique	Sites measured	Advantages	Disadvantages
DEXA	Central and peripheral	Precise measurements Minimal radiation Rapid Noninvasive	Machine is large (not portable) Expensive
QCT	Central and peripheral	Selectively measures trabecular bone Volumetric density Not influenced by degenerative disease	Poor precision Less reproducible High radiation Expensive
QUS	Peripheral	Portability Lack of radiation exposure Lower expense	Lack of precision Not useful in monitoring
RA	Peripheral	Uses conventional x-ray machinery	Measures bone density in a largely cortical site

DEXA, dual energy x-ray absorptiometry; QCT, quantitative computed tomography; QUS, quantitative ultrasonometry; RA, radiographic absorptiometry.

monly reported secondary causes of osteoporosis in men are hypogonadism, alcoholism, hypercalciuria, and malabsorption syndromes.

Prevention & Treatment

Effective therapies for prevention and treatment of osteoporosis are now available. The goal of therapy is to decrease osteoporosis-related morbidity and mortality by reducing the risk of fracture through maintaining or increasing bone strength.

A. NONPHARMACOLOGICAL THERAPY

Nonpharmacological therapy is an important adjunct to pharmacological management of osteoporosis. This includes elimination or reduction of potentially modifiable risk factors along with exercise and calcium and vitamin D supplementation.

1. Reduction of modifiable risk factors—Alcohol and tobacco use can be decreased and physical activity

Table 27–4. Serum markers.

Bone formation	Bone resorption
Serum bone-specific alkaline phosphatase	Urinary hydroxyproline
Serum osteocalcin	Urinary total deoxypyridinoline
Serum procollagen type I carboxyterminal pro-peptide	Urinary collagen type I cross-linked N-telopeptide
Serum procollagen type I N-terminal propeptide	Urinary collagen type I cross-linked C-telopeptide

increased in most elderly patients. Physical activity such as resistance training and weight-bearing exercises may have a 2-fold contribution to reducing fracture risk. First, it may enhance bone strength by optimizing BMD and improving bone quality. Second, it has the potential to reduce the risk of falling. Low-impact exercises, such as walking, have beneficial effects on other aspects of health and function, although their effects on BMD have been minimal. The emphasis of physical exercise programs in elderly patients with osteoporosis should not be on increasing bone mass but on improving muscle strength and balance. Older patients should be encouraged to participate safely in any activity in a frequent, regular, and sustained manner. The exercise should be weight bearing and easy to complete and should fit into their daily routine. A program of walking, sitting and standing exercises, and low-impact or water aerobics can be recommended initially and then gradually increased to more rigorous activity.

Reducing the use of medications that increase the risk of falls and making adjustments to the home environment can decrease the incidence of falls leading to fracture. Hip protectors can reduce the risk of hip fractures in nursing home residents. Hip protectors consist of a hard or soft shell with a soft padding that covers the area over the greater trochanter of the hip. Their use should be encouraged for patients at increased risk (ie, those with osteoporosis and high risk of falling), particularly those in nursing homes. However, compliance may be a problem.

2. Calcium & vitamin D—Bone loss in the elderly may be accelerated by calcium deficiency leading to secondary hyperparathyroidism. Deficiency of calcium and vitamin D contributes to alterations of bone re-

Table 27–5. Laboratory evaluation for secondary causes of osteoporosis.

Disease	Laboratory tests
Hypogonadism (men only)	Serum testosterone, prolactin
Malabsorption syndrome	Potential tests such as stool for fat or xylose breath test
Primary hyperparathyroidism	Ionized calcium, intact PTH (if calcium elevated)
Multiple myeloma	Serum and urine protein electrophoresis
Hyperthyroidism or excess thyroid hormone replacement	T_4, TSH
Osteomalacia	Alkaline phosphatase, 25(OH)D, 24-h urine calcium

PTH, parathyroid hormone; T_4, levothyroxine; TSH, thyroid-stimulating hormone; 25(OH)D, 25-hydroxyvitamin D.

modeling and bone integrity. Low calcium intake and vitamin D deficiency have been repeatedly observed in the elderly population. Vitamin D or calcium supplementation alone have little effect on bone mass in the early menopausal years but can have substantial effects on bone mass and fragility fractures in the elderly population.

a. Side effects—Risks of calcium supplementation are minimal. Older patients may suffer from constipation, rebound gastric hyperacidity, and dyspepsia, especially with calcium carbonate. Persons with personal or family histories of kidney stones must be screened with 24-h urinary calcium. Because most stones are calcium oxalate, and because calcium binds oxalate in the gastrointestinal (GI) tract, in most cases calcium is not contraindicated in stone disease. Calcium citrate is the preferred calcium supplementation in these patients because it decreases urine pH.

b. Recommended dose—The optimal effective dose of vitamin D is 400–800 IU/day. The recommended dose of calcium for elderly women and men is 1500 mg/day; women on hormone replacement therapy (HT) need 1000 mg/day. Dairy products are a good source of calcium, but they may not be tolerated in individuals with lactose intolerance, which is common in the elderly. Because the recommended dose of calcium and vitamin D usually is not obtained through diet alone, calcium supplementation is recommended. There is little evidence that one form of calcium supplementation is better than another. However, calcium citrate may be better tolerated in persons unable to tolerate other forms of calcium supplement and is better absorbed in the achlorhydric stomach.

A. Pharmacological Treatment

1. Bisphosphonates—These compounds bind avidly to hydroxyapatite crystals on bone surfaces and are potent inhibitors of bone resorption. Bisphosphonates significantly reduce vertebral fracture rates after only 1 year of treatment, making them ideal for patients with high short-term fracture risk.

a. Alendronate—

(1) Efficacy—Alendronate has been shown to prevent bone loss and increase BMD at the spine and hip by 5–10%. Also, alendronate therapy has been well tolerated. Elderly women with osteoporosis were shown to have significant gains in BMD at the lumbar spine and trochanter. It has been found that the magnitude of the fracture reductions with alendronate are similar in women who meet the WHO BMD criterion for osteoporosis without vertebral fracture and in those who have existing vertebral fracture with low BMD.

Treatment with alendronate also has significant effects on the physical disability resulting from osteoporotic fractures.

(2) Intermittent dosing—The efficacy of once-weekly compared with daily dosing of alendronate has been validated. The incidence of clinical and laboratory adverse effects, including GI intolerance, between the 2 regimens is also similar. However, rare but serious GI adverse events (perforation, ulcers, and bleeds) might be less with the once-weekly regimen. In addition, it is more convenient and has been approved by the Food and Drug Administration (FDA) for treatment of osteoporosis.

(3) Adverse effects—GI side effects (eg, heartburn, indigestion, pain while swallowing, and substernal discomfort) have been described, and a small number of patients have been reported to have experienced erosive esophagitis with alendronate. Because of this potential problem, it is important that patients take the medication in the morning with a full glass of water (6–8 oz) and remain upright (sitting or standing) for at least 30 min after the dose. An interval of 30 min before taking any liquid other than water is necessary to ensure absorption.

(4) Contraindications—Alendronate is contraindicated in patients with esophageal stricture or motility disorders and in those who are unable to remain upright for at least 30 min after ingestion of the drug. Alendronate should also be used with caution in patients with severe renal insufficiency (creatinine clearance < 35 mL/min).

(5) Recommended dose—The approved dose of alendronate for prevention of osteoporosis in recently menopausal women is 5 mg daily or 35 mg weekly. For treatment of postmenopausal osteoporosis, 10 mg daily or 70 mg weekly is the approved dose.

(6) Duration of use—The duration of alendronate therapy is not yet clear. One of the major determinants is what happens when therapy is discontinued. Seven-year follow-up of patients using alendronate showed that spinal BMD continued to increase through 7 years of alendronate treatment and BMD remained stable at other sites after rising during the first few years. After the withdrawal of treatment, there was a small increase in biochemical markers of bone turnover, but this was well below pretreatment levels 2 years after discontinuation. It appears that skeletal benefits may be preserved for at least 1–2 years after cessation, but long-term follow-up studies are needed.

b. Risedronate—

(1) Efficacy—Risedronate (5 mg/day) has been shown to increase lumbar spine BMD.

(2) Adverse effects—It is not known whether the GI side effects are different from alendronate.

(3) Contraindications—Contraindications to risedronate include esophageal stricture and motility disorders, hypocalcemia, and hypersensitivity to risedronate.

(4) Recommended dose—The approved dose for prevention and treatment of osteoporosis is 5 mg daily. BMD increases are equivalent with 5 mg once-daily and 35 mg once-weekly dosages.

c. Other bisphosphonates—Intermittent cyclical etidronate has been shown to significantly increase spinal bone mass and decrease the risk of vertebral fractures, especially among high-risk individuals. Cyclical etidronate is approved for treatment of osteoporosis in many countries. Although not approved by the FDA for treatment of osteoporosis, etidronate is often used off-label for patients who would benefit from a bisphosphonate but cannot tolerate other oral bisphosphonates. It is less expensive than alendronate or risedronate.

Zoledronic acid has also been shown to increase BMD at the spine and hip. The medication had similar effects on bone turnover and BMD when given as 1 mg every 3 mo or 4 mg every 12 mo. These increases were similar to those seen with risedronate and alendronate. Pamidronate has also been used, but no fracture data are available.

2. Hormone Therapy

a. Efficacy—The beneficial effects of HT on BMD at different skeletal sites have been documented. Conjugated estrogens have been shown to increase BMD by almost 6% in the spine and 2.8% in the hip after 3 years. The addition of progesterone did not alter the effect of estrogen. Estrogen and medroxyprogesterone acetate have produced a 1.4–3.9% increase in BMD at skeletal sites.

b. Duration & timing—The timing of initiation and duration of HT is the topic of much debate. It is suggested that women be started on estrogen within 2–7 years of menopause, but this guideline is being disputed. Several studies have shown that HT begun before 60 years of age prevents nonvertebral, hip, and wrist fractures, but there is insufficient evidence that fracture risk is reduced when HT is begun after age 60. Estrogen may have a positive effect on BMD even when started ≥ 20 years after menopause. Estrogen begun and continued after age 60 years appears to maintain and in some cases increase BMD. There is growing evidence, however, for an attenuation of the beneficial skeletal effects of HT after the withdrawal of treatment. The duration of therapy necessary to protect women against fragility fractures is indefinite.

c. Side effects—Compliance with HT is typically poor because of common side effects and concern about increased incidence of breast or endometrial cancer. Women who have not undergone hysterectomy should have progestins added to the estrogen regimen to prevent endometrial neoplasia. HT also increases the risk of venous thromboembolism and cholelithiasis. One major reason why elderly women discontinue therapy is irregular uterine bleeding. Low-dose HT can reduce the amount of uterine bleeding as well as the incidence of fluid retention, mastalgia, and headaches, making estrogen therapy much easier to tolerate. Concerns about cardiovascular risks (stroke and myocardial infarction) will limit the use of HT for treatment of osteoporosis in older women. See Chapter 36 for recommended doses of HT and contraindications to use.

3. Raloxifene—Selective estrogen receptor modulators (SERMs) are compounds that bind to and activate estrogen receptors but cause differential estrogenic or antiestrogenic responses in different tissues. Raloxifene was the first SERM approved by the FDA for the prevention and treatment of osteoporosis.

a. Efficacy—Raloxifene has been shown to reduce the incidence of new vertebral fracture in women with low BMD and no prevalent vertebral fracture by 55%. Among women with prevalent vertebral fractures, raloxifene reduced the incidence of new vertebral fracture by 30%.

b. Side effects—Women receiving raloxifene may be at increased risk of venous thromboembolism (~3/1000), a risk similar to estrogen. Hot flashes and leg cramps may also occur.

c. **Extraskeletal effects**—Raloxifene is associated with a 76% overall reduction of breast cancer and a 90% reduction in estrogen receptor-positive breast cancer. In addition, a post hoc analysis suggested that women may be at a significantly lower risk of cardiovascular events. A randomized controlled trial is ongoing to answer this question.

d. **Contraindications**—Raloxifene is contraindicated in patients with history of venous thromboembolic disease.

e. **Recommended dose**—The dosage for prevention of osteoporosis in recently menopausal women and treatment of established osteoporosis is 60 mg daily.

4. **Calcitonin**—Calcitonin, an endogenous hormone secreted by the parafollicular C cells of the thyroid gland, helps to maintain normal calcium homeostasis. Calcitonin acts directly on osteoclasts, with inhibitory effects on bone resorption.

a. **Efficacy**—Salmon calcitonin nasal spray (200 IU/day) has been shown to significantly reduce the risk of new vertebral fractures by 33–36% in women with prevalent vertebral fractures. It does not appear to reduce the risk of nonvertebral fractures.

b. **Side effects**—Common side effects of injectable calcitonin include nausea, local inflammatory reactions at the site of injection, and generalized flushing. Nasal calcitonin is well tolerated; the major side effect is nasal discomfort, including rhinitis and occasional epistaxis.

c. **Contraindications**—The major contraindication to the use of both forms of calcitonin is hypersensitivity.

d. **Recommended dose**—Injectable calcitonin is administered subcutaneously or intramuscularly at a dose of 50–100 IU daily; the recommended dose of nasal calcitonin is 200 IU daily, administered in alternate nostrils. In some patients, calcitonin has an analgesic effect, making it suitable for patients with acute vertebral fracture who are bedridden and may need to avoid bisphosphonates because of risk of esophageal injury or avoid estrogen because of risk of venous thromboembolism.

5. **Alternative therapies**—Phytoestrogens are a diverse group of compounds found in a wide variety of plant foods believed to have both estrogenic and antiestrogenic activity. Phytoestrogens may have a role in preventing osteoporosis. However, ipriflavone has not been shown to prevent bone loss or affect biochemical markers of bone metabolism.

6. **Anabolic agents**—In contrast to the currently available drugs that slow bone turnover, thereby allowing bone formation to exceed bone resorption, anabolic agents, like parathyroid hormone (PTH), actually stimulate remodeling, preferentially increasing formation over resorption.

PTH (20 μg subcutaneously once daily) has been shown to achieve a 65% reduction in vertebral fractures. New nonvertebral fragility fractures were reduced by 54%. Nausea and headache are the most common, but infrequent, side effects. PTH injection is now available for treatment of osteoporosis.

7. **Combination therapy**—More than 5% of women continue to lose bone density while receiving HT alone and require additional therapy for osteoporosis. Some nonresponse may be due to noncompliance or underdosing. Estrogen and bisphosphonates together have produced greater gains in BMD than either agent used alone, but no data on fracture reduction exist with combination therapy.

Patients treated with PTH who had previously been treated with alendronate for 18–36 mo had a blunted bone density response. Previous treatment with raloxifene and estrogen do not appear to blunt the BMD response. Sequential therapy with PTH first followed by an antiresorptive agent seems to be preferable, giving an additive effect on BMD. No fracture data are available.

C. FOLLOW-UP

Once patients have been identified and treatment is initiated, they should be monitored to evaluate the response to treatment and assess compliance. The response may be monitored by use of biochemical markers such as serum NTx 3–4 mo after initiating treatment with antiresorptive drugs. In most patients, these markers decrease by at least 40–70% compared with pretreatment levels. BMD should be repeated after 2 years of therapy. If BMD is stable at 2 years, it need not be repeated every 2 years as long as the patient continues the treatment and the medical condition is stable. Early follow-up may be required in patients who have a fracture while on drug treatment or if there is a change in the patient's medical condition or steroid dose.

 EVIDENCE-BASED POINTS

- *Osteoporosis is a major health problem in the elderly. The prevalence of osteoporosis increases with age from 15% in 50- to 59-year-olds to 70% in women aged 80 years.*

- *Osteoporosis has no clinical manifestations until there is a fracture. Vertebral spine and hip are the most common sites of fracture.*

- Low bone density is a major risk factor for fracture.
- BMD can be assessed by noninvasive techniques. DEXA is the most commonly used method to diagnose osteoporosis and identify candidates for intervention.
- Secondary causes of osteoporosis should be excluded in individuals with very low bone mineral density (Z scores ≤ 1.5).
- Physical exercise helps to maintain bone density; slow rate of bone loss; improve muscle coordination, mobility, and balance; and reduce incidence of falls.
- The combination of calcium and vitamin D reduces the risk of fractures.
- Supplementation with calcium and vitamin D is often required in the elderly.
- The bisphosphonates, alendronate and risedronate, inhibit bone resorption, increase spine and hip density, and significantly decrease the incidence of vertebral and hip fractures in postmenopausal women with osteoporosis.
- The evidence for antifracture efficacy of HT comes primarily from observational studies. The WHI (a randomized controlled trial) demonstrated a 34% reduction in hip and fractures.
- Raloxifene, a selective estrogen receptor modulator, mimics the beneficial effects of estrogen on bone while avoiding the adverse effects on the uterus and breast. It reduces the risk of vertebral fractures but not nonvertebral fractures.
- Calcitonin has weak antifracture efficacy at the vertebral spine.
- PTH has been demonstrated to reduce both vertebral and nonvertebral fractures.

REFERENCES

Black DM et al: Randomised trial of effect of alendronate on risk of fracture in women with existing vertebral fractures. Fracture Intervention Trial research group. Lancet 1996;348:1535. [PMID: 8950879]

Cauley JA et al: Estrogen replacement therapy and fractures in older women. Study of osteoporotic fractures research group. Ann Intern Med 1995;122:9. [PMID: 7985914]

Chapuy MC et al: Vitamin D₃ and calcium to prevent hip fractures in the elderly women. N Engl J Med 1992;327:1637. [PMID: 1331788]

Chesnut CH III et al: A randomized trial of nasal spray salmon calcitonin in postmenopausal women with established osteoporosis: the prevent recurrence of osteoporotic fractures study. PROOF study group. Am J Med 2000;109:267. [PMID: 10996576]

Cooper C et al: Population-based study of survival after osteoporotic fractures. Am J Epidemiol 1993;137:1001. [PMID: 8317445]

Cummings SR et al: Bone density at various sites for prediction of hip fractures. The Study of Osteoporotic Fractures Research Group. Lancet 1993;341:72. [PMID: 8093403]

Cummings SR et al: Effect of alendronate on risk of fracture in women with low bone density but without vertebral fractures: Results from the fracture intervention trial. JAMA 1998; 280:2077. [PMID: 9875874]

Dawson-Hughes B et al: Effect of calcium and vitamin D supplementation on bone density in men and women 65 years of age or older. N Engl J Med 1997;337:670. [PMID: 9278463]

Ettinger B et al: Contribution of vertebral deformities to chronic back pain and disability. The study of osteoporotic fractures research group. J Bone Min Res 1992;7:449. [PMID: 1535172]

Ettinger B et al: Reduction of vertebral fracture risk in postmenopausal women with osteoporosis treated with raloxifene: results from a 3-year randomized clinical trial. Multiple outcomes of raloxifene evaluation (MORE) investigators. JAMA 1999;282:637. [PMID: 10517716]

Gold DT: The clinical impact of vertebral fractures: quality of life in women with osteoporosis. Bone 1996;18(3 Suppl):185S. [PMID: 8777086]

Harris ST et al: Effects of risedronate treatment on vertebral and nonvertebral fractures in women with postmenopausal osteoporosis: A randomized controlled trial. Vertebral efficacy with risedronate therapy (VERT) study group. JAMA 1999;282: 1344. [PMID: 10527181]

Hulley S et al: Randomized trial of estrogen plus progestin for secondary prevention of coronary heart disease in postmenopausal women. Heart and estrogen/progestin replacement study (HERS) research group. JAMA 1998;280:605. [PMID: 9718051]

Kannus P et al: Prevention of hip fracture in elderly people with use of a hip protector. N Engl J Med 2000;343:1506. [PMID: 11087879]

Lindsay R et al: Prevention of spinal osteoporosis in oophorectomised women. Lancet 1980;2:1151. [PMID: 6107766]

McClung MR et al: Effect of risedronate on the risk of hip fracture in elderly women. Hip intervention program study group. N Engl J Med 2001;344:333. [PMID: 1172164]

Neer RM et al: Effect of parathyroid hormone (1-34) on fractures and bone mineral density in postmenopausal women with osteoporosis. N Engl J Med 2001;344:1434. [PMID: 11346808]

Orwoll E et al: Alendronate for the treatment of osteoporosis in men. N Engl J Med 2000;343:604. [PMID: 10979796]

Osteoporosis: Review of the evidence for prevention, diagnosis, and treatment and cost-effective analysis. Osteoporosis Int 1998: 8(Suppl 4):S7. [PMID: 10197173]

Reginster J et al: Randomized trial of the effects of risedronate on vertebral fractures in women with established postmenopausal osteoporosis. Vertebral efficacy with risedronate therapy (VERT) study group. Osteoporos Int 2000;11:83. [PMID 10663363]

Villareal DT et al: Bone mineral density response to estrogen replacement in frail elderly women: a randomized controlled trial. JAMA 2001;286:815. [PMID: 11497535]

Writing Group for the PEPI Trial: Effects of estrogen or estrogen/progestin regimens on heart disease risk factors in postmenopausal women. The postmenopausal estrogen/progestin interventions (PEPI) trial. JAMA 1995;273:199. [PMID: 7807658]

Pressure Ulcers

28

David R. Thomas, MD, FAGS, FACP

ESSENTIALS OF DIAGNOSIS

- Pressure ulcers are caused by pressure applied to susceptible tissues. Tissue susceptibility may be increased in the presence of maceration and by friction and shear forces.
- Comorbid conditions, especially immobility and decreased tissue perfusion, increase the risk of pressure ulcers.
- Most pressure ulcers develop over bony prominences, most commonly the sacrum, heels, and trochanteric areas.
- Most pressure ulcers develop in acute hospitals; the risk is greatest in orthopedic and intensive care unit patients.
- Pressure ulcers can be stage I (blanchable hyperemia), stage II (extension of the ulcer through the epidermis), stage III (full-thickness skin loss with damage or necrosis of subcutaneous tissue), or stage IV (full-thickness wounds with extensive destruction, tissue necrosis, or damage to muscle, bone, or supporting structures).
- Pressure ulcers do not necessarily progress from stage I through stage IV.

General Considerations

A. CAUSES

Pressure ulcers are the visible evidence of pathological changes in the blood supply to dermal tissues. The chief cause is pressure, or force per unit area, applied to susceptible tissues. Comorbid conditions, especially those resulting in immobility or reducing tissue perfusion, greatly increase the risk of pressure ulcers.

B. MANAGEMENT

Therapy for pressure ulcers is generally empiric, based on anecdotal experience, or borrowed from the treatment of patients with acute wounds. It is problematic because of multiple comorbidities, chronic duration of pressure ulcers, and frequently the physician's relative unfamiliarity with options.

Recognition of risk, relief of pressure, and optimizing nutritional status are components of both prevention and management guidelines. For persons with identified pressure ulcers, assessing the wound and implementing strategies for local wound care are paramount.

Thomas DR: Issues and dilemmas in the prevention and treatment of pressure ulcers: a review. J Gerontol Biol Sci Med Sci 2001;56:M328. [PMID: 11382790]

Thomas DR: Prevention and treatment of pressure ulcers: what works? What doesn't? Cleve Clin J Med 2001;68:704. [PMID: 11510528]

Thomas DR, Kamel HK: Wound management in postacute care. Clin Geriatr Med 2000;16:783. [PMID: 10984756]

C. INCIDENCE

The primary source of pressure ulcers appears to be the acute hospital. Among patients who experience pressure ulcers, 57–60% do so in the acute hospital. Incidence in hospitalized patients ranges from 3–30%; common estimates range from 9–13%. The incidence differs by hospital location; intensive care unit (ICU) patients and orthopedic patients are at greatest risk. Up to 66% of orthopedic patients have pressure ulcers of varying severity. Pressure ulcers develop early in the course of hospitalization, usually within the first week. The incidence of pressure ulcers in nursing homes is difficult to quantitate.

After discharge from the hospital, pressure ulcers remain a major problem in community care settings. Characteristics associated with pressure ulcers include recent institutional discharge, functional impairment, incontinence, and having had a previous ulcer. Pressure-relieving devices and other wound care strategies appeared to be underused and often indiscriminately applied.

D. RISK ASSESSMENT & RISK FACTORS

In theory, persons who are at high risk for pressure ulcers can be identified, and an increased effort can be directed to preventing ulcers. The classical risk assessment scale is the Norton Score, developed in 1962 and still widely used. Patients are classified using 5 risk factors graded from 1–4. Scores range from 5–20; higher scores indicate lower risk. The generally accepted at-risk score is ≤ 14; patients with scores < 12 are at particularly high risk.

A commonly used risk assessment instrument in the United States is the Braden Scale. This instrument assesses 6 items: sensory perception, moisture exposure, physical activity, mobility, nutrition, and friction/shear force. Each item is ranked from 1 (least favorable) to 3 or 4 (most favorable), with a maximal total score of 23. A score of ≤ 16 indicates a high risk.

Both the Norton Score and the Braden Scale have good sensitivity (73–92% and 83–100%, respectively) and specificity (61–94% and 64–77%, respectively) but poor positive predictive value (~37% at a pressure ulcer incidence of 20%). In populations with a lower incidence of pressure ulcers, such as those in nursing homes, the same sensitivity and specificity produce a positive predictive value of 2%. The net effect of poor positive predictive value means that many patients who will not develop pressure ulcers will receive expensive and unnecessary treatment.

In clinical practice, risk assessment has been problematic for 2 reasons. First, risk assessment is not universally applied. Less than 50% of the high-risk elderly persons admitted to acute care with a hip fracture had any sort of risk assessment performed. It is possible that resistance to implementing risk assessment models is due to recognition by clinicians that the instruments are inadequate. Second, no risk assessment study has demonstrated that persons identified at risk or who have a plan of care based on risk assessment are less likely to develop a pressure ulcer.

Because most pressure ulcers develop in the acute hospital, risk assessment in this setting is particularly important. In an ICU, 5 factors contribute to the risk of pressure ulcer after adjusting for 18 univariately significant risk factors: norepinephrine infusion, APACHE II score, fecal incontinence, anemia, and length of stay in the ICU. Independent risk factors for the development of a pressure ulcer after admission to a surgical service include emergency admission (which increased the risk 36-fold), age, days in bed, and days without nutrition.

Risk factors for the prevalence of pressure ulcers at admission include the presence of a fracture (increasing the risk 5-fold), fecal incontinence (increasing the risk 3-fold), and decreased serum albumin level (increasing the risk 3-fold). Applied prospectively to at-risk patients without pressure ulcers, these factors were associated with development of a pressure ulcer.

In functionally limited (bed or chair-confined) hospitalized patients, 9 factors were associated with the development of pressure ulcers, including nonblanchable erythema (increasing the risk 7-fold), lymphopenia (increasing the risk almost 5-fold), and immobility, dry skin, and decreased body weight (each of which increase the risk 2-fold).

Not surprisingly, risk factors in long-term care populations differ. In this population, the factors associated with development of pressure ulcers are facility dependent. In low-risk nursing homes, difficulty in ambulation, difficulty feeding oneself, and male gender were associated with a 2- to 4-fold risk of pressure ulcer. In high-risk nursing homes, difficulty with ambulation, fecal incontinence, difficulty feeding oneself, and diabetes mellitus predicted pressure ulcer development.

The risk of pressure ulcer may include a history of cerebrovascular accident (5-fold increase), bed or chair confinement (3.8-fold increase), and impaired nutritional intake (2.8-fold increase). In data derived from the Minimal Data Set, logistic regression analysis determined that dependence in transfer or mobility, confinement to bed, history of diabetes mellitus, and a history of pressure ulcer were significantly associated with an existing stage II–IV pressure ulcer.

In community-dwelling persons aged 55–75, the presence of a pressure ulcer was predicted by self-assessed poor health, current smoking, dry or scaly skin on examination, and decreased activity level.

The importance of these epidemiological risk predictors lies in understanding which factors are amenable to correction. Risk factor predictors from various sites suggest that immobility, dry skin, and nutritional factors are potentially modifiable. Efforts have centered on correction of these problems.

Prevention

A. QUALITY OF CARE

Pressure ulcers are increasingly used as indicators of quality of care. Whether or not pressure ulcers are preventable remains controversial. When aggressive measures for prevention of pressure ulcers have been applied, a "floor effect" for incidence has been noted. Pressure ulcers often occur in terminally ill patients, for whom the goals of care may not include prevention of pressure ulcers. Pressure ulcers also occur in severely ill patients, such as orthopedic patients or ICU patients, for whom the necessity for immobilization may preclude turning or the use of pressure-relieving devices.

Systematic efforts at education, heightened awareness, and specific interventions by interdisciplinary wound teams suggest that a high incidence of pressure ulcers can be reduced. Over time, reductions of 25–30% have been reported. The reduction may be transient, unstable over time, vary with changes in personnel, or occur as a result of random variation. Development of pressure ulcers can be, but is not always, a measure of quality of care.

B. PRESSURE RELIEF

The first efforts toward prevention should be to improve mobility and reduce the effects of pressure, friction, and shear forces. The theoretical goal is to reduce tissue pressure below capillary closing pressure of 32 mm Hg. If the target pressure reduction is unachievable, then pressure must be intermittently relieved to allow time for tissue recovery.

The most expedient method for reducing pressure is frequent turning and positioning. A 2-h turning schedule for spinal injury patients was deducted empirically in 1946. However, turning the patient to relieve pressure may be difficult to achieve despite best nursing efforts and is very costly in terms of staffing. The exact interval for optimal turning in prevention is unknown. The interval may be shortened or lengthened by host factors. Despite commonsense approaches to turning, positioning, and improving passive activity, no published data support the view that pressure ulcers can be prevented by passive positioning.

Because of the limitations and cost of turning schedules, a number of devices have been developed to prevent pressure injury. Devices can be defined as pressure relieving (consistently reducing interface pressure < 32 mm Hg) or pressure reducing (less than standard support surfaces but not < 32 mm Hg). The majority of devices are pressure reducing. Pressure-reducing devices can be further classified as static or dynamic. Static surfaces attempt to distribute local pressure over a larger body surface. Examples include foam mattresses and devices filled with water, gel, or air. Dynamic devices use a power source to alternate air currents and promote uniform pressure distribution over body surfaces. Examples include alternating pressure pads, air suspension devices, and air-fluid surfaces.

Some pressure-reducing devices have been proven more effective than "standard" hospital foam mattresses in moderate- to high-risk patients. Pressure-relieving mattresses in the operating theater have reduced the incidence of pressure sores postoperatively. Limited evidence suggests that low-air-loss beds reduce the incidence of pressure sores in ICUs. The differences among devices are unclear and do not demonstrate a superior device compared with other devices. Seat cushions and simple, constant-low-pressure devices have not been adequately evaluated. There is good evidence that air-fluid beds and low-air-loss beds improve healing rates.

Clark M: Repositioning to prevent pressure sores—what is the evidence? Nurs Standard 1998;13:56. [PMID: 9847811]

C. NUTRITIONAL INTERVENTIONS

One of the most important reversible factors contributing to wound healing is nutritional status. Of newly hospitalized patients with stage III or stage IV pressure ulcers, most were below their usual body weight, had a low prealbumin level, and were not taking in enough nutrition to meet their needs.

The results of trials to increase nutrient intake have been disappointing. It has been suggested that nutritional supplements have no effect on prevention of pressure ulcers. In addition, overnight supplemental enteral feeding has not been shown to affect development of pressure ulcers and severity.

Dietary intake, especially of protein, is important in healing pressure ulcers. An optimum dietary protein intake in patients with pressure ulcers is unknown but may be much higher than current adult recommendations of 0.8 g/kg/day. Half of chronically ill elderly persons are unable to maintain nitrogen balance at this level. Increasing protein intake beyond 1.5 g/kg/day may not increase protein synthesis and may cause dehydration. A reasonable protein requirement is, therefore, between 1.2–1.5 g/kg/day.

The deficiency of several vitamins has significant effects on wound healing. However, supplementation of vitamins to accelerate wound healing is controversial. There is insubstantial evidence to support use of a daily vitamin C supplement for healing pressure sores.

Zinc supplementation has not been shown to accelerate healing except in zinc-deficient patients. High serum zinc levels interfere with healing, and supplementation > 150 mg/day may interfere with copper metabolism.

Immune function declines with age, which increases risk for infection, and is thought to delay wound healing. Arginine supplementation has not been shown to enhance the proliferative response or pressure ulcer outcome.

Houston S et al: Adverse effects of large-dose zinc supplementation in an institutionalized older population with pressure ulcers. J Am Geriatr Soc 2001;9:1130. [PMID: 11555083]

Thomas DR: Improving outcome of pressure ulcers with nutritional interventions: a review of the evidence. Nutrition 2001;17:121. [PMID: 11240340]

Thomas DR: The role of nutrition in prevention and healing of pressure ulcers. Clin Geriatr Med 1997;13:497. [PMID: 9227941]

Clinical Findings

Several differing scales have been proposed for assessing the severity of pressure ulcers. The most common staging, recommended by the National Pressure Ulcer Task Force, is derived from a modification of the Shea Scale. Under this schematic, pressure ulcers are divided into 4 clinical stages.

The first response of the epidermis to pressure is hyperemia. Blanchable erythema occurs when capillary refilling occurs after gentle pressure is applied to the area. Nonblanchable erythema exists when pressure of a finger in the reddened area does not produce a blanching or capillary refilling. A stage I pressure ulcer is defined by nonblanchable erythema of intact skin. Nonblanchable erythema is believed to indicate extravasation of blood from the capillaries. A stage I pressure ulcer always understates the underlying damage because the epidermis is the last tissue to show ischemic injury. Diagnosing stage I pressure ulcers in darkly pigmented skin is problematic.

Stage II ulcers extend through the epidermis or dermis. The ulcer is superficial and presents clinically as an abrasion, blister, or shallow crater. With stage III pressure ulcers, there is full-thickness skin loss involving damage or necroses of subcutaneous tissue that may extend down to, but not through, underlying fascia. The ulcer presents clinically as a deep crater with or without undermining of adjacent tissue. Stage IV pressure ulcers are full-thickness wounds with extensive destruction, tissue necrosis, or damage to muscle, bone, or supporting structures. Undermining and sinus tracts are frequently associated with stage IV pressure ulcers. Stage I pressure ulcers occur most frequently, accounting for 47% of pressure ulcers, followed by stage II ulcers (33%). Stage III and IV ulcers comprise the remaining 20%.

This staging system for pressure ulcers has several limitations. The primary difficulty lies in the inability to distinguish progression between stages. Pressure ulcers do not progress absolutely through stage I to stage IV but may appear to develop from the inside out as a result of the initial injury. Healing from stage IV does not progress through stage III to stage I; rather, the ulcer heals by contraction and scar tissue formation. Second, clinical staging is inaccurate unless all eschar is removed, because the staging system reflects only depth of the ulcer.

Because pressure ulcers heal by contraction and scar formation, reverse staging is inaccurate in assessing healing. No single measure of wound characteristics has been useful in measuring healing. Several indexes of ulcer healing have been proposed but lack validation studies. The Pressure Ulcer Status for Healing (PUSH) tool (Figure 28–1) was developed and validated by the National Pressure Ulcer Advisory Panel to measure healing of pressure ulcers. The tool measures 3 components—size, exudate amount, and tissue type—to arrive at a numerical score for ulcer status. The PUSH tool adequately assesses ulcer status and is sensitive to change over time.

Stotts NA et al: An instrument to measure healing in pressure ulcers: development and validation of the pressure ulcer scale for healing (PUSH). J Gerontol Biol Sci Med Sci 2001;56:M795. [PMID: 11723157]

Complications

Colonization of chronic wounds with bacteria is common and unavoidable. All chronic wounds become colonized, usually with skin organisms followed in 48 h by gram-negative bacteria. The presence of micro-organisms alone (colonization) does not indicate an infection in pressure ulcers. The primary source of bacterial infections in chronic wounds appears to be the result of suprainfection resulting from contamination. Therefore, protection of the wound from secondary contamination is an important goal of treatment.

Evidence suggests that occlusive dressings protect against clinical infection, although the wound may be colonized with bacteria. Occlusive dressings very rarely cause a clinical infection.

It is often difficult to determine the presence of an infection in chronic pressure ulcers. The diagnosis of infection in chronic wounds must be based on clinical signs: advancing erythema, edema, odor, fever, or purulent exudate. When there is evidence of clinical infection, topical or systemic antimicrobials are required. Topical treatment may be useful when the wound is failing to progress toward healing. Systemic antibiotics are indicated when the clinical condition suggests spread of the infection to the bloodstream or bone.

Wounds with extensive undermining create pockets for infection with an increased likelihood for infection with anaerobic organisms. Obliteration of dead space reduces the possibility of infection.

Treatment

Maintaining a moist wound environment increases the rate of healing. Moist wound healing allows experimentally induced wounds to resurface up to 40% faster than air-exposed wounds. Any therapy that dehydrates the wound such as dry gauze, heat lamps, air exposure, or liquid antacids is detrimental to chronic wound healing.

Dressings allow moisture to escape from the wound at a fixed rate measured by the moisture vapor transmission rate (MVTR). An MVTR of < 35 g of water vapor/m^2/h is required to maintain a moist wound environment. Woven gauze has an MVTR of 68 g/m^2/h, and impregnated gauze has an MVTR of 57 g/m^2/h. In comparison, hydrocolloid dressings have an MVTR of 8 g/m^2/h.

Dressings that maintain a moist wound environment are occlusive, describing the propensity of a dressing to transmit moisture vapor from the wound to the external atmosphere. The available dressings differ in their properties of permeability to water vapor and in wound protection.

Patient Name:_____ Patient ID#:

Ulcer Location: _____ Date:

DIRECTIONS: Observe and measure the pressure ulcer. Categorize the ulcer with respect to surface area, exudate, and type of wound tissue. Record a subscore for each of these ulcer characteristics. Add the subscore to obtain the total score. A comparison of total scores measured over time provides an indication of the improvement or deterioration in pressure ulcer healing.

Length	0 0 cm^2	1 <0.3 cm^2	2 0.3–0.6 cm^2	3 0.7–1.0 cm^2	4 1.1–2.0 cm^2	5 2.1–3.0 cm^2	
x Width		6 3.1–4.0 cm^2	7 4.1–8.0 cm^2	8 8.1–12.0 cm^2	9 12.1–24.0 cm^2	10 >24.0 cm^2	**Subscore**
Exudate amount	0 None	1 Light	2 Moderate	3 Heavy			**Subscore**
Tissue type[a]	0 Closed	1 Epithelial tissue	2 Granulation tissue	3 Slough	4 Necrotic tissue		**Subscore**
							Total score

Length x Width: Measure the greatest length (head to toe) and the greatest width (side to side) using a centimeter ruler. Multiply these two measurements (length × width) to obtain an estimate of surface area in square centimeters (cm^2). Caveat: Do not guess! Always use a centimeter ruler and always use the same method each time the ulcer is measured.

Exudate Amount: Estimate the amount of exudate (drainage) present after removal of the dressing and before applying any topical agent to the ulcer. Estimate the exudate (drainage) as none, light, moderate, or heavy.

Tissue Type: This refers to the types of tissue that are present in the wound (ulcer) bed. Score as a "4" if there is any necrotic tissue present. Score as a "3" if there is any amount of slough present and necrotic tissue is absent. Score as a "2" if the wound is clean and contains granulation tissue. A superficial wound that is reepitheliazing is scored as a "1". When the wound is closed, score as a "0".

[a]**Necrotic tissue (eschar):** black, brown, or tan tissue that adheres firmly to the wound bed or ulcer edges and may be either firmer or softer than surrounding skin. **Slough:** yellow or white tissue that adheres to the ulcer bed in strings or thick clumps or is mucinous. **Granulation tissue:** pink or beefy red tissue with a shiny, moist, granular appearance. **Epithelial tissue:** for superficial ulcers, new pink or shiny tissue (skin) that grows in from the edges or as islands on the ulcer surface. **Closed/resurfaced:** wound is completely covered with epithelium (new skin).

Figure 28–1. PUSH tool version 3.0.

A. TOPICAL DRESSINGS

Occlusive dressings can be divided into broad categories of polymer films, polymer foams, hydrogels, hydrocolloids, alginates, and biomembranes. Each has several advantages and disadvantages. The choice of a particular agent depends on the clinical circumstances. The agents differ in the ease of application. This difference is important in pressure ulcers in unusual locations or when considering their use for home care. Dressings should be left in place until wound fluid is leaking from the sides, a period of days to 3 weeks.

1. Polymer films—Polymer films are impermeable to liquid but permeable to both gas and moisture vapor. Because of low permeability to water vapor, these dressings are not dehydrating to the wound. Nonpermeable polymers such as polyvinylidine and polyethylene can be macerating to normal skin. Polymer films are not absorptive and may leak, particularly when the wound is highly exudative. Most films have an adhesive backing that may remove epithelial cells when the dressing is changed. Polymer films do not eliminate dead space and do not absorb exudate.

2. Hydrogels—Hydrogels are 3-layer hydrophilic polymers that are insoluble in water but absorb aqueous solutions. They are poor bacterial barriers and do not adhere to the wound. Because of their high specific heat, these dressings are cooling to the skin, aiding in pain control and reducing inflammation. Most of these dressings require a secondary dressing to secure them to the wound.

3. Hydrocolloid dressings—Hydrocolloid dressings are complex dressings similar to ostomy barrier products. They are impermeable to moisture vapor and gases (their impermeability to oxygen is theoretically a disadvantage) and are highly adherent to the skin. In addition, they offer bacterial resistance. Their adhesiveness to surrounding skin is higher than some surgical tapes, but they do not adhere to wound tissue and do not damage epithelialization of the wound. The adhesive barrier is frequently overcome in highly exudative wounds. Hydrocolloid dressings cannot be used over tendons or on wounds with eschar formation. Several of these dressings include a foam padding layer that may reduce pressure to the wound.

4. Alginates—Alginates are complex polysaccharide dressings that are highly absorbent in exudative wounds. This high absorbency is particularly suited to exudative wounds. Alginates do not adhere to the wound; however, if the wound is allowed to dry, damage to the epithelial tissue may occur with removal.

5. Biomembranes—Biomembranes offer bacterial resistance but are very expensive and not readily available. These dressings could be problematic in wounds contaminated by anaerobes, but this effect has not been demonstrated clinically.

6. Saline-soaked gauze—Saline-soaked gauze that is not allowed to dry is an effective wound dressing. Moist saline gauze and occlusive-type dressings have similar pressure ulcer-healing abilities. The use of occlusive-type dressings has been shown to be more cost effective than traditional dressings primarily because of a decrease in nursing time for dressing changes. Table 28–1 provides a comparison of dressing types. General guidelines are presented in Table 28–2.

7. Phenytoin—Topical phenytoin therapy has been associated with a shorter time to complete healing and formation of granulation tissue.

B. Growth Factors

Acute wound healing proceeds in a carefully regulated fashion that is reproducible from wound to wound. A number of growth factors have been demonstrated to mediate the healing process, including transforming growth factor-α and β, epidermal growth factor, platelet-derived growth factor, fibroblast growth factor,

interleukin-1 and interleukin-2, and tumor necrosis factor-α. Accelerating healing in chronic wounds using these acute wound factors is attractive. Several of these factors have been favorable in animal models; however, they have not been as successful in human trials.

In pressure ulcers, recombinant platelet-derived growth factor (rhPDGF-BB) failed to improve the rate of complete healing, although a 15% difference in percentage of initial volume of ulcers has been shown with PDGF-BB. One report showed that more subjects had >70% wound closure with basic fibroblast growth factor. Sequential application of growth factors to mimic wound-healing progression has not been effective in pressure ulcers.

C. Adjunctive Therapies

Alternative or adjunctive therapies include electrical therapy, electromagnetic therapy, ultrasound therapy, low-level light therapy/laser therapy, and vacuum-assisted closure. None of these interventions has been clearly proven effective despite widespread clinical use.

D. Débridement

Necrotic debris increases the possibility of bacterial infection and delays wound healing. The preferred method of débriding pressure ulcers remains controversial. Options include mechanical débridement with dry gauze dressings, autolytic débridement with occlusive dressings, application of exogenous enzymes, or sharp surgical débridement. Surgical sharp débridement produces the most rapid removal of necrotic debris and is required in the presence of infection. Mechanical débridement can be easily accomplished by allowing a saline gauze dressing to dry before removal. Remoistening of gauze dressings in an attempt to reduce pain can defeat the débridement effect. Both surgical and mechanical débridement can damage healthy tissue or fail to clean the wound completely. Débridement with a dry gauze should be stopped as soon as a clean wound bed is obtained because dry dressings have been associated with delayed healing.

Thin portions of eschar can be removed by occlusion under a semipermeable dressing. Both autolytic and enzymatic débridement require periods of several days to several weeks to achieve results. Enzymatic débridement can dissolve necrotic debris, but whether it harms healthy tissue is debated. Penetration of enzymatic agents is limited in eschar and requires either softening by autolysis or cross-hatching by sharp incision before application.

Three enzyme preparations are currently marketed in the United States for débridement: collagenase, papain/urea, and a papain/urea-chlorophyll combination. Collagenase reduced necrosis, pus, and odor compared with inactivated control ointment and produced débridement in 82% of pressure ulcers at 4 weeks compared with petrolatum. Papain produced measurable débridement in 4 days compared with a control ointment. The issues of when to débride and which method to use remain controversial. Whether débridement improves the rate of healing remains undetermined.

E. SURGICAL THERAPY

Surgical closure of pressure ulcers results in a more rapid resolution of the wound. The chief problems are frequent recurrence of ulcers and inability of frail patients to tolerate the procedure.

The efficacy of surgical repair of pressure ulcers is high in the short term; however, its long-term efficacy has been questioned. Problems with surgical repair include suture line dehiscence, nonhealing, and recurrence. It has been shown, however, that growth factor treatment may improve the outcome of surgical repair.

Bradley M et al: Systematic reviews of wound care management: dressings and topical agents used in the healing of chronic wounds. Health Tech Assess 1999;3:1. [PMID: 10683589]

Prognosis

Pressure ulcers have been associated with increased mortality rates in both acute and long-term care settings. Death has been reported during acute hospitalization in 67% of patients who develop a pressure ulcer compared with 15% of at-risk patients without pressure ulcers. Patients who develop a new pressure ulcer within 6 weeks after hospitalization are 3 times as likely to die as those who do not develop a pressure ulcer. In long-term care settings, development of a pressure ulcer within 3 mo among newly admitted patients was asso-

ciated with a 92% mortality rate compared with 4% among residents who did not subsequently develop a pressure ulcer. Residents in a skilled nursing facility who had pressure ulcers experienced a 6-mo mortality rate of 77.3% compared with 18.3% in those without pressure ulcers. Patients whose pressure ulcers healed within 6 mo had a significantly lower mortality rate (11% vs. 64%) than those whose pressure ulcers did not heal.

Despite this association with death rates, it is not clear how pressure ulcers contribute to increased mortality. Patients with stage II pressure ulcers have been equally as likely to die as those with stage IV pressure ulcers. In the absence of complications, it is difficult to imagine how stage I or II pressure ulcers contribute to death. Pressure ulcers may be associated with mortality because of their occurrence in otherwise frail, sick patients.

Thomas DR: Are all pressure ulcers avoidable? J Am Med Direct Assoc 2001;2:297.

 EVIDENCE-BASED POINTS

- *Risk assessment for pressure ulcers remains problematic because of its infrequent use in health care settings and the lack of an association with improved outcomes. The floor effect in prevention of pressure ulcers may be due to the inability to correct all risk predictors.*
- *Pressure-reducing devices are superior to a standard hospital mattress in preventing pressure ulcers. Pressure-reducing devices appear to be ef-*

Table 28–1. Comparison of occlusive wound dressings.

Variables	Moist saline gauze	Polymer films	Polymer foams	Hydrogels	Hydrocolloids	Alginates, granules	Biomembranes
Pain relief	+	+	+	+	+	±	+
Maceration of surrounding skin	±	±	–	–	–	–	–
O$_2$ permeable	+	+	+	+	–	+	+
H$_2$O permeable	+	+	+	+	–	+	+
Absorbent	+	–	+	+	±	+	–
Damage to epithelial cells	±	+	–	–	–	–	–
Transparent	–	+	–	–	–	–	–
Resistant to bacteria	–	–	–	–	+	–	+
Ease of application	+	–	+	+	+	+	–

Adapted from Helfman T, et al: Occlusive dressings and wound healing. Clin Dermatol 1994;12:121; Witkowski JA & Parish LC: Cutaneous ulcer therapy. J Dermatol 1986;25:420. Used with permission.

Table 28–2. Therapeutic recommendations for treatment of pressure ulcers.

Stage	Needs	Dressing options
I and II	Clean, moist surface Protection from environment	Wet-to-moist saline gauze Thin-film polymer Hydrocolloid dressing
III and IV		
With deadspace, exudate	Clean, moist surface Protection from environment Adsorption of exudate Elimination of deadspace	Wet-to-moist saline gauze Hydrocolloid dressing Synthetic adsorption dressing Hydrogel
With necrosis	Clean, moist surface Protection from environment Débridement	 Surgical Mechanical Enzymatic Autolytic
Heel pressure ulcers	Protection from environment	Pressure reduction

fective in improving the healing rate of pressure ulcers. However, it is difficult to distinguish among various devices.

- Dietary protein intake seems linked to improved rates of healing, but the results of nutritional interventions to prevent pressure ulcers have been disappointing.
- Local wound treatment should aim at maintaining a moist wound environment. Choice of a particular dressing depends on wound characteristics such as exudate, dead space, and wound location.
- Débridement may improve time to a clean wound bed, but the effect of débridement on time to healing remains to be demonstrated. Surgical closure in elderly persons has been associated with a high recurrence rate.

Common Skin Disorders

29

Daniel S. Loo, MD, & Barbara A. Gilchrest, MD

SEBORRHEIC KERATOSIS

ESSENTIALS OF DIAGNOSIS

- Seborrheic keratosis is the most common benign epithelial tumor of adulthood.
- The trunk is affected more than the extremities, head, and neck.
- Primary lesions are 5–20 mm light brown to dark brown–black papules and plaques with a rough, warty surface (Figure 29–1).

Differential Diagnosis

Solar lentigo, melanocytic nevus, and verruca vulgaris are included in the differential diagnosis. If the diagnosis is uncertain, histopathological examination is strongly recommended.

Complications

Friction, pressure, and trauma to these lesions may cause irritation or inflammation.

Treatment

Irritated or inflamed lesions can be treated with cryotherapy (Box 29–1), curettage, or shave removal.

EPIDERMAL INCLUSION CYST

ESSENTIALS OF DIAGNOSIS

- This cutaneous cyst is an epithelium-lined sac filled with keratin and located within the dermis.
- Distribution is more common on the trunk than the face and extremities.
- Primary lesions are 0.5–4 cm flesh-colored to yellow dermal to subcutaneous nodules (Figure 29–2).

- Cysts are freely mobile on palpation. With pressure, cheese-like keratin can often be expressed through a central punctum.
- Differential diagnosis includes lipoma.

Complications

Rupture of the cyst wall leads to extrusion of keratin debris into the dermis and a foreign body inflammatory response. The area becomes tense, tender, and painful.

Treatment

These cysts do not resolve spontaneously. Permanent removal can be achieved only by excising the entire cyst wall. Incision and drainage (I&D) may temporarily relieve pressure but is not curative. In the case of a ruptured cyst, the use of antibiotics is controversial because this is not a true infection (abscess) but rather an inflammatory reaction to foreign material. However, tetracycline has an anti-inflammatory effect, and a dosage of 500 mg twice daily may be helpful. If there is no improvement within 1 week, I&D followed by infiltration of the area with triamcinolone acetonide, 10 mg/mL, will provide relief. Surgery of inflamed tissue is not recommended. If any portion of the cyst wall remains after treatment, recurrence is likely.

WARTS (VERRUCA VULGARIS & VERRUCA PLANTARIS)

ESSENTIALS OF DIAGNOSIS

- These human papillomavirus-induced growths are found most frequently on the hands and feet followed by the extremities and the trunk.
- Primary lesions are 5–15 mm flesh-colored papules and plaques with a verrucous or filiform surface. Reddish-brown punctate dots (thrombosed capillary loops) are diagnostic (Figure

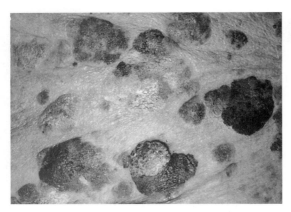

Figure 29–1. Seborrheic keratoses. Waxy, stuck-on papules and plaques, with varying shades of brown and a verrucous surface. Courtesy Neill Peters, MD.

29–3). The lesion may require paring with a no. 15 blade to visualize the capillary loops.

Differential Diagnosis

The differential diagnosis of verruca vulgaris includes flat warts and seborrheic keratosis. The differential diagnosis of verruca plantaris includes callus and clavus (corn).

Treatment

Multiple plantar warts are often stubborn regardless of the treatment modality. Several treatments may be needed before significant improvement occurs. Immunocompromised patients may have widespread involvement and are refractory to standard treatment modalities.

A. CRYOTHERAPY (SEE BOX 29–1)

Two to 3 freeze–thaw cycles are recommended to induce blistering. Treatment is repeated every 3–4 weeks. Plantar warts are thicker and often require paring with a no. 15 blade before freezing.

B. CANTHARADIN

Cantharadin 0.7% (Cantharone) can be used in the office setting. It is applied to the wart, allowed to dry, and covered for 8–12 h. A blister develops within 1–2 days. Treatment is repeated every 3–4 weeks.

C. SALICYLIC ACID

Salicylic acid 40% plasters can be used at home. The plaster is cut to fit over the wart and left in place for

---

BOX 29–1. CRYOTHERAPY

A. Indications
   Liquid nitrogen can be used to treat
      Actinic keratosis
      Seborrheic keratosis (irritated)
      Warts
B. Dipstick technique
   1. Roll extra cotton over the tip of the cotton applicator.
   2. Dip tip into liquid nitrogen.
   3. Apply tip of applicator to lesion until 1–2 mm of normal surrounding skin turns white.
   4. Wait until lesion completely thaws back to normal color.
   5. Repeat (number of freeze–thaw cycles depends on the lesion being treated).
C. Open-spray technique
   (Requires hand-held nitrogen unit and C-tip aperture)
   1. Nozzle should be 1–2 cm from target lesion and perpendicular to it.
   2. Squeeze trigger to emit continuous burst of spray.
   3. The lesion and not more than 1–2 mm of surrounding normal skin should be frosted.
   4. Wait until lesion completely thaws back to normal color.
   5. Repeat (number of freeze–thaw cycles depends on the lesion being treated).
D. Adverse effects
   Patients must be informed that
   1. During application treated area will sting or burn followed by throbbing.
   2. Treated area will become erythematous and edematous and will vesiculate or blister within hours.
   3. Hypopigmentation is common in darkly pigmented individuals.

---

24 h. This is repeated daily. Between treatments, the superficial macerated debris can be removed with a pumice stone or emery board.

ONYCHOMYCOSIS

 ESSENTIALS OF DIAGNOSIS

- *Characteristic features include distal thickening of the nail plate, yellow discoloration, and subungual debris (Figure 29–4).*

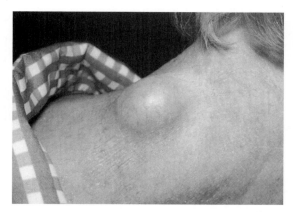

Figure 29–2. Epidermal inclusion cyst. This large 4 × 5-cm cyst on the left shoulder is tense but freely mobile over underlying tissues.

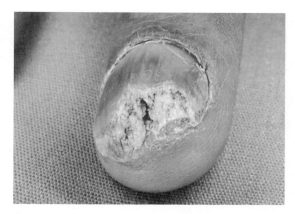

Figure 29–4. Onychomycosis. This fingernail demonstrates the characteristic thick subungual hyperkeratosis and debris.

- Because visual appearance is insufficient to make a diagnosis, microscopy is necessary.
- Differential diagnosis includes pincer nails, onychogryphosis, psoriasis, lichen planus, and repeated trauma.

General Considerations

Yeast or dermatophyte infection of the nail plate requires laboratory confirmation. Nail dystrophy alone is not sensitive or specific for onychomycosis. The average cost of systemic antifungal therapy is $400–$600. Thus, treating all patients with nail dystrophy for pre-

sumed onychomycosis is expensive. There are 3 diagnostic tests.

A. DIRECT MICROSCOPY

Trim back the distal edge of the involved nail. Use a small 1-mm curet or no. 15 blade to scrape the undersurface of the nail plate and nail bed. Place the sample on a glass slide and add 1 drop of potassium hydroxide (KOH) 20% with dimethylsulfoxide (DMSO). Demonstration of hyphae after a few minutes confirms the diagnosis. Sensitivity is highly variable and dependent on experience.

B. CULTURE

Obtain sample as just described and place on Sabouraud's dextrose agar containing chloramphenicol and cycloheximide (Mycosel or Mycobiotic agar). Nail clippings are poor specimens for culture. If there is no growth within 3 weeks, the test is negative. Sensitivity is 50–60%.

C. PATHOLOGY

Send a nail clipping in a formalin container for periodic acid-Schiff (PAS) stain. Sensitivity is > 90%.

Pathogenesis

Public exercise facilities and pools are common sites for transmission of dermatophytes, usually via the feet. Tinea pedis can spread to the adjacent nail and often precedes onychomycosis. Toenails are affected more often than fingernails.

Prevention

Treatment of tinea pedis with topical antifungals can prevent onychomycosis and decrease risk of recurrence.

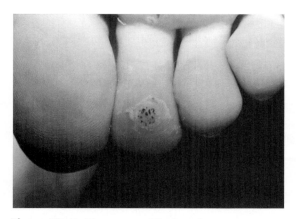

Figure 29–3. Plantar wart. The 2- to 3-mm punctate brown papules are thrombosed capillary loops.

Treatment

Before initiating therapy, patients should be informed that toenails grow very slowly, approximately 1 mm/mo. Thus, if half of the nail is involved, it will take 6–9 mo to clear. If the entire nail is involved, it will take 12–15 mo to clear. Systemic antifungals maintain an effective concentration in the nail matrix for 6–9 mo after therapy is discontinued.

A. SYSTEMIC ANTIFUNGALS

See Table 29–1 for comparison of dosing regimens, mycological cure, and cost.

Terbinafine—This is the treatment of choice for dermatophyte onychomycosis, providing superior long-term clinical efficacy and lower rates of relapse compared with pulse itraconazole. Terbinafine may increase levels of theophylline, nortriptyline, and caffeine and decrease the level of cyclosporine. Rifampin, cimetidine, and terfenadine may alter serum levels of terbinafine. Terbinafine is best avoided in patients with active hepatitis B or C, cirrhosis, or other chronic hepatic disorders. In healthy individuals, baseline liver function tests are optional.

Itraconazole—This is the treatment of choice for onychomycosis caused by yeast (*Candida*) or molds. Itraconazole is contraindicated in patients taking astemizole, terfenadine, triazolam, midazolam, cisapride, lovastatin, and simvastatin. Itraconazole may increase drug levels of oral hypoglycemic agents, immunosuppressants, HIV-1 protease inhibitors, and anticoagulants. Anticonvulsants, antituberculosis agents, revirapine, H_2 antihistamines, proton pump inhibitors, and didanosine may alter serum levels of itraconazole. Itraconazole is best avoided in patients with active hepatitis B or C, cirrhosis, or other chronic hepatic disorders. In healthy individuals, baseline liver function tests are optional.

B. CICLOPIROX NAIL LACQUER SOLUTION

Ciclopirox nail lacquer solution 8% may be effective in patients with only 1–2 nails affected and minimal involvement of the distal nail plate. It is brushed onto affected nails daily for 6 mo. Nails should be trimmed, with regular removal of the unattached infected nail.

Prognosis

With the use of systemic antifungals, relapse rates range from 20–50%. Prophylactic weekend application of topical antifungals may prevent recurrences.

Sigurgeirsson B et al: Long-term effectiveness of treatment with terbinafine vs itraconazole in onychomycosis. Arch Dermatol 2002;138:353. [PMID: 11902986]

DRY SKIN, PRURITUS, & ASTEATOTIC DERMATITIS

 ESSENTIALS OF DIAGNOSIS

- *Dry skin is a common problem and manifests itself predominantly as pruritus.*
- *More than 80% of elderly persons have symptoms related to skin problems; the most frequent complaint is pruritus from dry skin.*
- *Symptoms are more common in the winter.*
- *Indoor heat and low humidity combined with hot showers and overuse of soaps result in dryness and cracking of the skin.*
- *Dry skin may lead to asteatotic dermatitis, with erythematous patches and slightly raised plaques on the anterior shins and extensor surfaces of the arms and less involvement of the trunk. Cracking and dry scaling may also be seen.*

Prevention

A humidifier in the bedroom is helpful. Daily use of moisturizers, especially those containing lactic acid or urea, is recommended to heal dry skin. Moisturizers should be used after bathing while the skin is still slightly moist. Use of bath oils should be avoided because of the risk of slipping.

Table 29–1. Systemic antifungal treatment of toenails.

Drug	Dosing regimen	Mycological cure (18 mo)	Cost
Terbinafine	Continuous: 250 mg/day × 3–4 mo	75–80%	$510–$680
Itraconazole	Continuous: 200 mg/day × 3 mo	70%	$1000
	Pulse: 400 mg/day × 1 week/mo × 3–4 mo	40–50%	$470–$630
Fluconazole	150 mg × 1 day/week × 6 mo	50%	$260

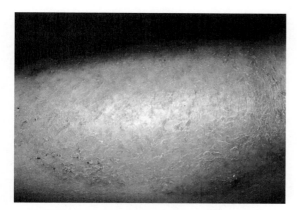

Figure 29–5. Asteatotic dermatitis. This plaque on the left lateral shin demonstrates fine crackling or fissuring.

Differential Diagnosis

Atopic dermatitis, contact dermatitis, and irritant dermatitis can resemble dry skin or asteatosis. Dry skin and asteatotic dermatitis (Figure 29–5) may also coexist with these conditions. Pruritus in the elderly can be caused by a variety of dermatological and systemic conditions, but the most common cause is dry skin.

Treatment

Patient education about preventing dry skin includes

- Reducing use of soaps and rinsing well.
- Application of hydrophilic petrolatum or urea 10% cream to moist skin immediately after bath or shower.
- Reducing vigorous rubbing of the skin with towels, which may exacerbate pruritus.
- In asteatotic dermatitis, in addition to measures used for dry skin, applying a class 4 topical steroid ointment to eczematous patches twice daily for 2–3 weeks or until inflammation and pruritus have resolved. (See Table 29–2 for topical steroid potency rating.)

SEBORRHEIC DERMATITIS

ESSENTIALS OF DIAGNOSIS

- *The face (especially between the eyebrows and nasolabial folds), scalp, and chest are affected (Figure 29–6).*
- *Primary lesions are erythematous patches and plaques with secondary changes of greasy scales.*

Table 29–2. Steroid cream potency rating.

Class	Trade name	Generic
1	Temovate 0.05%	Clobetasol proprionate
	Ultravate 0.05%	Halobetasol proprionate
2	Lidex 0.05%	Fluocinonide
	Psorcon 0.05%	Diflorasone diacetate
3	Aristocort A 0.5%	Triamcinolone acetonide
	Topicort LP 0.05%	Desoximetasone
4	Elocon 0.1%	Mometasone furoate
	Kenalog 0.1%	Triamcinolone acetonide
5	Westcort 0.2%	Hydrocortisone valerate
	Dermatop 0.1%	Prednicarbate
6	Desowen 0.05%	Desonide
	Aristocort A 0.025%	Triamcinolone acetonide
7	Hytone 1%	Hydrocortisone
	Hytone 2.5%	Hydrocortisone

A. Steroid ranking from
Class 1 (strongest) → class 7 (weakest)
1. Most steroids come in both a cream and ointment. For the same concentration, the ointment is slightly more potent than the cream (fluocinonide .05% ointment is stronger than fluocinonide .05% cream).
2. Most topical steroids are applied twice daily.
3. Class 1 steroids should be used in severe inflammatory or pruritic skin conditions (psoriasis, contact dermatitis, scabies).

B. Adverse effects
1. Atrophy, telangiectasias, and striae may occur with prolonged use of potent topical steroids (classes 1 and 2). For instance, clobetasol cream applied twice daily for > 1 mo may result in atrophy. The FDA limits the duration of use of all class 1 steroids to 2 weeks.
2. The face, genitals, intertriginous areas, and mucosal surfaces absorb steroids more readily and are more prone to these side effects. Potent topical steroids should not be used > 2 weeks on the face, genitals, intertriginous areas, and mucosal surfaces.
3. Potent topical steroids applied to > 50% total body surface area may have systemic effects.

FDA, Food and Drug Administration.

- *Rosacea, eczema, lupus, and photosensitivity disorders must be considered in the differential diagnosis.*

General Considerations

Overgrowth of a commensal yeast, *Malassezia furfur*, results in this common dermatitis.

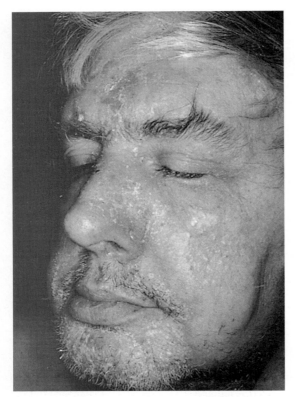

Figure 29–6. Seborrheic dermatitis. Abundant scale distributed over the medial eyebrows, nasolabial folds, mustache, and beard.

STASIS DERMATITIS

 ESSENTIALS OF DIAGNOSIS

- Chronic venous insufficiency results from pooling of venous blood in the lower extremities and increased capillary pressure.
- Chronic venous insufficiency is most commonly associated with varicose veins.
- Anterior shins are affected most, followed by calves, dorsal feet, and ankles.
- Primary lesions are red-brown to brown hyperpigmented macules and patches (Figure 29–7), often with pedal edema.
- Erythematous patches with fine crackling and scales can be seen as secondary changes.
- Ulceration may occur in up to 30% of patients.
- Pigmented purpuric dermatosis, minocycline hyperpigmentation, and contact dermatitis are included in the differential diagnosis.

Prevention

Compression stockings and leg elevation in patients with varicose veins may help prevent stasis changes.

Treatment

A. ANTIDANDRUFF SHAMPOOS

Over-the-counter zinc pyrithione 1%, selenium sulfide 1%, or ketoconazole 1% shampoo can be applied to the scalp every day for 1 week and then tapered to once or twice weekly to prevent recurrence. The lather should be massaged on the face for a few minutes before rinsing. Ketoconazole 2% shampoo may be more effective.

B. TOPICAL TREATMENT

Topical treatment may be needed for patients unresponsive to shampoos alone.

1. Facial involvement—Apply ketoconazole 2% cream twice daily for 2–3 weeks or class 6 steroid cream twice daily for 2–3 weeks.

2. Scalp pruritus—A class 5 steroid solution can be applied daily as needed.

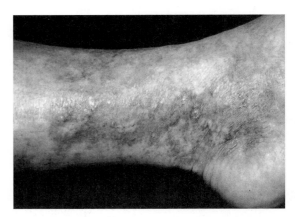

Figure 29–7. Stasis dermatitis. Hyperpigmented macules and patches involving the left medial malleolus.
Courtesy of Neill Peters, MD.

Treatment

Compression stockings at 20–30 mm Hg can be applied. Elevation of the legs above the level of the heart whenever sitting or lying down will reduce venous pooling. Class 5 steroid ointment applied twice daily will relieve any eczematous patches or plaques.

PSORIASIS

ESSENTIALS OF DIAGNOSIS

- *This is a hereditable T cell-mediated inflammatory dermatosis; 33% of those affected have a positive family history.*
- *Psoriasis may be precipitated by streptococcal pharyngitis (guttate psoriasis).*
- *There is symmetric involvement of extensor surfaces (elbows, knees, lumbosacral) and scalp. The flexures and genitals may also be involved (inverse psoriasis).*
- *Primary lesions are erythematous papules and plaques with secondary changes of thick micaceous scale (Figure 29–8).*
- *Nails may demonstrate yellow-brown oil spots, pitting (Figure 29–9), and onycholysis.*
- *Differential diagnosis includes eczema, seborrheic dermatitis, and lichen planus.*

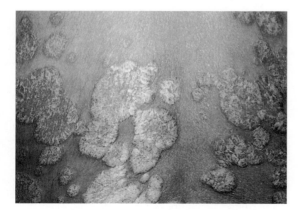

Figure 29–8. Psoriasis. Plaques with thick micaceous scale on the lower back.

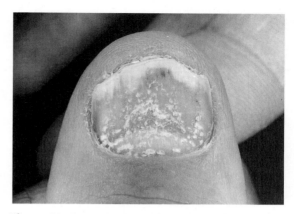

Figure 29–9. Nail psoriasis. This thumbnail demonstrates pitting and distal onycholysis.

Complications

Arthritis of the small and large joints may accompany psoriasis. Generalized pustular psoriasis and erythrodermic psoriasis may be life threatening and require hospitalization.

Treatment

Choice of therapy is dependent on disease severity. For individuals with < 30% total body surface area affected, topical therapies are generally effective.

A. TOPICAL CORTICOSTEROIDS

1. Trunk & extremities—Class 1 steroid ointment is applied to plaques twice daily for 2–3 weeks or until flattening of lesional skin occurs.

2. Face, intertriginous sites—Class 5 steroid cream is applied to plaques twice daily for 2–3 weeks or until flattening of lesional skin occurs.

B. CALCIPOTRIENE

Calcipotriene, .005% ointment applied twice daily, has a slower onset of action compared with topical steroids and is effective for moderate plaque psoriasis. Irritation is the most common side effect.

C. NATURAL SUNLIGHT

Natural sunlight, when practical, is often very helpful. Before 10 AM and after 2 PM, the patient should lie flat for 15–20 min on each side 2–3 times a week. For those patients with > 30% total body surface area affected, referral to a dermatologist for phototherapy or systemic agents should be considered.

Prognosis

Psoriasis is a chronic disease characterized by exacerbations and remissions. A positive family history, early onset, and extensive involvement are poor prognostic factors.

ROSACEA

ESSENTIALS OF DIAGNOSIS

- Sometimes referred to as adult acne, rosacea is most common in women aged 40 to 50 and is characterized by flushing.
- Lesions affect the central face (nose, cheeks, forehead, and chin).
- Primary lesions are erythematous papules and pustules (Figure 29–10).
- Secondary changes include confluent telangiectasias with erythema.
- Differential diagnosis includes acne, perioral dermatitis, and systemic lupus erythematosus.

Pathogenesis

Although the cause of rosacea is unknown, any stimulus that increases skin temperature of the head and neck can trigger flushing, including sunlight, hot showers, exercise, alcohol, hot beverages, and spicy foods.

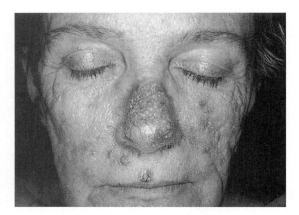

Figure 29–10. Rosacea. Papules and pustules of the central face with enlarged nose and telangiectasias.

Complications

Some cases can progress to rhinophyma (enlarged bulbous nose). Ocular involvement (blepharitis, conjunctivitis) may occur in up to 50% of patients.

Treatment

A. SUNSCREEN

Patients may be able to reduce symptoms by avoiding triggers and applying sunscreen with a sun protection factor of ≥ 15 daily.

B. TOPICAL ANTIBIOTICS

Topical antibiotics include metronidazole, 0.75% cream or gel applied twice daily, and sodium sulfacetamide 10%/sulfur 5% lotion applied twice daily.

C. SYSTEMIC ANTIBIOTICS

Systemic antibiotics include tetracycline, 500 mg orally twice daily on an empty stomach, and doxycycline, 100 mg orally twice daily.

D. LASER TREATMENT

For telangiectasias, the patient can be referred to a dermatologist for pulsed dye laser treatment. This is most effective, although it does not prevent development of new telangiectasias.

CONTACT DERMATITIS

ESSENTIALS OF DIAGNOSIS

- Contact dermatitis is a delayed-type hypersensitivity reaction to an antigen (allergen) that contacts the skin and causes severe pruritus.
- Symptoms can be acute or chronic.

Prevention

Patients should be advised to avoid sources of known allergens. Table 29–3 lists the most frequent contact allergens and their sources.

Differential Diagnosis

Acute contact dermatitis can be localized to 1 region or generalized and has linear or artificial patterns (Figure 29–11). Primary lesions include vesicles and erythema-

Table 29–3. Most frequent contact allergens & their sources.

Contact allergens	Common sources
Nickel	Jewelry
Fragrance mix	Skin or hair care products
Thimerosal	Vaccines, eye and nasal medications
Quaternium-15	Cosmetics
Neomycin	Antibiotic ointment
Formaldehyde	Nail polish, cosmetics
Bacitracin	Antibiotic ointment
Thiuram	Latex gloves, shoes (rubber products)
Balsam of Peru	Fragrance in cosmetics
Cobalt	Metal-plated objects (buckles, button, zippers)
P-paraphenylenediamine	Hair dye
Carba mix	Rubber elastic of underwear

tous, edematous plaques. Secondary changes include erosions, exudates, and crusts.

Chronic contact dermatitis can be localized to 1 region or generalized and occurs in linear or artificial patterns (indicative of external contact). Primary lesions appear as lichenified plaques. Secondary changes include hyperpigmentation.

Atopic dermatitis, scabies, and irritant dermatitis must be considered in the differential diagnosis.

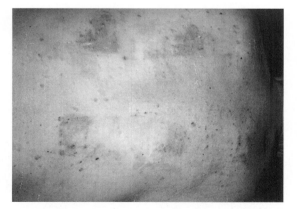

Figure 29–11. Contact dermatitis. These square-shaped, itchy plaques resulted from electrode adhesive pads from a transcutaneous electrical nerve stimulation unit.

Complications

Left untreated, dermatitis may spread, causing debilitating pruritus.

Treatment

If < 10% of the surface area is involved, a class 1 steroid ointment can be applied 3 times a day for 2–3 weeks or until the dermatitis and pruritus resolves. If > 10% of body surface area is affected, a prednisone taper is appropriate (Box 29–2).

DRUG ERUPTION (MORBILLIFORM)

ESSENTIALS OF DIAGNOSIS

- *Maculopapular eruptions, the most common type of drug eruption, usually occur during the first 2 weeks of a new medication.*
- *The most common drugs implicated in drug eruptions are penicillins (ampicillin, amoxicillin), sulfonamides (trimethoprim-sulfamethoxazole), nonsteroidal anti-inflammatory drugs (naproxen,*

BOX 29–2. PREDNISONE TAPER

A. Indications
   (severe pruritus from a variety of conditions)
   1. Contact dermatitis > 10% surface area
   2. Scabies
   3. Severe eczema
   4. Drug eruption
B. Dosing
   start with 1 mg/kg and then taper by 5 mg each consecutive day.
   1. For 130-lb patient, start with 60 mg and taper by 5 mg each day for 12-day course.
   2. Severe cases may require a higher starting dose or a prolonged taper over 2–3 weeks.
   3. Medrol dosepaks are inadequate for most adults.
C. Side effects
   (review patient's history for hypertension, diabetes, glaucoma)
   1. Water retention
   2. Weight gain
   3. Increased appetite
   4. Mood swings
   5. Restlessness

piroxicam), anticonvulsants (carbamazepine, phenytoin), and antihypertensives (captopril, diltiazem).

- *Distribution of drug eruptions is bilateral and symmetric, usually beginning on the head and neck or upper trunk and progressing down the limbs.*
- *Primary lesions are erythematous macules and papules with areas of confluence (Figure 29–12).*
- *Pruritus is occasionally present.*
- *Differential diagnosis includes viral exanthem, bacterial infection, and collagen vascular disease.*

Complications

Drug hypersensitivity syndrome is potentially life threatening and presents as a triad of fever, skin eruption (80% morbilliform), and internal organ involvement (hepatitis, nephritis, lymphadenopathy). This occurs on first exposure to the drug, with symptoms starting 1–6 weeks after exposure. Laboratory tests to evaluate potential asymptomatic internal organ involvement include transaminases, complete blood cell count, urinalysis, and serum creatinine.

Treatment

The drug most likely to have caused the eruption should be stopped along with any unnecessary medications.

Topical and oral steroids provide symptomatic relief. Regimens include class 1 steroid cream twice daily for 2–3 weeks or prednisone taper (see Box 29–2) if creams are ineffective. Resolution usually occurs within 1–2 weeks.

Sullivan JR, Shear NH: Drug eruptions and other adverse drug effects in aged skin. Clin Geriatr Med 2002:18;21. [PMID: 11913737]

HERPES ZOSTER (see also Chapter 34: Common Infections)

 ESSENTIALS OF DIAGNOSIS

- *Herpes zoster is caused by reactivation of varicella-zoster virus in the dorsal root ganglion.*
- *Distribution of grouped vesicular lesions is unilateral (Figure 29–13) and within 1–2 adjacent dermatomes (ophthalmic branch of trigeminal nerve, thoracic, and cervical are most commonly affected).*
- *Primary lesions are vesicles (Figure 29–14) on an erythematous base. Secondary changes consist of pustules and crusts.*
- *Immunosuppression, especially hematological malignancy and HIV infection, substantially increase the risk for herpes zoster as well as dissemination.*

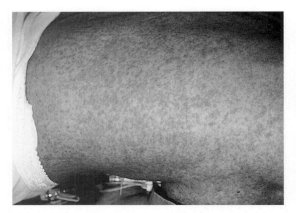

Figure 29–12. Morbilliform drug eruption. Macules and papules of the right flank and back with areas of confluence. Courtesy Melvin Lu, MD.

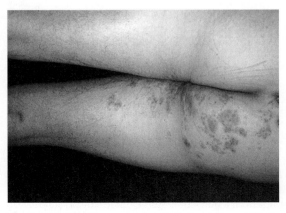

Figure 29–13. Herpes zoster. Unilateral S1 and S2 distribution.

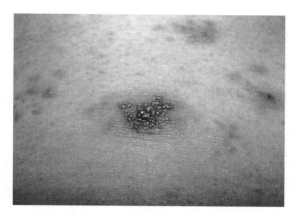

Figure 29–14. Herpes zoster. The same patient as in Figure 29–13 has grouped vesicles on an erythematous base.

General Considerations

Pain precedes the eruption in > 90% of cases. Rarely, the eruption does not develop, and neuralgia is the only manifestation of zoster (zoster sine herpete). In most cases, grouped vesicles in a dermatomal distribution are enough to establish the diagnosis. A positive Tzanck smear cannot distinguish between herpes simplex and varicella-zoster virus. Viral cultures identify herpes simplex within 2–3 days; however, varicella-zoster culture can take 1–2 weeks with frequent false-negative results.

Differential Diagnosis

Herpes simplex, eczema herpeticum, varicella, and acute contact dermatitis are included in the differential diagnosis.

Complications

Patients with cutaneous involvement of the V_1 branch of the trigeminal nerve may experience ocular complications (keratitis, acute retinal necrosis) and need to undergo immediate slit-lamp examination by an ophthalmologist, particularly if skin lesions involve the side and tip of the nose (Hutchinson's sign). Immunocompromised patients are at risk for dissemination, defined as > 20 vesicles outside the primary and immediately adjacent dermatomes. Cutaneous dissemination may be followed by visceral involvement (lung, liver, brain) in 10% of these high-risk patients.

Postherpetic neuralgia is pain that persists after resolution of the cutaneous eruption. This most common complication is age dependent, affecting at least 50% of patients older than 60, and most frequently involves the face.

Treatment

The systemic antiviral drugs (acyclovir, famciclovir, valacyclovir) are effective in the acute phase of zoster and should be used within 48–72 h of rash onset. These drugs have been shown to reduce acute pain, accelerate healing, prevent scarring, and reduce the incidence of postherpetic neuralgia. Systemic corticosteroids (prednisone) may help to reduce acute pain but have no effect on incidence or severity of postherpetic neuralgia. Although the safety profile for the antiviral drugs is excellent, headache, nausea, diarrhea, and central nervous system (CNS), renal, and hepatic dysfunction can occur. In more severe cases, especially in disseminated zoster, initial intravenous acyclovir should be considered. Studies indicate that oral therapy is as effective as intravenous therapy in ophthalmic zoster.

Prognosis

The affected dermatome usually heals within 3–4 weeks and occasionally may scar. Postherpetic neuralgia is the major cause of morbidity.

SCABIES

 ESSENTIALS OF DIAGNOSIS

- The Sarcoptes scabiei *mite inhabits the human stratum corneum. Characteristic initial lesions are 3–8 mm linear or serpiginous ridges (burrows; Figure 29–15), often with a gray dot at one end (mite).*

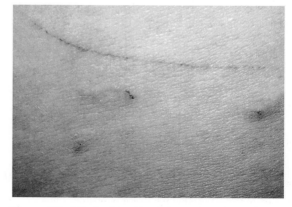

Figure 29–15. Scabies. Serpiginous 3- to 8-mm burrows above a linear excoriation.

- *The interdigital web spaces of the hands, volar wrists, penis shaft, and areolae are commonly involved.*
- *Secondary changes include papules and nodules (nodular scabies), diffuse eczematous dermatitis, thick hyperkeratotic crusted plaques (crusted or Norwegian scabies), and vesicles or bullae (bullous scabies).*
- *Pruritus is intractable and debilitating.*

General Considerations

Close body contact is the most common mode of transmission. Fomite transmission is rare because the female mite cannot survive away from the host for > 24–36 h. Risk factors include nursing home residence, HIV and AIDS, and crowded living conditions.

Clinical Findings

Diagnosis is confirmed (finding mites, eggs [Figure 29–16], or feces) using direct microscopy in a simple bedside test.

1. Specimen collection—Place a drop of mineral oil on the center of a glass slide. Touch the sharp part of a no. 15 blade to the drop (so that the specimen will adhere to the blade). Holding the blade perpendicular to the skin, scrape an epidermal burrow to remove the stratum corneum. Pinpoint bleeding indicates the correct depth. Wipe contents onto the center of the glass slide. Choose 2 other burrows, and repeat steps 2–4 to increase the yield. Place coverslip over specimen and gently press down.

2. Microscope settings—Use ×4 objective to scan the slide.

Differential Diagnosis

The differential diagnosis includes atopic dermatitis, contact dermatitis, drug eruption, and urticarial bullous pemphigoid.

Complications

Nodular scabies is a pruritic hypersensitivity reaction to remnants of the mite. The lesions are firm erythematous to red-brown nodules occurring on the genitals and the axillae. Patients who are immunocompromised may develop crusted or Norwegian scabies with extensive yellow crusting. Norwegian scabies is extremely contagious because each crust contains hundreds of mites. Epidemics of scabies in nursing homes are relatively common and often go undetected for long periods.

Treatment

Goals of therapy include mite eradication, alleviation of pruritus, and prevention of transmission.

A. SCABICIDE

The patient and all close contacts should be treated simultaneously, including those who are asymptomatic.

1. Permethrin—Permethrin 5% cream is the most effective topical treatment. A 60-g tube is prescribed for whole-body application. Patients can be instructed to take a bath or shower and completely dry before application. Cream should be applied to the entire skin surface (from the neck down), with particular attention to finger web spaces, feet, genitals, and intertriginous sites. The cream should be washed off in 8 h. This regimen is repeated in 1 week. Compliance will result in > 90% cure rate.

2. Lindane—Lindane 1% lotion application instructions are identical to those for permethrin. Lindane is safe if used appropriately. Overexposure to lindane (excessive cutaneous applications, ingestion, application to excoriated or infected skin) can cause CNS toxicity, convulsions, and rarely death. Thus, patients with extensively eroded skin or crusted scabies should not be treated with lindane.

3. Ivermectin—Ivermectin, 0.2 mg/kg as an oral dose and repeated at 10–14 days, should be considered in cases resistant to topical treatment, crusted scabies, and the immunocompromised host (eg, HIV patients). Al-

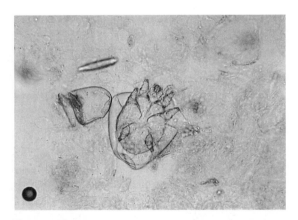

Figure 29–16. Direct microscopy. Scabies mite hatched from an egg. Courtesy Neill Peters, MD.

though more research is needed to determine the safety and efficacy of ivermectin compared with topical scabicides, this is a practical option for nursing home epidemics in which proper application of permethrin or lindane may be difficult to achieve.

B. Pruritus

Even after successful mite eradication, severe pruritus can persist for 3–4 weeks. This often debilitating symptom is frequently overlooked and leads to unnecessary discomfort and suffering. Patients may receive repeated treatment for scabies in the mistaken belief that infestation persists.

Class 1 steroid ointment can be applied 2–3 times daily for 2–4 weeks or until complete resolution of pruritus. Prednisone taper (see Box 29–2) may be needed.

C. Transmission Prevention

All clothes worn within 2 days of treatment, towels, and bed sheets should be machine washed in hot water or dry cleaned. Management of nursing home outbreaks requires clinical and epidemiological expertise and possibly involvement of public health experts.

Prognosis

Immunocompetent individuals do well with standard therapy. Crusted scabies, usually in the immunosuppressed, may require > 2 applications of topical scabicides or ivermectin or a combination.

Meinking TL, Elgart GW: Scabies therapy for the millennium. Pediatr Dermatol 2000;17:154. [PMID: 10792811]

Walker GJ, Johnstone PW: Interventions for treating scabies. Cochrane Database Syst Rev 2000;2:CD000320. [PMID: 10796527]

ACTINIC KERATOSIS

ESSENTIALS OF DIAGNOSIS

- *Actinic keratosis is a precursor lesion to squamous cell carcinoma.*
- *Distribution of lesions includes the face, lips, ears, dorsal hands, and forearms (photodistribution).*
- *Primary lesions are 3–10 mm rough, adherent, scaly white papules and plaques (Figure 29–17), often on an erythematous base.*
- *Palpation reveals a gritty, sandpaper-like texture. Lesions are often more readily palpated than visualized.*

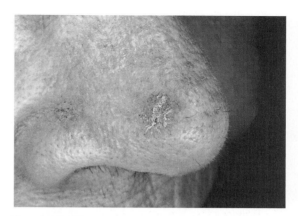

Figure 29–17. Actinic keratosis. This is a rough, adherent, scaly papule on the right nasal bridge.

- *Differential diagnosis includes dry seborrheic keratosis and retention hyperkeratosis.*

General Considerations

Actinic keratoses are more common in whites and are directly related to cumulative lifetime sun exposure. Immunosuppressed patients, particularly transplant recipients, are at higher risk for actinic keratoses. Daily sunscreen, long-sleeve shirts, broad-brimmed hats, and avoidance of sun can prevent these lesions.

Complications

Various studies cite a < 1–20% risk of transformation to squamous cell carcinoma (SCC) for an individual lesion over the course of a year.

Treatment

Cryotherapy (see Box 29–1) with 2 freeze–thaw cycles is recommended for actinic keratoses. 5-Fluorouracil 5% cream can be applied to affected areas twice daily for 3 weeks. Patients must be informed that treated areas will become severely irritated, inflamed, and eroded.

The patient should return in 1–2 weeks for assessment of side effects. Compliance may be improved by dividing the affected area into smaller subunits and treating 1 subunit at a time to minimize the inflammatory reaction.

Patients with actinic keratoses should be examined annually and are also at risk for basal cell carcinoma (BCC), SCC, and melanoma.

BASAL CELL CARCINOMA

ESSENTIALS OF DIAGNOSIS

- *Basal cell carcinoma is the most common skin cancer (~75%) and is related to chronic ultraviolet light exposure.*
- *Basal cell carcinoma is derived from stem cells in the basal layer of the epidermis.*
- *The head and neck are most frequently involved; the nose is the most common site.*
- *Primary lesions are translucent or pearly papules or nodules (Figure 29–18), often with visible telangiectasias. Secondary changes include central ulceration or crusting.*
- *The lesion may break down or bleed and does not heal.*
- *Biopsy (rolled shave or punch technique) is required to confirm the diagnosis.*
- *Squamous cell carcinoma, keratoacanthoma, and sebaceous hyperplasia are included in the differential diagnosis.*

Complications

Although BCC rarely metastasizes, if left untreated, it may become locally invasive and extend to underlying cartilage, fascia, muscle, and bone.

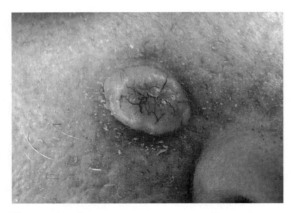

Figure 29–18. Basal cell carcinoma. A 1.5-cm shiny nodule with telangiectasias adjacent to the right nasal ala.

Treatment

Electrodesiccation and curettage (ED&C) and excision have comparable cure rates of 90% for low-risk tumors.

Mohs' surgery is the most effective technique (98–100% cure rate) and is indicated for high-risk tumors.

Prognosis

BCC patients determined to be at high risk for recurrence and metastasis have ≥ 1 of the following: recurrent tumor, tumor on the trunk and extremities > 2 cm, tumor on the head and neck > 1 cm, tumor with poorly defined borders, tumor with immunosuppressed host, and tumor occurring at a site of prior radiation. Recurrence rate with standard modalities (ED&C or excision) is > 10%.

For patients with a prior BCC, the 3-year cumulative risk for BCC recurrence is ~44%. For most patients, an annual skin exam is sufficient for detecting new BCCs. Because the number of previous skin cancers is a strong risk factor for subsequent skin cancers, patients with multiple BCCs should be seen more frequently.

Marcil I, Stern RS: Risk of developing a subsequent nonmelanoma skin cancer in patients with a history of nonmelanoma skin cancer. Arch Dermatol 2000;136:1524. [PMID: 11115165]

Miller SJ: The National Comprehensive Cancer Network (NCCN) guidelines of care for nonmelanoma skin cancers. Dermatol Surg 2000;26:289. [PMID: 10759812]

SQUAMOUS CELL CARCINOMA

ESSENTIALS OF DIAGNOSIS

- *SCC is derived from keratinocytes above the basal layer of the epidermis, often with actinic keratoses as precursor lesions.*
- *The head, neck, dorsal hands, and forearms are affected.*
- *Primary lesions are firm indurated papules, plaques, or nodules (Figure 29–19). Secondary changes include rough adherent scale, central erosion, or ulceration with crust.*
- *The lesion does not heal and breaks down or bleeds.*
- *Biopsy with rolled shave or punch technique is required to confirm the diagnosis.*
- *Differential diagnosis includes basal cell carcinoma and keratoacanthoma.*

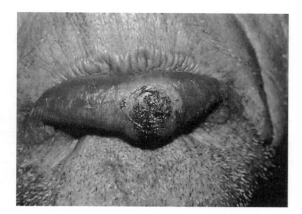

Figure 29–19. Squamous cell carcinoma. This hard 2.5 × 2.5-cm nodule with overlying dry hemorrhagic crust is at risk for spread to cervical nodes. Courtesy Melvin Lu, MD.

General Considerations

SCC comprises ~20% of all skin cancers and has the capacity to metastasize. If SCC is suspected, palpation of regional lymph nodes is recommended. SCC should be suspected in any persistent nodule, plaque, or ulcer, especially when occurring in sun-damaged skin, on the lower lip, in areas of prior radiation, in old burn scars, or on the genitals. Immunosuppressed patients (eg, transplant recipients) are at higher risk for SCC because of impaired cell-mediated immunity.

Complications

SCC on the lips or ears has a 10–15% risk of spread to cervical nodes. The overall rate of metastasis from all skin sites ranges from < 1–5%.

Treatment

ED&C and excision have comparable cure rates of 90% for low-risk tumors. Mohs' surgery is the most effective technique (98–100% cure rate) and is indicated for high-risk tumors.

Prognosis

SCC patients considered to be at high risk for recurrence and metastasis have 1 or more of the following: recurrent tumor; tumor on the trunk and extremities > 2 cm; tumor on the head and neck > 1 cm; tumor occurring on the genitals, lips, ears, site of prior radiation, or scar; tumor with poorly defined borders; and tumor with immunosuppressed host. Recurrence rate with standard modalities (ED&C or excision) is > 10%.

For patients with a prior SCC, the 3-year cumulative risk for another SCC is ~18%. Annual follow-up examinations for at least 3 years is recommended. Because the number of previous skin cancers is a strong risk factor for subsequent skin cancers, patients with multiple SCCs should be seen more frequently.

Marcil I, Stern RS: Risk of developing a subsequent nonmelanoma skin cancer in patients with a history of nonmelanoma skin cancer. Arch Dermatol 2000;136:1524. [PMID: 1115165]

Miller SJ: The National Comprehensive Cancer Network (NCCN) guidelines of care for nonmelanoma skin cancers. Dermatol Surg 2000;26:289. [PMID: 10759812]

MELANOMA

 ### ESSENTIALS OF DIAGNOSIS

- *Melanoma, derived from melanocytes, has the greatest potential for metastasis.*
- *The trunk and legs are affected more than the face and neck, although the face and neck are more likely to be affected in the elderly.*
- *The primary lesion is a brown–black macule, papule, plaque, or nodule with ≥ 1 of the following features (Figure 29–20): asymmetry, border irregularity, color variegation, diameter > 6 mm.*
- *Patients may notice an increase in size (diameter) of a pigmented lesion and bleeding.*

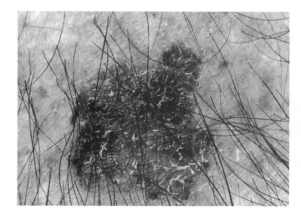

Figure 29–20. Melanoma. 2 × 2-cm plaque on the chest with varying shades of brown to black, asymmetry, and irregular borders.

• *Lesions should be excised with a margin of clinically normal skin down to subcutaneous fat.*

General Considerations

The incidence of melanoma is increasing faster than any other cancer. The lifetime risk of melanoma in an individual in the United States born in 2001 is estimated at 1 in 71. Melanoma is the most common cancer in women aged 25–29 and the second most common, after breast cancer, for women aged 30–34.

Older men have the highest incidence of melanoma and the highest mortality rates from melanoma. In the United States, the incidence of thick tumors (> 4 mm) has continued to increase in men 60 years of age and older. Nearly 50% of all melanoma deaths involve white men 50 years of age and older.

Risk factors include light complexion (red–blond hair), blistering sunburns during childhood, tendency to tan poorly and sunburn easily, and a positive family history. Additional risk factors in the middle-aged population include age > 50 years, male sex, and a history of actinic keratoses or nonmelanoma skin cancers.

Differential Diagnosis

Seborrheic keratosis, solar lentigo, dysplastic nevus, and pigmented BCC are included in the differential diagnosis.

Complications

Untreated melanoma has a high risk of metastasis to lymph nodes, liver, lungs, and brain.

Treatment

Melanoma is treated by surgical excision with margins determined by histological tumor thickness (Breslow depth). Evaluation of nodal involvement with sentinel lymph node biopsy is recommended for primary melanomas deeper than 1.0 mm and for tumors ≤ 1 mm when histological ulceration is present. Frequency of follow-up, laboratory tests, and imaging studies depends on stage of disease.

Prognosis

Tumor thickness and presence or absence of histological ulceration are the most important prognostic factors. Patients with thin melanomas (< 1.0 mm) have the best prognosis (> 90% 5-year survival rate), whereas those with thick tumors (> 4 mm) have a 50% 5-year survival rate. For patients with nodal involvement, the number of affected nodes determines the overall prognosis.

Balch CM et al: Final version of the American Joint Committee on Cancer staging system for cutaneous melanoma. J Clin Oncol 2001;19:3635. [PMID: 11504745]

Jemal A et al: Recent trends in cutaneous melanoma incidence among whites in the United States. J Natl Cancer Inst 2001;93:678. [PMID: 11333289]

Sober AJ et al: Guidelines of care for primary cutaneous melanoma. J Am Acad Dermatol 2001;45:579. [PMID: 11568750]

Cancers in the Geriatric Population   30

Joanne E. Mortimer, MD, & Janet McElhaney, MD

General Considerations

Elderly patients with cancer provide a unique challenge to the oncologist, whether the intent is cure or palliation of symptoms. Curative therapy may require aggressive and potentially morbid operations, radiation therapy, or chemotherapy. Such aggressive approaches are more toxic in the elderly, who tend to be less resilient.

Cancers in the elderly may demonstrate a distinct natural history that differs from that of younger patients. For example, breast cancers tend to have a more favorable prognosis in the elderly, whereas acute leukemias have a worse prognosis. In addition, because toxicities from therapeutic intervention may be more frequent in the elderly, more severe modifications in therapy may be required. Although radiation therapy is generally well tolerated, alterations in the radiation fields and doses may be necessary to decrease toxicity without significantly compromising efficacy.

Most of the antineoplastic agents are cytotoxic to rapidly dividing cells and are not specific for cancer cells. This lack of specificity results in myelosuppression, mucositis, and hair loss. In general, older patients experience more frequent and more severe normal tissue toxicities. Both the peripheral neuropathy from vincristine and the cardiotoxicity from doxorubicin develop at lower cumulative doses than is typically seen in younger patients. Similarly, mucositis from the combination of 5-fluorouracil (5-FU) and leucovorin is also more common and more severe in the elderly. Alterations in renal and, to a lesser extent, hepatic function occur with age and should be considered in the selection and dosing of chemotherapy. Agents such as methotrexate, cisplatin, and bleomycin are normally excreted by the kidney and may produce excessive toxicity in the elderly if administered in conventional doses. With an awareness of the normal aging physiology and knowledge of the pharmacology of antineoplastic agents, chemotherapy may be safely administered.

Treatment

Once it has been determined that the cancer is not curable or that the patient is physically unable to tolerate aggressive therapy, the goal becomes palliation of cancer-related symptoms. Palliative care may involve the management of symptoms related to the cancer and its spread (eg, pain or shortness of breath from a pleural effusion) or may require preemptive therapy to avoid a more morbid complication resulting from untreated cancer. Radiation therapy to the spine to prevent spinal cord compression is an example.

It has consistently been shown that pain is not managed well in the elderly, especially women and minority populations. Cancer pain management should be tailored to the individual patient's pain needs. Initially, scheduled doses of acetaminophen (650 mg 4 times/day) combined with a short-acting opioid analgesic, such as oxycodone, may provide pain relief for 4–6 h. Acetaminophen potentiates the effect of the opioid analgesic when given in regular doses, so that lower doses of an opioid may be effective. Thus, acetaminophen/opioid combinations should be avoided unless they simplify pain management without disrupting the scheduled acetaminophen regimen. As the need for pain medications increases, short-acting opioid analgesics should be used for dose titration and then converted to a long-acting medication equivalent such as sustained-release morphine, oxycodone, and fentanyl to provide effective control of pain.

Complications

Constipation is an expected side effect of opioid analgesics, which cause paralysis of the myenteric plexus. A daily dose of a laxative is recommended for all patients when an opioid analgesic is initiated. Delirium and agitation are additional complications of opioid use that may be confused with adequate pain control. Sedative medications such as benzodiazepines can often paradoxically increase agitation as a result of worsening delirium. This problem can be minimized with lower and more frequent dosing of the opioid analgesics.

Fentanyl patches may provide more rapid drug delivery because of age-related atrophy of the skin; thus, lower dose patches may help to avoid delirium. Combinations of medications may be required, depending on the type of cancer pain being treated, and include antidepressant drugs and gabapentin, especially for neuralgic pain.

BREAST CANCER

The incidence of breast cancer increases with age and plateaus in the seventh decade. In 1973, 37% of breast cancers were diagnosed in women older than 65; in 1995, that number increased to 46.7%. The natural history of breast cancer in the elderly is unique. When prognostic factors such as estrogen receptor (ER), histological grade, ploidy, p53, epithelial growth factor receptor (EGFR), and c-*erb*-b2 status are assessed, it appears that tumors become less aggressive with advancing age. Despite this, 60% of breast cancer-related deaths involve women 65 years of age and older. The high mortality rate may be explained by several factors. First, breast cancer is a common disease in this age group, and patients have life-threatening comorbid conditions. Second, physicians tend to treat the elderly less aggressively than younger individuals.

Primary Breast Cancer

Treatment

Treatment recommendations should be made on an individual basis, taking into consideration comorbid conditions and expectations of therapy. Whenever possible, patients should be encouraged to participate in trials designed to assess how cancers can best be managed.

A. BREAST CONSERVATION THERAPY

Although modified radical mastectomy and breast conservation therapy with lumpectomy and radiation share similar survival rates, elderly women are less likely to undergo breast conservation therapy. Possibly some women chose mastectomy because they find the 6–7 weeks of daily radiation treatments for breast conservation cumbersome. It has also been shown that physicians are less likely to offer breast conservation therapy to older women.

Data suggest that, after surgical removal of the primary cancer, tamoxifen without radiation therapy may be adequate in select patients. However, by eliminating breast irradiation, ipsilateral breast cancer recurrences are more common and are generally treated by mastectomy for local control of the primary cancer. Despite the higher rate of "in-breast" recurrences, the survival for women treated with this less aggressive approach is identical to that among women treated with conventional surgery and radiation therapy. Resection of the primary tumor and administration of tamoxifen may be appropriate for select women with small, ER+ breast cancers, and a finite life expectancy. Older women with a favorable long-term outlook should be treated as aggressively as younger women.

B. ADJUVANT THERAPY

For women with localized ER+ breast cancers, 5 years of adjuvant tamoxifen decreases the recurrence rate and incidence of contralateral breast cancers. In older women on tamoxifen, the incidence of venous thromboemboli and uterine cancer is higher than in younger women; however, the benefits of adjuvant tamoxifen outweigh the risks. An aromatase inhibitor such as anastrozole may be substituted in women for whom tamoxifen is contraindicated. When chemotherapy is indicated, the reduction in recurrence and survival advantage is identical to that observed in younger women.

Although one must weigh comorbid conditions when making treatment recommendations, appropriately administered adjuvant therapy has been shown to be cost effective. In the absence of severe comorbidities, the guidelines for adjuvant therapy are identical to those used to treat younger women. Women with ER+ breast cancers should receive adjuvant hormonal therapy, usually with tamoxifen. Chemotherapy should be considered for those women whose primary cancers are > 1 cm and ER– or her-2 positive and those with multiple node involvement.

Metastatic Disease

Treatment

Because the majority of breast cancers are ER+, hormonal therapy is the mainstay of treatment for advanced breast cancers. The aromatase inhibitors (anastrozole, letrozole, and exemestane) have achieved a higher rate of tumor regression and a longer duration of efficacy and have replaced tamoxifen as first-line therapy for metastatic disease. In ER– disease and cancers that are hormone resistant, chemotherapy may provide effective palliation. Newer, less toxic single agents such as oral capecitabine have been shown to be as effective as combination chemotherapy. The humanized monoclonal antibody trastuzumab (Herceptin) is reserved for those patients whose cancers overexpress the her-2 protein. Trastuzumab is effective as a single agent and, when combined with initial chemotherapy, offers better a survival rate compared with chemotherapy alone.

Prevention

Screening mammography have been shown to decrease breast cancer mortality in women aged 70–79. Screening mammography identifies early lesions in older women as effectively as in younger women. A single decision analysis and cost-effective study of mammography in women older than 69 demonstrated that survival may be favorably affected by screening mammography. The American Geriatrics Society recommends annual screening mammography for women up to age 85, provided that their life expectancy is > 3 years.

LUNG CANCER

General Considerations

Lung cancer is the leading cause of cancer death in both men and women. The majority of patients are older than 65. Cancers arising from lung parenchyma are categorized as either small cell or non-small cell (adenocarcinoma, large cell, squamous cell, bronchoalveolar cell, or mixed histologies). Although older individuals are less likely to be referred for aggressive surgical procedures, a tissue confirmation of cancer and determination of histology provides important diagnostic and prognostic information. Prognosis is also related to the stage of disease, performance status, gender, and patient's ability to tolerate adequate treatment. Although age is not an independent prognostic factor, elderly patients do experience more side effects from the chemotherapy used to treat lung cancer. This is especially true of myelosuppression.

Treatment

Treatment is determined by the primary tumor histology (small cell or non-small cell) and disease stage (limited or extensive). Lung cancer confined to the primary tumor site and regional nodal drainage is considered to be limited stage. Spread outside this area is extensive stage and is incurable.

A. SMALL CELL LUNG CANCER

Small cell lung cancers comprise 15–20% of all lung cancer histologies. Thirty-three percent of patients have limited-stage disease, and treatment with both chemotherapy and radiation therapy is the standard of care. Concurrent chemotherapy and radiation produces a prolongation in survival. Median survival is 20 mo, and 20% of patients remain free of disease after 5 years. Because anthracycline-based chemotherapy regimens appear to be more toxic and are probably less effective, etoposide with cisplatin or carboplatinum is administered every 21 days for 4–6 cycles. The optimal time for initiation of radiation therapy is the subject of some debate. However, overall survival and local control of the primary tumor are greater when radiation is initiated with the first cycle of chemotherapy. It has been shown that elderly patients are more likely to require delays in chemotherapy or dose reductions as a result of toxicity. Yet, despite the need to modify chemotherapy, the likelihood of response to treatment and overall survival are

similar to that for younger patients treated with higher doses of chemotherapy. The efficacy of treatment does not appear to be compromised by these alterations in therapy.

For patients with extensive-stage disease, chemotherapy prolongs the median survival from 6–8 weeks to 8–10 mo. Patients who are able to receive ≥ 4 cycles of chemotherapy appear to have a better survival than those who receive fewer cycles. Such data should be viewed with caution because it is possible that the patients who were able to tolerate "more" chemotherapy had a better prognosis. New regimens that are less dose intensive and toxic are being tested in the elderly. The survival rates reported with these regimens appear comparable to those for younger patients using more toxic regimens.

B. NON-SMALL CELL LUNG CANCER

Most newly diagnosed lung cancers are of non-small cell histology. Rarely, patients have a solitary nodule that may be removed surgically for cure. Appropriate staging includes a mediastinoscopy with nodal sampling before removal of the primary tumor. If nodal metastases are identified, the patient is diagnosed with limited-stage disease and treated accordingly. Similar to small cell cancers, limited-stage non-small cell lung cancers are treated with combined platinum-based chemotherapy and radiation therapy. Combined-modality therapy results in an improved survival compared with radiation alone, and elderly patients derive the same survival benefit from the combined modality approach as younger patients. In older patients, chemotherapy doses are often attenuated because of declining performance status or because of an increased incidence of mucositis or myelosuppression.

In metastatic non-small cell lung cancer, chemotherapy may provide palliation. Chemotherapy has been compared with best supportive care (pain management and radiation therapy to painful areas of disease). A small but significant survival advantage has been realized with chemotherapy. Newer agents such as vinorelbine and gemcitabine may be effective and are better tolerated than platinum-containing regimens. Single-agent vinorelbine has been shown to produce significant improvement in median survival, overall survival, and quality of life compared with best supportive care. Results are further improved when vinorelbine is administered in combination with gemcitabine. Chemotherapy should be offered to patients with extensive-stage non-small cell lung cancer, especially in those who have not lost weight and have a good performance status. Although lung cancer is most often fatal, meaningful improvement in survival and quality of life can be achieved. By modifying chemotherapy doses and schedule, toxicity can be minimized without compromising efficacy.

COLORECTAL CANCER

Rectal Cancer

The natural history of rectal cancer differs from colon cancer. Because the rectum lies in close proximity to the sacral plexus, uterus, bladder, and prostate, a wide radial margin is often difficult to obtain with surgery, and local recurrences are common. To prevent local disease recurrence, 5-FU in conjunction with radiation therapy is administered either before or after surgical resection. In the Medicare population, the advantages of combined-modality treatment of rectal cancer are similar to those observed in younger patients.

Metastatic Colorectal Cancer

Although most large bowel cancers metastasize to the liver, the pattern of disease recurrence differs somewhat depending on whether the primary tumor arises from the colon or rectum. The drainage of the colon is via the portal vein, and the liver is the most common site, and possibly the only site, of metastasis. Because the inferior mesenteric vein receives drainage from the rectum, systemic metastasis to sites in addition to the liver may develop.

Metastatic colorectal cancer is generally incurable. However, resection of liver metastases may provide long-term disease-free survival for select patients. 5-FU-based regimens may provide both improved quality of life and prolongation in survival. Although only palliative, the addition of irinotecan to 5-FU and leucovorin produces a greater likelihood of tumor regression and possibly a longer survival than achievable with 5-FU and leucovorin alone. Oxaliplatin is the newest active agent used to palliate metastatic colorectal cancer. Neither irinotecan nor oxaliplatin-containing regimens have been specifically tested in the elderly population.

Complications

If the primary tumor is not removed, perforation, bleeding, and obstruction may develop, requiring emergency surgical intervention. Emergency operations performed in patients age 70 and older are associated with higher than expected morbidity and mortality.

Treatment

The treatment of colorectal cancers in the elderly does not differ from that for younger individuals. Surgical resection of the primary tumor has been the mainstay of treatment, even in patients with metastatic disease.

For patients with newly diagnosed cancers, the resection specimen provides important staging information.

When the regional nodes are involved, 32 weeks of adjuvant 5-fluorouracil (5-FU) and leucovorin is recommended. In this setting, the leucovorin is administered not to "rescue" the patient from chemotherapy toxicity (as with methotrexate) but to potentiate the antitumor effect of 5-FU. In the Medicare population, a regimen of adjuvant 5-FU and leucovorin has been shown to reduce the risk of death by 27%, an advantage equivalent to that demonstrated in younger patients. Possibly because this regimen is relatively nontoxic, adjuvant chemotherapy is appropriately administered to elderly patients.

Prevention

Colonoscopy has been established as a cost-effective screening tool. The initial screening should begin at age 50 and is repeated every 10 years until age 85 years. If polyps are identified, the procedure should be repeated every 3–5 years.

Prognosis

Prognosis is related to the depth of invasion of the primary tumor, involvement of regional structures (eg, bladder or uterus), and nodal involvement.

PANCREATIC CANCER

General Considerations

More than 66% of pancreatic cancers develop in individuals 65 years of age and older. Even when it appears that the disease is confined to the organ, few patients survive 5 years.

Treatment

Pancreaticoduodenectomy may provide long-term survival for a small percentage of patients. However, the complications of the procedure are significantly higher in patients 70 years of age and older.

Pain is a common and debilitating problem in patients with pancreatic cancer. Even if the patient is found to have unresectable disease at the time of surgical exploration, palliation of pain and prevention of future pain may be achieved by neurolysis of the celiac ganglion.

If the disease is localized to the pancreas but not resectable, combined chemotherapy and radiation therapy may provide both palliation and a slight survival advantage. Candidates for such an approach should be carefully selected because this therapy is toxic. Once the disease has metastasized, palliation is the goal of any intervention. Single-agent gemcitabine has been shown to improve quality of life, with superior pain control and a modest survival advantage.

OVARIAN CANCER

General Considerations

The incidence of ovarian cancer increases with age, peaking at 80–84 years.

Treatment

Most women present with advanced stages of the disease and are treated with surgery and chemotherapy. Ideally, patients should undergo surgery for both staging and treatment. A total abdominal hysterectomy with bilateral salpingo-oophorectomy and surgical debulking of visible tumor should be performed. Staging also includes nodal sampling, and cytological examination of smears obtained from the cul-de-sac and diaphragms bilaterally.

The most effective initial chemotherapy combines paclitaxel with cisplatin or carboplatinum. Although chemotherapy is effective and relatively nontoxic, older women are less likely to receive treatment. The serum marker CA-125 is an excellent indicator of disease and is of value in monitoring the efficacy of chemotherapy and identifying disease recurrence after initial treatment.

LEUKEMIA

Chronic Lymphocytic Leukemia

Although chronic lymphocytic leukemia (CLL) is very responsive to chemotherapy and radiation therapy, early treatment intervention has never been shown to alter the survival. Therefore, treatment should be initiated only when symptoms are manifested: either B-symptoms (fever, night sweats, 10% weight loss over 6 mo) or symptoms from enlarged nodes. Symptoms referable to nodal enlargement may also be palliated with chemotherapy or localized radiation therapy. Oral alkylating agents combined with prednisone provide effective palliation of fever, night sweats, and weight loss.

Acute Nonlymphocytic Leukemia

General Considerations

The incidence of acute nonlymphocytic leukemia (ANL) increases with age and the prognosis is inversely related.

Treatment

Overall, 75% of all patients receiving induction chemotherapy with cytarabine and an anthracycline will achieve complete remission; however, durable remissions are observed in only 30–40%. ANL in patients older than 40 is more aggressive and less amenable to therapy. In the elderly, ANL frequently develops after a history of myelodysplasia and cytogenetic abnormalities, such as deletions of chromosome 5 or 7. Leukemic cells from older patients are also more likely to express genes that confer drug resistance. These factors predict resistance to conventional induction regimens. Furthermore, treatment-related mortality during induction is as high as 25%. Thus, complete remissions are achieved in only 45% of older patients, and long-term remissions are rare. When lower doses of chemotherapy are used to minimize treatment-related complications, the remission rate is significantly less as well.

Patients and their families should understand that the treatment for ANL is toxic and relatively ineffective. Whenever possible, patients should be referred to oncologists who enter patients in clinical studies that address improved methods of supportive care and innovative regimens. For frail and elderly patients with significant comorbidities, it is reasonable not to offer induction therapy and to provide only palliative care.

LYMPHOMA

Indolent Histologies

General Considerations

Lymphomas with an indolent natural history based on the Revised European-American Classification of Lymphoid Neoplasms (REAL Classification) are listed in Table 30–1. As with CLL, treatment of low-grade lymphomas does not appear to alter the natural history of the disease, even though the disease is sensitive to treatment.

Treatment

Chemotherapy and radiation therapy are reserved for the treatment of symptoms produced by the disease.

Aggressive Histologies

General Considerations

The aggressive histologies are summarized in Table 30–1. More than 50% of the aggressive histologies develop in individuals older than 60, and age > 60 years has been identified as a poor prognostic factor by the International Prognostic Factors Project.

Treatment

Patients with stage I and stage II disease are treated with chemotherapy and radiation therapy and, regard-

Table 30–1. Lymphoma pathology.

B cell	T cell	NK cell
Indolent histologies		
Small lymphocytic/CLL	Mycosis fungoides	
Lymphoplasmacytic	Large granular lymphocytosis	
Follicular, any type	Cutaneous anaplastic large cell (CD30+)	
Marginal zone		
MALT		
Nodal (monocytoid B cell) splenic		
Aggressive histologies		
Mantle cell	Peripheral T cell, unspecified	NK, unspecified
Diffuse large cell, any type	Anaplastic large cell	Nasal T/NK type
Burkitt like	Angioimmunoblastic	
	Intestinal enteropathy associated	
	Subcutaneous panniculitic	
	Hepatosplenic	

CLL, chronic lymphocytic leukemia; NK, natural killer.

less of age, have a favorable prognosis. Patients with more advanced-stage disease, stage III and stage IV, are treated with chemotherapy alone.

For more than 2 decades, the combination of cyclophosphamide, doxorubicin, vincristine, and prednisone (CHOP) has been the standard chemotherapy. Patients older than 60 are more likely to experience neutropenia and fever than younger patients. However, when doxorubicin has been deleted from the regimen or the dose has been attenuated, the efficacy has been significantly compromised. After the first cycle of chemotherapy, the use of colony-stimulating factors will decrease the incidence of neutropenia. However, neither the complete response rate nor survival is improved by the administration of these costly agents.

It is expected that chemotherapy will produce complete remission of disease in the majority of patients, with 30–40% remaining disease free after 5 years. The benefits of chemotherapy are somewhat less for patients who are older than 60 or who have 1 or more comorbid medical conditions. Thus, conventionally administered CHOP chemotherapy remains the chemotherapy of choice in the elderly. Rituximab (Rituxan) is a chimeric monoclonal antibody directed against CD-20, a cell surface protein found on all non-Hodgkin's lymphomas that arise from B cells. The addition of rituximab to CHOP has achieved higher complete remissions and 2-year event-free and overall survivals compared with CHOP alone. Although rituximab is relatively nontoxic, it is extremely expensive. Before considering the combination of rituximab and CHOP chemotherapy as the new standard, additional data from confirmatory trials are needed. As we learn more about the biology of the malignant diseases, it is likely that such targeted therapies will produce a significant impact.

PROSTATE CANCER

General Considerations

The diagnosis and treatment of prostate cancer has changed dramatically over the past 15 years as a result of prostate-specific antigen (PSA) measurement. This glycoprotein is produced almost entirely by the epithelial cells of the prostate. The Food and Drug Administration first approved the measurement of PSA in 1986 as a method for monitoring progression of prostate cancer. PSA declines after effective treatment for prostate cancer and increases with ineffective therapy. Similarly, recurrent or persistent elevations of PSA after initial treatment of localized disease are predictive of disease recurrence.

Screening & Prevention

Controlled trials to address the efficacy of PSA as a screening test are ongoing, and results are not expected for many years. Yet annual or biannual measurement of PSA has become part of a routine annual exam for men; the incidence and prevalence of prostate cancer has increased because of better detection. With screening, the lifetime risk for prostate cancer is 16%, and the risk of dying of the disease is 3.4%.

The American Cancer Society and American Urologic Society support annual screening, whereas others suggest that the decision to measure PSA be made on a case-by-case basis after discussion of the potential benefits and harms of treatment if a cancer is diagnosed. Until data from the controlled trials are available, the use of PSA as a screening test is likely to continue.

The 5α-reductase inhibitor, finasteride has been shown to prevent or delay the onset of prostate cancer, especially low grade prostate cancers. Men assigned finasteride experienced fewer urinary symptoms but more frequent problems with sexual functioning. In weighing the risk and benefits, finasteride cannot be routinely recommended as chemoprevention.

Treatment

The approach to men with PSA elevations and prostate cancer is summarized in Figure 30–1. PSA levels > 4.0 ng/mL are considered abnormal and should be followed by 4-quadrant transrectal biopsies. Because PSA elevations may be seen with any process that distorts the gland, including benign prostatic hypertrophy and prostatitis, only 25% of men with PSA elevations between 4–10 ng/mL will ultimately be diagnosed with prostate cancer. The probability that the patient has

cancer increases with higher elevations of PSA. The PSA is extremely sensitive but lacks specificity. It is important to discuss the impact of making a cancer diagnosis in the asymptomatic patient whose PSA is elevated, because the normal tissue damage from surgery and radiation therapy may be greater than that produced by an indolent cancer.

As a result of PSA screening, most prostate cancer is diagnosed at an early stage when it is still confined to the gland. Treatment with radical prostatectomy or radiation therapy appears to provide comparable rates of local disease control and overall survival. It may be argued that nerve-sparing prostatectomy offers the advantage of preserving potency and providing an accurate pathological stage, and radiation therapy may be reserved for "salvage therapy" in the event of a local recurrence.

Watchful waiting is appropriate for men who have a limited survival. Treatment may be initiated when symptoms develop. Results achieved with watchful waiting are equivalent to those of radical prostatectomy. However, patients treated with surgery are less likely to die of prostate cancer.

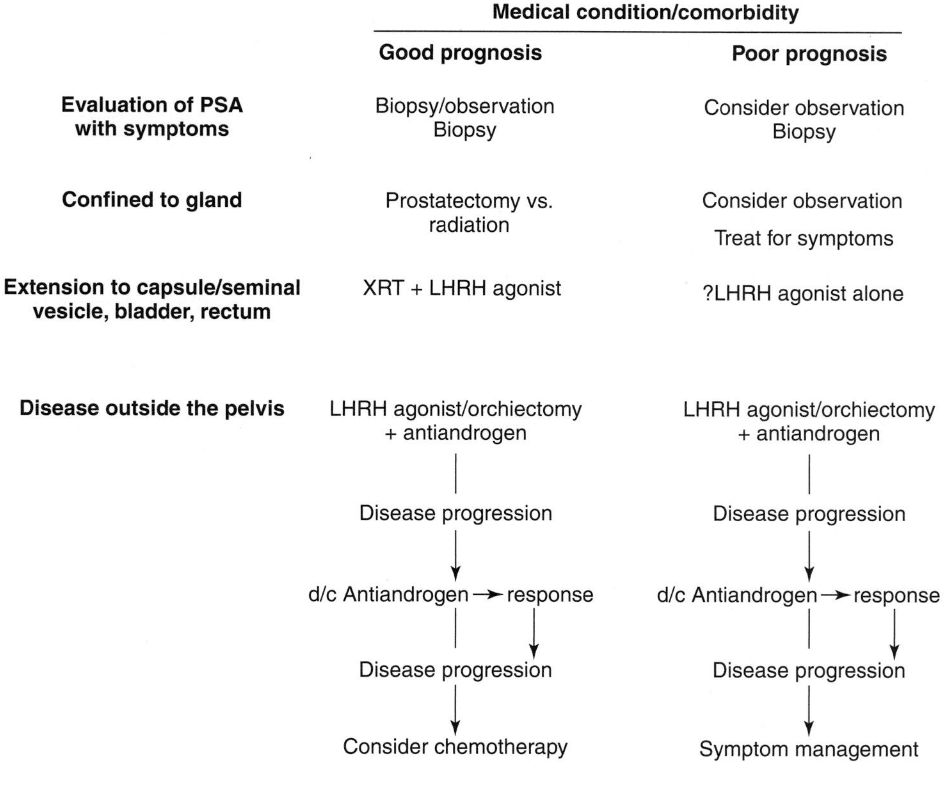

	Medical condition/comorbidity	
	Good prognosis	**Poor prognosis**
Evaluation of PSA with symptoms	Biopsy/observation Biopsy	Consider observation Biopsy
Confined to gland	Prostatectomy vs. radiation	Consider observation Treat for symptoms
Extension to capsule/seminal vesicle, bladder, rectum	XRT + LHRH agonist	?LHRH agonist alone
Disease outside the pelvis	LHRH agonist/orchiectomy + antiandrogen ↓ Disease progression ↓ d/c Antiandrogen → response ↓ Disease progression ↓ Consider chemotherapy	LHRH agonist/orchiectomy + antiandrogen ↓ Disease progression ↓ d/c Antiandrogen → response ↓ Disease progression ↓ Symptom management

Figure 30–1. General schema for prostate cancer treatment.

Patients with large tumors and those with symptoms of urinary obstruction should be offered surgery or radiation therapy.

For cancers that have advanced locally through the capsule or into the seminal vesicles, rectum, bladder sphincter (T3, T4), the combination of radiation with a luteinizing hormone-releasing hormone (LHRH) agonist may produce superior local control of disease and possibly a longer survival than radiation therapy alone. Similarly, patients with yet more advanced disease to pelvic nodes also benefit from the combination of radiation and hormonal therapy.

Widespread prostate cancer is initially managed with combined hormonal therapies. The addition of a 5α-reductase inhibitor such as flutamide in combination with bilateral orchiectomy or an LHRH agonist is more likely to control the disease and may prolong survival. A slight survival advantage has been achieved with the addition of an antiandrogen. With disease progression, cessation of flutamide may produce a hormone withdrawal response. Once the patient's disease has become resistant to hormonal therapy, chemotherapy may offer palliation. Single agents such as mitoxantrone or docetaxel provide palliation in select patients.

Complications

Complications associated with nerve-sparing prostatectomy include impotence and urinary incontinence. Definitive radiation therapy to control disease confined to the prostate gland is associated with bowel and bladder dysfunction, which slowly resolve over time; impotence; urinary incontinence; and diarrhea or urgency. Newer radiation therapy techniques that restrict the radiation field to the prostate gland (eg, brachytherapy implants) may offer effective local control with less toxicity than conventional whole pelvis external beam radiation.

Men undergoing radical prostatectomy are more likely to experience erectile dysfunction and urinary leakage but less likely to have urinary obstruction than patients treated with watchful waiting.

REFERENCES

American Geriatric Society Panel on Persistent Pain in Older Persons: The management of persistent pain in older persons. J Am Geriatr Soc 2002;50;S205. [PMID: 12067390]

ATAC (Arimidex, Tamoxifen Alone or in Combination) Trialists' Group: Anastrozole alone or in combination with tamoxifen versus tamoxifen alone for adjuvant treatment of postmenopausal women with early breast cancer: the first results of the ATAC randomised trial. Lancet 2002;359:2131. [PMID: 12090977]

Barry MJ: Prostate-specific-antigen testing for early diagnosis of prostate cancer. N Engl J Med 2001;344:1373.

Bernabai R et al: Management of pain in elderly patients with cancer. JAMA 1998;279:1877. [PMID: 11333995]

Chan JKC: The new World Health Organization classification of lymphomas: the past, the present and the future. Hematol Oncol 2001;19:129. [PMID: not available]

Cleeland CS: Undertreatment of cancer pain in elderly patients. JAMA 1998;279:1914. [PMID: 9634265]

Coiffer B et al: CHOP chemotherapy plus rituximab compared with CHOP alone in elderly patients with diffuse large-B-cell lymphoma. N Engl J Med 2002;346:235. [PMID: 11807147]

Diab SG et al: Tumor characteristics and clinical outcome of elderly women with breast cancer. J Natl Cancer Inst 2000; 92:550. [PMID: 10749910]

Dighiero G et al: Chlorambucil in indolent chronic lymphocytic leukemia. N Engl J Med 1998;338:1506. [PMID: 9593789]

Early Breast Cancer Trialists' Collaborative Group: Tamoxifen for early breast cancer: an overview of the randomised trials. Lancet 1998;351:1451. [PMID: 9605801]

Elderly Lung Cancer Vinorelbine Italian Study Group: Effects of vinorelbine on quality of life and survival of elderly patient with advanced non-small cell lung cancer. J Natl Cancer Inst 1999;91:66. [PMID: 9890172]

Etzioni R et al: Overdiagnosis due to prostate-specific antigen screening: lessons from the U.S. prostate cancer incidence trends. J Natl Cancer Inst 2002;94:981. [PMID: 12096083]

Extermann M et al: What threshold for adjuvant therapy in older breast cancer patients? J Clin Oncol 2000;18:1709. [PMID: 10764431]

Frasci G et al: Gemcitabine plus vinorelbine versus vinorelbine alone in elderly patients with advanced non-small-cell lung cancer. J Clin Oncol 2000;18:2529. [PMID: 10893283]

Frazier AL et al: Cost-effectiveness of screening for colorectal cancer in the general population. JAMA 2000;284:1954. [PMID: 11035892]

Fyles A et al: Preliminary results of a randomized study of tamoxifen ± breast radiation in T1/2 N0 disease in women over 50 years of age. Proc Am Soc Clin Oncol 2001;21:92. [PMID: not available]

Holmberg L et al: A randomized trial comparing radical prostatectomy with watchful waiting in early prostate cancer. N Engl J Med 2002;347:781. [PMID: 12226148]

Hughes KS et al: Comparison of lumpectomy plus tamoxifen with and without radiotherapy in women 70 years of age or older who have clinical stage I estrogen receptor positive breast cancer. Proc Am Soc Clin Oncol 2001;21:93. [PMID: not available]

Ires L et al: SEER cancer statistics review, 1973–1999. National Cancer Institute, 2002.

Iwahyna TJ, Lamont EB: Effectiveness of adjuvant fluorouracil in clinical practice: a population-based cohort study of elderly patients with stage III colon cancer. J Clin Oncol 2002; 20:3992. [PMID: not available]

Kaufmann M et al: Exemestane is superior to megestrol acetate after tamoxifen failure in postmenopausal women with advanced breast cancer: results of phase III randomized double-blind trial. J Clin Oncol 2000;18:1399. [PMID: 10735887]

Kerlikowske K et al: Continued screening mammography in women aged 70 to 79 years: impact on life expectancy and cost-effectiveness. JAMA 1999;282:2156. [PMID: 10591338]

Kouroukis CT et al: Chemotherapy for older patients with newly diagnosed, advanced-stage, aggressive-histology non-Hodgkin lymphoma: a systematic review. Ann Intern Med 2002; 136:144. [PMID: 11790067]

Miller TP et al: Chemotherapy alone compared with chemotherapy plus radiotherapy for localized intermediate- and high-grade non-Hodgkin's lymphoma. N Engl J Med 1998;339:21. [PMID: 9647875]

Mouridsen H et al: Superior efficacy of letrozole versus tamoxifen as first-line therapy for postmenopausal women with advanced breast cancer: results of a phase III study of the international letrozole breast cancer group. J Clin Oncol 2001; 19:2596. [PMID: 11352951]

National Cancer Institute: Surveillance and end results program (Public use CD-Rom 1973–1995). Cancer Statistics Branch, National Cancer Institute, 1998.

Neugut AI et al: Use of adjuvant chemotherapy and radiation therapy for rectal cancer among the elderly: a population-based study. J Clin Oncol 2002;20:2643. [PMID: 12039925]

O'Mahony S et al: Current management of opioid-related side effects. Oncology 2001;15:61. [PMID: 11271983]

Poen JC et al: Chemoradiotherapy in the management of localized tumors of the pancreas. Ann Surg Oncol 1999;6:117. [PMID: 10030424]

Prostate Cancer Trialists' Collaborative Group: Maximum androgen blockade in advanced prostate cancer: an overview of the randomised trials. Lancet 2000;355:1491. [PMID: 10801170]

Sargent DJ et al: A pooled analysis of adjuvant chemotherapy for resected colon cancer in the elderly. N Engl J Med 2001; 345:1091. [PMID: 11596588]

Slamon D et al: Use of chemotherapy plus a monoclonal antibody against her2 for metastatic breast cancer that overexpressed her2. N Engl J Med 2001;344:783. [PMID: 11248153]

Sonnenberg A et al: Cost-effectiveness of colonoscopy in screening for colorectal cancer. Ann Intern Med 2000;133:573. [PMID: 11033584]

Stanford JL et al: Urinary and sexual function after radical prostatectomy for clinically localized prostate cancer. JAMA 2000; 283:354. [PMID: 10647798]

Sundararajan V et al: Variations in the use of chemotherapy for elderly patients with advanced ovarian cancer: a population-based study. J Clin Oncol 2001;20:173. [PMID: 11773167]

Thompson IM et al: The influence of finasteride on the development of prostate cancer. N Engl J Med 2003;349:215. [PMID: 12824459]

Warren JL et al: Costs of treatment for elderly women with early-stage breast cancer in fee-for-service settings. J Clin Oncol 2001;20:307. [PMID: 11773184]

Westeel V et al: New combination of old drugs for elderly patients with small cell lung cancer: a phase II study of the PAVE regimen. J Clin Oncol 1998;16:1940. [PMID: 9586913]

RELEVANT WORLD WIDE WEB SITE

http://seer.cancer.gov/csr/1973-1999.

Anemia

31

Pearl Toy, MD

ANEMIA

ESSENTIALS OF DIAGNOSIS

- *For euvolemic men, hemoglobin concentration < 13 g/dL.*
- *For euvolemic women, hemoglobin concentration < 12 g/dL.*
- *Hemoglobin concentrations may be higher in those living at high altitude and in those who smoke.*
- *Hemoglobin concentrations are 0.5–1.0 g/dL lower in blacks of both sexes and all ages.*

General Considerations

Anemia in elderly people is due to disease and not aging. Conditions that cause anemia are more common in the elderly (eg, malignancy, infection, and gastrointestinal bleeding). Even if there is no apparent clinical disease, anemia in the elderly deserves investigation.

Izaks GJ et al: The definition of anemia in older persons. JAMA 1999;281:1714. [PMID: 10328071] (A study of anemia in 755 patients older than 85.)

Prevention

- Judicious blood testing in hospitalized patients would minimize anemia resulting from blood loss for laboratory testing, especially in intensive care unit patients.
- Specific nutritional anemias are prevented by adequate iron, folate, and vitamin B_{12} intake and replacement.

Clinical Findings

A. SYMPTOMS & SIGNS

Symptoms of anemia increase with severity, beginning with mild fatigue and progressing to decreased mobility, dyspnea on exertion, angina, loss of concentration, cognitive impairment, and confusion. Even in the nor-

movolemic young and healthy adult, acute anemia below a hemoglobin (Hgb) of 7 g/dL impairs cognitive function and memory. If blood loss leads to hypovolemia, patients may have dizziness on standing.

A sign of anemia is tachycardia. Electrocardiography may show ischemic changes. With hypovolemia, orthostatic hypotension occurs. Pallor, although common, is not a reproducible sign among different observers.

Weiskopf RB et al: Acute severe isovolemic anemia impairs cognitive function and memory in humans. Anesthesiology 2000;92:1646. [PMID: 10839915]

World Health Organization: Nutritional anaemias: report of a WHO scientific group. World Health Organization, 1968.

B. LABORATORY FINDINGS

In the anemic patient, initial tests should include Hgb, hematocrit (Hct), red blood cell count and indices, reticulocyte count, white blood cell count and differential, and platelet count.

To assess whether the marrow has increased red cell production in response to anemia, calculate the reticulocyte production index:

$$\text{Reticulocyte production index (RPI)} = \% \text{Reticulocytes} \times \text{Hct}/45 \times 0.5.$$

Reticulocyte production index (RPI) = % Reticulocytes × Hct/45 × 0.5.

The RPI corrects for the degree of anemia (normalized to a Hct of 45%) and for the doubling in survival of shift reticulocytes. Normal RPI is approximately 1.0. Values > 2.0 indicate increased marrow response to anemia.

C. SPECIAL TESTS

Bone marrow examination is usually not needed in the evaluation of anemia. Indications for bone marrow aspirate and biopsy include pancytopenia or blast cells in the circulation.

Differential Diagnosis

A. NORMOCYTIC ANEMIA (MEAN CORPUSCULAR VOLUME) [MCV] 80–100 FL)

- Blood loss.
- Early microcytic or macrocytic anemias (see following discussion).

B. Microcytic Anemia (MCV < 80 fL)

- Inadequate iron availability: iron deficiency, anemia of chronic disease, rarely copper deficiency.
- Inadequate heme synthesis: lead poisoning, sideroblastic anemia.
- Inadequate globin synthesis: thalassemia minor

C. Macrocytic Anemia (MCV > 100 fL)

- Reticulocytosis.
- Alcoholism.
- Lipid disorders: liver disease, hypothyroidism, hyperlipidemia.
- Hypothyroidism.
- Folate or vitamin B_{12} deficiency.
- Drugs that interfere with nucleic acid synthesis (eg, zidovudine, cytosine arabinoside, methotrexate).
- Abnormal red cell maturation (eg, myelodysplastic syndromes).

D. Blood Loss

Blood loss is most commonly from the gastrointestinal or genitourinary tract. Iron deficiency implies chronic occult blood loss. Common sources include carcinoma, ulcer, atrophic gastritis, gastritis from drug ingestion, bleeding hemorrhoids, angiodysplasia of the colon, and vaginal bleeding.

E. Anemia of Chronic Disease

Anemia of chronic disease is the most common normocytic anemia in the elderly but becomes microcytic in later stages. Chronic diseases include inflammation and cancer. Anemia is also associated with chronic renal insufficiency and liver disease.

Serum ferritin is normal or elevated in anemia of chronic disease as a result of inflammation or cancer. Subcutaneous erythropoietin is used to treat anemic patients with renal insufficiency or cancer when the Hgb is < 10 g/dL. For cancer patients on chemotherapy with anemic symptoms, subcutaneous erythropoietin 3 times/week (150 U/kg) for a minimum of 4 weeks improves quality of life. Dosage should be titrated once the Hgb concentration reaches 12 g/dL. If there is no response, no benefit is observed beyond a 6- to 8-week trial.

Rizzo JD et al: Use of epoietin in patients with cancer: evidence-based clinical practice guidelines of the American Society of Clinical Oncology and the American Society of Hematology. Blood 2002;100:2303. [PMID: 12239138]

F. Iron Deficiency

Iron deficiency anemia is characterized by small, pale red cells and depleted iron stores. Serum ferritin reflects iron stores, and a level < 10 µg/L is diagnostic of iron deficiency. However, serum ferritin levels are increased in inflammation, liver disease, and states of increased red cell turnover. Iron deficiency implies blood loss if the patient does not have malabsorption and has not had total gastrectomy.

Oral iron therapy is inexpensive, safe, and convenient. Iron sulfate 300 mg (60 mg elemental iron) orally 3 times/day between meals should increase the Hgb concentration approximately 2 g/dL over 3 weeks. Addition of 250 mg ascorbic acid at the time of iron administration enhances iron absorption. For elderly patients, iron sulfate is often given only once daily to minimize gastrointestinal side effects. Gastrointestinal side effects relate to the amount of elemental iron ingested. Patients with gastric side effects may titrate to a tolerable dose with elixir of ferrous sulfate (45 mg of elemental iron per 5 mL). If full replenishment of iron stores is desired, therapy can continue for 6 mo after the Hgb becomes normal.

G. Vitamin B_{12} & Folate Deficiency

Both vitamin B_{12} and folate deficiency cause a macrocytic anemia. Deficiency of either vitamin should be suspected with macrocytosis (with or without anemia), pancytopenia, and unexplained neurological and psychiatric signs and symptoms in the elderly as well as in those with alcoholism and malnutrition. An important distinction is that vitamin B_{12} causes neurological disease such as dorsal column peripheral neuropathy, incontinence, and dementia, whereas folate does not. Low stomach acidity is present in 15% of elderly persons and is the major cause of vitamin B_{12} deficiency. Other causes include gastrectomy, small bowel disease of surgery, prolonged use of antacids, and a strict vegan diet. Folate deficiency can be caused by malabsorption, poor nutrition, alcoholism, and chronic hemolysis.

In making a diagnosis, if serum folate is > 4 ng/mL and vitamin B_{12} concentration is > 300 pg/mL, deficiencies of the 2 vitamins are unlikely, and additional testing is not required. If the patient has low or low–normal (< 300 pg/mL) vitamin B_{12} levels, deficiency can be diagnosed by elevated homocysteine and methylmalonic acid (MMA) levels in patients without renal failure. Among the elderly, estimates of the prevalence of vitamin B_{12} deficiency, defined as increased MMA, vary from 15–44%. Serum or even red blood cell folate levels fluctuate and do not necessarily reflect body stores. In folate deficiency, serum homocysteine is elevated but MMA levels are normal. Because folate does not reverse neurological damage of vitamin B_{12} deficiency, B_{12} deficiency must be ruled out before treatment with folate.

Both deficiencies can be easily repleted: folate deficiency with folic acid, 1 mg/day, and vitamin B_{12} deficiency with a regimen of vitamin B_{12}, 1000 μg/day for the first week, 1000 μg/week for 4 weeks or until the Hct is normal, and then 1000 μg/mo for life. Treatment is somewhat controversial in patients with low–normal vitamin B_{12} but elevated MMA levels (0.40–2.00 μmol/L). Treatment improves test results and neurological symptoms in patients with MMA levels > 0.60 μmol/L, but objective neurological tests do not improve.

Hvas AM et al: Vitamin B_{12} treatment normalizes metabolic markers but has limited clinical effect: a randomized placebo-controlled study. Clin Chem 2001;47:1396. [PMID: 11468228] (In patients with mildly to modestly increased P-MMA [0.40–2.00 μmol/L] not previously treated with vitamin B_{12}, vitamin B_{12} treatment was associated with improved neurological symptoms but not improved neurological tests in patients with MMA > 0.60 μmol/L or homocysteine > 15 μmol/L.)

H. RED BLOOD CELL TRANSFUSION

Whereas young patients can tolerate low Hgb concentrations, the elderly cannot because of underlying cardiopulmonary disease. The red blood cell transfusion trigger is not clear; however, among patients 65 years of age and older with acute myocardial infarction, blood transfusion is associated with a lower short-term mortality rate if the hematocrit on admission is ≤ 30% (Hgb 10 g/dL). In addition, it may be effective in patients with a hematocrit as high as 33% (Hgb 11 g/dL) on admission.

Elderly patients are especially susceptible to fluid overload, and each unit of red blood cell transfusion should be given slowly over 4 h if the patient is not acutely bleeding. In addition, diuretics may be indicated.

Wu WC et al: Blood transfusion in elderly patients with acute myocardial infarction. N Engl J Med 2001;345:1230. [PMID: 11680442]

Prognosis

The mortality risk in elderly anemic patients with or without obvious clinical disease is about twice that of nonanemic patients.

Izaks GJ et al: The definition of anemia in older persons. JAMA 1999;281:1714. [PMID: 10328071] (A study of anemia in 755 older than 85.)

 EVIDENCE-BASED POINTS

- *Although anemia is common in the elderly, it is never normal.*
- *Transfuse red blood cells slowly to prevent fluid overload.*
- *Erythropoietin treatment improves quality of life in cancer patients undergoing chemotherapy who have anemia of chronic disease with Hgb concentrations < 10 g/dL.*

Endocrine Disorders

32

Steven R. Gambert, MD, & Myron Miller, MD

■ DISEASES OF THE THYROID GLAND

ESSENTIALS OF DIAGNOSIS

- Many thyroid disorders occur with increasing frequency with advancing age. Normal age-related changes must be distinguished from diseases that occur with greater frequency.
- The aging thyroid gland develops both micro- and macronodules and increasing amounts of fibrous tissue and lymphocytes. There is a reduction in follicle size and colloid. The thyroid may lie more retrosternal and may become smaller in size.
- Less thyroxine (T_4) is produced as a function of normal aging, and the half-life of T_4 half-life increases from approximately 6–9 days over the life span. Levels of T_4 and free T_4 remain constant in the absence of disease.
- The more metabolically active thyroid hormone T_3 is produced in greater quantities by the thyroid gland itself with increasing age. Although levels of free T_3, in the absence of disease, remain constant, fewer elderly persons maintain T_3 levels at the upper range of normal.
- TSH production by the pituitary is not diminished by the aging process; the upper limit of normal, 5 mU/L, is not affected by age.
- Low levels of antithyroglobulin antibodies, with titers < 1:100, may be present in individuals without clinical signs of a thyroid disorder. Moderate to high titers, 1:1600 to 1:25,600, can be found in patients with nonthyroid autoimmune disorders. High serum antithyroglobulin or antithyroid peroxidase antibody titers, an elevated serum TSH,

with or without reduced levels of serum T_4, is consistent with autoimmune thyroiditis.
- Serum T_3 is reduced in many nonthyroidal illnesses and may accompany a low T_4 concentration. This is referred to as euthyroid sick syndrome. Free T_4 and TSH are usually normal. With severe illness, however, there can be a marked reduction of both total and free T_4. Although serum TSH is usually normal, it may be low, raising the question of secondary hypothyroidism.

SUBCLINICAL HYPOTHYROIDISM

ESSENTIALS OF DIAGNOSIS

- Reduced feeling of general well-being.
- Minimally reduced psychomotor skills.
- Reduced intelligence.
- Normal serum T_4, free T_4, T_3, free T_3.
- Increased serum TSH.
- Dyslipidemia.

General Considerations

Both subclinical hypothyroidism and subclinical hyperthyroidism affect a relatively large number of elderly persons. Although a small percentage of these cases will progress to overt clinical hypothyroidism each year, individuals with high levels of antimicrosomal antibodies are at greater risk of decline in thyroid function. Several studies have observed beneficial effects of T_4 therapy in patients with subclinical hypothyroidism; no studies have specifically addressed this question in older patients.

Clinical Findings

Elderly patients with subclinical hypothyroidism may present with few or no complaints. Elderly women with atherosclerosis and an even higher percentage of those with a history of myocardial infarction have a higher incidence of subclinical hypothyroidism. Treatment with L-thyroxine compared with placebo has been shown to result in an overall improvement in general well-being. In addition, noninvasive indexes of myocardial contractility also improved, as did memory, psychomotor speed, and serum cholesterol levels. Subclinical hypothyroidism progresses to frank hypothyroidism in 5–8% of affected persons each year, with higher rates in those with high levels of antimicrosomal antibodies.

Treatment

Although some physicians advocate replacement therapy for all persons with subclinical hypothyroidism, many believe that treatment is best reserved for those individuals with TSH levels > 10 mU/L or for those with serum TSH levels between 5–10 mU/L with coexisting high levels of antimicrosomal antibodies. If treatment is not initiated, careful follow-up is essential because a percentage of these individuals will develop hypothyroidism each year. The goal of treatment, when initiated, is to normalize serum TSH values as long as the dose of thyroid hormone that is required produces no unwanted clinical effects.

Canaris GJ et al: The Colorado thyroid disease prevalence study. Arch Intern Med 2000;160:526. [PMID: 10695694]

Cooper DS: Clinical practice. Subclinical hypothyroidism. N Engl J Med 2001;345:260. [PMID: 11474665]

Helfand M, Redfern CC: Screening for thyroid disease: an update. Ann Intern Med 1998;129:144. [PMID: not available]

Ladenson PW et al: American Thyroid Association guidelines for detection of thyroid dysfunction. Arch Intern Med 2000; 160:1573. [PMID: 10847249]

SUBCLINICAL HYPERTHYROIDISM

ESSENTIALS OF DIAGNOSIS

- *Atrial fibrillation.*
- *Osteopenia/osteoporosis.*
- *Shortened systolic time interval.*
- *Suppressed level of serum TSH.*
- *Normal T_4, free T_4, T_3, free T_3.*

General Considerations

Subclinical hyperthyroidism is a term used to identify individuals with suppressed levels of serum TSH with normal levels of circulating thyroid hormones.

Clinical Findings

Subclinical hyperthyroidism may occur as a consequence of thyroid hormone replacement for hypothyroidism. Although still maintaining circulating levels of T_4 within normal range, these individuals are taking higher doses than necessary to normalize serum TSH. Shorter systolic time intervals, atrial fibrillation, and osteopenia have been associated with this entity. Epidemiological data suggest that this problem affects 4–7% of persons older than 60 not on thyroid hormone therapy. Unfortunately, there is little in the literature to help determine whether treatment is indicated. Most agree that treatment should be initiated if there are clearly associated symptoms, such as a worsening of cardiovascular function or cardiac arrhythmias, excessive wasting of muscle, anorexia, depression, or significant osteoporosis. Atrial fibrillation has been described in 10% of these patients. Patients with subclinical hyperthyroidism have been shown to be at increased risk of both cardiovascular and all-cause mortality.

Treatment

Varied outcomes are reported for affected individuals; 47–61% have normal serum TSH levels on retesting within 1 year without any intervention, and 1.5–13% develop hyperthyroidism. It remains unclear exactly when to treat subclinical hyperthyroidism because therapy has the potential for toxicity and expense, and in some patients the problem may resolve on its own. Treatment is best considered on an individual basis with careful follow-up because hyperthyroidism in the elderly often presents in a nonspecific manner and may lead to a decline in functional capacity before or without more classic signs or symptoms of hyperthyroidism. Treatment of subclinical hyperthyroidism may improve bone mineral density and atrial fibrillation if identified. If treatment is selected, ablation therapy with iodine 131 is the preferred modality.

Parle JV et al: Prediction of all-cause and cardiovascular mortality in elderly people from one low serum thyrotropin result: a 10-year cohort study. Lancet 2001;358:861. [PMID: 11567699]

Sawin CT et al: Low serum thyrotropin concentrations as a risk factor for atrial fibrillation in older persons. N Engl J Med 1994; 331:1249. [PMID: not available]

Toft AD: Clinical practice. Subclinical hyperthyroidism. N Engl J Med 2001;345:512. [PMID: 11519506]

HYPOTHYROIDISM

ESSENTIALS OF DIAGNOSIS

- *Dry skin.*
- *Increased weakness.*
- *Paresthesias.*
- *Memory loss and depression.*
- *Constipation.*
- *Cold intolerance.*
- *Cardiomegaly.*
- *Anemia.*
- *Elevated serum TSH.*
- *Low serum T_4, free T_4, T_3, free T_3.*
- *Radioiodine uptake usually low.*
- *Hyponatremia.*

General Considerations

Hypothyroidism is a common disease of the elderly, with a reported prevalence of 0.9–17.5%. Hypothyroidism in the elderly most commonly results from an autoimmune thyroiditis. Prior radioiodine treatment and subtotal thyroidectomy are also potential causes. The risk of hypothyroidism is > 50% after the first year of radioiodine treatment, with an additional annual incidence of 2–4% each year thereafter. Hypothyroidism may also be the natural end point to previous Graves' disease. Medications may also lead to hypothyroidism, particularly in persons with autoimmune thyroiditis. The most common medications associated with hypothyroidism include iodine-containing radiographic contrast agents, lithium, amiodarone, and iodine-containing cough medicines. Hypothyroidism may also result from a secondary cause: either a pituitary or hypothalamic abnormality.

Clinical Findings

Many of the presenting complaints are confused with other age-prevalent disorders. This problem is further compounded by the often insidious onset of illness. Whereas younger patients commonly present with weight gain, cold intolerance, paresthesias, and muscle cramps, older patients may not. However, fatigue and weakness are common. Many persons who are later discovered to be hypothyroid are unable to identify exactly when the symptoms actually began. Neurological find-

ings may include dementia, ataxia, and carpal tunnel syndrome.

Classic symptoms of dry skin, paresthesias, constipation, hypothermia, and cold intolerance among others are often present in older persons without a thyroid abnormality. On physical examination, a delay in the relaxation of deep tendon reflexes may not be easily apparent in a person of advancing age. Hypercholesterolemia may be more common in both circumstances as well. For these reasons, the examining physician should maintain a high index of suspicion of hypothyroidism when evaluating any older person, especially women and those with a personal or family history of some form of thyroid disease.

Primary hypothyroidism is associated with an elevated serum TSH concentration. Changes in protein binding may reduce the level of total T_4; T_3 may be reduced in persons with significant medical illness or malnutrition. Even measures of free T_4 may be misleading; T_4 may be suppressed in individuals with T_3 toxicosis. For these reasons, an increase in serum TSH remains the best way to detect primary failure of the thyroid gland regardless of age. During the recovery phase after an acute nonthyroidal illness, however, an elevation of serum TSH level may not represent true clinical hypothyroidism; in this case, the serum TSH returns to the range of normal within 4–6 weeks. Although uncommon in the elderly, hypothyroidism can be secondary to pituitary or hypothalamic failure, with low serum TSH and T_4 levels. Although antithyroid antibodies are detectable in the circulation of many persons with hypothyroidism, these tests are not indicated in the workup of every patient suspected of being hypothyroid. TSH screening is indicated in those older patients with cognitive problems, goiter, hypercholesterolemia, family history of thyroid illness, or history of thyroid abnormality.

Differential Diagnosis

Many of the presenting signs and symptoms of hypothyroidism in persons of any age resemble findings common to many other age-prevalent disorders, notably congestive heart failure and unexplained ascites resulting from cardiac or hepatic abnormalities. A thick tongue may result from primary amyloidosis. Anemia may result from vitamin B_{12}, folate, or iron deficiency or volume expansion. Depression may be present, and other alterations in cognition may be due to medication toxicity or dementia.

Treatment

L-Thyroxine is the preferred medication to treat hypothyroidism. In general, brand names are suggested to minimize variability that may occur with generic preparations. It is also easier for the elderly person to identify the medication with a consistent color and shape. Elderly patients generally require a smaller amount of L-thyroxine to normalize their thyroid status, on average, 110 μg/day. Because of the age-related increase in T_4 half-life, it will take longer to reach a steady state. A longer time between dose increases is necessary to reduce unwanted side effects.

The commonly adage of "start low and go slow" should be followed when starting any elderly patient on thyroid hormone replacement therapy. Because many elderly patients with hypothyroidism may have underlying cardiovascular disease, therapy should start with 25 μg/day, with gradually increasing increments of 25 μg every 4–6 weeks. Individuals with significant cardiac disease may require dose changes as low as 12.5 μg and should even be started at that dose. Once a dosage of 75 μg/day is achieved without side effects, increments of 12.5 μg are advised. The final dose required is the amount of L-thyroxine that reduces the serum TSH into the range of normal and does not have associated side effects.

A euthyroid state is not always desirable for patients with significant coronary artery disease. In this circumstance, the use of a β-adrenergic blocking agent may allow a clinically euthyroid state to be reached without induction of symptoms of myocardial ischemia. Monitoring of TSH is necessary to avoid inducing iatrogenic subclinical hyperthyroidism from excessive doses of replacement thyroid hormone.

Prognosis

With early treatment, return to a normal state of health is expected. Complete response to thyroid treatment, however, may take months, and patients will require replacement therapy with thyroid hormone for life.

MYXEDEMA COMA

ESSENTIALS OF DIAGNOSIS

- *Alteration in mental state or coma.*
- *Hypothermia.*
- *History of hypothyroidism.*
- *Elevated serum TSH.*
- *Low serum T_4 and free T_4.*
- *Hyponatremia.*

General Considerations

Myxedema coma is a serious consequence of untreated or inadequately treated hypothyroidism. Although rare, it almost exclusively occurs in the older patients. Coma is seen in the most severe cases; more common features include alteration in cognition, lethargy, seizures, psychotic symptoms, and confusion and disorientation. In most cases, the affected individual has had a precipitating event such as a severe infection, cold exposure, alcoholism, or the use of psychoactive medications, sedatives, or narcotics.

Clinical Findings

A history of increased fatigue and somnolence is common as is a history of treatment of a thyroid disorder or use of narcotic, sedative, or antipsychotic medication. Infections, particularly pneumonia and urosepsis, are common. Physical examination may demonstrate classic signs and symptoms of hypothyroidism, including dry, scaly skin, bradycardia, and edema. Profound hypothermia as well as hypoventilation and hypotension may exist. Headaches, ataxia, nystagmus, psychotic behavior, muscle spasms, and sinus bradycardia may precede the coma. There may also be a pericardial effusion, ileus, megacolon, and easy bruising.

Laboratory findings classically include a markedly elevated serum TSH and reduced total and free serum T_4. Hypoglycemia and hyponatremia are common. Autoimmune deficiency states, including diabetes mellitus and adrenal insufficiency, are sometimes associated with hypothyroidism and other autoimmune disorders. Creatine phosphokinase of muscle origin is often elevated. Myocardial infarction can occur in the presence of myxedema coma and may complicate the initiation of thyroid hormone therapy. In rare circumstances, myoglobinuria and rhabdomyolysis may occur. Arterial blood gases usually demonstrate a decrease in partial pressure of oxygen and an increase in partial pressure of carbon dioxide, indicating acute or impending respiratory failure. Anemia is also a common finding and is often normochromic, normocytic, or macrocytic. Cardiomegaly is often seen on chest x-ray film. Evoked potentials may have abnormal amplitude or latency, and electroencephalogram may demonstrate triphasic waves that disappear with thyroid replacement.

Differential Diagnosis

Included in the differential diagnosis are dementia, sepsis, intracranial bleed or tumor, hepatic encephalopathy, congestive heart failure, and hypothyroidism.

Treatment

In most cases, patients with severe illness and coma are started on thyroid hormone replacement based on clinical suspicion before obtaining confirming laboratory data. When deciding on therapy, the following principles should be considered:

1. Myxedema coma has a very high mortality rate if treatment is delayed or is inadequate.

2. The uncertainty of diagnosis before receiving laboratory results must be balanced with empiric therapy, especially if the patient is later found not to be hypothyroid.

3. Supportive therapy must be provided and includes ventilatory support for respiratory failure, antibiotics for infection as indicated, and management of hypothermia by external rewarming. Hypotension may be treated with fluid replacement, although dopamine infusion might be required. Hyponatremia must be treated, although thyroid hormone replacement in itself will result in a decrease in antidiuretic hormone (ADH) and produce a brisk diuresis. Hypoglycemia and anemia will need to be monitored carefully and treated on the basis of individual needs. Care must be taken to prevent aspiration, fecal impaction, pressure sores, and urinary retention.

4. Prompt initiation of thyroid hormone replacement is essential. The initial dose for treatment of myxedema coma is between 300 and 500 μg of L-thyroxine given intravenously. This high dose is necessary to occupy hormone-binding sites that have been left free as a result of significant and prolonged hormone deficiency. In addition, precipitating factors such as infection may increase the turnover of T_4 and thus warrant a higher initial replacement dose. High doses can increase myocardial oxygen consumption and the potential for myocardial infarction. Once there is evidence of a clinical response, usually noted by a diuresis and increase in body temperature and heart rate, the daily dose of L-thyroxine should be reduced to 50–100 μg and can be given orally and adjusted as necessary. The use of T_3 or combinations of T_4 and T_3 are not recommended.

5. Because adrenal insufficiency may coexist with myxedema coma, suspicion of cortisol deficiency should be high. A suggestive history, physical examination, or electrolyte abnormalities calls for administration of intravenous glucocorticoids. Initiating glucocorticoid therapy for all patients with myxedema coma is controversial. In life-threatening situations, blood for measurement of plasma cortisol should be drawn, and intravenous stress doses of corticosteroids should be administered and continued until there is laboratory confirmation of adrenal status and a decision can be made to continue, taper, or stop the corticosteroids.

Prognosis

Myxedema coma is a serious condition that occurs largely in elderly hypothyroid persons. Aggressive supportive therapy and thyroid hormone therapy is essential while possible contributing factors are evaluated and treated as necessary. Close monitoring is required when treatment is initiated to avoid toxicity from the relatively large starting doses of thyroid hormone. Even under the best of circumstances, there is considerable mortality related to delay in diagnosis and presence of coexisting morbidities.

Yamamoto T et al: Factors associated with mortality of myxedema coma: report of eight cases and literature survey. Thyroid 1999;9:1167. [PMID: 10646654]

HYPERTHYROIDISM

 ESSENTIALS OF DIAGNOSIS

- *Weight loss.*
- *Cardiac arrhythmias, angina, or heart failure.*
- *Change in bowel habits.*
- *Muscle wasting.*
- *Functional decline.*
- *Change in cognition.*
- *Suppressed TSH.*
- *Increased T_4, free T_4, T_3, free T_3.*

General Considerations

Hyperthyroidism is the result of an excessive amount of circulating thyroid hormone either from endogenous production or iatrogenic sources. Clinically, this disorder is accompanied by a broad spectrum of signs and symptoms that vary among individuals and can differ markedly between young and old persons. A greater percentage of affected individuals are older than 60. Several studies of prevalence indicate the presence of hyperthyroidism in 1–3% of community-residing elderly persons. Hyperthyroidism is far more common in women than in men, with estimates ranging from 4:1 to 10:1.

Graves' disease remains the most common cause of hyperthyroidism in young persons and may still be present in elderly patients. With increasing age, however, more cases of hyperthyroidism result from multinodular toxic goiter. Although multinodular goiters are commonly found in the elderly and are not usually associated with clinical disease, they may evolve into toxic multinodular thyroid goiters. A toxic adenoma may cause hyperthyroidism and is usually identified on thyroid scan as a solitary hyperfunctioning nodule with suppression of activity in the remaining portion of the thyroid gland.

Hyperthyroidism may rarely result from ingestion of iodide or iodine-containing substances. Iodine may be introduced from seafood, although this problem is more common after exposure to iodinated radiocontrast agents and to amiodarone. Up to 40% of patients taking amiodarone will have serum T_4 levels above the normal range as a result of the drug's effect on T_4 metabolism; far fewer (5%) will develop clinically apparent thyrotoxicosis. The hyperthyroidism can be of rapid onset and severe in magnitude.

Hyperthyroidism must always be considered in the elderly person who is already receiving thyroid hormone therapy. This is particularly important if the dose is > 0.15 mg of L-thyroxine daily, although even smaller doses may be excessive, especially in small individuals of advanced age. Persons taking the same dose of thyroid hormone for many years may become hyperthyroid simply because of an age-associated decline in the body's ability to degrade T_4.

Although extremely rare, a TSH-producing pituitary tumor may be the cause of hyperthyroidism. Nonsuppressed levels of serum TSH in the presence of increased amounts of circulating thyroid hormone are seen with these tumors. Hyperthyroidism may also rarely result with overproduction of thyroid hormone from a widespread metastatic follicular carcinoma.

Transient hyperthyroidism may occur in patients with silent or subacute thyroiditis as a result of increased release of thyroid hormone into the circulation during the inflammatory phase of the illness. Radiation injury, which may be caused by radioactive iodine therapy for hyperthyroidism, may also result in an outpouring of thyroid hormone.

Hyperthyroidism is usually accompanied by elevated levels of both T_4 and T_3. However, a subgroup of elderly hyperthyroid individuals have isolated elevations of T_3 alone. T_4 is either within the normal range or may, in fact, be suppressed. This circumstance is referred to as T_3 toxicosis. Although it can occur with any type of hyperthyroidism, it is most commonly seen in older patients with toxic multinodular goiter or solitary toxic adenomas. The diagnosis is made on clinical grounds and measurements demonstrating an elevated level of serum T_3 and a suppressed level of serum TSH. T_4 toxicosis, or an isolated increase in serum T_4 without an elevation in serum T_3, most commonly occurs in a sick elderly person with hyperthyroidism. Disease or malnutrition interferes in the normal removal of iodine from the 5' position of T_4 and thus a decreased ability to convert T_4 to T_3.

Clinical Findings

A. SYMPTOMS & SIGNS

Clinical findings associated with hyperthyroidism in the elderly vary greatly. In general, the clinical presentation of hyperthyroidism at this time of life differs from the more classic findings noted earlier in life (Table 32–1). The presenting feature may be a decline in functional capacity. There may be increased fatigue, muscle weakness, cognitive changes, loss of appetite, weight loss, cardiac arrhythmias, and congestive heart failure. Eye findings associated with the hyperthyroidism are less commonly noted in the elderly. Rather than frequent bowel movements, more commonly there is a return to normal from preexisting constipation. Anemia and hyponatremia are often noted and thought to be due to other coexisting illnesses. Although this relative lack of the classic findings of hyperthyroidism does not occur in every older person with hyperthyroidism, a subgroup develops an apathetic hyperthyroid state. In this circumstance, the patient lacks the hyperactivity, irritability, and restlessness common to young patients who are hyperthyroid and presents instead with severe weakness, lethargy, listlessness, depression, and the appearance of a chronic wasting illness. Often the person is incorrectly diagnosed as having a malignancy or severe depression.

Symptoms less common in the elderly patients include nervousness, increased diaphoresis, increased ap-

Table 32–1. Frequency of signs & symptoms of hyperthyroidism in young versus elderly patients.

Symptom/sign	Young (%)	Elderly (%)[a]
Palpitation	100	61.5
Goiter	98	61.0
Tremor	96	63.0
Excessive perspiration	92	52.0
Weight loss	73	77.0
Eye signs	71	42.0
Arrhythmias	4.6	39.0

[a]Data represent a compilation of several studies.

petite, and increased frequency of bowel movements. More common symptoms include marked weight loss, present in > 80% of elderly patients, poor appetite, worsening angina, agitation, confusion, and edema.

Similarly, physical findings differ in elderly patients. Hyperreflexia, palpable goiter, and exophthalmos are usually absent, although lid lag and lid retraction may be present. The pulse rate tends to be slower. Cardiac manifestations are particularly important in the elderly person who may have coexisting heart disease. An increased heart rate with a related increase in myocardial oxygen demand, stroke volume, cardiac output, and shortened left ventricular ejection time underlie the clinical consequences of palpitations. There is also an increased risk of atrial fibrillation (often with slow ventricular response), exacerbation of angina in patients with preexisting coronary artery disease, and precipitation of congestive heart failure that responds less readily to conventional therapy.

Gastrointestinal problems may occasionally include abdominal pain, nausea, and vomiting. Diarrhea and increased frequency of bowel movements resulting from the effect of the thyroid hormone on intestinal motility can occur, but these symptoms are often absent and constipation is still common. There may be an alteration in liver enzymes, including elevation of alkaline phosphatase and gamma-glutamyltranspeptidase levels, which become normal after a return to the euthyroid state. Weakness, especially of proximal muscles, is a major feature of hyperthyroidism in the elderly and is often accompanied by muscle wasting and functional decline. Disorders of gait, postural instability, and falling may be noted. Tremor is noted in > 70% of elderly persons with hyperthyroidism. The tremor is usually more coarse than in other common tremors. A rapid relaxation phase of the deep tendon reflex is difficult to identify in the older thyrotoxic individual. Central nervous system (CNS) manifestations may be prominent and include confusion, depression, changes in short-term memory, agitation and anxiety, and a decreased attention span. Other findings that have been associated with hyperthyroidism include worsening of glucose tolerance, mild increases in serum calcium, and osteoporosis resulting from increased bone turnover.

B. Laboratory Tests

The altered and often atypical presentation of hyperthyroidism in the elderly patient warrants a high degree of suspicion among clinicians and the initiation of appropriate laboratory studies. Serum free T_4 and a measurement of serum TSH are the preferred tests for diagnosing thyroid dysfunction. The findings of a normal or low serum free T_4 with a suppressed serum TSH raises the possibility of T_3 toxicosis and warrants a measurement of serum T_3 by radioimmunoassay. Although the finding of anti-TSH receptor antibodies confirms the diagnosis of Graves' disease, it is rarely necessary to obtain this test.

C. Special Tests

Thyroid scanning with technetium and measurement of 24-h ^{131}I uptake can be useful in distinguishing Graves' disease from toxic multinodular goiter. Scanning may also demonstrate the presence of a small, diffusely active goiter that could not be detected on physical examination. Very low ^{131}I uptake in a patient with elevated circulating thyroid hormone levels suggests exogenous thyroid hormone ingestion, the hyperthyroid phase of painless or subacute thyroiditis, or iodine-induced hyperthyroidism.

Differential Diagnosis

Patients with hyperthyroidism in later life commonly have coexisting illness, and it is important not to attribute all presenting signs and symptoms to the hyperthyroid state itself. The most common differential diagnoses to consider include anxiety, malignancy, depression, diabetes mellitus, menopause, and pheochromocytoma.

Treatment

Therapy should be directed at the specific cause of the hyperthyroid state. Therefore, the underlying cause must be determined to exclude the possibility of one of the transient forms of illness, such as excessive hormone ingestion, iodine exposure, or subacute thyroiditis. The majority of older patients with either Graves' disease or multinodular toxic goiter can be treated with antithyroid medications, radioactive iodine, or surgery. The preferred treatment, however, is radioactive iodine.

A useful initial step in treating suspected hyperthyroidism is to administer a β-adrenergic blocking agent such as long-acting propranolol, metoprolol, nadolol, or atenolol. These agents quickly control associated palpitations, angina, tachycardia, and agitation. Caution is advised, however, in persons with congestive heart failure, chronic obstructive pulmonary disease, or diabetes mellitus being treated with insulin.

Once a diagnosis of Graves' disease or toxic nodular goiter is confirmed, treatment should be initiated with one of the antithyroid drugs: propylthiouracil or methimazole. These agents impair biosynthesis of thyroid hormone, thus depleting intrathyroidal hormone stores and ultimately leading to decreased hormone secretion. A decline in serum T_4 concentration is usually seen within 2–4 weeks after initiation of antithyroid drug therapy, and the dose should be tapered once thyroid hormone levels reach the normal range to avoid hypothyroidism. In 1–5% of patients, the antithyroid medications may result in fever, rash, and arthralgias. A drug-induced agranulocytosis may be more common in elderly patients and will most likely occur within the first 3 mo of treatment, especially in those who receive > 30 mg/day of methimazone. Periodic white blood cell count monitoring should be considered, with discontinuation of the antithyroid medication if there is evidence of neutropenia.

Long-term antithyroid medication use can be effective in patients older than 60 with Graves' disease, who appear to respond fairly quickly and have a greater likelihood of a long-lasting remission. Because these medications rarely will provide a long-lasting effect for those with a toxic multinodular goiter, more definitive therapy is needed once the patient returns to a euthyroid state on medication. The recommended treatment in most elderly persons with hyperthyroidism is thyroid gland ablation with ^{131}I. Once the patient achieves a euthyroid status on antithyroid medication, these agents should be stopped for 3–5 days, after which ^{131}I is given orally. Therapy with β- blockers can be maintained and antithyroid agents restarted 5 days after radiotherapy and should be continued for 1–3 mo until the major effect of radioiodine is achieved. Although some physicians attempt to calculate a specific dose that will render the patient euthyroid without subsequently developing hypothyroidism, many patients will still develop permanent hypothyroidism. For this reason, most clinicians advocate treating the older person with hyperthyroidism with a relatively large dose of ^{131}I to ensure ablation of thyroid tissue and thus avoid the possibility of hyperthyroidism recurrence.

After treatment, the patient is closely monitored in order to start replacement doses of thyroid hormone, because hypothyroidism may develop in as few as 4 weeks after treatment. Regardless of dosing regimen used, 40–50% of patients will be hypothyroid within 12 mo of ^{131}I administration, with 2–5% developing hypothyroidism each year thereafter.

Prior treatment with antithyroid medication prevents the possibility of radiation-induced thyroiditis after ^{131}I therapy. However, in some circumstances, when clinical and laboratory features suggest a mild case of hyperthyroidism and no cardiac problems are noted, it may be appropriate to treat the hyperthyroid patient with ^{131}I without antithyroid medication pretreatment. When this option is chosen, the patients should be started on a β-blocker and continue with it until thyroid hormone levels return to normal.

Surgery is not recommended as a primary treatment for hyperthyroidism in the elderly patients. Coexisting illness, particularly cardiac, increases operative risk. In addition, postoperative complications of hypoparathyroidism and recurrent laryngeal nerve damage are sig-

nificant risks. Surgery may be indicated in the rare patient with tracheal compression secondary to a large goiter.

Atrial fibrillation occurs in 10–15% of hyperthyroid patients. Treatment of the underlying disease is essential; cardioversion and anticoagulation are considered on an individual basis. The longer the hyperthyroid period, the less likely is the return to normal sinus rhythm; most benefit is found in those who become euthyroid within 3 weeks. Cardioversion is usually reserved for those patients who still remain in atrial fibrillation after 16 weeks of euthyroidism. Many older individuals with hyperthyroidism who develop atrial fibrillation are at greater risk of thromboembolic events, especially those with a history of thromboembolism, hypertension, or congestive heart failure and those with evidence of left atrial enlargement or left ventricular dysfunction. In the absence of contraindications, anticoagulant therapy should be given with warfarin in a dose that will increase the international normalization ratio to 2.0–3.0. Warfarin should be continued until the patient is euthyroid and normal sinus rhythm has been restored.

Allahabadia A et al: Age and gender predict the outcome of treatment for Graves' hyperthyroidism. J Clin Endocrinol Metab 2000;85:1038. [PMID: 10729936]

Trivalle C et al: Differences in the signs and symptoms of hyperthyroidism in older and younger patients. J Am Geriatr Soc 1996;44:50. [PMID: 8537590]

NODULAR THYROID DISEASE & NEOPLASIA

 ESSENTIALS OF DIAGNOSIS

- Thyroid nodule(s).
- Occasional compressive symptoms of dyspnea, dysphagia, pain in neck.
- Cervical adenopathy.

General Considerations

Multinodular thyroid glands occur more commonly in individuals who have lived in areas of iodine deficiency. Often there is a history of goiter dating to childhood or young adulthood. Very large multinodular goiters, particularly those with a significant substernal component, may compress the trachea and lead to problems of dyspnea and wheezing or problems with swallowing. All patients with thyroid nodules should be questioned regarding prior exposure to external radiation of the head, neck, and upper thorax. Radiation to these areas markedly increases the risk of thyroid malignancy. Radiation increases the risk of thyroid malignancy as well as benign nodules and parathyroid adenomas. Approximately 16–29% of persons who received low-dose radiation to the head and neck as children will develop palpable thyroid nodules; approximately 33% become malignant and clinically detected only after 10–20 years, reaching a peak incidence 20–30 years after radiation exposure.

Clinical Findings

A. Symptoms & Signs

Thyroid nodules usually remain asymptomatic, being discovered by the patient inadvertently or by the physician during a routine physical examination. On occasion, a thyroid nodule may result in an acute onset of neck pain and neck tenderness. This may be an acute or subacute thyroiditis or hemorrhage into a preexisting nodule. Although a single thyroid nodule is more commonly associated with malignancy than a multinodular thyroid gland, only 5% of clinically apparent solitary nodules will be malignant. The vast majority of thyroid nodules are benign and include follicular and colloid adenomas, Hashimoto's thyroiditis, and thyroid cysts.

Malignant thyroid neoplasms may be papillary, follicular, medullary, or anaplastic carcinomas; lymphoma; or, in rare cases, metastatic disease to the thyroid. Nonthyroid lesions may appear as nodules on physical examination; these include lymph nodes, aneurysms, parathyroid cysts and adenomas, and thyroglossal duct cysts. The risk that a solitary thyroid nodule will prove to be malignant is increased by a history of radiation exposure, age > 60, rapid increase in size, hoarseness of the voice suggesting an impingement of the recurrent laryngeal nerve, and hardness on palpation. Age is also a factor in predicting the histological type of malignancy. The overall histological distribution of all thyroid cancer is 79% papillary, 13% follicular, 3% Hürthle cell, 3.5% medullary, and 1.7% anaplastic. In patients older than 60, papillary carcinoma accounts for 67% of thyroid cancers. Follicular carcinoma peaks in frequency between the fourth and sixth decades of life (mean age at diagnosis, 44). Together with Hürthle cell carcinoma, these cancers account for 20% of thyroid malignancies in the over-60 population. Medullary carcinoma has a peak incidence during the fifth and sixth decades of life and represents approximately 5% of thyroid cancers in the elderly (Table 32–2). Anaplastic carcinomas occur almost exclusively in elderly people and account for ~6% of thyroid cancers in older patients. Anaplastic car-

Table 32–2. Thyroid malignancy in the older patient.

Cancer type	Patients affected (%) > Age 40	> Age 60	10-Year survival > Age 60 (%)
Papillary/mixed	79	64	< 65
Follicular	13	20	< 57
Medullary	3	5	< 63
Anaplastic	2	6	0
Lymphoma	3	5	99+

cinoma is characterized by rapid growth, rock-hard consistency, and local invasiveness. Involvement of the recurrent laryngeal nerve and compression of the trachea are common. Lymphoma and metastatic cancers occur infrequently in the older patient. Lymphoma usually presents with a rapidly enlarging painless neck mass that may cause compressive symptoms. Coexisting Hashimoto's thyroiditis is common.

B. Laboratory Tests

The major objective in evaluating an elderly person with a thyroid nodule is to rule out the presence of a malignancy. Blood tests of thyroid function will usually be normal unless there is a hyperfunctioning adenoma or toxic multinodular goiter. An elevated serum TSH may be noted in persons with subclinical hypothyroidism and nodular disease, as may result from long-standing Hashimoto's thyroiditis. Serum thyroglobulin is often elevated in the setting of thyroid cancer but cannot differentiate malignancy from benign nodules or thyroiditis with any degree of certainty. It is, therefore, more commonly used as a marker for recurrence or metastasis in patients with papillary or follicular carcinoma who have undergone total thyroidectomy. An elevation of serum calcitonin concentration is indicative of a medullary carcinoma but is not part of the initial evaluation unless there is a family history of multiple endocrine neoplasia (MEN).

C. Special Tests

Fine-needle aspiration (FNA) of the thyroid remains the best way to obtain tissue for cytological or histological examination. FNA is indicated in any patient with a solitary nodule and when there is suspicion of thyroid malignancy based on clinical evaluation, ultrasonography, or thyroid scan. This procedure, when performed by a skilled clinician, has proven to be safe, inexpensive, and capable of determining presence or absence of malignancy with an accuracy of close to 95% and even greater with sonographic guidance. In general, cytopathological findings from FNA are divided into 4 categories: positive for malignancy, suspicious for malignancy, negative for malignancy, and nondiagnostic. A repeat FNA is indicated for a nondiagnostic but clinically suspicious nodule. Malignant cells found on FNA indicate the need for surgery. The combination of suspicious cytology by FNA and a cold-appearing nodule on thyroid scan also indicates the need for surgical excision of the suspicious nodule. Benign cytology in either a solid or cystic nodule warrants observation. If the FNA is suggestive of a lymphoma, a repeat biopsy using a large-needle or even a surgical biopsy is indicated.

Isotopic scanning is no longer considered the initial diagnostic test in evaluating a suspicious nodule because of its relatively high false-positive and false-negative rates and high cost. Isotope imaging is best used when evaluating a patient with a thyroid nodule who has had a nondiagnostic result from FNA. Because malignant tissue is more likely unable to take up iodine, the identification of a nodule as hot on ^{123}I or technetium scanning makes malignancy in the nodule less likely, although clearly still possible. Scanning may also reveal an apparent single nodule that is, in fact, part of a multinodular thyroid gland, again decreasing the risk of malignancy. The presence of a nonfunctioning or a cold nodule is not proof of a malignancy because 95% of thyroid nodules will prove to be cold; the frequency of malignancy in cold nodules is 5%. Hot nodules associated with normal circulating levels of thyroid hormone and no compressive symptoms should be observed with repeat examinations performed at 6- to 12-mo intervals. These nodules may eventually result in hyperthyroidism; thus, clinical correlation is also warranted. High-resolution ultrasonography can detect thyroid lesions as small as 2 mm and can also permit classification of a nodule as solid, cystic, or mixed solid-cystic. It will often identify multinodularity in a gland even when a single nodule is palpated clinically. This technique cannot be used to distinguish with any degree of certainty malignant from benign nodules because there is a great deal of overlap in the characteristics identified using ultrasonography. Ultrasonography is best used to detect recurrent or residual thyroid cancer as well as to screen persons with a history of radiation exposure earlier in life.

Computed tomography (CT) and magnetic resonance imaging (MRI) are expensive and add little to the initial assessment of malignancy. They may be useful in evaluating the extent of disease in patients found to have anaplastic carcinoma or lymphoma and may provide useful information regarding compression of neck structures and the size and substernal extent of nodules and goiters.

Medullary carcinoma of the thyroid gland can be monitored using blood calcitonin measurements both in the basal state and after stimulation. Blood levels of carcinoembryonic antigen may also be elevated in patients with residual or recurrent medullary carcinoma.

Differential Diagnosis

The differential diagnosis includes thyroid duct cysts, benign adenomas, toxic thyroid nodule, thyroid malignancy, hemorrhage, and multinodular thyroid gland.

Treatment

Although the basic principles for treating thyroid cancer do not differ significantly between the young and old, older individuals need to be more carefully evaluated for comorbid conditions and risk of surgery. Surgery for thyroid cancer should be performed only by an experienced surgeon. Papillary or follicular carcinoma is usually treated with near-total thyroidectomy because of the high frequency of multicentricity of malignancy and the need to remove functional thyroid tissue to monitor the patient with total-body radioiodine scanning. Thyroid remnants detected postoperatively are ablated with ^{131}I. At 6 mo and subsequently at yearly intervals, scanning should be obtained and serum thyroglobulin measured to determine whether residual functional tissue exists. If active tissue is found, large ablative doses of ^{131}I should be administered. This approach has reduced the recurrence rate of both papillary and follicular carcinomas and prolonged survival.

Patients treated for malignancy are treated judiciously with suppressive doses of L-thyroxine as tolerated with the desired objective of reducing serum TSH to below normal as measured by third-generation TSH assays. The administration of suppressive doses of L-thyroxine carries a substantial risk of precipitating or aggravating ischemic heart disease and arrhythmias as well as accelerating bone turnover. The older patient will need to be monitored closely and the dose of thyroid hormone reduced if cardiac symptoms develop. An acceleration of bone loss will occur and necessitate treatment with antibone resorption agents in some circumstances (eg, in osteopenic women). Medullary carcinoma of the thyroid gland is best treated with a total thyroidectomy because the disease is often multicentric. The majority of medullary carcinomas do not respond to ^{131}I treatment; therefore, palliative therapy is recommended using external irradiation if residual thyroid tissue or recurrent disease is detected. Thyroid lymphoma should be clinically staged using CT or MRI. External irradiation in combination with chemotherapy has been associated with a survival rate close to 100%.

Prognosis

Age at diagnosis is an important factor in predicting cancer aggressiveness and mortality from differentiated thyroid cancer. Individuals diagnosed after the age of 50 have a higher rate of recurrence and death (see Table 32–2). The 10-year survival for patients with papillary carcinoma is ~97% in those younger than 45 and < 65% for those older than 60 at diagnosis. The 10-year survival rate for persons with follicular carcinoma is 98% for those younger than 45 and < 57% for those older than 60 at diagnosis. The older the person is when a follicular carcinoma is diagnosed, the greater is the risk of recurrence and death.

The 10-year survival rate for persons with medullary carcinoma is 84% for individuals younger than 45 and decreases with advancing age. Persons in the seventh decade of life have a high rate of persistent disease even after surgery. Anaplastic carcinoma of the thyroid gland is rarely associated with more than a 1-year survival after diagnosis because of its rapid progression and high propensity to metastasize. Palliative treatment of compressive symptoms may be achieved by surgery followed by high-dose external radiation. Chemotherapy with doxorubicin or cisplatin, or a combination, may be beneficial in combination with surgery and external irradiation.

Mazzaferri EL: An overview of the management of papillary and follicular thyroid carcinoma. Thyroid 1999;9:421. [PMID: 10365671]

■ DISEASES OF THE ADRENAL CORTEX

Old age is associated with a reduced metabolic clearance rate of cortisol but with a compensatory decrease in secretion rate. Consequently, basal levels of serum cortisol are unaffected over the life span. Basal adrenocorticotropic hormone (ACTH) levels are unchanged or slightly increased with age in healthy individuals. Diurnal cortisol rhythm is reported to show a significant age-related phase advance (earlier peak and nadir level) similar to that observed in depressed patients. This is thought to be related to changes in sleep patterns.

The adrenal androgen precursor dehydroepiandrosterone (DHEA) reaches peak blood levels in both men and women by age 20–30 and then declines steadily so that, after age 70, levels are < 20% of the peak. Although early reports and popular lay literature have attributed a number of antiaging properties to DHEA, more recent studies in which DHEA has been administered for 6–12 mo have shown little or no effect on objective measures of physiological function. Some studies, however, suggest a beneficial effect on mood and sense of general well-being.

Hypothalamic-pituitary-adrenal axis response to known major stimuli remains intact with increasing age. Stimulation tests of this axis using insulin-induced hypoglycemia or metyrapone administration result in a normal or slightly longer period of cortisol and ACTH secretory response in older persons. Peak cortisol response to stress is also greater, and both cortisol and ACTH levels remain elevated for a longer period in elderly compared with younger persons. Moreover, dexamethasone causes less inhibition of cortisol in older patients. It is unknown whether this age-related hyperresponsiveness of the pituitary-adrenal axis to stressful situations contributes to age-prevalent illness, including osteoporosis, glucose intolerance, muscle atrophy, and immunosuppression. Adrenal cortical response to exogenous ACTH, measured by circulating cortisol levels, is unaffected by aging.

ACUTE ADRENAL INSUFFICIENCY

 ESSENTIALS OF DIAGNOSIS

- *Weakness.*
- *Abdominal pain.*
- *Nausea and vomiting.*
- *Low blood pressure.*
- *Hyperkalemia.*
- *Hyponatremia.*
- *Inappropriate response of plasma cortisol to cosyntropin (ACTH 1–24).*

General Considerations

Acute adrenal insufficiency results from a deficiency in cortisol secretion and, in elderly people, occurs most often as a result of failure of the adrenal gland rather than a pituitary gland disorder. The adrenal gland may be unable to produce an adequate amount of corticosteroids and mineralocorticoids because of an autoimmune process involving the entire adrenal gland or from a replacement of healthy adrenal tissue with tumor or infection, such as in tuberculosis. Adrenal crisis may also result from an increased demand for glucocorticoids in an individual unable to increase output sufficiently. This occurs most commonly as a result of chronic adrenal suppression from exogenous corticoid use and less often from stress from trauma, surgery, hemorrhage, or infection. Rarely, this may result from a sudden increase in the metabolic turnover of corticosteroids, as can occur when a patient with both adrenal insufficiency and hypothyroidism is treated with thyroid hormone. Corticosteroid-induced adrenal suppression can occur after as few as 3–4 weeks of exogenous steroid treatment with doses > 15 mg of prednisone or the equivalent dose of other glucocorticoids. In general, individuals on long-term glucocorticoid therapy who have stopped treatment before the return of function of the suppressed adrenal glands or who need a higher dose will have a less clear picture because of the ability of renin and angiotensin to maintain aldosterone function despite suppression of glucocorticoid activity in the adrenal gland.

Clinical Findings

A. SYMPTOMS & SIGNS

Patients with adrenal insufficiency often have nausea and vomiting and abdominal pain and may have an altered mental state and fever. In general, blood pressure is low. Signs of primary adrenal insufficiency may include hyperpigmentation and evidence of dehydration. Elderly persons commonly have sparse or absent pubic and axillary hair; therefore, this is less commonly noted as an abnormality during later life.

B. LABORATORY TESTS

Laboratory findings may include hyponatremia or hyperkalemia. Hypoglycemia and elevation of blood urea nitrogen (BUN) and creatinine are common. Eosinophilia may be noted as well. Cultures may be positive if there is an underlying infection. The cosyntropin (ACTH 1–24) stimulation test is abnormal, and plasma ACTH is usually elevated in persons with primary failure of the adrenal gland. With this test, patients are given 0.25 mg of cosyntropin intravenously over 2–3 min, and serum cortisol is measured immediately before and 30 and 60 min after administration. Under normal circumstances, serum cortisol rises by at least 7 μg/dL to at least 20 μg/dL. Hydrocortisone administration will interfere with the test results, but other glucocorticoids such as dexamethasone or prednisone do not interfere with the specific assay for cortisol.

Differential Diagnosis

Although adrenal insufficiency should be considered in any patient who presents with hyperkalemia and hypotension, other possible causes for these findings should be considered.

Other causes of hypotension in particular include sepsis, hemorrhage, and cardiogenic diseases. Renal insufficiency may cause hyperkalemia as may gastrointestinal bleeding, rhabdomyolysis, and medications such as spironolactone and angiotensin-converting enzyme inhibitors. Hyponatremia may occur in hypothyroidism, with diuretic use, in drug and disease states associated with inappropriate ADH secretion, and with malnutrition, cirrhosis, and vomiting. Eosinophilia may be associated with blood dyscrasias, allergies, medication reactions, and parasitic infections. The associated gastrointestinal findings of nausea, vomiting, and abdominal pain may, in fact, be due to other gastrointestinal tract disorders common during later life. Hyperpigmentation may not be noted in older persons of dark complexion or who have sun-induced skin damage.

Treatment

Replacement of both glucocorticoids and mineralocorticoids is needed in severe cases of adrenal insufficiency. Because hydrocortisone has some mineralocorticoid activity, it is the corticosteroid of choice for patients with mild cases and is effective in doses of 25–37.5 mg orally; two thirds of the dose is given in the morning and one third in the late afternoon or evening. If salt-retaining effects from this therapy are insufficient, fludrocortisone is added to the daily regimen in dosages of 0.05–0.3 mg orally each day or every other day. The exact dose required will vary with the individual and, therefore, should be clinically adjusted in relation to postural blood pressure changes, level of potassium, and body weight. The dose is reduced if hypokalemia, hypertension, or edema occur, especially when fluid and electrolyte management is complicated by cardiac disease or renal insufficiency. Underlying factors that may have contributed to the onset of adrenal insufficiency, particularly infections, should be sought. The dosage of hydrocortisone may need to be adjusted upward to a stress dosage as high as 300 mg/day, although usually 50 mg intravenously or intramuscularly every 6 h will be sufficient, even for the most stressful situations.

Prognosis

With adequate replacement therapy, adrenal insufficiency is a treatable illness. When accompanied by other illnesses the risk mortality is increased. If the underlying cause is an autoimmune disease, other endocrine problems such as diabetes mellitus and hypothyroidism as well as pernicious anemia may be present.

Parker CR et al: Effects of aging on adrenal function in the human: responsiveness and sensitivity of adrenal androgens and cortisol to adrenocorticotropin in premenopausal and postmenopausal women. J Clin Endocrinol Metab 2000;85:48. [PMID: 10634362]

CUSHING'S SYNDROME

ESSENTIALS OF DIAGNOSIS

- Central obesity.
- Diabetes mellitus.
- Muscle wasting.
- Easy bruising.
- Purple striae.
- Hypertension.
- Poor wound healing.
- Elevated serum cortisol and urinary free cortisol.
- Lack of normal suppression of serum cortisol with dexamethasone.

General Considerations

Cushing's syndrome is caused by an excessive amount of circulating corticosteroids. In elderly patients, it most commonly results from exogenous exposure to corticosteroids given for a variety of medical disorders. The most frequent endogenous cause is ectopic production of ACTH by neoplasms, especially small cell carcinoma of the lung and carcinoid tumor. Cushing's disease (ie, oversecretion of ACTH by a pituitary tumor) is less common in elderly than younger patients, is usually associated with a small benign adenoma, and occurs more often in women than men. Approximately 15% of cases of endogenous Cushing's syndrome are non-ACTH dependent and result from an adrenal adenoma, carcinoma, or bilateral nodular adrenal hyperplasia. Although adrenal adenomas are generally small and produce mostly glucocorticoids, carcinomas tend to be larger on presentation and more commonly produce excessive amounts of both glucocorticoids and androgens, often resulting in virilization and hirsutism.

Clinical Findings

A. SYMPTOMS & SIGNS

Although central obesity, thin arms and legs, and a round "moon face" are classic findings, these may be harder to detect in older patients. For example, the "buffalo hump" deposition of fat at the back of the neck may, in older women, be confused with a kyphosis resulting from osteoporosis. Thin, transparent skin, bruising, muscle atrophy and weakness, diabetes melli-

tus, and hypertension are other common findings easily confused with many other age-prevalent disorders. Thirst is less often reported by elderly compared with younger patients. Polyuria may result from increases in blood sugar from glucocorticoid-induced diabetes. Blood glucose is often elevated, and glycosuria may be present. Occasionally, there is a leukocytosis and hypokalemia. Wound healing may be impaired, and changes in mental function, including anxiety, psychosis, and depression, may occur.

B. LABORATORY TESTS

A low-dose dexamethasone suppression test can be used to screen for hypercortisolism. Dexamethasone, 1 mg, is given orally at 11 PM, and serum is collected at 8 AM the next morning for cortisol. A cortisol level < 5 μg/dL is considered normal and excludes a diagnosis of Cushing's syndrome. If there is failure of suppression, further evaluation should include a 24-h urine collection for free cortisol and creatinine. A high 24-h urine free cortisol or a free cortisol–creatinine ratio of > 95 μg/g creatinine is suggestive of hypercortisolism. A 2-mg dexamethasone suppression test using 0.5 mg of dexamethasone administered orally every 6 h for 48 h can also be used as a screening test. Urine is collected on day 2, and excretion of urinary free cortisol > 20 μg/24 h or urinary 17-hydroxycorticosteroid > 4.5 mg/day helps confirm hypercortisolism.

Once hypercortisolism is confirmed, plasma ACTH should be determined. A level of ACTH below the normal range indicates a probable adrenal tumor; an elevated level indicates overproduction by either the pituitary or an ectopic ACTH-secreting tumor. MRI of the pituitary can identify a pituitary adenoma with considerable accuracy. Selective inferior petrosal venous sampling for ACTH can be done to confirm a pituitary source of ACTH and to help distinguish its origin from other sites. A CT or MRI scan of the chest and abdomen to look for ectopic sources of ACTH is indicated and can localize a tumor of the adrenal glands.

Differential Diagnosis

Hypercortisolism can result from iatrogenic use of steroid medications. Alcoholic patients and those with depression may also have increased levels of cortisol. Abnormal dexamethasone suppression tests have been described in patients with morbid obesity, depression, and a variety of CNS disorders. In these patients, urine free cortisol should be measured and an attempt made to assess diurnal variation in cortisol secretion because these tests are usually within normal limits in the setting of obesity. Hypertension resulting from other causes is common in the elderly, and estrogen replacement therapy may alter normal dexamethasone suppressibility.

Treatment

Cushing's disease is best treated by removing the pituitary adenoma responsible for the increase in ACTH secretion. After its removal, the adrenal gland remains unable to respond to normal stimulation for a prolonged time, and there is an altered ability to respond under conditions of stress. Hydrocortisone replacement therapy is necessary until normal pituitary-adrenal axis function returns, often taking as long as 6–24 mo. Radiation therapy has also been used to treat Cushing's disease, with an approximate cure rate of 25%. For patients who are not surgical candidates, inhibition of adrenal steroid biosynthesis can be useful in controlling symptoms and has been achieved with metyrapone, 500 mg every 6 h, in combination with aminoglutethimide, 250–500 mg every 6 h, and ketoconazole, 200 mg every 6 h. Physiological replacement doses of a glucocorticoid may be necessary to avoid drug-induced adrenal insufficiency.

Adrenal neoplasms secreting cortisol should be resected when possible and often can be removed laparoscopically. Because the nonaffected adrenal gland is usually suppressed, once again hydrocortisone replacement is indicated until the gland returns to normal function. Metastatic adrenal carcinoma can be managed with the medications just mentioned or with mitotane, 2–10 mg daily in divided doses. Ectopic ACTH-secreting tumors should be surgically resected. If this is not possible, once again, medications may be used to suppress the high levels of cortisol. The somatostatin analogue octreotide has been used to suppress ACTH secretion successfully in as many as 33% of cases in which it has been attempted.

Prognosis

Patients who have hypercortisolism as a result of iatrogenic use of corticosteroids can usually expect a return to normal after discontinuation of the steroid therapy. In hypercortisolism, the best prognosis for total recovery is seen when a benign adrenal adenoma is easily removed. Pituitary adenomas are more difficult to treat and, even in the best of hands, have a failure rate of 10–20%. Even those who respond have a 15–20% recurrence rate over the next decade. The prognosis of patients with ectopic ACTH-producing tumors depends on the underlying type and degree of tumor involvement.

Papanicolaou DA et al: A single midnight serum cortisol measurement distinguishes Cushing's syndrome from pseudo-Cushing states. J Clin Endocrinol Metab 1998;83:1163. [PMID: 9543134]

DYSLIPIDEMIA

 ESSENTIALS OF DIAGNOSIS

- *Hypercholesterolemia.*
- *Hypertriglyceridemia.*

General Considerations

Dyslipidemia is a major health risk regardless of age. The absolute risk of coronary heart disease increases dramatically with age in both men and women. Nearly 50% of all deaths in men older than 65 are thought to result from coronary heart disease, and the rate is even higher for women. Longitudinal studies show that total cholesterol levels increase in men after the onset of puberty until the sixth decade of life. This is followed by a plateau until the eighth decade, after which serum levels of cholesterol fall. In women, serum cholesterol concentrations are slighter higher than in men before age 30. Between 30 and 55 years, serum cholesterol increases although at a slower rate than in men. By age 60, cholesterol levels in women are equal to that of men and thereafter increase at a faster rate. The age-related changes in serum cholesterol concentration are primarily due to an increase in the low-density lipoprotein (LDL) cholesterol component. High-density lipoprotein (HDL) cholesterol levels do not vary greatly with age and are ~10 mg/dL higher on average in women than in men. This age-related increase in LDL cholesterol is thought to result from a diminished activity of hepatic LDL receptors.

Clinical Findings

A. SYMPTOMS & SIGNS

Although heart disease mortality has declined consistently since the 1960s, coronary heart disease remains the leading cause of death for both men and women in the United States; hypercholesterolemia is a major modifiable risk factor regardless of age. The incidence of dyslipidemia is highest in patients with early-onset coronary heart disease before 55 years of age in men and 65 years of age in women. The prevalence of coronary artery disease in this population exceeds 80% compared with 40–50% in the general population of similar age. Dyslipidemia is defined as a serum total cholesterol, LDL cholesterol, triglyceride, apo-B, or Lp(a) concentration > the 90th percentile or HDL-cholesterol or apo-A-1 concentration < the 10th percentile. High concentrations of LDL are particularly associated with atherosclerosis. A low level of HDL cholesterol is also highly correlated with coronary heart disease. The total cholesterol–HDL ratio is suggested as a better predictor of future coronary heart disease. In men, a ratio > 6.4 is associated with a greater risk; among women, a ratio > 5.6 is considered to be a significant risk of coronary disease. The optimal level of LDL cholesterol is considered to be a value < 100 mg/dL in both men and women. HDL cholesterol appears to have a protective effect with the goal of achieving levels > 40 mg/dL in men and 51 mg/dL in women. The role of isolated elevation of triglycerides as a risk factor for heart disease is controversial, although they appear to be an independent predictor for coronary disease in women.

B. LABORATORY TESTS

Lipids are insoluble in plasma and circulate bound to lipoproteins, which transport the lipid to various tissues for energy, steroid hormone production, bile acid formation, and lipid deposition. The lipoprotein consists of esterified and unesterified cholesterol, triglycerides, phospholipids, and protein. The protein components of lipoprotein are referred to as apoproteins or apolipoproteins. These serve as cofactors for enzymes and ligands for receptors. Lipoproteins are classified into 5 major groups, each with a different identifiable function.

Chylomicrons are very large particles that carry dietary lipid. They are associated with a variety of apolipoproteins, including A-1, A-11, A-lV, B-48, C-1, C-11, C-111, and E.

Very low-density lipoproteins (VLDLs) carry endogenous triglycerides and cholesterol. The major apolipoproteins associated with VLDLs are B-100, C-1, C-11, C-111, and E. Intermediate-density lipoproteins (IDLs) carry cholesterol esters and are associated with apolipoprotein B-100. LDLs carry cholesterol esters and

are associated with apolipoprotein B-100. HDLs carry cholesterol esters and are associated with apolipoproteins A-l, A-11, C-1, C-11, C-111, D, and E.

Classically, patients can be classified into 1 of 6 subtypes of dyslipidemias, referred to as the Fredrickson Classification (Table 32–3). A serum lipid profile generally includes measurements of total cholesterol, triglycerides, and HDL cholesterol. A lipoprotein analysis is best done after a 12- to 15-h fast. The serum cholesterol is ~3% lower than that obtained from plasma. The total cholesterol can vary by 4–10% within an individual because of a variety of factors, including illness (eg, myocardial infarction), infection, trauma, or surgery. There is also some variability between laboratories. For these reasons, more than 1 measurement of total cholesterol should be obtained before initiating treatment. Tissue injury may generate acute-phase proteins, which may impair hepatic lipoprotein production and metabolism, thus reducing serum concentrations of total cholesterol, HDL cholesterol, LDL cholesterol, and apolipoproteins B and A-1; triglyceride and lipoprotein(a) levels may rise under these circumstances.

Several categories of primary lipoprotein disorders lead to dyslipidemia. Most of these are detected early in life, but some may be noted for the first time later in life. Familial hypertriglyceridemia is associated with a decrease in the ability to remove serum triglycerides. This is caused by a decrease in lipoprotein lipase activity and an increased hepatic secretion of triglyceride-rich VLDLs. Although evidence of a relationship of triglycerides to coronary heart disease is unclear, persons with triglyceride levels > 2000 mg/dL are at high risk for pancreatitis.

Familial combined hyperlipidemia is associated with increased hepatic secretion of apolipoprotein B containing VLDL that is converted to LDL. Depending on the ability to remove particles, VLDL or LDL or both accumulate. This is associated with a high risk of coronary heart disease, peripheral vascular disease, and stroke.

Table 32–3. Fredrickson classification of dyslipidemias.

Phenotype	Chylomicron concentration	Total cholesterol concentration	Triglyceride cholesterol	1 VLDL Cholesterol concentration
I	⇑⇑⇑	⇔	⇑⇑⇑	⇔
IIa	⇔	⇑⇑⇑	⇑	⇔
IIb	⇔	⇑⇑⇑	⇑	⇑
III	⇑	⇑	⇑	⇑
IV	⇔	⇑ or ⇔	⇑⇑⇑	⇑⇑⇑
V	⇑⇑⇑	⇑ or ⇔	⇑	⇑⇑⇑

1, very low-density lipoproteins; 2, low-density lipoproteins; 3, high-density lipoproteins.

Familial dysbetalipoproteinemia, or remnant removal disease, is associated with an increased secretion of VLDL and an impaired ability to remove remnant lipoproteins. This results from either a homozygous or heterozygous pattern for apolipoprotein E-2. This is also associated with a significant risk of vascular disease. Familial or polygenic hypercholesterolemia is associated with a decrease in LDL receptor activity. A defect in apolipoprotein B renders identification by the LDL receptor difficult. Once again, this disorder is associated with a high risk of vascular events, particularly myocardial infarction and stroke. Familial hypoalphalipoproteinemia, or low HDL syndrome, is associated with a decrease in apolipoproteins, increased removal, and increased cholesterol-ester transfer protein or hepatic lipase activity. This disorder commonly is associated with elevated levels of triglycerides and is associated with both peripheral vascular disease and coronary heart disease.

Treatment

Cholesterol-lowering therapy may have positive effects on patients with atherosclerotic plaques and those with severe hypercholesterolemia who are still free of clinical heart disease. Patients should be stratified according to presumed risk. Recommendations for treatment are based on LDL cholesterol levels and are influenced by the presence of coronary heart disease and other cardiac risk factors. Treatment considerations include cost-effectiveness, patient compliance, and side effects. Discontinuation rates for lipid therapy in long-term studies regardless of age approach 40% for treatment with bile acid sequestrants, 46% for nicotinic acid, 37% for gemfibrozil, and ~15% for statins.

Treatment guidelines have not been established for elderly patients. Individual considerations must be made and careful thought given to patient choice, comorbidities, and expected life span. Age itself should not be a factor in deciding against treatment. It has been estimated that > 40% of persons older than 65 will meet the criteria for primary prevention. Treatment appears to be reasonable for elderly patients at highest risk, such as for those with an LDL cholesterol > 160 mg/dL with additional cardiac risk factors who have failed at dietary modification.

Prognosis

Persons with homozygous patterns of familial hyperlipidemia, primarily effecting LDL cholesterol, usually present with associated medical problems early in life and have significant morbidity and mortality despite best efforts of treatment. Elderly individuals who first present for treatment of dyslipidemia often have advanced coronary artery, cerebrovascular, or peripheral vascular disease as a result of years of lipid abnormalities. Although the goals of treatment may be the same regardless of age, medication side effects and patient acceptance may result in a less satisfactory outcome. The best way to achieve an optimal outcome is to initiate risk factor modification and appropriate drug therapy before vascular diseases develop.

Aronow WS: Underutilization of lipid lowering drugs in older persons with prior myocardial infarction and a serum low-density lipoprotein cholesterol > 125 mg/dL. Am J Cardiol 1998;82:668. [PMID: not available]

National Cholesterol Education Program (NCEP) Expert Panel: Executive summary of the THIRD Report of the NCEP Expert Panel on detection, evaluation, and treatment of high blood cholesterol in adults (Adult Treatment Panel lll). JAMA 2001;285:2486. [PMID: not available]

■ ANTERIOR PITUITARY

The ability to secrete growth hormone is impaired with aging, which can reduce muscle mass and alter body composition. The normal nocturnal surges of growth hormone secretion are diminished with age. After stimulation of growth hormone secretion by insulin-induced hypoglycemia, growth hormone increases in both young and old. This response, however, is diminished in some elderly patients, leading to the concept of reduced reserve. A significant effect of age on arginine-induced growth hormone secretion has not been observed.

The ability to produce luteinizing hormone (LH) and follicle-stimulating hormone (FSH) appears to be preserved into old age; elevations occur in response to primary failure of end-organs. Age-related alterations have been described on the feedback in inhibition of gonadotropin secretion by sex steroids. Age has also been associated with changes in plasma levels of prolactin. Until age 45, the mean value for men is ~66% of that found in women; levels become more equal with age. Blood levels of ACTH and TSH are within normal limits in healthy older people.

PITUITARY DISORDERS/ HYPOPITUITARISM

 ESSENTIALS OF DIAGNOSIS

- *Low blood pressure.*
- *Visual field defects.*

- *Headaches.*
- *Elevated prolactin, growth hormone, ACTH.*
- *Low levels of FSH and LH.*
- *Low TSH and T$_4$.*
- *Deficient cortisol response to stimulation.*

Clinical Findings

A. SYMPTOMS & SIGNS

Major clinical manifestations of pituitary tumors are due to mass effects or alterations in pituitary hormone production. Most pituitary tumors in elderly persons are nonfunctional adenomas found during CT or MRI imaging of the brain done for other CNS problems. Mass effects include retro-orbital headaches and visual field deficits. Prolactin-producing micro- and macroadenomas are the most common of the functional tumors and can present with galactorrhea. Much less common are ACTH-secreting adenomas with Cushing's syndrome and growth hormone-secreting tumors with acromegaly.

Pituitary adenomas can result in loss of normal pituitary hormone production and present clinically with features of hypopituitarism. Many of the findings noted in younger persons with hypopituitarism are not readily apparent in the elderly because of age-related changes that make it more difficult to note a difference in libido, pubic and axillary hair, menstrual irregularity, and even such constitutional symptoms as weakness, cold intolerance, and impotence. Manifestations of hypopituitarism resulting from adenoma will vary depending on its size and location and the specific hormones affected. A deficiency of TSH results in hypothyroidism. ACTH deficiency causes diminished cortisol secretion and may lead to symptoms of weakness, weight loss, and hypotension. Deficiencies in FSH and LH in men may be associated with a diminished libido, reduced body hair including beard growth, reduced muscle mass, and impotence.

B. LABORATORY FINDINGS

Laboratory findings are related to the specific deficiency noted. Fasting blood glucose may be low. Hyponatremia resulting from cortisol deficiency may be present. TSH, T$_4$, and free T$_4$ will be low if TSH secretion is reduced. Elevated prolactin levels are present in persons with prolactinomas and often in patients with acromegaly. The ACTH stimulation (cosyntropin stimulation) test has an inadequate response; 0.25 mg given intravenously results in < 20 μg/dL rise within 30–60 min. Baseline ACTH is usually low or normal.

Growth hormone deficiency is often found but difficult to detect clinically or with laboratory testing because of age-related effects. Stimulation tests, including hypoglycemia and exercise, are difficult and even dangerous in the elderly patient and are best avoided. Visual field impairments may be found. Rarely, hemorrhage in the pituitary may result in a complete loss of pituitary function with dramatic onset of symptoms. The pituitary and sellar region is visualized with CT or MRI.

Differential Diagnosis

In addition to pituitary adenoma, hypopituitarism can result from metastatic lesions to the pituitary and from ischemia causing necrosis of the hypothalamus or pituitary itself, most often in association with severe prolonged hypotension and cerebral anoxia. Severe illness can also cause suppressed pituitary function, especially TSH. Exogenous administration of corticosteroids reduces adrenal reserve and the normal pituitary-adrenal axis.

Treatment

Hypopituitarism requires prompt treatment with replacement hormone therapy given for thyroid and adrenal insufficiency. If the patient is hypothyroid, L-thyroxine should be started but only after any coexisting cortisol deficiency has been corrected. Testosterone levels in men should be determined and replaced as necessary to alleviate related symptoms. Estrogen replacement should be considered as with any postmenopausal woman.

Depending on the size and extent of the adenoma, surgery or radiation may be indicated to treat manifestations of mass effect, most importantly visual field defects resulting from compression of the optic chiasm. Prolactin-producing adenomas can be managed medically with the dopamine agonists bromocriptine or cabergiline. Prolactin levels are usually reduced to normal, and galactorrhea, if present, resolves. Tumor size will decrease in some patients. Similarly, patients with acromegaly can be treated with somatostatin analogues with consequent reduction in levels of growth hormone and insulin-like growth factor as well as shrinkage of tumor size.

Pinzone JJ et al: Primary medical therapy of micro- and macroprolactinomas in men. J Clin Endocrinol Metab 2000;85:3053. [PMID: 10999785]

Schmidt DN, Wallace K: How to diagnose hypopituitarism. Learning the features of secondary hormonal deficiencies. Postgrad Med 1998;104:77. [PMID: 9676563]

DIABETES INSIPIDUS

ESSENTIALS OF DIAGNOSIS

- Polyuria.
- Polydipsia.
- Dehydration.
- Urine specific gravity < 1.006 in the setting of ad libitum fluid intake.
- Urine osmolality hypotonic relative to plasma osmolality.
- Response of polyuria and urine osmolality to exogenous vasopressin administration (if from pituitary causes).

General Considerations

Diabetes insipidus is associated with an increased thirst and large volumes of urine with low specific gravity or urine osmolality resulting from deficiency of or resistance to the action of ADH. Most commonly, in elderly patients, diabetes insipidus is due to a hypothalamic or pituitary disorder resulting in an inadequate ability to secrete ADH. It can result from trauma, infection, sarcoidosis, metastases, anoxic damage, and, rarely, pituitary adenoma. Nephrogenic diabetes insipidus results from a defect in the kidney that interferes with water reabsorption; the polyuria is unresponsive to the action of exogenous ADH, and ADH secretion is not impaired. Acquired forms of ADH-resistant diabetes insipidus are most common during later life and may be less severe than congenital forms. A variety of medical conditions, including pyelonephritis, renal amyloidosis, acute tubular necrosis, potassium deficiency, multiple myeloma, Sjögren's syndrome, and chronic hypercalcemia, can cause this problem. Medications, notably lithium and demeclocycline, can also cause a renal-resistant state.

Clinical Findings

A. SYMPTOMS & SIGNS

Thirst is a hallmark of this disorder, although fewer elderly complain of this compared with younger patients until much later in the course of illness. Polyuria may lead to dehydration unless the elderly person is able to keep up with the need for increased amounts of volume. Other presenting symptoms and signs include in-continence, hypernatremia, dehydration, altered mental status, hypotension, and hyperuricemia in association with a central cause of diabetes insipidus resulting from reduced clearance of urate, which accompanies this disorder.

B. LABORATORY TESTS

A 24-h urine collection should be obtained for volume, creatinine, and glucose. Serum sodium, glucose, urea nitrogen, calcium, uric acid, and potassium should also be measured. In nephrogenic diabetes insipidus, serum ADH levels will be high.

Differential Diagnosis

Polyuria may result from other disorders in the older person, including diabetes mellitus, excess circulating levels of corticosteroid (as with Cushing's syndrome or with exogenous administration), lithium use, diuretic use, and excess fluid intake).

Treatment

Central diabetes insipidus responds to ADH preparations given under carefully supervised conditions. Desmopressin acetate can be given intranasally every 12–24 h as required for thirst and polyuria. Treatment is usually begun with 0.05–0.1 mL (100 µg/mL solution) every 12–24 h with individual titration thereafter. Because many elderly patients will not complain of excessive thirst until they are significantly hyperosmolar, monitoring is essential to determine proper dose requirements in a given patient. Desmopressin can also be given intravenously, intramuscularly, or subcutaneously, and an oral preparation is available but with more variable response. Potential side effects of the oral preparation include GI symptoms and elevated hepatic enzymes. Nasal preparations may cause nasal irritation and occasional agitation. Overtreatment may lead to water retention and hyponatremia.

Prognosis

Transient cases of diabetes insipidus may follow pituitary surgery and will usually remit within days to several weeks. Occasionally, permanent diabetes insipidus will remain and require lifelong treatment. Chronic diabetes insipidus can be successfully managed with appropriate desmopressin treatment and in itself should not result in increased morbidity or mortality. Elderly patients frequently have electrolyte disturbances that require careful monitoring.

Bichet DG: Nephrogenic diabetes insipidus. Am J Med 1998;105: 431. [PMID: 9831428]

SYNDROME OF INAPPROPRIATE ADH SECRETION

ESSENTIALS OF DIAGNOSIS

- *Fatigue, lethargy, confusion, seizures, coma.*
- *Increased free water intake.*
- *Hyponatremia, plasma hypo-osmolality.*
- *Urine osmolality hypertonic relative to plasma.*
- *Urine sodium excretion > 20 mEq/L.*
- *Low serum BUN, creatinine, uric acid.*

General Considerations

Age is associated with alterations in the secretion of ADH from the hypothalamic-neurohypophysial system and in the renal response to ADH. Basal blood levels of ADH may be increased with advancing age. More importantly, elderly persons have an enhanced secretory response of ADH to the stimuli of plasma hypertonicity and plasma volume reduction. Renal changes associated with normal aging can lead to impaired ability to dilute urine and excrete a water load. As a consequence, the elderly person is at increased risk for water retention and dilutional hyponatremia, characterized as the syndrome of inappropriate ADH secretion (SIADH). Hyponatremia resulting from SIADH has been observed in 7–10% of community-residing older persons and as many as 20% of elderly nursing home residents.

Clinical Findings

A. SYMPTOMS & SIGNS

The clinical presentation is related to the effects of hyponatremia on the CNS. There is a general relationship between level of serum sodium and severity of symptoms; however, the more important factor is the rapidity of onset of hyponatremia. Mild symptoms, generally seen with serum sodium in the range of 120–130 mEq/L, are headache, fatigue, and lethargy. With more severe hyponatremia, confusion is often present and can progress to seizures, obtundation, and coma when serum sodium falls to $\leq$ 105–110 mEq/L. The more rapid the decline in serum sodium, the more severe the symptoms are likely to be for any given level of serum sodium. Typically, patients with SIADH do not have edema.

There are many potential underlying causes, including CNS disease of any type, the use of any number of

classes of drugs, pulmonary diseases, malignancies, and enteral tube feeding (Table 32–4). Idiopathic SIADH (no evident underlying cause), has been observed in ~2% of elderly individuals older than 80; whites are at higher risk than blacks. A common factor is the precipitation of SIADH by the administration of free water through hypotonic intravenous fluids (eg, 0.45% saline and 5% dextrose in water), encouragement of large unspecified amounts of oral fluid intake, or excessive water administered with tube-fed diets.

B. LABORATORY TESTS

The diagnosis of SIADH requires differentiation of dilutional from depletional hyponatremia. This can usually be accomplished by careful history of diet, fluid intake, and fluid losses (eg, fever, tachypnea, vomiting, diarrhea, polyuria) and drugs. Commonly available laboratory measures such as hematocrit, BUN, creatinine, and uric acid are often helpful in distinguishing between types of hyponatremia. The hallmark of SIADH is the combination of low serum sodium and osmolality, urine osmolality inappropriately concentrated for level of serum osmolality, and excretion of sodium in the urine at a concentration > 20 mEq/L.

Differential Diagnosis

The diagnosis of SIADH requires the exclusion of other disorders that can cause dilutional hyponatremia, including hypothyroidism, adrenal insufficiency, congestive heart failure, cirrhosis, and renal failure. Pseudohyponatremia can be seen with marked hyperlipidemia or paraproteinemia and can be recognized by measurement of serum osmolality, which will be normal at the same time that serum sodium is reduced. Hyperglycemia is accompanied by a reduction in serum sodium, which corrects when blood glucose level is restored to normal.

Treatment

Initial treatment is directed at determining and addressing the underlying cause of the SIADH where possible. Mildly symptomatic hyponatremia can be treated with fluid restriction, usually at a level of 1000–1200 mL/24 h. More symptomatic hyponatremia requires the administration of hypertonic (3%) saline intravenously at a rate sufficient to increase serum sodium by 0.5–1.0 mEq/L/h with the objective of increasing serum sodium by no more than 12–15 mEq/L in the first 24 h and to a level no higher than 125 mEq/L to avoid inducing central pontine myelinolysis. The patient with seizures or coma and very low serum sodium may require intravenous furosemide in a dose of 1 mg/kg

Table 32–4. Causes of the syndrome of inappropriate antidiuretic hormone secretion in elderly patients.

Central nervous system disorders
   Vascular diseases (thrombosis, embolism, hemorrhage, vasculitis)
   Trauma (subdural hematoma, subarachnoid or intracranial hemorrhage)
   Tumor
   Hydrocephalus
   Infection (meningitis, encephalitis, brain abscess)
   Lupus erythematosus
   Postoperative transsphenoidal hypophysectomy
   Schizophrenia
Neoplasms with ectopic hormone production
   Small cell carcinoma of the lung
   Pharyngeal carcinoma
   Pancreatic carcinoma
   Thymoma
   Lymphoma, Hodgkin's disease, reticulum cell sarcoma
   Bladder carcinoma
Pulmonary diseases
   Pneumonia
   Lung abscess
   Bronchiectasis
   Tuberculosis
Drugs
   CNS active drugs
      Antipsychotics
      Antidepressants (tricyclics, selective serotonin reuptake inhibitors)
      Anticonvulsants (carbamazepine)
      Narcotics
      Hallucinogenics (MDMA/"ecstasy")
   ACE inhibitors
   Antineoplastic agents (vincristine, vinblastine, cyclophosphamide)
   ADH analogues (desmopressin, lysine vasopressin)
   Sulfonylurea (chlorpropamide)
   Hypolipidemic (clofibrate)
Endocrine diseases
   Pituitary tumor
   Hypothyroidism
   Adrenal insufficiency
Other
   Positive pressure ventilation
   Acquired immune deficiency syndrome
   Idiopathic SIADH

CNS, central nervous system; MDMA, N-methyl-3,4-methylene-dioxyamphetamine; ACE, angiotensin-converting enzyme; ADH, antidiuretic hormone; SIADH, syndrome of inappropriate ADH secretion.

body weight to induce a rapid loss of water in excess of sodium. In this circumstance, diuretic-induced potassium and magnesium losses need to be monitored and replaced. Chronic SIADH can often be managed with fluid restriction. If this is not successful, demeclocycline, 600–1200 mg/day, can be given to induce renal resistance to ADH action with consequent enhanced water loss.

Prognosis

Long-term outcome is depends on the underlying cause of the SIADH. CNS disease is often chronic with resultant chronic SIADH. Drug-induced SIADH will usually resolve rapidly with discontinuation of the drug. SIADH resulting from malignancy will depend on the ability to treat the malignancy. Severe hyponatremia is often a marker for the severity of underlying illness and is associated with a high level of morbidity and mortality, especially when accompanied by cachexia.

Gross P et al: The treatment of severe hyponatremia. Kidney Int 1998;64(suppl):S6. [PMID: 9475480]

Miller M: Syndromes of excess antidiuretic hormone release. Critical Care Clin 2001;17:11. [PMID: 11219224]

PRIMARY HYPERPARATHYROIDISM

 ESSENTIALS OF DIAGNOSIS

- *Fatigue.*
- *Depression.*
- *Vertebral fracture.*
- *Polydipsia and polyuria.*
- *Renal calculi.*
- *Hypercalcemia.*
- *Hypophosphatemia.*
- *Elevated serum parathyroid hormone (PTH).*
- *Osteopenia on radiological examination.*

General Considerations

Hyperparathyroidism is a common disorder that affects predominantly postmenopausal women, with an incidence of approximately 2 per 1000. At least 50% of patients have no or minimal nonspecific symptoms or signs (eg, hypertension). The most frequent underlying disease is a single benign parathyroid adenoma. Occasionally, 2 or more glands may be involved. Less commonly, primary hyperparathyroidism is due to 4-gland hyperplasia. A small number of patients have hyperparathyroidism as a component of MEN type 1 (MEN-1) or MEN-2 syndromes when it is familial and may be accompanied by pancreatic and pituitary tumors (MEN-1) or medullary carcinoma of the thyroid and pheochromocytoma (MEN-2).

Clinical Findings

A. SYMPTOMS & SIGNS

The most common clinical circumstance is the unanticipated finding of hypercalcemia during a routine screening, biochemical assessment, or initial evaluation of suspected osteoporosis. Mild nonspecific complaints include fatigue, lack of energy, and generalized weakness. CNS symptoms of depression or mild cognitive impairment may be present. Questioning may disclose increased thirst and polyuria, which is due to the antagonistic effect of hypercalcemia on the renal action of ADH. A history of renal calculi is rare. However, a history of fracture, loss of height, and disproportionately low-for-age bone mineral density on dual energy x-ray absorptiometry scan calls for measurement of serum calcium.

B. LABORATORY FINDINGS

When serum calcium is minimally or only intermittently increased, measurement of ionized serum calcium can establish the presence of hypercalcemia. Other common laboratory findings that support the diagnosis are elevated serum chloride and alkaline phosphatase levels. Serum BUN and creatinine should be measured because secondary hyperparathyroidism is often found in the presence of renal insufficiency. The diagnosis is confirmed by measuring serum PTH using an assay for the intact form of the hormone. Levels are almost always elevated above the upper limit of normal but may occasionally be in the upper normal range, when comparison with simultaneously measured serum calcium will demonstrate failure of PTH to be appropriately suppressed by the hypercalcemia.

Differential Diagnosis

The findings of hypercalcemia along with low–normal or low serum phosphorus suggest the diagnosis of primary hyperparathyroidism. Other causes of hypercalcemia will usually be associated with lowered levels of PTH and include a number of malignancies with or without bone metastases (squamous cell carcinoma of the lung, breast cancer, renal cell carcinoma, multiple myeloma, lymphoma). Hypercalcemia in many of these malignancies may be mediated by tumor-secreted PTH-related protein. Other causes of hypercalcemia include thiazide diuretics, vitamin D toxicity, sarcoidosis, hyperthyroidism, and hypocalciuric hypercalemia.

Parathyroid adenoma can be localized with a high degree of sensitivity and specificity by means of isotopic scanning with technetium 99m sestamibi. Other imaging procedures, including CT, MRI, and ultrasonography, are less helpful. Selective sampling of veins draining the parathyroid glands for step-up in PTH levels can be done in patients who have had previous parathyroid surgery with failure to identify abnormal parathyroid tissue.

Treatment

Parathyroid surgery is often recommended despite uncertainties regarding the benefit of parathyroidectomy in patients with no or only mild symptoms and mild elevation of serum calcium. Elderly patients are at risk for sudden elevation of serum calcium if they become dehydrated. Alleviation of CNS symptoms may become evident after parathyroidectomy, even in those patients thought to be asymptomatic. The increased risk of fracture in the elderly woman with significant osteoporosis can be reduced by correction of the hyperparathyroidism. Surgery should be performed only by a surgeon experienced in parathryoidectomy to reduce the risk of damage to the recurrent laryngeal nerves and of permanent postoperative hypoparathyroidism. In the case of parathyroid adenoma, identification and removal of the adenoma will be curative. If parathyroid hyperplasia is found, 3½ of 4 identified glands must be removed. The availability of intraoperative rapid PTH assays can confirm in the operating room that the surgeon has successfully removed the abnormal tissue.

Medical management can be used in patients who are not candidates for surgery. Acute hypercalcemia can be treated with intravenous infusion of the bisphosphonate pamidronate in doses of 60–90 mg or with intravenous mithramycin in a dose of 25 µg/kg body weight. Chronic hypercalcemia can be controlled by oral or intravenous bisphosphonates, but elevated PTH levels are not lowered and may even rise further with the potential for adverse effect on bone. Calcium receptor agonists capable of suppressing PTH secretion are under investigation.

Marx SJ: Hyperparathyroid and hypoparathyroid disorders. N Engl J Med 2000;343:1863. [11117980]

Silverberg SJ et al: A 10 year prospective study of primary hyperparathyroidism with or without parathyroid surgery. N Engl J Med 1999;341:1249. [PMID: 1052803]

Diabetes in the Elderly

33

Rossana D. Danese, MD, & David C. Aron, MD, MS

ESSENTIALS OF DIAGNOSIS

- Fasting (no caloric intake for ≥ 8 h) plasma glucose ≥ 126 mg/dL (7.0 mmol/L) or symptoms of diabetes plus casual plasma glucose concentration ≥ 200 mg/dL (11.1 mmol/L) or
- 2-h plasma glucose ≥ 200 mg/dL (11.1 mmol/L) during a 75-g oral glucose tolerance test confirmed on a subsequent day.

General Considerations

Aging is associated with declining beta cell function and relative insulinopenia independent of insulin resistance as well as insulin resistance itself. Furthermore, the risk of developing diabetes mellitus (DM) type 2 increases with obesity, lack of physical activity, and loss of muscle mass, all of which can occur with aging. The prevalence of DM (diagnosed and undiagnosed) in the elderly U.S. population has been estimated at 7 million, or 20% of all people 65 years of age and older. Native Americans, Hispanics, and blacks are at particularly high risk. The prevalence seems to decline slightly in those older than 75 compared with those 65–74 years old and decreases further in those older than 85. The dysmetabolic syndrome (syndrome X) consisting of the association among insulin resistance (DM type 2), hyperlipidemia, hypertension, and obesity increases in those 65–74 years old.

Boyle JP et al: Projection of diabetes burden through 2050: impact of changing demography and disease prevalence in the U.S. Diabetes Care 2001;24:1936. [PMID: 11679460]

Franse LV et al: Type 2 diabetes in older well-functioning people: who is undiagnosed? Data from the Health, Aging, and Body Composition study. Diabetes Care 2001;24:2065. [PMID: 11723084]

Rockwood K et al: Incidence and outcomes of diabetes mellitus in elderly people: report from the Canadian Study of Health and Aging. Can Med Assoc J 2000;162:769. [PMID: 10750461]

Shorr RI et al: Glycemic control of older adults with type 2 diabetes: findings from the Third National Health and Nutrition Examination Survey 1988–1994. J Am Geriatr Soc 2000;48:264. [PMID: 10733051]

National Center for Chronic Disease Prevention and Health Promotion: National diabetes fact sheet: www.cdc.gov/diabetes/pubs/estimates.htm

Pathogenesis

DM type 1 is an autoimmune disease that expresses a bimodal distribution (ie, an increased incidence in the very young and the old). Pancreatic beta cells are destroyed, resulting in absolute insulinopenia and subsequent hyperglycemia. Ketoacidosis may occur. Other autoimmune diseases such as vitamin B_{12} deficiency, vitiligo, thyroid disease, or rheumatoid arthritis may be present. Exogenous insulin is required for survival and glucose control.

DM type 2 is less well understood, but it results from relative insulinopenia secondary to insulin resistance (in peripheral tissues). Early in insulin resistance, insulin production is increased to levels greater than normal to maintain euglycemia, a condition known as dysmetabolic syndrome. Associated features include acanthosis nigricans, central obesity, hypertension, dyslipidemia, and an increase in coronary heart disease risk. Over time, relative insulinopenia with hyperglycemia results. Exercise, carbohydrate control, and oral glucose-lowering agents with or without insulin are required for glucose control.

Secondary causes of DM type 2 include pancreatic disease (including pancreatic carcinoma), endocrinopathies (most commonly thyrotoxicosis), infection, and drugs (glucocorticoids, niacin, phenytoin, thiazides, protease inhibitors, and the newer atypical antipsychotic drugs and newer immunosuppressive agents).

Blackburn D et al: Quantification of the risk of corticosteroid-induced diabetes mellitus among the elderly. J Gen Intern Med 2002;17:717. [PMID: 12220369]

Prevention

An increasing incidence of diabetes and the introduction of safe medications with less adverse hypoglycemia have spurred studies in the prevention of DM type 2. In the Diabetes Prevention Program, a nationwide study sponsored by the National Institutes of Health,

338

lifestyle modification (7% weight loss and minimum 150 min physical activity per week) achieved a reduction in incidence of diabetes of 58% compared with placebo, whereas metformin, 850 mg twice daily, reduced this incidence of diabetes by 31%. Among patients ≥ 60 years, the advantage of lifestyle modification over metformin was even greater. This landmark study will likely affect future recommendations for screening and prevention of DM type 2.

Clinical Findings

A. SYMPTOMS & SIGNS

The classic symptoms of diabetes mellitus—polyuria (worsening incontinence), polydipsia, and polyphagia—exist mainly with plasma glucose > 200 mg/dL. Weight loss, blurred vision, and dehydration may also be present. Patients with lesser degrees of hyperglycemia may be asymptomatic or may present with weight loss or signs and symptoms of chronic infection, especially of the genitourinary tract, skin, or mouth. Diabetes is associated with reduced cognitive function in elderly patients, and the decline correlates with glucose control. Findings of other autoimmune disease may be present in patients with DM type 1; findings of the dysmetabolic syndrome may be present in those with DM type 2. On occasion, patients may present not with symptoms of hyperglycemia but with macrovascular complications (atherosclerotic disease) or signs and symptoms of microvascular complications, especially retinopathy or neuropathy. Restless leg syndrome, perhaps mimicking (or caused by) diabetic neuropathy, has an increased prevalence in diabetics.

In DM type 2 patients treated with insulin, sulfonylureas, or meglitinides, it is important to assess for symptoms of hypoglycemia as well as hyperglycemia and micro- and macrovascular complications. Both adrenergic (sweating, palpitations, tremors) and neuroglycopenic (confusion, nightmares, violence) symptoms should be sought because they are less often spontaneously reported by elderly diabetics. Severe hypoglycemia may present as transient hemiparesis or coma. Severe hypoglycemia may also precipitate angina. When appropriate (eg, when there is a significant risk for hypoglycemia), patients should be encouraged to check their fingerstick glucose before driving.

Sinclair AJ et al: Cognitive dysfunction in older subjects with diabetes mellitus: impact on diabetes self-management and use of care services. Diab Res Clin Prac 2000;50:203. [PMID: 11106835

B. LABORATORY FINDINGS

The diagnosis of DM can be established in a symptomatic patient by a random glucose > 200 mg/dL or a fasting glucose ≥ 126 mg/dL. If required, a 75-g glucose tolerance test may be performed. In addition to hyperglycemia, hyponatremia (pseudohyponatremia), findings of dehydration, and hypomagnesemia and hypokalemia (resulting from osmotic diuresis) may also be present. The hemoglobin (Hgb) A_{1C} should be obtained as a baseline value even though it is not used as a diagnostic test. Total cholesterol, particularly in poorly controlled DM type 2, is commonly elevated. The lipid profile commonly displays elevated triglycerides and low levels of high-density lipoproteins (HDLs). The low-density lipoprotein (LDL) cholesterol is not always elevated but consists of a higher proportion of small dense LDL, which is more atherogenic.

C. SCREENING TESTS

The American Diabetes Association (ADA) recommends screening with fasting plasma glucose every 3 years beginning at age 45. Hemoglobin A_{1C} is not recommended for screening because of lack of standardization among laboratories, but alternative approaches have been suggested. Those with risk factors for diabetes, including obesity, inactivity, hypertension, and dyslipidemia, all of which are increasingly common in the elderly, should be screened more frequently. Screening for DM is indicated in the elderly to relieve symptoms, improve quality of life, and prevent or delay subsequent complications.

Knowler WC et al: Diabetes Prevention Program Research Group. Reduction in the incidence of type 2 diabetes with lifestyle intervention or metformin. N Engl J Med 2002;346:393. [PMID: 11832527]

D. DIAGNOSTIC CRITERIA

The ADA criteria were developed to emphasize fasting glucose values in the diagnosis of DM and to ease establishing a diagnosis. Diagnostic criteria established by the World Health Organization in 1985 set a fasting plasma glucose ≥ 140 mg/dL but emphasized a 2-h plasma glucose ≥ 200 mg/dL. Because glucose intolerance is a characteristic of aging, the ADA criteria (with emphasis on fasting glucose) have been questioned for underestimating the incidence of DM in the elderly. Currently, a state of prediabetes or impaired glucose homeostasis is recognized and furthermore associated with cardiovascular disease. The ADA defines impaired fasting glucose as a fasting plasma glucose ≥ 110 mg/dL but < 126 mg/dL; impaired glucose tolerance is defined as 2-h glucose ≥ 140 mg/dL and ≤ 200 mg/dL.

American Diabetes Association: Clinical practice recommendations 2002. Diabetes Care 2002;25(suppl 1).

Barr RG et al: Tests of glycemia for the diagnosis of type 2 diabetes mellitus. Ann Intern Med 2002;137:263. [PMID: 12186517]

Expert Committee on the Diagnosis and Classification of Diabetes Mellitus: Report of the Expert Committee on the Diagnosis and Classification of Diabetes Mellitus. Diabetes Care 2002;25:S5. [PMID: 12017675]

Sinclair AJ et al: Prevalence of diabetes in care home residents. Diabetes Care 2001;24:1066. [PMID: 11375372]

Wahl PW et al: Diabetes in older adults: comparison of 1997 American Diabetes Association classification of diabetes mellitus with 1985 WHO classification. Lancet 1998;352:1012. [PMID: 9759743]

American Diabetes Association: Clinical practice recommendations 2002:
http://care.diabetesjournals.org/content/vol25/suppl_1/

Complications

A. Acute Complications

Acute complications are metabolic and infectious. Chronic complications include the microvascular (retinopathy, neuropathy, nephropathy) and macrovascular (cardiovascular disease) complications.

Ketoacidosis occurs in DM type 1 and results from a lack of insulin action in the presence of glucagon. Predisposing factors include infection, stroke, and myocardial infarction as well as missed insulin doses. Typically, patients present with symptoms of the precipitating factor, acidosis/hyperosmolality, and abdominal pain. Coma and mental status alteration may be present. Insulin is the mainstay of treatment in addition to fluid replacement. Identification and management of the precipitating factor are critical (eg, treatment of acute infection). Mortality rates are highest for the oldest patients, especially those with coexisting renal disease and infection. Ketoacidosis is rare in DM type 2.

Nonketotic hyperosmolar coma occurs predominantly in elderly patients with DM type 2 and results from osmotic diuresis caused by hyperglycemia and consequent dehydration. Predisposing factors include dementia, infection, stroke, and myocardial infarction. A decrease in the glomerular filtration rate promotes further hyperglycemia and dehydration through a vicious cycle. Glucose levels commonly reach $\geq$ 600 mg/dL, and serum osmolality often exceeds 320 mOsm/L. A fluid deficit of 5–10 L is typical. Fluids are thus the mainstay of treatment, usually given as normal saline if hemodynamic instability is present or 50% normal saline otherwise (because free water is typically lost in an osmotic diuresis). Insulin is also required as well as treatment of the precipitating factors. The coma/mental status alterations may take several days to clear, lagging behind correction of the serum osmolality. Mortality rates are relatively high; severe hyperosmolarity, advanced age, and nursing home residence are the major prognostic factors associated with death.

Elderly patients with diabetes are at particularly increased risk of severe and unusual infections, particu-larly malignant external otitis. Necrotizing infection resulting from *Pseudomonas aeruginosa* initially involves the external ear canal and progresses to the mastoid air cells, skull base, or temporal bone. The clinical presentation consists of fever, otalgia, otorrhea, and, less commonly, cranial nerve palsy. Treatment involves surgical débridement and antibiotics. Other infections associated with diabetes include rhinocerebral mucormycosis, necrotizing fasciitis, emphysematous cholecystitis, and emphysematous pyelonephritis. Elderly patients with diabetes are also at increased risk for renal papillary necrosis, presenting as insidious renal failure.

Kitabchi AE et al: Management of hyperglycemic crises in patients with diabetes. Diabetes Care 2001;24:131.

Malone ML et al: Characteristics of diabetic ketoacidosis in older versus younger adults. J Am Geriatr Soc 1992;40:1100. [PMID: 1401693]

B. Chronic Complications

1. Retinopathy—The major predictor of risk for retinopathy is the duration of diabetes mellitus. In addition to being the most threatening of the chronic microvascular complications associated with DM, diabetic retinopathy is a leading cause of blindness in the United States. Ischemia is believed to be the major culprit of diabetic retinopathy, and glucose control has been shown to be of major benefit.

The classification of retinopathy includes nonproliferative disease (NPDR), preproliferative disease, and proliferative retinopathy. NPDR includes microaneurysms (small outpouchings of the capillary vessel wall, which appear as small red dots on exam), hard exudates (shiny yellow deposits caused by damage of the blood retinal barrier and leakage of lipids, carbohydrates, and proteins), intraretinal hemorrhages, and macular edema. Preproliferative retinopathy, signifying an increased likelihood of proliferative retinopathy, includes cotton wool spots (white feathery spots resulting from capillary closure) and irregular and narrowed retinal arterioles and veins. Proliferative retinopathy is neovascularization at the disk or elsewhere, which can leak or bleed into the vitreous leading to visual loss. Fibrous tissue may also occur with neovascularization, possibly leading to retinal detachment.

Proliferative retinopathy is treated with panretinal photocoagulation, which is believed to decrease oxygen demand and induce regression of retinal neovascularization. Laser is also used to treat macular edema. Vitrectomy is undertaken if neovascularization leads to vitreous hemorrhage without adequate resorption or if retinal detachment occurs. In addition to good glycemic control, management of hypertension and dyslipidemia may reduce progression of retinopathy because each has been shown to be a risk factor for retinopathy. Hypertension is an independent risk factor for any retinopathy, and its tight control reduces progression of retinopathy. Aspirin has been shown to be of no risk or benefit.

Diabetics are also at increased risk of cataracts and glaucoma. Cataracts and glaucoma are 2 and 3 times more likely, respectively, in diabetic patients older than 65 than in their nondiabetic counterparts. On the basis of this increased risk of visual loss as a result of retinopathy, cataracts, and glaucoma and the subsequent effect of this loss on quality of life and risk of accidents, it has been recommended that elderly patients undergo a dilated eye exam by an ophthalmologist at diagnosis and yearly thereafter.

Vijan S et al: Cost-utility analysis of screening intervals for diabetic retinopathy in patients with type 2 diabetes mellitus. JAMA 2000;283:889.

2. Neuropathy—Neuropathy is a distressing complication of DM and can lead to loss of sleep, limitation of activity, and depression. Diabetic neuropathies include focal neuropathies, polyneuropathy, and autonomic neuropathy. Focal neuropathies include entrapment syndromes and mononeuropathies. The most common entrapment syndrome is carpal tunnel syndrome, which may produce symptoms limited to the hand or the entire arm. The ulnar nerve and nerves of the feet may also be involved with entrapment syndromes, which generally are of slow onset and persist until treated. Focal neuropathies caused by mononeuritis, in contrast, are acute in onset, resolve spontaneously, and may be multiplex. These neuropathies are caused by vasculitis and subsequent ischemia. The most commonly involved nerves are cranial nerves III, IV, VI, and VII, but thoracic and peripheral nerves may be involved as well. Physical therapy may be necessary, but the neuropathy resolves spontaneously.

Proximal motor neuropathy (diabetic amyotrophy) primarily affects elderly patients. It begins with thigh pain, initially unilateral and then bilateral, which progresses to proximal muscle weakness and wasting. It may coexist with distal symmetric polyneuropathy. Treatment includes glycemic control (usually insulin) and physical therapy. Some forms of amyotrophy respond to immunotherapy. Distal symmetric polyneuropathy, more commonly recognized as "glove and stocking" sensory symptoms, is the most common neuropathy of elderly diabetics. Pain, which can interrupt sleep and limit activity, can be treated with multiple agents, including anticonvulsants (gabapentin, phenytoin, and carbamazepine) and antidepressants (tricyclics). However, the anticholinergic effects of the tricyclics limit their usefulness in the older patient. Dysesthesia of a burning quality is sometimes treated with topical capsaicin or oral mexiletine, although their role in treatment of older patients is not well established.

Patients with distal sensory polyneuropathy are predisposed to Charcot joints, which may mimic gout or degenerative joint disease. A plain film of the foot will usually differentiate the Charcot joint. Distal sensory polyneuropathy also predisposes to neuropathic foot ulcer, which remains the leading cause of foot amputation in the United States. The feet should be inspected at each office visit and daily self-examination encouraged. A monofilament identifies patients with sensory neuropathy. Therapeutic shoes, prescribed by a podiatrist and individually designed to prevent blisters, calluses, and ulcers, are covered by Medicare for peripheral neuropathy if any of the following conditions coexist: callus formation, poor circulation, foot deformity, or history of foot callus, ulcer, or amputation (partial or complete). One pair of shoes plus 3 pairs of inserts are covered annually.

Autonomic neuropathy can be the most life-threatening form of diabetic neuropathy. Tachycardia carries an increased risk of sudden death, whereas postural hypotension imparts an increased risk of syncope and falling with injury. Other forms of autonomic neuropathy include neurogenic bladder, sexual dysfunction, gastropathy (which is particularly sensitive to glycemic control), enteropathy, and gustatory sweating. Patients with autonomic neuropathy are more likely to have hypoglycemic unawareness.

Vinik AI: Diagnosis and management of diabetic neuropathy. Advances in the care of older people with diabetes. Clin Geriatr Med 1999;15:293. [PMID: 10339635]

Wheeler SG et al: Prospective study of autonomic neuropathy as a predictor of mortality in patients with diabetes. Diab Res Clin Pract 2002;58:131. [PMID: 12213355]

3. Nephropathy—Elderly diabetics are at particular risk for development or progression of nephropathy. Independent risk factors for the development of proteinuria and renal insufficiency include degree and duration of glycemic control, hypertension, longer duration of diabetes, male sex, and higher total cholesterol levels. Smoking increases the risk of progression of nephropathy. Nephropathy progresses from microalbuminuria to overt proteinuria to renal insufficiency and end-stage renal disease (ESRD), although the course may be shorter than the typical 10–20 years observed in a younger population. Elderly patients are at risk for acute renal failure from renal insults such as administration of intravenous contrast agents in the course of radiological procedures, nephrotoxic drugs, and comorbid illness (eg, congestive heart failure).

The diagnosis of diabetic nephropathy is usually made clinically and not by renal biopsy. Diabetic nephropathy is defined as a urinary albumin excretion

> 300 mg/day and an appropriate time course in the absence of other obvious secondary causes of renal disease in diabetes, with specificities of nearly 100% in DM type 1 and > 85% in DM type 2. Screening for microalbuminuria, the precursor of frank proteinuria and renal insufficiency, may be accomplished by measuring the urinary albumin–creatinine ratio on a spot urine specimen.

In DM types 1 and 2, good glycemic control reduces the risk of microalbuminuria, progression of albuminuria, and development of renal insufficiency. Lowering of blood pressure reduces the decline in glomerular filtration rate and albuminuria. Angiotensin-converting enzyme (ACE) inhibitors reduce the rate of progression of proteinuria and the rate of ESRD, although the data are stronger in patients with DM type 1. Similarly, angiotensin receptor blockers (ARBs) reduce proteinuria and loss of GFR in type 2 diabetes. Blood pressure should be controlled to reduce stroke and cardiovascular complications regardless of the presence or absence of microalbuminuria. Adverse events with ACE inhibitors and ARBs include renal insufficiency in patients with renal artery stenosis and hyperkalemia in the presence of type IV renal tubular acidosis (hyporeninemic hypoaldosteronism).

ESRD in elderly diabetics is increasing in number. The nephropathy in older diabetics is different from that seen in young diabetics. The pathological findings may suggest ischemia and hypertension, whereas the classic Kimmelstiel-Wilson lesions may be absent. As a clinical correlation, many patients present with ESRD typically after an episode of acute renal failure that does not resolve.

4. Cardiovascular disease—Diabetes imparts at least a 2-fold risk in coronary heart disease. The conventional risk factors of hypertension, hyperlipidemia, smoking, and diabetes persist through old age. The role of glycemic control is well established for microvascular complications but less well established for macrovascular complications. Still, the data from the UKPDS and elsewhere suggest a benefit, and glycemic control should be optimized in the elderly. Aspirin therapy has been shown to be beneficial in secondary prevention of coronary events. It has been broadly recommended that all adults with diabetes take at least low-dose aspirin daily (81 mg) unless there is a specific contraindication (ADA guidelines).

Bonora E, Muggeo M: Postprandial blood glucose as a risk factor for cardiovascular disease in type 2 diabetes: the epidemiological evidence. Diabetologia 2001;44:2107. [PMID: 11793012]

DECODE Study Group on behalf of the European Diabetes Epidemiology Group: Glucose tolerance and cardiovascular mortality: comparison of fasting and 2-hour diagnostic criteria. Arch Intern Med 2001;161:397. [PMID: 11176766]

Treatment

The pathophysiological and psychosocial principles underlying management are similar for both young and elderly patients. Consideration is given to the patient's preferences, commitment, health beliefs, coexisting illnesses, and economic issues. Some factors, including life expectancy, functional status, and availability of support services, strongly impact the treatment goals for the elderly diabetic. Age-associated changes in cognitive function, visual function, physical functioning, dentition, and taste perception can affect the ability to implement various management approaches. The elderly diabetic may be at greater risk for hypoglycemia but can be taught to monitor for and treat hypoglycemia appropriately (Table 33–1). In addition, the frequent hospitalizations among the elderly can disrupt outpatient regimens.

A. GLYCEMIC CONTROL

Aggressive glucose control in patients with DM type 1 is extremely important to reduce the risk of microvascular and macrovascular complications.

The ADA currently recommends goal HgbA$_{1C}$ levels < 7.0% with action suggested at levels > 8.0%. Premeal and bedtime home glucose monitoring should be maintained at 90–130 mg/dL and 110–150 mg/dL, respectively. The American College of Clinical Endocrinologists recommends preprandial glucose levels < 110 mg/dL, postprandial and bedtime glucose < 140 mg/dL, and HgbA$_{1C}$ < 6.5%. The benefits of this degree of control must be balanced against the risks, namely hypoglycemia and weight gain.

Age itself is an important factor in hypoglycemia. The Department of Veterans Affairs/Department of Defense guidelines recommend different HgbA$_{1C}$ targets based on the individual's risk of microvascular complications. Less stringent treatment goals may be

Table 33–1. Risk factors for hypoglycemia in the elderly diabetic.

Therapy with sulfonylureas or insulin
Renal insufficiency
Hepatic dysfunction
Cognitive impairment
Autonomic neuropathy and adrenergic blocking agents
Poor nutrition
Alcohol
Sedative agents
Complex regimens
Polypharmacy
Tight glycemic control
Recent hospitalization

appropriate in those with limited life expectancies and hypoglycemic unawareness and in individuals with co-morbid conditions such as seizure, dementia, psychiatric illness, alcoholism, and coronary artery disease.

Glycemic control in the hospital has traditionally been designed primarily to maintain safe levels of glucose (ie, 90–200 mg/dL to prevent hyperglycemia-induced dehydration and catabolism while avoiding hypoglycemia). Some studies have shown a benefit of good glycemic control in terms of in-hospital mortality.

The complex nature of geriatric patients and diabetes management requires a team approach. The physician, in conjunction with a certified diabetes educator, dietitian, social worker, and pharmacist, can best address the lifestyle modifications that diabetes management requires in the face of multiple comorbidities, difficult social situations, and polypharmacy. Moreover, careful attention to comorbid illness is essential. For example, many elderly patients with diabetes are depressed. Fluoxetine has been demonstrated to improve glycemic control in obese elderly patients who are depressed presumably because it results in weight loss. Because mortality in diabetes is primarily related to cardiovascular disease, the overall regimen should aim at reducing cardiovascular risk (eg, controlling blood pressure, lipid levels, and glucose levels) rather than focusing solely on management of glucose. In fact, blood pressure and lipid level control has been thought to confer greater benefit in terms of mortality than glucose control.

Diabetes Control and Complications Trial Research Group: The effect of intensive treatment of diabetes on the development and progression of long-term complications in insulin-dependent diabetes mellitus. N Engl J Med 1993;329:977. [PMID: 8366922]

Earnshaw SR et al: Optimal allocation of resources across four interventions for type 2 diabetes. Med Decision Mak 2002; 22;S80.

Eastman RC et al: Model of complications of NIDDM: I. Model construction and assumptions. Diabetes Care 1997;20:725. [PMID: 9135934]

Eastman RC et al: Model of complications of NIDDM: II. Analysis of the health benefits and cost-effectiveness of treating NIDDM with the goal of normoglycemia. Diabetes Care 1997;20:735. [PMID: 9135935]

Metchick LN et al: Inpatient management of diabetes mellitus. Am J Med 2002;113:317.

Van den Bergh G et al: Intensive insulin therapy in critically ill patients. N Engl J Med 2001;345:1359. [PMID: 11794168]

Vijan S et al: Estimated benefits of glycemic control in microvascular complications in type 2 diabetes. Ann Intern Med 1997;127:788. [PMID: 11028137]

1. Nonpharmacological therapy—Consistent carbohydrate intake can help maintain euglycemia in some patients with DM type 2 and can be essential to maximize glycemic control in DM type 1. In elderly diabetics, malnutrition can be more of a concern than obesity, and dietary restrictions may be harmful. This is especially true for patients in long-term health care facilities who may be malnourished. These patients should be given unrestricted menus with consistent amounts of carbohydrate at meals and snacks and medications adjusted to control glucose if necessary. For community-dwelling patients, individualization of dietary therapy by a dietitian is recommended and, as of 2002, is covered by Medicare if at least 1 of the following criteria are met: newly diagnosed, HgbA$_{1C}$ > 8.5%, recent initiation of medication, or high risk for complications. Eligible beneficiaries receive up to 10 h of diabetes education with a certified diabetes educator or registered dietitian within a 12-mo period.

Exercise is of benefit in DM because it improves insulin resistance, increases muscle mass, reduces adiposity, improves weight, and improves lipids and blood pressure. Both aerobic and nonaerobic activity has been shown to be beneficial. The best time to exercise is 1–2 h after a meal when glucose levels tend to be highest. Both hypo- and hyperglycemia may be seen up to 24 h after exercise and medication adjustments must be advised. In short-term studies (up to 6 mo) the effect on glycemic control has been variable.

2. Pharmacological therapy (Table 33–2)—

a. Sulfonylureas—The sulfonylureas in common use include glipizide (Glucotrol), glyburide (Diabeta, Micronase, Glynase), and glimepiride (Amaryl). Sulfonylureas reduce glycated hemoglobin by 1–2% (which corresponds to a reduction in mean blood glucose values of 30–60 mg/dL). Generally, most of the therapeutic effect occurs with half of the maximum recommended dose. Because sulfonylureas act predominantly by increasing pancreatic insulin secretion, weight gain is common and hypoglycemia may occur. In addition to advanced age, risk factors for drug-induced hypoglycemia include renal dysfunction, missed or smaller meals, alcohol, infection, recent hospitalization, and use of other drugs that potentiate hypoglycemia, including salicylates, sulfonamides, and warfarin. Glyburide has shown a 2-fold relative risk of hypoglycemia compared with glipizide. Patients on β-blockers should be cautioned regarding the possible lack of warning (adrenergic) symptoms such as tachycardia. Sulfonylureas should be avoided or used cautiously in the elderly diabetic, especially those with renal insufficiency (because of increased risk of hypoglycemia with accumulation of active metabolites), liver disease, or sulfa allergy. If implemented, starting doses should be low, perhaps half that for younger patients, and education regarding hypoglycemia provided.

Table 33–2. Oral glucose-lowering agents.

Agent	Expected decrease HgbA1c (%)	Plasma half-life (h)	Contraindications	Side effects	Cost
Sulfonylureas	1–2		Renal insufficiency	Hypoglycemia	
Glipizide		2–4	Sulfa allergy	Weight gain	$
Glyburide		10	Hepatic insufficiency		$
Glimepiride		~9			$$
Meglitinides	1–2		Hepatic insufficiency	Hypoglycemia	
Repaglinide		1			$$$$
Nateglinide		1.5			$$$$
α-Glucosidase Inhibitors	0.5–1		Small bowel disease	Flatulence	
			Severe renal insufficiency	Diarrhea/GI upset	
Acarbose					$$$
Miglitol		6			
Biguanides	1–2		Lactic acidosis predisposition	Lactic acidosis (rare)	
Metformin			Renal insufficiency	GI symptoms	$$
			Hepatic insufficiency/alcohol		
Thiazolidinediones	1–2		Congestive heart failure	Fluid retention/edema	
Rosiglitazone		3–4	Liver disease	Hepatotoxicity	$$$$
Pioglitazone		6–24			$$$$

$, lowest; $$$$, highest, GI, gastrointestinal.

Ben-Ami H et al: Drug-induced hypoglycemic coma in 102 diabetic patients. Arch Intern Med 1999;159;281. [PMID: 9989540]

Jollis JG et al: Relation between sulfonylurea therapy, complications, and outcome for elderly patients with acute myocardial infarction. Am Heart J 1999;138:S376. [PMID: 10539800]

Shorr RI et al: Incidence and risk factors for serious hypoglycemia in older persons using insulin or sulfonylureas. Arch Intern Med 1997;157:1681. [PMID: 9250229]

b. Biguanides—Metformin (Glucophage) is the only available biguanide in the United States. Metformin likely acts by decreasing hepatic glucose production and improving peripheral (muscle) insulin sensitivity. Because insulin production is not augmented but actually lessened, hypoglycemia does not occur with monotherapy. Weight loss is often an added benefit of biguanide use in obese diabetics.

Metformin lowers glycated hemoglobin by 1–2%. It should not be used in conditions with an increased tendency to lactic acidosis, such as renal or hepatic insufficiency, alcohol abuse, or poor peripheral perfusion and hypoxic states. In properly selected elderly patients, the risk for lactic acidosis is low with metformin use. However, it should be used with caution because the elderly are at increased risk for other conditions that predispose to lactic acidosis (eg, pneumonia, heart failure) or renal insufficiency (dehydration, stroke, myocardial infarction). In addition, patients with low muscle mass but normal creatinine may have reduced renal clearance. More commonly, the limiting side effect has been gastrointestinal distress (nausea, diarrhea). This can be minimized by taking the tablet at the end of a meal, gradually increasing the dosage, and using the extended-release formulation. Vitamin B_{12} deficiency has also been reported.

Gregorio F et al: Poorly controlled elderly type 2 diabetic patients: the effects of increasing sulfonylureas dosages or adding metformin. Diab Med 1999;16:1016. [PMID: 10656230]

c. Meglitinides—The main effect of meglitinides is on postprandial hyperglycemia, which may be of particular benefit in the elderly, although definitive studies are lacking. Repaglinide (Prandin) and nateglinide (Starlix) increase pancreatic response to meal-related glucose loads; premeal dosing and a short duration of action promote glucose-dependent insulin release (by a mechanism different than sulfonylureas) that diminishes with low blood glucose concentrations. In clinical trials, however, the incidence of hypoglycemia in patients treated with repaglinide was comparable to that among patients treated with sulfonylureas. Likewise, glycated hemoglobin can be expected to improve 1–2%. The meglitinides do not contain a sulfur moiety and may be useful in patients who are allergic to sulfonylureas. They can also be used in renal insufficiency with dosage adjustment but should be used with caution in hepatic insufficiency because of extensive metabolism by the liver.

d. α-glucosidase inhibitors—The main effect of the α-glucosidase inhibitors acarbose (Precose) and miglitol (Glyset) is on postprandial hyperglycemia.

Taken with the first bite of a meal, these agents interfere with brush-border enzymes in the gut that digest disaccharides/polysaccharides to monosaccharides, thus reducing the rise in postprandial glucose. They do not augment insulin secretion and, when used as monotherapy, do not cause hypoglycemia or weight gain. Each reduces glycated hemoglobin by 0.5–1.5% and decreases postprandial glucose by ~50 mg/dL. Because α-glucosidase inhibitors are not absorbed at usual doses (in particular acarbose), they generally can be safely used in elderly patients and with either renal or hepatic insufficiency (although rare cases of dose-dependent elevated transaminases have been reported). Flatulence and diarrhea are the predominant side effects but diminish with continued use over several months. To minimize gastrointestinal distress, initial doses are low and gradually increased over several weeks. Miglitol has been shown to be useful and safe compared with sulfonylureas.

Johnston PS et al: Advantages of alpha-glucosidase inhibition as monotherapy in elderly type 2 diabetic patients. J Clin Endocrinol Metab 1998;83:1515. [PMID: 9589648]

e. **Thiazolidinediones**—The thiazolidinediones (TZDs) rosiglitazone (Avandia) and pioglitazone (Actos) act as insulin sensitizers. They bind to and activate specific nuclear receptors (peroxisome proliferator activator receptors), which enhance the transcription of a number of genes involved in glucose metabolism. The initial effects of the glitazones may not be seen for 2–3 weeks, and maximal effects may require 3 mo of use. The overall efficacy is comparable to that of sulfonylureas and metformin, with a 1–2% improvement in glycated hemoglobin and a mean reduction in fasting plasma glucose of 30–60 mg/dL. Patients also using exogenous insulin are able to decrease insulin doses significantly. Troglitazone, a TZD removed from the market, was found to be effective in elderly diabetics. The TZDs may be of benefit in elderly diabetics; because they do not cause hypoglycemia when used as monotherapy, they are dispensed once daily and can be used with safety in renal failure. However, they should be avoided in hepatic insufficiency. The TZDs have also been recognized to cause fluid retention, resulting in lower extremity edema in up to 15% of patients and congestive heart failure in up to 3%. These agents should be avoided or used with caution at a low dose in patients with a history of congestive heart failure. Fluid retention, decreased glycosuria, and an increased differentiation and proliferation of adipocytes may be contributing factors to the weight gain not uncommonly associated with these agents.

Because the oral agents work to lower glucose levels through different mechanisms, combinations of agents are quite effective at lowering blood glucose. When combination therapy is used, the effect of each agent on glucose control is additive.

f. **Insulin**—Insulin is required in all patients with DM type 1. Insulin is also generally required in any patient with moderate or severe hyperglycemia, especially in the presence of renal or hepatic insufficiency. The trend in insulin use is to give smaller doses more frequently, allowing for better control of hyperglycemia (in particular postprandial hyperglycemia) and less hypoglycemia. In addition to human NPH and regular insulin (Table 33–3), newer insulin analogues with differing pharmacokinetics are available and offer increased flexibility of dosing and reduced risk of hypoglycemia. They have not been studied in elderly patients alone. Lispro (Humalog) and Aspart (Novolog) are genetically engineered human insulins with rapid absorption and onset of action within 15 min. The peak effect is reached by 120 min, and duration of action is ~4–5 h. These rapid-acting insulins are injected immediately before a meal and reduce the risk of late hypoglycemia seen with regular insulin. For patients with varying oral intake, these insulins are advantageous in that they can also be effectively administered after a meal and the dose can be adjusted for the carbohydrate eaten.

Glargine (Lantus) is marketed as a peakless, once-daily 24-h basal insulin, which can be used in place of twice-daily human NPH insulin or Ultralente. It is used as a basal insulin in patients uncontrolled despite

Table 33–3. Insulin products in common use.

Type	Onset of action	Peak action	Duration	Cost
Lispro	15 min	30–90 min	2–4 h	$$
Aspart	15 min	30–90 min		$$
Regular	30–60 min	2–3 h	4–6 h	$
NPH	2–4 h	6–10 h	10–16 h	$
Glargine	–	–	22–24 h	$$

$, lowest; $$, highest.

double or triple oral therapy and in insulinopenic patients using premeal rapid-acting insulin boluses. It can be an ideal insulin in patients receiving a consistent amount of carbohydrate over 24 h (eg, continuous tube feeds). Glargine cannot be mixed in a syringe with any other insulin. Currently, the only disadvantage to its use is its cost. If fasting hyperglycemia is the main consideration and daytime glucoses can be controlled with oral agents, bedtime human NPH insulin in amounts necessary to normalize the morning glucose is safe, convenient, efficacious, and less expensive than glargine. If fasting glucose is controlled but the values rise in daytime, glargine is the better choice.

For simplicity, insulin mixtures such as 70/30 (70% human NPH, 30% regular insulin or 70% human NPH, 30% Aspart), 50/50 (50% human NPH, 50% regular insulin), and 75/25 (75% human NPH, 25% Lispro) may be particularly useful. The premixed insulins have been shown to be more accurate and acceptable in elderly patients with fewer errors and increased ease of use, although metabolic control and rate of hypoglycemia are unchanged. However, some patients may not achieve adequate glucose control with these fixed-dose regimens, and basal split-dose human NPH or glargine with regular insulin or rapid-acting insulin may be needed.

Elderly patients can learn insulin administration, especially with premixed insulins and pen-delivery systems. The majority of insulins are available in pen-delivery systems as well as vials. The pen systems, available as reusable pens with refillable cartridges or as prefilled disposable pens, require the user to attach a needle, set the dose by a dial, and depress the plunger to administer the dose. They are quick and easy to use and can be more precise than insulin syringes and vials. The pen systems are more acceptable, more efficacious, and as safe as conventional syringes. If conventional syringes are used, low-dose syringes (which hold up to 30 units or 50 units compared with 100 units and have more visible unit markings) should be prescribed whenever possible. Magnifying devices that attach to a syringe are also available.

Agurs-Collins TD et al: A randomized controlled trail of weight reduction and exercise for diabetes management in older African-American subjects. Diabetes Care 1997;200:1503. [PMID: 9314625]

Ligtenberg PC et al: Effects of physical training on metabolic control in elderly type 2 diabetes mellitus patients. Clin Sci 1997;93:127. [PMID: 9301427]

UK Prospective Diabetes Study (UKPDS) Group: Effect of intensive blood-glucose control with metformin on complications in overweight patients with type 2 diabetes (UKPDS 34). Lancet 1998;352:854. [PMID: 9742977]

UK Prospective Diabetes Study (UKPDS) Group: Intensive blood-glucose control with sulphonylureas or insulin compared with conventional treatment and risk of complications in patients with type 2 diabetes (UKPDS 33). Lancet 1998;352:837. [PMID: 9742796]

B. INSULIN SELF-MANAGEMENT

Ideally, the best way to tailor an insulin regimen is by home glucose monitoring done pre- and postprandial and at bedtime. Elderly diabetics can be taught to reliably self-monitor blood glucose without adverse effects on quality of life. Currently, Medicare reimburses once-daily testing for non-insulin-treated patients and 3 times daily for insulin-treated patients. Newer glucometers and test strips, which use smaller amounts of blood and capillary action as well as alternate-site testing (forearm, upper arm, thigh, or calf), have made glucose monitoring significantly easier. The FreeStyle (Therasense), One Touch Ultra (Lifescan), and Soft Tac (Medisense) meters are approved for use with blood secured from alternate sites. The Soft Tac lances skin and automatically transfers blood to the test strip for ease of use. Talking glucometers are also available for blind patients. Devices that aid in the management of diabetes in the elderly are outlined in Table 33–4.

Harris MI: National Health and Nutrition Examination Survey (NHANES III). Frequency of blood glucose monitoring in relation to glycemic control in patients with type 2 diabetes. Diabetes Care 2001;24:979. [PMID: 11375356]

Heisler M et al: The relative importance of physician communication, participatory decision making, and patient understanding in diabetes self-management. J Gen Intern Med 2002; 17:243. [PMID: 11972720]

Hirsch IB et al: A multifaceted intervention in support of diabetes treatment guidelines: a controlled trial. Diab Res Clin Pract 2002;58:27. [PMID: 12161054]

Langa KM et al: Informal caregiving for diabetes and diabetic complications among elderly Americans. J Gerontol B Psychol Sci Soc Sci 2002;57:S177. [PMID: 11993744]

Prognosis

Diabetes imparts an ~2-fold risk of death in the elderly. Approximately 50% of patients die from cardiovascular disease. Otherwise, elderly patients have an ~1.5 relative risk of admission to an institution. This is likely

Table 33–4. Devices to aid diabetes management in the elderly.

Insulin pen-delivery systems, especially premixed insulins
Low-dose syringes
Syringe-attached magnifying devices
Comfort Curve (Accucheck) test strips
Alternate site monitors (see text)
Talking glucometers for the blind

due to microvascular complications of diabetes, which increase in incidence with the duration of diabetes. With target diabetes control and management of co-morbid conditions, many patients may prevent or delay the onset of these complications and lead a quality life. Treatment of hypertension with diuretics and calcium channel blockers reduces mortality and risk of macro-vascular complications in elderly patients with DM type 2.

Gerstein H, Haynes RB (eds): Evidence-based diabetes care. BC Dekker, 2001.

RELEVANT WORLD WIDE WEB SITES

American Association of Clinical Endocrinologists: www.aace.com

American Diabetes Association: www.diabetes.org

Diabetes Monitor: www.diabetesmonitor.com

Diabetes UK (formerly British Diabetic Association): www.diabetes.org.uk

International Diabetes Federation: www.idf.org

Veterans Health Administration Diabetes Program: www.va.gov/diabetes

Common Infections

34

Robert A. Bonomo, MD, & Mary Anne Johnson, MD

ESSENTIALS OF DIAGNOSIS

- The most common infections in the elderly are urinary tract infections, respiratory tract infections, gastroenteritis, and skin and soft tissue infections.
- Diagnosing infections in the elderly may be challenging because of atypical presentations and the frequent presence of cognitive impairment.
- Delirium, falls, or functional decline may be the presenting or only sign of an infection. Fever may be absent.
- Viral respiratory infections, especially if caused by influenza or respiratory syncytial virus, are associated with significant morbidity and mortality.
- Screening for latent tuberculosis in high-risk elderly and treating those with positive skin tests with isoniazid significantly reduces the risk of active tuberculosis.
- Chronic medical conditions increase the risk of bacterial pneumonia in the elderly; nursing home residents are at greatest risk.
- Asymptomatic bacteriuria is common in the elderly and requires no treatment.
- Gastroenteritis in the community and nursing home can be caused by viruses or bacteria; mortality from gastroenteritis and dehydration is higher in the elderly than in any other age group.
- Antibiotics are overused in nursing homes, contributing to antibiotic resistance.
- Treatment of infections in the elderly may be complicated by comorbid conditions, which alter pharmacokinetics of antibiotics, and by the possibility of drug interactions.

General Considerations

Despite the significant progress that has been made with the development of highly potent antibacterial agents and life-saving therapies, infectious diseases are among the major causes of morbidity and mortality in the elderly. Pneumonia, influenza, and bacteremia are the most frequent fatal infections. Many other infections, including HIV infection, can also cause significant morbidity and mortality.

Atypical presentations of infection are common in the elderly and may lead to delays in therapy. Functional decline, delirium, weight loss, or falls may be the only clues to a serious underlying infection. Fever is absent in 20–30% of elderly patients harboring a serious infection. For example, > 20% of patients older than 65 will not develop fever in the setting of pneumococcal bacteremia.

Pathogenesis

The elderly are at increased risk for infection predominantly because of comorbid conditions (eg, diabetes mellitus, chronic obstructive pulmonary disease, congestive heart failure, malnutrition), which decrease resistance. In addition, age-related changes in organ function and a decline in immune function, predominantly cell-mediated immunity, also contribute. Another risk factor is disruption of normal barriers with use of invasive devices and procedures. Institutionalization increases risk, especially for epidemic infections, because of group living.

Prevention

Although few data exist on specific nutritional interventions to prevent infections, ensuring adequate overall nutrition should decrease risk. Optimal management of chronic illnesses such as diabetes, prevention of pressure ulcers, and avoidance of indwelling catheters are recommended to reduce risk of infection. Immunization with influenza and pneumococcal vaccines reduces infection and severity of illness. Nosocomial infections can often be avoided when caregivers routinely practice hand washing. Appropriate use of antibiotics in the hospital and nursing home can decrease the risk of infections with resistant organisms, such as *Clostridium difficile*. Community-dwelling elderly should be educated regarding hand washing and safe food practices as well as avoidance of contact with symptomatic persons.

Treatment

Treatment of infections, once diagnosed, is challenging in the elderly. Older persons have reduced renal clearance of antibiotics, an increased risk of medication interactions and adverse drug effects, and problems with compliance because of cognitive impairment or financial and social problems.

Norman DC: Fever in the elderly. Clin Infect Dis 2000;31:148. [PMID: 10913413]

Stalam M, Kaye D: Antibacterial therapy. Antibiotic agents in the elderly. Infect Dis Clin North Am 2000;14:357. [PMID: 10829260]

Yoshikawa TT: Epidemiology and unique aspects of aging and infectious diseases. Clin Infect Dis 2000;30:931. [PMID: 10880303]

■ COMMON INFECTIONS

URINARY TRACT INFECTIONS

General Considerations

Increased risk for UTI in the elderly is associated with changes of aging, including prostatic hypertrophy and loss of estrogen effect, neurogenic bladder from stroke or diabetes, incontinence, and use of indwelling and condom catheters.

Clinical Findings

Asymptomatic bacteriuria (> 100,000 colonies/mL on 2 consecutive specimens in an asymptomatic patient) is common, affecting 1–6% of men and 10–20% of women over age 60 in the community and 15–35% of men and 25–50% of women in nursing homes. The most common organisms isolated are *Escherichia coli, Klebsiella pneumoniae, Proteus mirabilis,* and staphylococci. Asymptomatic bacteriuria in nursing home residents, especially those with indwelling catheters, is more likely to be polymicrobial compared with that in community-dwelling elderly, and organisms are more likely to be antibiotic resistant.

Distinguishing asymptomatic from symptomatic infection may be difficult. Pyuria is almost always present in asymptomatic bacteriuria; therefore, its presence cannot be used to distinguish asymptomatic from clinical infection.

Reliance on clinical evidence of infection in making a decision to treat is compromised by the frequent absence of fever in infected elderly patients and by the inability of many patients to describe symptoms. However, in the absence of some objective evidence of infection, such as fever, flank pain, or change in cogni-

tive or functional status, treatment for a positive culture should be withheld and the patient observed.

Treatment

Asymptomatic bacteriuria should not be treated, except just before planned genitourinary tract surgery. Treatment of asymptomatic bacteriuria in nursing home residents has not been shown to alter mortality and may contribute to increased antibiotic resistance in nursing facilities.

Symptomatic UTIs in elderly women include cystitis and pyelonephritis. The infecting organisms are similar to those in asymptomatic bacteriuria. Cystitis in elderly women has traditionally been treated with 7 days of antibiotics; a shorter duration may also be effective, but more studies are needed. Men with UTI usually have a prostatic focus and require 2–6 weeks of treatment with an antibiotic such as trimethoprim-sulfamethoxazole or a quinolone, both of which penetrate well into the prostate. An ultrasound examination of the genitourinary system might be warranted.

Single-agent empiric antimicrobial therapy is appropriate for all patients with presumed UTI. In nursing home patients, breadth of coverage should be based on the antibiotic resistance pattern in the facility. Patients with suspected sepsis from UTI require hospitalization and treatment with a beta-lactam/beta-lactamase combination, a third-generation cephalosporin, or a quinolone such as ciprofloxacin. In catheterized patients, because of the possibility of infection with gram-positive organisms (ie, methicillin-resistant *Staphylococcus aureus* and enterococci in up to 20% of patients), it is also appropriate to consider using a beta-lactam/beta-lactamase inhibitor combination or adding vancomycin for empiric treatment. Once culture results are available, the empiric antibiotic regimen should be changed to an appropriate antibiotic with the narrowest spectrum. Recommended empiric therapy is included in Table 34–1.

Nicolle LE: Urinary tract infections in long-term-care facilities. Infect Control Hosp Epidemiol 2001;22:167. [PMID: 11310697]

RESPIRATORY TRACT INFECTIONS

Viral Infections

General Considerations

Older adults usually experience at least 1 upper respiratory tract infection (URI) per year. Although the incidence of URI is lower in older adults than in younger patients, the morbidity and mortality associated with viral URIs are significantly greater. The management of

Table 34–1. Empiric therapy.

Infections	Drug
Respiratory tract	
Influenza	Amantadine
	Rimantidine
	Oseltamivir
	Zanamivir
RSV	Ribavirin in selected cases
Tuberculosis (prophylaxis)	INH
Bronchitis exacerbation	
FEV$_1$ > 35% predicted	Amoxacillin/clavulanic acid
	or macrolide
FEV$_1$ < 35% predicted	Antipneumococcal fluoroquinolone (levofloxacin)
Pneumonia	
Community acquired, treated as outpatient	Levofloxacin
	or azithromycin
	or doxycycline
Community acquired, hospitalized	Ceftriaxone plus azithromycin
	or levofloxacin alone
Nursing home acquired, treated in nursing home	Levofloxacin ± clindamycin
	or moxifloxacin
	or levofloxacin
	or ceftriaxone
Nursing home-acquired, hospitalized	Beta-lactam/beta-lactamase inhibitor plus macrolide
	or ceftriaxone plus clindamycin
	or levofloxacin plus clindamycin
	or moxifloxacin
Infected pressure ulcers	Amoxacillin/clavulanic acid
	or piperacillin/tazobactam
	or ertapenem
	or levofloxacin/metronidazole
	or ciprofloxacin/clindamycin
Varicella-zoster virus	Famciclovir
	Valacyclovir
	Acyclovir
Gastroenteritis	Trimethoprim-sulfamethoxazole
	or ciprofloxacin
Urinary tract	Ciprofloxacin
	Levofloxacin
	Amoxacillin/clavulanic acid
	Ceftriaxone

RSV, respiratory syncytial virus; FEV$_1$, forced expiratory volume in 1S.

viral respiratory infections is problematic because it is often difficult to determine a cause and to distinguish viral from bacterial causes. Influenza types A and B, parainfluenza, coronavirus, and rhinovirus are the cause of most common viral respiratory infections. Influenza type A and respiratory syncytial virus (RSV) cause the greatest morbidity and mortality.

Influenza types A and B cause epidemics of disease almost every winter. In the United States, these winter influenza epidemics can cause illness in 10–20% of people and are associated with an average of 36,000 deaths and 114,000 hospitalizations every year, most frequently in the elderly. RSV is second to influenza as a cause of death from viral respiratory infections.

Prevention

Prevention of influenza is the most effective way to decrease morbidity and mortality. Hospitalization and mortality in both community-dwelling elderly and nursing home residents are reduced when vaccine is administered before the influenza season. Because the influenza virus undergoes minor antigenic change from year to year and significant antigenic change periodically, the composition of the vaccine changes annually. All at-risk individuals must, therefore, be immunized annually. The Centers for Disease Control (CDC) recommends influenza immunization for, among others, all those 50 years of age and older, those with chronic medical conditions or immunosuppression, and all nursing home residents. The recommendation to immunize those 50 years old and older is based on the fact that many individuals in this age group have undiagnosed high-risk conditions. To further protect those who may not mount a protective antibody response either because of age or immunosuppression, it is also recommended that caregivers for persons at risk be immunized. Physicians caring for the elderly should have an influenza immunization plan in place to ensure that all those at risk receive the vaccine each fall.

Side effects of the influenza vaccine are the same for the elderly as for younger individuals: local soreness, low-grade fever, and muscle aches. The risk of Guillain-Barré syndrome with recent vaccines has been extremely small. The potential for serious complications from influenza far outweighs this small risk. When influenza occurs in a nursing home, the CDC recommends antiviral prophylaxis for all residents to prevent an epidemic. A plan for instituting such prophylaxis should be in place in all nursing homes. Prophylaxis should be continued for at least 2 weeks or, if cases continue to occur, until 1 week after the outbreak has ended. Amantadine prophylaxis has been shown to control influenza outbreaks in nursing homes. Fewer data are available on use of the newer agents in institutional outbreak control.

Clinical Findings

A. SYMPTOMS & SIGNS

Classic influenza presents with abrupt onset of fever, chills, headache, and myalgias, which are accompanied by pharyngitis, nonproductive cough, and clear, watery nasal congestion. The fever accompanying influenza infection can last from 4–8 days. A characteristic symptom of influenza infection is retro-orbital eye pain. As patients age, they may have fewer symptoms of influenza infection and may present only with fever, cough, and confusion. The most common complications of influenza in the elderly are pneumonia (influenzal or bacterial) and exacerbation of underlying chronic lung disease.

Common symptoms of RSV infection include rhinorrhea, cough, sputum production, shortness of breath, and wheezing.

Parainfluenza virus, coronavirus, and rhinovirus cause the common cold, with symptoms of rhinorrhea, cough, and sneezing.

B. LABORATORY TESTS

Viral culture for influenza using nasopharyngeal swab, is useful in making an etiological diagnosis because the symptoms of influenza may be similar to those of other viruses such as RSV. Rapid antigenic tests, with 80–90% sensitivity and specificity (depending on sample quality), are commercially available to detect influenza types A and B.

Unfortunately, the sensitivity of culture for RSV is extremely poor because the shedding of RSV in the oropharynx is low. In addition, RSV is thermolabile and does not survive long in transit.

Treatment

Antiviral treatment for influenza should be administered within 48 h, and preferably within 12 h, of symptom onset. The earlier the antivirals are administered, the more effective they are in reducing symptoms and preventing complications. The older antivirals amantadine and rimantidine are active only against influenza type A. The neuraminidase inhibitors zanamivir (inhaled) and oseltamivir are effective against both influenza types A and B.

The treatment of RSV infection in the elderly is supportive, with hydration, oxygenation, and treatment of bronchospasm with bronchodilators. It is unclear whether aerosolized ribavirin affects symptoms in the elderly. Infection control measures are critical to stop the spread of RSV, especially in the institutional setting. RSV can survive for more than 6 h on environmental surfaces and is highly efficient in spreading among close contacts. Because compliance with hand washing in health care facilities is frequently poor, additional protective equipment such as gowns and gloves may decrease spread.

Treatment of the common cold is symptomatic with acetaminophen, decongestants, and antihistamines. However, many cold remedies contain medications that can cause adverse effects in the elderly or interact with prescription medications.

Tuberculosis

General Considerations

In the United States, ~12% of new cases of tuberculosis (TB) each year involve persons older than 65. Most TB in the elderly is a result of reactivation of latent infection and involves the lungs. However, extrapulmonary TB, including miliary disease, is more frequent in the elderly than in younger individuals. Reactivation is thought to occur because of a decline of cell-mediated immunity with age and the development of medical conditions. Malignancy, diabetes, lymphoreticular cancers, poor nutrition, renal insufficiency, and gastrointestinal surgeries as well as chronic institutionalization increase the risk of TB in the elderly.

Screening for Latent Disease

The tuberculin test is the best available screening test to detect previous infection. It is recommended that only those who have increased risk for TB be screened: residents and employees of nursing homes and other high-risk congregate living settings; persons with recent close contact with an active case; those who have immigrated within the past 5 years from a country with a high prevalence of TB; and those with certain medical conditions such as diabetes, renal disease, significant weight loss, some types of gastrointestinal surgery, and immunosuppression. In the elderly who have not received routine annual tests and in those admitted to nursing homes, a 2-step TB test should be done if the initial test is negative. A second test is performed a week after the first to detect the booster phenomenon. In many elderly persons who were infected at a young age, the delayed hypersensitivity has waned. The second test, if positive, will confirm that the first test has boosted this immunity. This is a positive test; it is not a conversion. Failure to perform a 2-step test initially, especially in nursing home residents, will result in an inability to discriminate the booster phenomenon from a conversion at the next annual test. A conversion requires evaluation for active disease, treatment, and an epidemiological investigation for a source case and other cases. Therefore, this distinction is critical.

Guidelines regarding criteria for positive tuberculin skin tests use ≥ 10 mm of induration as a positive test in most individuals; 5 mm of induration is considered positive in those with HIV infection, persons receiving immunosuppressive therapy, recent contacts of active cases, and patients with a chest x-ray film consistent with prior TB. Persons with positive skin tests should be evaluated for active TB with symptom review and chest x-ray film. If either of these indicate the possibility of TB, respiratory isolation, with transfer to the hospital for nursing home residents, and further evaluation are indicated. Clinicians should be aware of atypical presentations of TB in the elderly. Occasionally, pulmonary infiltrates will be located in the basal portions of the lung and be interpreted as aspiration pneumonia. Therefore, any pulmonary infiltrate in the presence of a positive skin test should be evaluated for the possibility of TB.

Treatment

If the chest x-ray film does not reveal evidence of active disease in a person with a positive skin test (ie, latent disease), it is recommended that isoniazid (INH) therapy be administered for 9 mo. Once-a-day dosing with 300 mg of INH has been shown to decrease the incidence of active TB by at least 60%. Elderly persons are at greatest risk for hepatotoxicity from INH, but the risk is low. Alcohol use may increase this risk. At least 1 study has shown no increased risk in those with chronic hepatitis, HIV infection or concurrent medication use. The use of rifampin and pyrazinamide for latent disease results in more hepatotoxicity than use of INH alone. In patients receiving treatment for latent disease, monthly clinical monitoring for symptoms is essential. In addition, patients must be instructed to stop INH and contact the clinician if unexplained nausea, anorexia, fatigue, fever, or right upper quadrant pain occurs.

Baseline liver function tests at the initiation of INH therapy are usually indicated in the elderly. Monthly laboratory monitoring of liver function tests is important in those who have cognitive impairment and who cannot report symptoms. It should also be done in those with baseline abnormalities in liver function tests, those receiving other hepatotoxic drugs, those who are positive for HIV, and those using alcohol. A rise in serum aminotransferase activity > 5 times normal or clinical evidence of hepatitis requires prompt discontinuation of INH therapy.

Some authorities suggest administering pyridoxine (vitamin B_6) to reduce risk of neuropathy from INH in those at greatest risk for neuropathy (eg, those with diabetes, uremia, alcoholism, HIV, and malnutrition).

Active TB should be treated in conjunction with a specialist to ensure appropriate medication prescription and public health follow-up of the patient and contacts.

Bronchitis

General Considerations

Acute bronchitis in an elderly person without chronic lung disease is a self-limited condition that is generally viral in origin and requires no antibiotic treatment.

Clinical Findings

Symptoms of bronchitis are similar to those of pneumonia with cough, sputum production and sometimes fever. Clinical findings are insufficient to rule out pneumonia; thus a chest x-ray is essential.

Treatment

During an influenza outbreak, bronchitis in the context of an influenza-like disease should be treated with influenza antiviral therapy. Bronchitis causing an exacerbation of chronic lung disease is frequently treated with antibiotics. However, evidence supporting efficacy is lacking despite the findings of increased numbers of pneumococci and *Haemophilus influenzae* in the sputum. The decision to use antibiotics in bronchitis should be based on forced expiratory volume in 1 s (FEV_1) and age. The more severely impaired patients ($FEV_1 < 35\%$) merit treatment for acute exacerbations.

Pneumonia

General Considerations

Pneumonia is the sixth most common cause of death in the United States; most of the deaths occur in the elderly. The mortality rate from pneumonia is 5 times greater in those older than 64 years than in those younger than 64.

The elderly possess many medical conditions that place them at risk for pneumonia: underlying chronic obstructive pulmonary disease or chronic bronchitis, alcoholism, dementia, neurological illness (strokes or parkinsonism), heart failure, diabetes, and renal disease.

Clinical Findings

A. SYMPTOMS & SIGNS

Symptoms of pneumonia usually include fever and cough with sputum production, but in the elderly symptoms may be more subtle.

B. LABORATORY TESTS

Sputum cultures are generally obtained for diagnosis. However, it is often difficult to obtain sputum cultures in the elderly and a satisfactory etiological diagnosis is not made. Blood cultures may be positive in a small percentage of patients.

Most studies in the elderly identify pneumococcus as the most prevalent pathogen. Other pathogens include *H. influenzae, S. aureus,* enteric gram-negative organisms, *Legionella* species, and *Chlamydia.* The most serious infections are due to *S. pneumoniae* and *Legionella.*

Treatment

Guidelines have been published for the empiric treatment of community-acquired pneumonia. Specific antibiotic recommendations for outpatient and inpatient treatment are in Table 34–1.

The severity of pneumonia often dictates site of care and has an impact on the choice of therapy. Guidelines for assessing severity of pneumonia in elderly outpatients are outlined in Table 34–2. In general, elderly

outpatients have significant comorbidities, which make hospitalization necessary. In those who are hemodynamically stable, have mild symptoms, and can comply with therapy, outpatient management may be successful but close follow-up is essential.

Elderly persons in nursing homes have a 10-fold greater incidence of pneumonia than those in the community, and pneumonia is the most common reason for transfer of nursing home residents to the hospital. Nursing home residents represent 10–18% of all patients hospitalized with pneumonia. The decision to transfer a patient with pneumonia from a nursing home to the hospital may be aided by published guidelines for predicting pneumonia mortality (Table 34–3). These guidelines predict 30-day mortality using clinical criteria: respiratory rate > 30/min, pulse > 125/min, acute change in mental status, and history of dementia. When 2 or more of these findings are present, mortality is 30%. Factors that have been associated with treatment failure in the nursing home include respiratory rate > 30, pulse > 90, temperature > 38.1 °C, oxygen saturation < 92%, use of a mechanically altered diet, feeding tube dependence, and altered level of consciousness.

The possibility of infection with penicillin-resistant pneumococci should be considered when choosing empiric antibiotic therapy for nursing home-acquired pneumonia. There have been several outbreaks of pneumococcal pneumonia in nursing homes, some of which have involved penicillin-resistant pneumococci. Because of the prevalence of the pneumococcus as a pathogen and because of increasing antibiotic resistance, immunization of the elderly with the 23-valent polysaccharide pneumococcal vaccine should be a priority in all settings. Recommendations for treating nursing home-acquired pneumonia are included in Table 34–1. No prospective studies have established the superiority of one antibiotic regimen over another.

Table 34–2. Severity assessment for lower respiratory tract infection in community-dwelling elderly.

Independent variables associated with mortality within 30 days
Acute aggravation of coexisting illness
Respiratory rate ≥ 25 breaths/min
Elevated C reactive protein (≥ 100 mg/L)

In one study, the mortality rate was 2.2% if the patients had none or only 1 of the independent risk factors and 20% if they had all 3 risk factors.

Table 34–3. Independent variables associated with mortality within 30 days in nursing home-acquired pneumonia.

Respiratory rate > 30 breaths/min
Pulse > 125 beats/min
Altered mental status
History of dementia

Bartlett JG et al: Practice guidelines for the management of community-acquired pneumonia in adults. Infectious Diseases Society of America. Clin Infect Dis 2000;31:347. [PMID: 10987697]

Centers for Disease Control: Prevention and control of influenza. MMWR Morb Mortal Wkly Rep 2002;51:1. [PMID: 12002171]

Centers for Disease Control: Targeted tuberculin testing and treatment of latent tuberculosis infection. American Thoracic Society. MMWR Morb Mortal Wkly Rep 2000;49:1. [PMID: 10881762]

Feldman C: Pneumonia in the elderly. Med Clin North Am 2001; 85:1441. [PMID: 11680111]

Fine MJ et al: A prediction rule to identify low-risk patients with community-acquired pneumonia. N Engl J Med 1997;336:243. [PMID: 8995086]

Johnson JC et al: Nonspecific presentation of pneumonia in hospitalized older people: age effect or dementia? J Am Geriatr Soc 2000;48:1316. [PMID: 11037021]

Koivula I et al: Risk factors for pneumonia in the elderly. Am J Med 1994;96:313. [PMID: 10421277]

Marrie TJ: Community-acquired pneumonia in the elderly. Clin Infect Dis 2000;31:1066. [PMID: 11049791]

Medina-Walpole AM, Katz PR: Nursing home-acquired pneumonia. J Am Geriatr Soc 1999;47:1005. [PMID: 10443864]

Muder RR: Management of nursing home-acquired pneumonia: unresolved issues and priorities for future investigation. J Am Geriatr Soc 2000;48:95. [PMID: 10642029]

Naughton BJ, Mylotte JM: Treatment guideline for nursing home-acquired pneumonia based on community practice. J Am Geriatr Soc 2000;48:82. [PMID: 10642027]

Naughton BJ et al: Outcome of nursing home-acquired pneumonia: derivation and application of a practical model to predict 30 day mortality. J Am Geriatr Soc 2000;48:1292. [PMID: 11037018]

Nuorti JP et al: An outbreak of multidrug-resistant pneumococcal pneumonia and bacteremia among unvaccinated nursing home residents. N Engl J Med 1998;338:1861. [PMID: 9637804]

Seppa Y et al: Severity assessment of lower respiratory tract infection in elderly patients in primary care. Arch Intern Med 2001; 161:2709. [PMID: 11732936]

GASTROENTERITIS

General Considerations

More than 75% of all deaths from diarrhea in the United States occur in those older than 55; 50% occur in those older than 74. The greatest risk to the elderly person with diarrhea is dehydration, which may lead to cardiac, renal, and cerebrovascular complications.

A decrease in gastric acidity as a result of medications, gastric atrophy, surgery, and systemic illnesses increases the risk of infection with gastrointestinal pathogens. Elderly patients living in nursing homes or other group settings are at particularly high risk because of shared bathrooms and dining facilities, the high prevalence of incontinence, and poor staff compliance with hand-washing practices.

The principal bacterial pathogens causing diarrhea in the elderly are *C. difficile, Campylobacter* species, *Escherichia coli, Salmonella* species, and *Shigella* species. When onset of symptoms is within 12 h of ingestion of contaminated food, the toxins of *Clostridium perfringens, Bacillus cereus,* or *S. aureus* may be responsible.

Antibiotic-associated diarrhea caused by *C. difficile* is common in the elderly because of more hospitalizations, nursing home stays, and antibiotic use. Up to 50% of patients older than 65 will develop *C. difficile*-associated diarrhea after hospitalization and antibiotic use. Much of the problem with *C. difficile* is due to poor infection control practices.

Clinical Findings

A. SYMPTOMS & SIGNS

The patient experiencing diarrhea may have crampy lower abdominal pain, anorexia, fever, malaise, and watery or bloody diarrhea. In general, symptoms are not specific enough to identify the causative pathogen.

C. difficile can cause severe diarrhea, fever and systemic toxicity.

B. LABORATORY TESTS

Cultures of stool and testing for *C. difficile* toxin in outpatients are indicated when there is a history of recent travel, recent hospitalization, inflammatory bowel disease, prior antibiotic use or unsafe food ingestion; when illness occurs in a cluster; when fever, dehydration, abdominal pain, or bloody diarrhea is present; when the patient is immunocompromised; when symptoms are severe or prolonged; and when fecal leukocytes or blood are present. Bacterial cultures for *Salmonella, Shigella, E. coli,* and *Yersinia* should always be obtained in patients hospitalized because of diarrhea and in nursing home patients with diarrhea. A stool examination for ova and parasites should be done when the patient is immunocompromised, has traveled recently, or has prolonged diarrhea. Identification of a pathogen helps tailor antibiotic therapy and assists in public health surveillance for actual or potential outbreaks.

Suspicion of *C. difficile* should be high in any hospital or nursing home-acquired diarrhea, especially with a history of antibiotic use. Diagnosis can be made by identifying the toxin in stool specimens. Flexible sigmoidoscopy or colonoscopy looking for pseudomembranes should be performed for persistent diarrhea with negative stool studies.

Treatment

In outpatients with diarrhea, viral pathogens are most common, and treatment focuses on rehydration and electrolyte replacement. Elderly patients, especially those who are frail, can become dehydrated after only 1 or 2 loose stools. Therefore, the first step in managing diarrhea is to ensure that patients have adequate oral or, if necessary, intravenous, replacement of fluids and electrolytes.

Patients with infectious inflammatory diarrhea, as evidenced by the presence of fecal leukocytes, may be started on empiric antibiotics before culture results. Antimotility drugs should not be given for inflammatory diarrhea. Where Shiga toxin-producing *E. coli* is suspected (nonbloody diarrhea without fever), antibiotics are not recommended because they may increase the risk of hemolytic uremic syndrome. In other causes of community-acquired or traveler's diarrhea, trimethoprim-sulfamethoxazole or a quinolone can be used. *Campylobacter* may be resistant to quinolones and require erythromycin.

C. difficile should be treated with oral metronidazole. Recurrent or severe disease may require oral vancomycin, but this should not be used as first-line therapy.

Guerrant RL et al: Practice guidelines for the management of infectious diarrhea. Clin Infect Dis 2001;32:331. [PMID: 1170940]

Slotwiner PK, Brandt LJ: Infectious diarrhea in the elderly. Gastroenterol Clin North Am 2001;30:625. [PMID: 11586549]

INFECTED PRESSURE ULCERS

Clinical Findings

A. Symptoms & Signs

Clinical evidence of infection includes warmth, tenderness, purulent discharge, foul odor and tissue crepitus.

B. Laboratory Tests

Determining whether a pressure ulcer is infected is a challenge. Superficial swab cultures collect surface-contaminating organisms, and a positive swab culture does not necessarily mean that the ulcer is infected. The ultimate decision is clinical, based on information obtained at the bedside and histopathological evidence. If there is clinical evidence of infection, superficial cultures do not effectively reveal the infecting organism. Tissue biopsy and culture and fluid irrigation/aspiration cultures are superior alternatives. However, tissue irrigation and aspiration may yield positive results even in noninfected ulcers.

The diagnosis of infection from deep tissue biopsy requires the finding of $> 10^6$ micro-organisms per gram of tissue. Often up to 4 isolates, including anaerobes 25% of the time, will be recovered from appropriately obtained samples. The most common aerobic isolates obtained from cultures are *Proteus mirabilis*, enterococci, *E. coli*, staphylococci, and *Pseudomonas*. The most common anaerobic isolates are peptostreptococci, *Bacteroides*, and *Clostridia*. Bacteremia from infected pressure ulcers is more frequently from anaerobes than aerobes and is associated with a high mortality.

C. Special Tests

Bone biopsy should be done if osteomyelitis is clinically suspected based on an elevated white blood cell count, elevated sedimentation rate, and positive radiographic findings.

Plain films should be obtained to look for evidence of osteomyelitis, but these are often nondiagnostic. Computed tomography scans have high specificity but limited sensitivity. Their role is to assess the size of the ulcer, presence of fistulas, and possible joint involvement. Magnetic resonance imaging has a sensitivity of 98% and a specificity of 89% in detecting osteomyelitis. Radionucleotide scintigraphy and gallium scanning have been shown to be sensitive but not specific. Indium-labeled white blood cell scanning has been shown to have a specificity of seventy-seven percent compared with bone biopsy. Indium studies are particularly helpful when there is associated soft tissue inflammation. However, this procedure has not been well studied in patients with pressure ulcers.

Treatment

Antibiotic therapy for infected pressure ulcers should be used in conjunction with débridement, appropriate wound dressings, and management of pressure ulcer risk factors. Empiric antibiotics often must be administered in very ill patients. The superiority of one empiric regimen over another has not been assessed. Because these infections are polymicrobial, the use of a beta-lactam/beta-lactamase inhibitor combination should be strongly considered. Quinolone combined with metronidazole or clindamycin is another option. Because of poor tissue perfusion of infected pressure ulcers, antimicrobial therapy should be administered intravenously in all patients who are extremely ill. Topical treatment is not effective for any infected pressure ulcer.

Livesley NJ, Chow AW: Infected pressure ulcers in elderly individuals. Clin Infect Dis 2002;35:1390 [PMID: 12439803]

HERPES ZOSTER

General Considerations

Herpes zoster (HZ) is a neurocutaneous reactivation disease, occurring only in those previously infected with the varicella-zoster virus (VZV). Almost all persons older than 65 have been previously infected. The incidence of HZ in the elderly is 7–11 cases per 1000 persons per year. Risk factors for the reactivation of VZV include increasing age, immunosuppression, chronic diseases, and use of some medications. Illnesses most frequently associated with VZV reactivation include lymphomas, leukemias, HIV infection, and autoimmune diseases such as lupus and rheumatoid arthritis.

Prevention

VZV can be transmitted to seronegative susceptible contacts, especially during the vesicular stage. Direct contact or airborne or droplet nuclei may transmit infection. Immunization of health care workers and appropriate isolation procedures should help prevent the spread of this infection in the institutional setting. If exposure of susceptible persons occurs in an institutional setting, consultation with an infection control expert is essential to prevent an outbreak.

Clinical Findings

A. SYMPTOMS & SIGNS

Clinicians should consider the possibility of zoster in any cutaneous syndrome involving acute unilateral dermatomal pain. Pain occurs 2–3 days before a rash develops and, in rare cases, may be the only manifestation of VZV infection. Dermatomal distribution of maculopapular followed by vesicular lesions on an erythematous base generally is sufficient to make the diagnosis, although laboratory studies may be needed in some instances to distinguish herpes simplex from varicella-zoster infection. Vesicle formation may continue for 5 days, and it usually takes 7–12 days for the vesicles to crust over.

B. LABORATORY TESTS

Direct fluorescent antibody testing for the detection of VZV antigens in vesicular fluid is extremely specific and sensitive.

Complications

The major complication of VZV is postherpetic neuralgia, a persistent burning, throbbing, or stabbing pain that can be severely incapacitating and lead to depression, dependence, and isolation. Postherpetic neuralgia occurs in up to 50% of untreated adults older than 50 and in 75% of those older than 70. Pain may last more than 1 year, especially in those older than 70. Other rare neurological complications may occur, such as focal motor paresis in the affected area. Ophthalmic HZ, presenting with periocular, forehead, and nasal pain and lesions, is an ophthalmologic emergency because vision loss may occur. Ophthalmic HZ can also cause granulomatous angiitis of the carotid artery, which may lead to stroke. Cutaneous dissemination and visceral involvement can occur in immunocompromised patients, but the risk of dissemination is decreased significantly with antiviral therapy. Bacterial superinfection with streptococci and staphylococci can also occur.

Treatment

Antiviral therapy with acyclovir, famciclovir or valacyclovir reduces acute inflammation and pain in most patients treated within 72 h of rash onset. Patients may also benefit from therapy begun after 72 h, especially if new vesicle formation continues. Because famciclovir and valacyclovir dosing schedules are simpler than that for acyclovir, these drugs may be preferable. The duration of postherpetic neuralgia is decreased by as much as 50% with antiviral therapy. Although steroids may improve acute pain, they do not decrease the incidence of postherpetic neuralgia. One study has shown that elderly persons (with no contraindications to steroids) treated with a short course of tapering prednisone in combination with acyclovir had improved quality of life, improved sleep, and more rapid return to normal activities than those treated with acyclovir alone. Steroid treatment had no effect on incidence or duration of postherpetic neuralgia. The role of steroids in combination with antiviral therapy in healthy elderly persons with HZ remains unclear but may be considered in those with no contraindications. In the treatment of VZV-induced facial paralysis, steroids may have a role in conjunction with antiviral therapy.

Because postherpetic neuralgia can be profoundly debilitating, early and aggressive pain management is essential. A number of medications have been used for the treatment of postherpetic neuralgia, including topical lidocaine, gabapentin, and tricyclic antidepressants. Unfortunately, none of these therapies has been prospectively studied. Opiates will be necessary in many patients to treat pain, although these medications may be associated with side effects in the elderly.

Gnann JW Jr, Whitley RJ: Herpes zoster. N Engl J Med 2002; 347:340. [PMID: 12151472]

O'Donnell JA, Hofmann MT: Skin and soft tissues. Management of four common infections in the nursing home patient. Geriatrics 2001;56:33. [PMID: 11641861]

Schmader K: Herpes zoster in older adults. Clin Infect Dis 2001;32:1481. [PMID: 11317250]

FEVER OF UNKNOWN ORIGIN

General Considerations

Fever of unknown origin (FUO) has been defined as a temperature > 101 °F persisting without diagnosis for at least 3 weeks despite at least 1 week of evaluation in the hospital. The definition has been revised to reflect the 4 different major causes, and hence different evaluation and treatment strategies: classic FUO, nosocomial FUO, immune-deficient FUO, and HIV-associated FUO. In the elderly, compared to younger persons, classic FUO is more likely to be caused by collagen vascular diseases such as temporal arteritis, by TB, or by malignancy (usually hematological). Other noninfectious causes include medications, alcoholic hepatitis, thyroiditis, hyperthyroidism, and venous thromboembolism. One third of FUOs in the elderly are caused by infection, the most common of which are infective endocarditis, tuberculosis, abscesses (usually intra-abdominal), and complicated urinary tract infections. The percentage of FUOs caused by abscesses has declined recently with the availability of more sophisticated diagnostic imaging tools.

Clinical Findings

Evaluation of an elderly patient with FUO should include a thorough history (eg, travel history; risk for immunosuppression, including HIV infection; medications; prior antibiotic use, procedures, or surgery; and TB history or exposure). Because patients with FUO have already had an extensive evaluation, further studies should be based on findings from those studies, additional information from repeated histories or examinations, and data published about the frequency of particular causes.

Treatment

Most FUOs in the elderly represent atypical presentations of common diseases, and many are treatable. Therefore, persistence in the evaluation is indicated, particularly in ruling out TB and temporal arteritis, which may require urgent treatment. In general, the recommendation is to delay therapy of the fever unless a cause is specifically identified or the patient is at im-

minent risk of dying. Initiating empiric antibiotics can lead to confusion in subsequent assessments.

Knockaert DC et al: Fever of unknown origin in adults: 40 years on. J Intern Med 2003;253:263. [PMID: 12603493]

Tal S et al: Fever of unknown origin in the elderly. J Intern Med 2002;252:295. [PMID: 12366602]

ANTIBIOTIC RESISTANCE

Antibiotic resistance in nursing homes is a serious concern and has resulted, in part, because of excessive use of antibiotics in this setting. In addition, patients admitted to nursing homes frequently come from hospitals and are colonized with resistant organisms from that setting. Nursing home residents may be colonized or become infected with vancomycin-resistant enterococci, methicillin-resistant *S. aureus,* penicillin-resistant pneumococci, multiresistant gram-negative bacilli, quinolone-resistant *Pseudomonas* species, and *Acinetobacter* species (Table 34–4). Blood stream infection with methicillin-resistant *S. aureus* poses a significant threat in the nursing home patient.

Guidelines have been published to help clinicians who work in nursing homes to diagnose and treat infections. Promoting appropriate antibiotic use through such guidelines, providing education, and monitoring

Table 34–4. Resistant pathogens found in long-term care facilities.

Multiresistant gram-negative bacilli
Extended spectrum beta-lactamase producing gram-negative bacilli (*Escherichia coli* and *Klebsiella pneumoniae*)
Inhibitor resistant beta-lactamase producing *E. coli, Klebsiella* spp, or *Proteus* spp.
Plasmid-mediated third-generation cephalosporin-resistant *Klebsiella pneumoniae,* and *E. coli*
Third-generation cephalosporin-resistant *Enterobacter* and *Citrobacter* spp
Quinolone-resistant *Pseudomonas aeruginosa*
TMP/SMX-resistant *E. coli*
Resistant gram-positive bacteria
Methicillin-resistant *Staphylococcus aureus*
Vancomycin-resistant enterococci (VRE)
Penicillin-resistant *Streptococcus pneumoniae* (resistant also to macrolides, clindamycin, sulfamethoxazole, and tetracyclines)

TMP, trimethoprim-sulfamethoxazole.

antibiotic use and antibiotic-resistance patterns are all measures designed to reduce inappropriate use of antibiotics and thereby reduce the emergence of resistant organisms

Bentley DW et al: Practice guideline for evaluation of fever and infection in long-term care facilities. J Am Geriatr Soc 2001;49:210. [PMID: 11207876]

Bonomo R: Multiple antibiotic-resistant bacteria in long-term care facilities: an emerging problem in the practice of infectious diseases. Clin Infect Dis 2000;31:1414. [PMID: 11096012]

Bradley SF: Issues in the management of resistant bacteria in long-term-care facilities. Infect Control Hosp Epidemiol 1999; 20:362. [PMID: 10349960]

Loeb M et al: Colonization with multiresistant bacteria and quality of life in residents of long-term-care facilities. Infect Control Hosp Epidemiol 2001;22:67. [PMID: 10968724]

Mody L et al: Prevalence of ceftriaxone- and ceftazidime-resistant gram-negative bacteria in long-term-care facilities. Infect Control Hosp Epidemiol 2001;22:193. [PMID: 1137907]

Nicolle LE et al: Antimicrobial use in long-term-care facilities. SHEA Long-Term-Care Committee. Infect Control Hosp Epidemiol 2000;21:537. [PMID: 10968724]

SECTION IV

Special Situations

Special Issues in Women's Health: Hormonal Health Issues of Early & Late Postmenopausal Women

35

Julie A. Elder, DO, Barbara J. Messinger-Rapport, MD, PhD, & Holly L. Thacker, MD, FACP

ESSENTIALS OF DIAGNOSIS

- *The interval of hormonal flux preceding menses cessation is the menopausal transition. During this time, many women experience signs and symptoms of estrogen deficiency, which may persist for 2–8 years before menopause.*

- *Menopause (cessation of estrogen production) is marked by the absence of menses for 1 year, typically occurring at age 51 (range, 40–55).*

- *The clinician identifies menopause by history and physical examination without laboratory or imaging studies.*

- *The early postmenopausal phase consists of the first 5 years after cessation of menses.*

- *The late postmenopausal phase constitutes the remainder of a woman's life.*

■ DIMINISHED ESTROGEN PRODUCTION

Diminished estrogen production, encountered during menopause, has long-term health implications. Many of the clinical signs and symptoms experienced during the menopausal and postmenopausal years can be directly and indirectly linked to hormonal deficiencies. Various body systems are affected, including vasomotor/neuroendocrine, skin/hair, urogenital, skeletal, and cardiovascular (Table 35–1).

VASOMOTOR/NEUROENDOCRINE SYSTEM

Symptoms & Signs

Women typically encounter hot flashes during the menopause transition and early postmenopausal phase. Other problems include cephalgia, flushing, nausea, and diaphoresis. Women may also experience palpitations, dizziness, and "skin-crawling" sensations. These symptoms of estrogen deficiency persist an average of 5 years. However, up to 25% of women will experience hot flashes beyond this period.

Although menopause does not cause depression, women with previously diagnosed panic disorder or depression may note exacerbations of their disease processes with the onset of the vasomotor symptoms as a result of estrogen deficiency. Appropriate identification of an underlying mood disorder is important because some form of depression occurs in 1–5% of community dwellers older than 65. Older women are more likely to be depressed than older men regardless of race, ethnic background, and economic status. Complaints of helplessness and hopelessness, symptoms of irritability, and findings of cognitive deficits may be more prominent than dysphoria. Left untreated, depression

Table 35–1. Menopausal signs & symptoms.

Vasomotor/neuroendocrine	Integument	Urogenital	Skeletal	Cardiovascular
Cephalgia/sleep disturbance	Decreased skin elasticity	Increased risk of UTIs	Osteopenia	Increased LDL-C
Exacerbation of depression and panic disorder	Hirsutism	Urinary incontinence	Loss of height	Decreased HDL-C
Hot flashes	Mucosal dryness	Dyspareunia	Osteoporosis	Increased body fat
Palpitations	Alopecia	Vaginal atrophy	Fractures	Atherothrombotic events
Sleep disturbances	Deepening of the voice	Pruritus vulvae	Frailty	
Memory/cognitive changes		Sexual dysfunction and decreased libido		

UTI, urinary tract infection, LDL-C, low-density lipoprotein cholesterol, HDL-C, high-density lipoprotein cholesterol.

can lead to cognitive and functional decline and increased overall morbidity.

Treatment

Systemic estrogen, either oral or transdermal, may relieve vasomotor symptoms. Higher doses of estrogen and, occasionally, the addition of androgens may be required to fully alleviate the symptoms in younger women who have been surgically castrated. Lower doses of estrogen typically suffice in older women, although some may experience inadequate symptom relief. These women may benefit from the addition of methyltestosterone (ie, a combination of esterified estrogen and methyltestosterone).

Estrogen therapy may augment antidepressive therapy and improve quality of life in appropriate candidates (ie, those whose vasomotor symptoms contribute to their depressive symptoms during the menopause transition and early postmenopausal phase). There is also evidence that unopposed estradiol may decrease symptoms of depression independent of vasomotor symptoms. The mechanism by which estradiol reduces depressive symptoms is unclear; however, it modulates neuronal function via noradrenergic, dopaminergic, and gamma-aminobutyric acid-mediated systems.

INTEGUMENT SYSTEM

Symptoms & Signs

Estrogen deficiency is responsible for mucosal dryness in the vagina and possibly in the eyes, nose, and mouth. Some women may complain of skin aging because decreased collagen and elastin production causes a loss of skin elasticity. Approximately 30% of skin collagen is lost within the first 5 years of menopause as a result of estrogen deficiency. Estrogen deficiency results in a relative androgen excess associated with a male-pattern alopecia, hirsutism, and deepening of the upper register of the voice.

Treatment

Hormone therapy (HT) during the transition and early postmenopausal phase enhances skin thickness, improves vascularization, and increases the life cycle of hair follicles. It also improves the quality and context of collagen. The overall effect may be an improvement in skin texture and enhancement of skin healing.

UROGENITAL SYSTEM

Symptoms & Signs

Loss of estrogen's stimulation of receptors in the urethra, vagina, and bladder may cause significant dysfunction of the urogenital system. Dysuria, urinary incontinence (UI), increased urinary frequency, and urinary tract infections may result from estrogen deficiency. These symptoms increase in incidence with age.

Sexual dysfunction resulting from dyspareunia and decreased libido may be a problem that women are hesitant to mention. Deficiency of estrogen and androgen may lead to thinning of the vaginal tissues, causing dyspareunia. In addition, the urethra and bladder can become irritated during intercourse and cause recurrent cystitis and urethritis.

Treatment

Either systemic or topical estrogen can control most urogenital symptoms related to hormone deficiency including dyspareunia, dysuria, urinary incontinence, and sexual dysfunction. Topical vaginal estradiol and estriol, however, are the only hormone regimens that demonstrate a reduction in the frequency of urinary tract infections. Addition of a vaginal estrogen to systemic estrogen therapy may augment the urogenital benefits without requiring an increased systemic dose.

SKELETAL SYSTEM

General Considerations

Estrogen plays an important role in the preservation of bone mineral density (BMD). Women begin losing bone mass gradually at ~30 years of age. This decline in bone mass continues with age and accelerates throughout the menopause transition and into the menopause years. In fact, postmenopausal women who are recently estrogen deficient can lose up to 4–5% of their bone mass annually, eventually leading to low bone mass and osteoporosis. Osteoporosis is responsible for 1.5 million low-trauma fractures each year, resulting in considerable morbidity and mortality in the older population. Osteoporosis must be prevented, if possible, and treated once it is diagnosed because the risk of recurrent osteoporotic fractures is high.

Prevention and Treatment

Prevention of osteoporosis begins in childhood with appropriate nutrition, exercise, and weight management. Continuation of appropriate lifestyle habits into midlife and beyond, including sufficient calcium and vitamin D intake, weight-bearing exercise, and avoidance of smoking and excessive caffeine consumption, helps maintain peak bone mass.

The National Osteoporosis Foundation recommends BMD screening for all women older than 65 regardless of race. The optimal interval for bone density screening has not yet been established. However, it is hoped that early intervention will reduce the risk of fractures. Medicare currently covers bone density screening every 2 years in women older than 65.

Calcium intake is an important component of nutrition. Replacement of calcium has been shown to increase bone density in young women and stabilize bone density in postmenopausal women. Postmenopausal women require at least 1200–1500 mg of calcium in split doses plus 400–800 IU of vitamin D daily. Daily ingestion of > 50,000 μg (10,000 IU) of vitamin A should be avoided because of an increased risk for hip fractures.

Oral and transdermal estrogens have been approved by the Food and Drug Administration (FDA) for the prevention of osteoporosis. Other medications that are FDA approved to prevent or treat osteoporosis include bisphosphonates (risedronate, alendronate), selective estrogen receptor modulators (raloxifene), and calcitonin nasal spray (treatment only). Bisphosphonate use is associated with a reduction in hip fractures. Women who begin estrogen in the early postmenopausal phase and continue the regimen for an average of 15 years have demonstrated an 80% decrease in hip fracture rate.

Discontinuation of estrogen may result in a loss of accumulated benefit. If HT is begun during the menopause transition and early postmenopausal phase, it maintains its benefit as long as it is continued. Consideration should, therefore, be given to continuing HT throughout the late postmenopausal phase if bone protection is the goal and the risk–benefit equation for the individual woman warrants long-term treatment. The initiation of estrogen therapy in the late postmenopausal phase has been shown to preserve and even increase bone density. Even low doses of estrogen (eg, 0.3–0.45 mg of conjugated estrogen or 0.5 mg of estradiol-17β) may improve bone density.

Women who are at increased risk for falling should consider wearing hip protector pads, which significantly decrease the incidence of hip fractures. Hip pads cost approximately $100 and can be ordered from Tytex Group. Currently, insurance companies do not cover the cost.

Tytex Group: www.safehip.com

VASCULAR/METABOLIC SYSTEM

Body fat increases and lean body mass decreases with aging. Fat is deposited centrally. Insulin resistance may also develop. These changes, accompanied by an increase in low-density lipoprotein cholesterol (LDL-C) and a decrease in high-density lipoprotein cholesterol (HDL-C), increase the risk of cardiovascular disease. HT decreases LDL-C, increases HDL-C, and decreases insulin resistance. Observational data favor HT in terms of preventing vascular disease and prolonging survival in women. However, it has been shown that a combination of conjugated equine estrogens, 0.625 mg, and medroxyprogesterone acetate, 2.5 mg, failed to reduce coronary artery disease (CAD), nonfatal myocardial infarctions (MIs), and CAD-related deaths in hormone users with known heart disease despite an 11% reduction in LDL-C.

In addition, estrogen and progestin therapies have not be shown to prevent coronary heart disease (CHD) in women with intact uteri. HT should not be used for cardiovascular risk reduction in late postmenopausal women. In fact, HT has been shown to increase the cardiovascular risk, primarily from nonfatal MIs. Currently, the American Heart Association advises against starting or using HT for the prevention of cardiovascular disease in women older than 50.

OTHER ISSUES

Systemic Lupus Erythematosus

Lupus is more common in women than in men and appears to have symptom variation with hormonal fluctuations (ie, with pregnancy and the menstrual cycle). It has been suggested that there is a 2.5- to 2.8-fold increased risk of lupus associated with postmenopausal estrogen use.

Osteoarthritis

The incidence and severity of osteoarthritis (OA) increase with age in postmenopausal women. HT may decrease the risk of OA in postmenopausal women, in part, by increasing BMD. High BMD has been associated with a decreased prevalence of knee OA. In addition, a high BMD and a gain in BMD have been associated with decreased risk of knee OA progression.

■ HORMONE THERAPY

The decision to begin or continue HT should be based on symptoms and patient preferences, including contemplation of anticipated risks, associated benefits, and choice of agent.

North American Menopause Society: www.menopause.org

Complications (Table 35–2)

A. THROMBOEMBOLISM

Systemic HT use increases a woman's relative risk of venous thromboembolism (VTE) by 2- to 4-fold. The absolute VTE risk is very low in young, healthy women and does not translate into a clinically significant risk with hormone therapy use in symptomatic young women. However, VTE risk increases with age and comorbidity. For example, women with an average age of 67 and known CAD have been shown to have ~1 VTE

Table 35–2. Risk & benefits of HT.

Risks	Benefits
Endometrial cancer	Improvement in vasomotor symptoms
Gallbladder disease	Improvement in vaginal atrophy
Thromboembolism	Prevention of osteoporosis and fracture reduction
Breast cancer diagnosis	May decrease risk of colon cancer
Lupus	May decrease risk of Alzheimer's dementia if started at the time of menopause (not when started in the late post-menopausal phase)
Stroke, diagnosis of nonfatal MI	

MI, myocardial infarction.

per year for every 260 women treated. Women with prior VTE are at a very high risk for recurrent events.

B. ENDOMETRIAL CANCER

Estrogen taken alone (unopposed estrogen) more than doubles the risk of endometrial adenomatous hyperplasia, a precursor for endometrial cancer, in women with intact uteri. The addition of progestin reduces the risk of endometrial cancer to slightly less than the spontaneous occurrence rate of endometrial cancer in non-HT users. Low-dose intravaginal forms of estrogen rarely stimulate the endometrium enough to require progestins. However, higher vaginal doses of estrogen may cause bleeding in 10% of cases, requiring progestin opposition therapy.

C. BREAST CANCER

Short-term use of HT (< 4 years) does not increase the risk of breast cancer. Epidemiological data suggest that estrogen therapy increases the relative risk of breast cancer after 5 years of therapy. This risk may be amplified with increasing duration of therapy and decreased to baseline after cessation of therapy, suggesting that HT is a growth promoter rather than a carcinogen. The WHI reported an increased risk of breast cancer in hormone-estrogen-progestin users with a hazard ratio of 1.26.

D. GALLBLADDER DISEASE

Gallbladder disease is associated with various risk factors, including older age, female gender, obesity, oral contraceptive use, estrogen therapy, and ethnicity. Adequate vitamin C intake may reduce the risk of gallstones in women.

Postmenopausal estrogen may increase the risk of gallbladder disease and cholecystectomy. It has been shown that women with coronary artery disease have a 40% increased risk for symptomatic gallbladder disease and an increased risk of biliary tract surgery while taking HT.

Treatment

Pregnancy, active venous thromboembolism, undiagnosed vaginal bleeding, active liver disease, unstable cardiovascular syndromes, active breast cancer, and active endometrial cancer are absolute contraindications to HT (Table 35–3).

Relative contraindications include previously treated breast cancer, previously treated uterine cancer, previous thromboembolism, gallbladder disease, uncontrolled hypertension, existing heart disease, migraines, uterine fibroids, seizure disorder, and marked hypertriglyceridemia (see Table 35–3).

Table 35–3. Contraindications to HT.

Absolute	Relative
Active breast cancer	Gallbladder disease
Active endometrial cancer	Hypertriglyceridemia
Active liver disease	Migraines
Active venous thromboembolism	Previous thromboembolism
Pregnancy	Previously treated breast cancer
Undiagnosed vaginal bleeding	Previously treated uterine cancer
Unstable cardiovascular syndromes	Seizure disorder
	Uncontrolled hypertension
	Coronary artery disease
	Uterine fibroids

A. ESTROGEN

Systemic estrogen is administered orally or transdermally (Tables 35–4 and 35–5). Intravaginal estrogen therapy with or without standard HT may augment the treatment of urogenital symptoms (Table 35–6). Intravaginal estrogen is available in the form of creams, tablets, and intravaginal estradiol rings. Women usually insert the rings themselves, but the health care provider can assist with insertion and removal if necessary. There is no significant systemic absorption of estradiol with the intravaginal estradiol ring, and it does not stimulate the endometrium. This is an advantage for women with intact uteri who are not using progestins and for those who are suffering from local genitourinary symptoms who do not want or cannot tolerate the systemic effects of estrogen.

The use of intravaginal estrogen creams and tablets may occasionally be associated with systemic absorption, thus stimulating endometrial growth. Evaluation of the endometrium with an endometrial pipelle biopsy is necessary if endometrial stimulation is suspected. A progestin must accompany systemic estrogen replacement to prevent endometrial hyperplasia in women with intact uteri and in some women using vaginal estrogens.

Oral estrogen is available in multiple forms with variations in the metabolic half-lives between preparations. Estradiol-17β has the shortest half-life and requires split dosing for symptom control. Transdermal estradiol in patch form may benefit women who cannot tolerate or take oral forms because of nausea. It is also beneficial in women with elevated triglycerides because transdermal estradiol does not increase triglyceride levels to the same degree as oral estrogen. A skin gel may soon be available.

The typical starting dose of oral conjugated equine estrogen (CEE) or synthetic conjugated estrogen is 0.3–0.625 mg daily. Doses can be adjusted higher or lower depending on the symptoms after 1 mo of therapy. Younger women who have been surgically castrated may need higher doses of estrogen. Increased use of ultra-low doses of estrogen (such as 0.3 or 0.45 mg of CEE combined with ultra-low doses of medroxyprogesterone acetate [MPA]) is the new standard based on the favorable results regarding control of vasomotor symptoms, metabolic effects, bone benefits, and endometrial bleeding profile in symptomatic early postmenopausal women.

Conjugated equine estrogen has been used clinically for > 6 decades and is commonly used by postmenopausal women. However, some women prefer synthetic forms of conjugated estrogens, or natural, plant-derived, lab-synthesized estrogens that are not derived from animal products. If a woman cannot tolerate conjugated estrogens, other forms of estrogen, such as estrone (E_3), micronized estradiol (E_2), esterified estrogen, or transdermal E_2 (estradiol) should be considered. The FDA has approved all postmenopausal estrogens for the treatment of vasomotor symptoms and local genitourinary atrophy. Only some estrogens, however, have been FDA approved to prevent postmenopausal

Table 35–4. Oral estrogens.

Oral estrogens	Low dose (mg)	Standard dose (mg)	Medium dose (mg)	Higher doses (mg)	Highest doses (mg)
Cenestin (synthetic conjugated estrogen)		0.625	0.9	1.25	
Estinyl (ethinyl estradiol)	0.02	0.05		0.5	
Estrace (estradiol-17β	0.5	1.0		2.0	
Menest/estratab (esterified estrogen)	0.3	0.625		1.25	2.5
Ogen (estrone)		0.625		1.25	2.5
Ortho-Est (estrone)		0.625		1.25	
Premarin (conjugated equine estrogen)	0.3 (0.45 mg)	0.625	0.9	1.25	2.5

Table 35–5. Transdermal estrogens (estradiol-17β).

Patch	Low dose (mg)	Standard dose (mg)	Medium dose (mg)	Higher doses (mg)	Highest doses
Alora (matrix patch)		0.05	0.075	0.1	q3.5 days
Climara (matrix patch)	0.025	0.05	0.075	0.1	Weekly
Esclim (matrix patch)	0.025 0.0375	0.05	0.075	0.1	q3.5 days
Estraderm (reservoir patch)		0.05		0.1	q3.5 days
Vivelle Dot (matrix patch)	0.025 0.0375	0.05	0.075	0.1	q3.5 days

osteoporosis. Examples include CEE, CEE/MPA, estradiol, and estropipate.

B. PROGESTERONE

Progesterone downregulates estrogen receptors. Progestins are synthetic formulations that are better absorbed than micronized progesterone (Table 35–7). Oral progestins can be taken cyclically (12 days/month) or continuously (daily) at lower doses. For cyclic therapy, 5–10 mg of MPA or 200 mg of micronized progesterone is taken 12 days each month. Micronized progesterone is taken in the evening because of its potentially sedating and hypnotic effects. It is also taken with food to enhance absorption. Heavier and younger women may require larger doses of progestins. Cyclic therapy is usually preferable for recently menopausal women. The goal of cyclic therapy is to switch eventually to continuous combined (daily estrogen and progestin) therapy to promote amenorrhea, which is favored by most women. For continuous estrogen-progestin therapy, 1.5, 2.5, or 5 mg of MPA is taken every day. If ultra-low doses of estrogen are used, lower doses of MPA can be used, such as 1.5 mg of MPA or 100 mg of micronized progesterone daily. The addition of MPA to CEE appears to further enhance the benefits of estrogen in vasomotor symptom control. Progestins and estrogen are also available in combined forms, including a transdermal patch and oral pills (Table 35–8). Cyclic regimens cause withdrawal bleeding in the majority of users, whereas continuous use over 6 mo induces amenorrhea, a desired effect. An endometrial biopsy or a transvaginal ultrasonogram should be performed to assess the endometrial thickness if amenorrhea is not induced after 6 mo of continuous therapy. Endometrial stripes measuring > 5 mm in postmenopausal women are suspicious. Heavy bleeding that lasts > 1 week per month also warrants evaluation of the endometrium. Saline infusion sonography (SIS) can be used to visualize local defects, such as endometrial polyps or asymmetric areas in the endometrium via ultrasonography. Performed in either the outpatient or operative setting by an experienced operator, hysteroscopy provides direct visual information of the endometrium and the uterine cornua. The cornua is not well seen with SIS.

Most nonmalignant postmenopausal bleeding can be treated with progestin therapy. There are certain circumstances, however, when a hysterectomy is indicated (eg, atypical hyperplasia in women older than 30 and adenomatous hyperplasia without atypia in women who have had persistent uterine bleeding or who have failed progestin therapy). Uterine leiomyomas, pelvic pain, moderate to severe idiopathic uterine bleeding, and uterine hypertrophy may also warrant a hysterectomy.

Table 35–6. Intravaginal estrogens.

Estrogen	Dose
Estrace cream (ethinyl estradiol)	2 g daily intravaginally for 2 weeks, then 1 g 1–3 ×/week
Estring intravaginal ring (estradiol)	Delivers 7.5 µg daily intravaginally for 90 days
Ogen cream (estropipate)	2 g daily intravaginally for 2 weeks, then 1 g 1–3 ×/week
Premarin cream (conjugated equine estrogen)	2 g daily intravaginally for 2 weeks, then 1 g 1–3 ×/week
Vagifem tablets (estradiol)	25 µg daily intravaginally for 2 weeks, then 25 µg 2 ×/week
Femring (estradiol)	Delivers systemic and local estradiol for 90 days

Table 35-7. Oral progestins.

Oral Progestins	Dose
MPA (ultra-low dose)	1.5 mg may be combined with 0.3 or 0.45 mg CEE
Prometrium (progesterone USP)	100 mg daily or 200 mg days 1–12 (taken at night with food)
Provera (MPA)	10 mg days 1–12 or 2.5–5.0 mg daily
Prochieve 4% or 8%	Vaginal gel applied intravenously every other night

CEE, conjugated equine estrogen; MPA, medroxyprogesterone acetate.

Controversies of Estrogen Therapy in the Late Postmenopausal Phase

Use of HT in older, asymptomatic women does not show any primary or secondary cardiovascular benefit, whereas symptomatic HT users have experienced cardiovascular risk reduction, primarily in VTE and stroke. Explanations may include inability to control for all variables in the epidemiological data, unknown pharmacogenetic contributions, and particularly the specific hormonal and life phase in which HT is initiated. The data and the controversial underlying issues make the physician's decision to initiate HT in the late postmenopausal phase much more difficult. For the older woman who wants bone protection but has some increased risk for cardiovascular disease, stroke, and breast cancer, other agents besides HT should be considered.

A. VASOMOTOR SYMPTOMS

A small percentage of women continue to have vasomotor symptoms in the late postmenopausal phase. Some women who never had perimenopausal symptoms may develop vasomotor symptoms in their 60s and 70s because of an age-related decrease in testosterone production. The aromatization of endogenous testosterone to estradiol may have protected these women from vasomotor symptoms in their early menopausal years. Ultra-low doses of estrogen, such as 0.3 mg of CEE or .025 mg of transdermal estradiol-17β, may be of benefit as a low-dose alternative to the standard dose that a woman is already taking or, if appropriate, as an initial HT regimen. Initiation of HT must be very gradual and in lower doses in postmenopausal women. In older women, hormone therapy can be discontinued when vasomotor symptoms resolve, providing there are no other systemic indications for its continued use.

Some women may require higher doses of estrogen for vasomotor symptom control beyond the perimenopausal phase, making it difficult to transition to a standard dose of estrogen. In these women, low-dose testosterone allows for maintenance of a relatively low dose of estrogen for symptom control. Continuing testosterone supplementation in the late postmenopausal phase is controversial but can be offered to women with significant vasomotor symptoms who are at lower than average risk for cardiovascular disease. Plasma lipid levels, liver function tests, and clinical evidence of virilization should be monitored periodically during follow-up exams.

B. OSTEOPOROSIS

Bisphosphonates are the initial therapy of choice for hip fracture prevention in older, late postmenopausal women, although an 80% risk reduction for hip fractures has been demonstrated in women 75 years and older on long-term estrogen therapy. This risk reduction has not been equaled by any other medications, including bisphosphonates.

HT must be continued indefinitely to maintain its benefits. Ideally, the lowest dose of estrogen should be used to minimize long-term VTE and breast cancer risks and maintain osteoporosis protection. Raloxifene, 60 mg daily, may be considered for women with spinal osteopenia or osteoporosis who are at greater-than-average risk for breast cancer. Raloxifene appears to maintain bone density while possibly lowering the risk

Table 35-8. HT combination therapy.

HT combinations	Dose
Activella	1.0 mg estradiol-17β plus 0.5 mg NA
CombiPatch	0.05 mg estradiol-17β + 0.25 or 0.14 mg NA
Femhrt	5 μg ethinyl estradiol plus 1.0 mg NA
Ortho-Prefest	1.0 mg estradiol-17β for 3 days alternating with 1.0 mg estradiol-17β plus 0.09 mg NA for 3 days
Premphase	0.625 mg CEE alone days 1–14 followed by 0.625 mg CEE plus 5.0 mg MPA days 15–28
Prempro	2.5 or 5.0 mg MPA + 0.625 mg CEE (or 1.5 MPA and 0.45 CEE)

NA, norethindrone acetate; MPA, medroxyprogesterone acetate; CEE, conjugated equine estrogen.

for breast cancer. The VTE risk of raloxifene is equivalent to that of estrogen; however, there is no vasomotor benefit and no positive effect on skin or vaginal atrophy. Preliminary data on cognition do not show any increased risk of memory loss associated with raloxifene.

C. COGNITION

The prevalence of Alzheimer's Disease (AD) increases with age to nearly 50% in ≥ 85 years. Epidemiological studies of HT users compared with nonusers have demonstrated a reduction in risk or a delay in the clinical manifestations of dementia, particularly AD. However, a benefit of HT in women with established AD has not been established, and women who start hormone therapy in the late postmenopausal period may actually have an increased risk of dementia and stroke.

D. PHARMACOGENETICS

Pharmacogenetics may influence how women respond to HT. The prothrombin gene mutation variant is one example. HT users with hypertension who have this genetic variant have a 10- to 20-fold greater risk for myocardial infarction than HT users who do not carry this genetic variant. Factor V Leiden is another example of a genetic variant that may affect vascular events associated with HT use. However, ~188 women would need to be screened for the factor V Leiden variant and have HT withheld to prevent 1 VTE.

Genetic typing, particularly in combination with BMD testing, may also help identify women at high and low risk of fragility fractures. This insight would help risk-stratify long-term HT use in the late postmenopausal phase for osteoporotic protection. In addition, genetic differences in the estrogen receptor gene have been shown to affect lipids. Women with a specific estrogen receptor-α variant have markedly increased HDL cholesterol and no increase in ultra-sensitive C-reactive protein. It is hoped that pharmacogenetics will help identify women who will benefit the greatest and the least from long-term HT.

EVIDENCE-BASED POINTS

- *The routine well-care visit of the older woman should assess the stage of menopause and determine the physical, emotional, and sexual impact of estrogen deficiency.*
- *The impact of associated risks, such as heart disease, breast cancer, thromboembolism, uterine cancer, colon cancer, dementia, arthritis, skin aging, and osteoporosis as well as the relative risks and benefits of initiating, maintaining, or discontinuing HT should be discussed.*
- *A healthy lifestyle that includes good nutrition with adequate calcium and vitamin D is essential. Exercise must be emphasized to maintain strength and flexibility and minimize cardiovascular and osteoporosis risks.*

REFERENCES

Barrett-Connor E: Postmenopausal estrogen therapy and selected (less-often-considered) disease outcomes. Menopause 1999; 6:14. [PMID: 10100175]

Brincat MP: Hormone replacement therapy and the skin. Maturitas 2000;35:107. [PMID: 10924836]

Cauley JA et al: Estrogen replacement therapy and fractures in older women. Study of Osteoporotic Fractures Research Group. Ann Intern Med 1995;122:9. [PMID: 7985914]

Grady D et al: Postmenopausal hormone therapy increases risk for venous thromboembolic disease. The Heart and Estrogen/ Progestin Replacement Study. Ann Intern Med 2000;132: 689. [PMID: 10787361]

Henderson VW et al: Estrogen for Alzheimer's disease in women: randomized, double-blind, placebo-controlled trial. Neurology 2000;54:295. [PMID: 10668686]

Herrington DM et al: Common estrogen receptor polymorphism augments effects of hormone replacement therapy on E-selectin but not C-reactive protein. Circulation 2002;105: 1879. [PMID: not available]

Herrington DM et al: Estrogen-receptor polymorphisms and effects of estrogen on HDL-C in women with CAD. N Engl J Med 2002;346:967. [PMID: not available]

Hoibraaten E et al: Increased risk of recurrent venous thromboembolism during hormone replacement therapy–results of the randomized, double-blind, placebo- controlled estrogen in venous thromboembolism trial (EVTET). Thromb Haemost 2000;84:961. [PMID: 11154141]

Hulley S et al: Randomized trial of estrogen plus progestin for secondary prevention of coronary heart disease in postmenopausal women. Heart and Estrogen/Progestin Replacement Study (HERS) Research Group. JAMA 1998;280:605. [PMID: 9718051]

Kannus P et al: Prevention of hip fracture in elderly people with use of a hip protector. N Engl J Med 2000;343:1506. [PMID: 11087879]

O'Meara ES et al: Hormone replacement therapy after a diagnosis of breast cancer in relation to recurrence and mortality. J Natl Cancer Inst 2001;93:754. [PMID: 11353785]

Petri M: Exogenous estrogen in systemic lupus erythematosus: oral contraceptives and hormone replacement therapy. Lupus 2001;10:222. [PMID: 11315357]

Schairer C et al: Menopausal estrogen and estrogen-progestin replacement therapy and breast cancer risk. JAMA 2000;283: 485. [PMID: 10659874]

Shlipak MG et al: Hormone therapy and in-hospital survival after myocardial infarction in postmenopausal women. Circulation 2001;104:2300. [PMID: 11696469]

Simon JA et al: Effect of estrogen plus progestin on risk for biliary tract surgery in postmenopausal women with coronary artery disease. The Heart and Estrogen/Progestin Replacement Study. Ann Intern Med 2001;135:493. [PMID: 11578152]

Soules MR et al: Executive summary: Stages of Reproductive Aging Workshop (STRAW) Park City, Utah, July 2001. Menopause 2001;8:402. [PMID: not available]

Utian WH et al: Relief of vasomotor symptoms and vaginal atrophy with lower doses of conjugated equine estrogens and medroxyprogesterone acetate. Fertil Steril 2001;75:1065. [PMID: 11723411]

Villareal D et al: Bone mineral density response to estrogen replacement in frail elderly women: a randomized controlled trial. JAMA 2001;286:815. [PMID: 11497535]

Wang PN et al: Effects of estrogen on cognition, mood, and cerebral blood flow in AD: a controlled study. Neurology 2000;54:2061. [PMID: 10851363]

Women's Health Initiative Study Group: Risks and benefits of estrogen plus progestin in healthy postmenopausal women. Principal results from the Women's Health Initiative randomized controlled trial. JAMA 2002;288:321. [PMID: 12117397]

RELEVANT WORLD WIDE WEB SITE

National Osteoporosis Foundation: Osteoporosis Clinical Practice Guideline, B120: www.nof.org/professionals/clinical/clinical.htm

Health Issues of the Aging Male

Hosam Kamel, MD, & Laurie Dornbrand, MD

Life expectancy today is 74 years for men and 80 years for women, a remarkable rise in longevity from 100 years ago, when men lived an average of 48 years and women an average of 51 years. Men aged 65 currently have a life expectancy of another 16 years compared with another 19 years for women. In the past 10 years, life expectancy at birth has increased more for males than females, narrowing the gender gap in longevity. It has been postulated that the improvement in longevity can be ascribed to advances in medicine, healthier lifestyles, improved access to health care, and generally better health before age 65.

HYPOGONADISM & HORMONAL CHANGES OF THE AGING MALE

 ## ESSENTIALS OF DIAGNOSIS

- Testosterone as well as free and bioavailable testosterone levels tend to decline with age, and circadian fluctuation in testosterone also appears to decline with age.
- The hypogonadism associated with aging often appears to be hypothalamic/pituitary in origin and most often not accompanied by a rise in luteinizing hormone.
- Signs of testosterone deficiency include decreased libido, decreased sense of well-being, fatigue, osteoporosis, and loss of muscle mass.

General Considerations

Many but not all males undergo hormonal changes with age. Controversy exists regarding the terminology of male hormone change with age (eg, male menopause, andropause, male climacteric) and its clinical meaning. What is clear is that testosterone and the more clinically relevant forms bioavailable testosterone and free testosterone decline with age. Free testosterone measures the non-sex hormone-binding globulin (SHBG) non-albumin-bound testosterone, whereas bioavailable testos-

terone measures the non-SHBG-bound fraction (testosterone that is both free and albumin bound). The circadian rhythm of both free and bioavailable testosterone is blunted with age. Between the ages of 50 and 70, ~50% of healthy males will have bioavailable testosterone concentrations below the lowest level seen in men aged 20–40.

The decline in testosterone seen with aging appears to be due to secondary (hypogonadotropic) hypogonadism rather than primary hypogonadism. Low androgen in aging males often fails to produce an associated increase in luteinizing hormone (LH), suggesting an age-associated hypothalamic pituitary dysfunction. It appears likely that deficits reside at the hypothalamic/pituitary level, with an alteration in gonadotropin-releasing hormone (GnRH) secretory function, a decreased stimulation of LH, and delayed feedback by testosterone.

Clinical Findings

A. SIGNS & SYMPTOMS

Signs and symptoms of testosterone deficiency may include decrease in libido, decreased strength and muscle mass, osteoporosis, anemia, and fatigue (Table 36–1).

B. SCREENING TOOL

A validated questionnaire as a hypogonadism screening tool has been developed.

C. LABORATORY TESTS

Total testosterone levels may be normal in androgen-deficient elderly men because SHGB increases with aging. Therefore, free or bioavailable testosterone measurements are preferred. However, as an initial screen, a total testosterone level of < 200 can also be considered as diagnostic of hypogonadism. If the result is in the borderline range, either free or bioavailable testosterone should be measured. LH levels are not helpful in diagnosing hypogonadism in older men: A low value does not contradict the diagnosis.

Treatment

Treatment with testosterone has been shown to result in a marked improvement in libido. In addition, feelings of well-being and improvement in mood can occur

Table 36–1. Signs & symptoms of gonadal deficiency in men.

Loss/decrease of libido
Decreased muscle mass
Decreased strength
Decreased visuospatial skills
Osteoporosis
Arthralgias
Diminished well-being, impaired mood
Fatigue
Anemia
Increased irritability
Lethargy

with testosterone replacement in hypogonadal men. Improvement in muscle strength, bone mass, and erectile function appears variable.

Testosterone is usually administered via intramuscular injection or as transdermal patches. Oral testosterone is relatively contraindicated, as no 17β testosterone is available in the United States, and 17α compounds are associated with hepatotoxicity. Intramuscular injections of either testosterone enanthate or cypionate have an onset of action of 2–3 days and a duration of efficacy of ~ 2 weeks. A therapeutic response is sometimes seen after the second or third injection, even if there has been no response initially; thus, a series of 3 injections 2–3 weeks apart constitutes a reasonable therapeutic trial. Typical dosage regimens of testosterone injections are 200–300 mg intramuscularly every 2–4 weeks. Doses and dosing intervals are adjusted based on the extent and duration of the effect; it is not necessary to monitor testosterone levels. If treatment is successful and therapy is continued, the patient or partner may be taught to self-administer the injections.

Typical transdermal dosage regimens are 2.5–10 mg administered daily, usually adjusted in 2.5-mg increments. As with injections, they are titrated to effect, not serum level; however, as with injections, supraphysiological levels of bioavailable testosterone are not recommended. The scrotal patch (Testoderm) has been associated with skin irritation and adherence problems; because of the latter, shaving of scrotal hair is recommended. The nonscrotal patch (Androderm) is applied to truncal skin and has less associated skin irritation. Testosterone gel (Androgel) is applied to truncal skin (shoulders and abdomen). Skin-to-skin transfer to a partner is possible, so wearing a shirt over the application site is recommended during intimate contact.

Testosterone therapy is contraindicated in men with known or suspected prostate cancer. A baseline prostate-specific antigen (PSA) should be obtained before starting treatment; rectal exam and prostate symptom assessment are also recommended. Men with elevated PSA levels or abnormal prostate exams should be referred for urological clearance before considering treatment. Because testosterone stimulates red blood cell production, a baseline hemoglobin (Hgb) or hematocrit (Hct) should also be obtained. PSA and Hgb or Hct levels should be checked after 3 mo of treatment. However, polycythemia is dependent on neither dose nor duration of administration. PSA should be monitored at 6-mo intervals thereafter, as should hematocrit in men with values at the upper limit of normal. PSA increases of > 1.4 ng/mL between 2 measurements is cause for urological evaluation. Hct levels > 52 should prompt modification of the regimen.

Morley JE et al: Validation of a screening questionnaire for androgen deficiency in aging males. Metabolism 2000;49:1239. [PMID: 11016912]

MALE SEXUAL FUNCTION & DYSFUNCTION

Sexual behavior and interest continue into old age, although the proportion of sexually active persons declines. Of community-dwelling elders older than 70, ~ 30% report recent sexual intercourse. As in all age groups, there is marked individual variation in sexual interest and capacity. Apart from the increased prevalence of medical illnesses that impair sexual function, impediments to sexual activity in older adults may include social factors, such as unavailability of a sexually functional partner, and negative attitudes toward sexuality and aging.

Individuals who stay sexually active are less likely to report changes in function and may note less intense changes compared with those whose activity has been minimal or interrupted. This may in part reflect gradual adaptation to normal physiological changes, such as the need for increased time and stimulation to achieve erection, decreased firmness of erections, and increased sensitivity to drugs, such as alcohol, which impair sexual responsiveness.

Erectile Dysfunction

 ESSENTIALS OF DIAGNOSIS

- *Inability to achieve and maintain an erection adequate for intercourse.*

General Considerations

Erectile dysfunction (ED) is the most common sexual dysfunction in men. Although this problem is often referred to as impotence, the latter term is imprecise and pejorative and thus preferably avoided. About 70% of men have ED by age 70, usually as the result of vascular disease. Vascular causes include atherogenic arterial disease (impaired inflow), venous disease (impaired outflow), or a combination of these. Other causes are listed in Table 36–2.

Clinical Findings

A. PATIENT ASSESSMENT

The goals of assessment are to identify the type and extent of dysfunction and contributing medical causes.

Chronic medical conditions, particularly diabetes and vascular and neurological disease, as well as prior surgical procedures in the abdominal-pelvic region should be identified. A complete list of medications should be obtained: Antihypertensive agents, including diuretics, and psychotropic medication are the drugs most likely to cause ED, but many other agents may be associated, including alcohol and drugs of abuse. Patients should be asked to describe the onset of symptoms, the relationship of symptoms to events or medications, whether erections occur under any circumstances, such as with manual stimulation or spontaneously, and the estimated firmness of the best erections obtainable. Libido is typically unaffected; loss of libido raises the index of suspicion for hypogonadism as well as for pharmacological or psychological precipitants. The ability to have orgasms and to ejaculate is frequently preserved in men with ED; the absence of ejaculation suggests a neurogenic cause.

B. VASCULAR ASSESSMENT

Vascular examination should include measurement of blood pressure, assessment of peripheral pulses, and auscultation for abdominal and inguinal bruits. Neurological exam should include deep tendon reflexes and motor-sensory exam of the legs. Integrity of the sacral plexus is assessed by perianal sensation (S2–S4), sphincter tone (S4–S5), and bulbocavernosus reflex, a contraction of the anal sphincter when the glans penis is squeezed (S2–S4). Secondary sexual characteristics (beard, body hair, and testicular size and consistency) as well as gynecomastia should be noted, but these are less sensitive indicators of hypogonadism in older men.

Testosterone should be tested in men with ED, although the diagnosis of hypogonadism in unlikely in a man with normal libido. Because of the strong association between diabetes and ED, and because ED can be the presenting complaint in type 2 diabetes mellitus, a fasting glucose level or HgbA$_{1C}$ should be obtained. Thy-

Table 36–2. Causes of erectile dysfunction.

Dysfunction	Cause
Vascular disorders	
	Arterial, venous leak syndrome, penile Reynaud's, trauma
Medication	
	Diuretics
	Antihypertensives (all classes)
	Tranquilizers, antidepressants, antipsychotics
	H$_2$ receptor blockers
	Digoxin
	Estrogens, antiandrogens
	Nonsteroidals
	Anticonvulsants
"Street" drugs	
	Tobacco
	Alcohol
	Opiates or marijuana
Endocrine or metabolic disorders	
	Diabetes
	Hyperproplactinemia
	Thyroid disease (both hypo and hyper)
	Hypogonadism
	Cushing's disease and syndrome
	Altered neurotransmitters
Neurological disorders	
	Autonomic dysfunction
	Sensory neuropathy
	Spinal cord injury
	Cerebrovascular accidents
	Temporal lobe epilepsy
	Multiple sclerosis
Systemic disorders	
	Renal failure
	Chronic obstructive pulmonary disease
	Cirrhosis
	Myotonia dystrophica
Psychological disorders	
	Depression
	Performance anxiety
	Widower's syndrome
	Stress
Miscellanous	
	Peyronie's disease

roid function tests and other baseline lab studies, such as complete blood cell count and chemistry panel with liver function tests should be performed if they have not already been done in the course of other medical care. When the index of suspicion is high, a prolactin level may be helpful but should not be ordered routinely.

Vascular studies, ranging from Doppler measurement of penile pulsation to more sophisticated assessments of flow, are useful principally when surgical interventions are being considered. Nocturnal penile tumescence testing does not add significant information to that available from the history and physical exam.

Treatment

A single cause for ED, such as a medication or hypogonadism, is identified in only a minority of older men. When a drug has been identified as the potential cause of ED, a period of 4–6 weeks off the agent may be necessary to detect improvement. In many situations, however, it is not practical to discontinue or change the offending medications. A trial of testosterone in hypogonadal men may be warranted if there are no contraindications. However, when the cause is multifactorial, testosterone treatment or adjusting medications alone may not be adequate to correct the problem.

The goal of treatment should be a satisfactory sexual experience rather than simply a firm erection. Choice among the available treatment options is influenced by patient and partner preferences. When possible, the patient's partner should be included in treatment decisions to clarify expectations and avoid misinformation.

A. Pharmacology

1. Testosterone—Testosterone may correct ED in hypogonadal men but is more effective at improving libido, energy, and sense of well-being. Its efficacy has not been demonstrated in men with normal testosterone levels and may be limited in hypogonadal men with other considerations for testosterone therapy.

2. Selective phosphodiesterase type 5 (PDE5) inhibitors—Sildenafil, vardenafil, and tadalafil are oral agents with response rates of ~ 50–80% in men with ED of various types. They have become the initial treatments of choice in most practice settings. These agents promote erection by inhibiting the degradation of cyclic guanosine monophosphate (cGMP). They potentiate the hypotensive efects of nitrates and are contraindicated in patients who take nitrates in any form. The cardiac risk appears to be related to the physiological effects of exertion rather than the drugs themselves; risk of untoward events may be unacceptably high in men with low cardiac output, resting hypotension, and other manifestations of severe cardiac compromise. These agents can interact with α-blockers and CYP 3A4 inhibitors such as ketoconazole. They should be used cautiously in men with impaired renal or hepatic function.

Sildenafil has the longest safety record of these drugs and is preferred for that reason. Side effects are dose related and include headache, flushing, dyspepsia, and transient visual changes. It is available in 25-, 50-, and 100-mg tablets, and a starting dose of 25 mg is recommended in older men. Sildenafil should be taken 1–2 h prior to sexual activity and has a duration of action of about 4 hours. Absorption is slowed if the pill is consumed in proximity to a high-fat meal.

Vardenafil is available in 2.5-, 5-, 10- and 20-mg tablets and is similar in price, onset, and duration of action of sildenafil. Tadalafil is available in 5-, 10-, and 20-mg tablets, has a slower onset of action (~ 45 min) and a longer duration of action (~ 36 h) than the other two agents. High fat meals do not impact its absorption.

Patients should understand that these medications potentiate rather than produce erections; achieving an erection will still require sexual stimulation. The price of these pills is about $10 per dose; the tablets may be broken to reduce the cost per dose.

3. Vasodilators—Intracorporeal injections or urethral suppositories of vasodilators, such as prostaglandin E_1 (Alprostadil) or papaverine (with or without phentolamine), can produce erections when self-administered just before intercourse. Papaverine is not approved for use for erectile dysfunction. Short-term side effects include local pain, burning sensation, bruising, and induration. Long-term effects may include fibrosis of the penile shaft, manifested by nodules, diffuse scarring, plaque, or curvature. The incidence of side effects is lower with prostaglandin E_1 than with papaverine; however, the cost (≥ $20 per dose) is at least twice as much. Injection therapy is best prescribed and supervised by a urologist, who can manage the rare complications (eg, priapism, hematoma) should they occur. Injection therapy has been far supplanted by use of sildenafil.

4. Other agents—Although many other agents are touted to improve male sexual function, including yohimbine and a number of herbal supplements, there is scant evidence to support their efficacy.

B. Mechanical Devices

Vacuum tumescence devices are highly effective in ED of almost all causes and have few side effects and contraindications. Erections are induced by negative pressure, which enhances the flow of blood into the penis. This is attained by placing a plastic tube over the penis, obtaining a seal, and creating a vacuum with a hand or battery-operated pump. The erection is maintained by a latex constriction ring, which is slid off the tube onto the penis and may be left in place for up to 30 min. Men with Peyronie's disease may have difficulty fitting a cylinder over the penile curvature, and caution is recommended in those taking coumadin, although serious bruising is rarely a problem. The erections achieved are not completely the same as a natural erection; patients and partners may describe a cold blue penis and hinge effect (the penis pivoting from the base). An unexpected benefit in a small proportion of men is the spontaneous return of natural erections after a period of using the device. Although this phenomenon has not been studied, it is theorized that the repeated stimulation increases regional vascularity.

Patient reluctance to use a mechanical device may be difficult to overcome. However, a skillful orientation to the use of the vacuum device enhances the chance of success. The cost of a set ranges from $150–400; a substantial proportion is reimbursed by Medicare. It is highly recommended that devices be dispensed from companies with strong customer support and preferably with available clinical instruction in using the system.

C. SURGICAL OPTIONS

Patient preference should dictate the therapeutic option chosen. Penile prosthetic devices are usually used as a last resort. Options include malleable, hinged, rigid, or inflatable devices. Ideally, the potential burdens and benefits of each option should be discussed extensively with a physician with expertise in the area before a decision is made.

Fink HA et al: Sildenafil for male erectile dysfunction: a systematic review and meta-analysis. Arch Intern Med 2002;162:1349. [PMID: 12076233] (This update concluded that sildenafil is safe and effective and is not associated with adverse cardiovascular outcomes in men who are not taking nitrates.)

Goldstein I et al: Oral sildenafil in the treatment of erectile dysfunction. N Engl J Med 1998;338:1397. [PMID: 9580646] (Sildenafil was safe and effective in a variety of causes of erectile dysfunction.)

Lue TF: Erectile dysfunction. N Engl J Med 2000;342:1802. [PMID: 10853004] (A thorough review of pathophysiology and treatment of erectile dysfunction.)

Ejaculatory Dysfunction

Ejaculation, the forceful emission of semen from the urethra, is distinct from orgasm, although the 2 processes typically occur together. The volume of ejaculate is decreased in normal aging, as are duration and intensity of orgasmic contractions.

Retrograde or absent ejaculation occurs in older men as a result of incomplete closure of the bladder neck during ejaculation. This condition may result from transurethral prostatectomy (TURP) or bladder neck incisions, diabetic autonomic neuropathy, α-blocker therapy for prostatism, as well as spinal cord injuries. Cloudiness of the first voided urine after ejaculation helps establish the diagnosis; microscopic examination of the urine for spermatozoa can be performed but is rarely necessary. Unless fertility is an issue, which is not

often the case for an older man, treatment to reverse retrograde ejaculation is rarely pursued, and reassurance may be the only treatment necessary. Premature ejaculation is the most common ejaculatory dysfunction in younger men but is unusual in the elderly.

Delayed or absent orgasm may be a side effect of antidepressant medications, notably the selective serotonin reuptake inhibitor (SSRI) class. Clinical surveys suggest that these effects are more common than is reported in the drug literature. Antidepressants with the lowest prevalence of side effects are reportedly bupropion (Wellbutrin), nefazodone (Serzone), and possibly mirtazepine (Remeron). Reasonable approaches to managing anti-depressant-induced sexual dysfunction are to reduce the drug dosage, wait for adaptation, and consider interrupting drug treatment or switching to a drug with presumed lower incidence of dysfunction. A number of pharmacological antidotes have been used, including sildenafil, buspirone, and psychostimulants, based largely on case reports rather than controlled studies.

BENIGN PROSTATIC HYPERPLASIA

 ESSENTIALS OF DIAGNOSIS

- Symptoms of obstruction and irritation on voiding.
- An elevated American Urologic Association score.
- Possible enlargement of prostate on exam.
- Absence of other diagnoses that might causes symptoms (eg, prostatitis)

General Considerations

The incidence of benign prostatic hyperplasia (BPH) increases in men after age 40. Approximately 50% of men between the ages of 51 and 60 in the United States have BPH. By the age of 80, the prevalence is 80%. Both genetic and environmental factors have been implicated in the development of BPH.

Clinical Findings

A. SYMPTOMS & SIGNS

Men with BPH often present with lower urinary tract symptoms, including increased urinary frequency, urgency, nocturia, intermittent urination, incomplete bladder emptying, straining on micturition, and weak urinary stream. Such symptoms may be caused by conditions other than BPH (eg, lower urinary tract infection, bladder cancer, bladder stone, or prostate cancer). Thus, initial assessment of a patient presenting with lower urinary tract symptoms should focus on ensuring that these symptoms are due to BPH and not other causes.

Assessment of the degree of the symptoms of BPH and their impact on the quality of life is easily achieved using a symptom score sheet developed by the American Urologic Association (AUA; Table 36–3). In this assessment tool, each symptom is assigned a score. Based on the total score, symptom severity is described as mild, moderate, or severe. This symptom score is not specific for BPH and thus should be corroborated with other signs from the history and physical.

B. Physical Examination

A comprehensive medical history and a focused clinical examination combined with targeted tests enable an accurate diagnosis of BPH in the majority of cases.

The digital rectal examination (DRE) is an important component of the physical examination of a man presenting with lower urinary symptoms. During this examination, prostate size, shape and consistency should be evaluated. The prostate gland in an individual with BPH is usually smooth, symmetrically enlarged, and rubbery in consistency, and the central sulcus can often be felt. A tender, firm prostate usually indicates prostatitis, whereas a hard, nodular prostate with loss of the central sulcus should raise the suspicion of prostate cancer (see Chapter 30 for a discussion of prostate cancer). However, it is the posterior portion that can be palpated. Urinalysis and a kidney function test should also be performed in men presenting with lower urinary symptoms. PSA testing is optional and depends on patient preferences and goals of care. Current recommendations include DRE and PSA assessment in men older than 50 with a life expectancy > 10 years. Risks and benefits of screening should be discussed.

Treatment

Treatment depends on severity of symptoms and patient preferences. Patients with mild symptoms (AUA scores

Table 36–3. Symptom score sheet to assess BPH symptoms.

Variable	Not at all	> 1 time in 5	< Half the time	Half the time	> Half the time	Almost always	Patient score
Incomplete emptying: Over the past month, how often have you had a sensation of not emptying your bladder completely after you finished urinating?	0	1	2	3	4	5	
Frequency: Over the past month, how often have you had to urinate again < 2 h after you finished urinating?	0	1	2	3	4	5	
Intermittency: Over the past month, how often have you found you stopped and started again several times when you urinated?	0	1	2	3	4	5	
Urgency: Over the past month, how often have you found it difficult to postpone urination?	0	1	2	3	4	5	
Weak stream: Over the past month, how often have you had a weak urinary stream?	0	1	2	3	4	5	
Straining: Over the past month, how often have you had to push or strain to begin urination?	0	1	2	3	4	5	
Nocturia: Over the past month, how many times did you most typically get up to urinate from the time you went to bed at night until the time you got up in the morning?	0	1	2	3	4	5	
Total score							

Adapted from Barry MJ et al: The American Urological Association Symptoms index for benign prostatic hyperplasia. J Urol 1992;148:1549. Used with permission.

< 8) usually do well with watchful waiting. Those with moderate to severe symptoms (AUA scores ≥ 8) should be counseled on the benefits and risks of watchful waiting, medical therapy, and surgery. Patients with moderate to severe symptoms may require additional testing, including urinary flow rates, postvoid residual urine, and ultrasonography. Men who have refractory urinary retention, recurrent urinary tract infection, recurrent or gross hematuria, bladder stones, or renal insufficiency related to BPH should be counseled to receive a more acute form of intervention such as surgery.

The α_1-receptors are situated on smooth muscle cells in prostatic stroma and capsule as well as in the urethra and bladder neck. Norepinephrine binds to the α_1-receptors and stimulates smooth muscle contraction, resulting in urinary outflow obstruction. Prazosin, a selective α_1-receptor blocker, was found to improve symptom scores and urine flow rates and decrease postvoid residual volume in patients with BPH. Other selective α_1-receptor blockers include doxazosin and terazosin. More recently, so-called uroselective inhibitors of the α_{1A}-adrenoreceptors (eg, tamsulosin) have been developed and are useful in men with lower blood pressure, orthostasis, or other cardiovascular side effects. The α-adrenergic receptor blockers have been shown to improve symptom scores and flow rates. These drugs have a rapid onset of action, with symptom improvement that may begin rapidly, and achieve full therapeutic benefit by 3 mo. Side effects of α-adrenergic receptor blockers were reported in 10–15% of cases and include orthostatic hypotension, fatigue, dizziness, headaches, falls, and, less frequently, asthenia, palpitations, and gastrointestinal disturbances such as nausea, vomiting, diarrhea, and constipation. Although the hypotensive effect of α_1-blockers may be desirable in some hypertensive patients with BPH, α-blockers are not associated with the beneficial cardiovascular effects seen with other antihypertensive classes and should not be considered as the most appropriate antihypertensive therapy. Dosages are as follows: prazocin, 1–5 mg orally twice daily; terazocin, 1–10 mg orally every day; doxazocin, 1–8 mg orally every day; and tamsulosin, .4–.8 mg orally every day. One should start with the lowest possible dose and increase slowly until the patient is satisfied or the maximum dose is reached. The physician should warn the patient about the potential of orthostatic hypotension, particularly with any increase in dose.

Finasteride, a drug that inhibits the 5 α-reductase enzyme, has been shown to reduce urinary retention and need for invasive therapy in men with BPH and demonstrated prostate enlargement. Combination therapy with an α-blocker and finasteride reduces the risk of overall clinical progression of BPH when compared to either therapy alone. Finasteride may decrease overall prostate cancer while increasing the risk of high-grade prostate cancer. Other side effects of finasteride include decreased libido and erectile dysfunction. Because of the potential risk associated with its use, physicians should counsel men about potential risks and benefits before beginning finasteride therapy. The dose is 5 mg orally daily.

Saw palmetto and other herbal supplements are commonly used by men as treatments for BPH. Data suggest that saw palmetto can improve symptoms but has no effect on urinary flow rates or quality of life. Side effects may include gastrointestinal distress, and decreased libido.

Surgical options include TURP, transurethral incision of the prostate (TUIP), and open prostatectomy. TURP achieves ≥ 75% chance of symptom improvement and ~85% reduction in symptom score. Complications include bleeding requiring transfusion in 8% of cases, urethral strictures and bladder neck stenoses requiring surgery in 5% of cases, and rarely the development of transurethral syndrome, which results from the absorption of irrigating fluid via the prostatic veins, resulting in hyponatremia and volume overload. In addition, 65% of men will have retrograde ejaculation after TURP. TURP does not, however, affect potency. Open prostatectomy is used when the prostate is too large for endoscopic removal or in the presence of other comorbid urological conditions, but it has a higher complication rate than TURP. TUIP is an option for some men with small prostates and moderate to severe symptoms and is associated with fewer complications than TURP. Other techniques include transurethral vaporization of the prostate, laser ablation, transurethral microwave thermotherapy, transurethral needle ablation, and balloon dilation.

EVIDENCE-BASED POINTS

- α-Adrenergic blockers or finasteride are effective in reducing symptoms in men with BPH.
- Combination therapy with an α-adrenergic blocker and finasteride reduces the risk of overall clinical progression of BPH more than either drug alone.
- Finasteride may delay or prevent prostate cancer overall, but may increase the risk of high-grade prostate cancer.
- Watchful waiting is a reasonable alternative to surgery in symptomatic men without complications of BPH.

REFERENCES

McConnell JD et al: The long-term effect of doxazocin, finasteride, and combinatin therapy on the clinical progression of benign prostatic hyperplasia. N Engl J Med 2003;349:2387. (This 4.5 year trial found that combination therapy with doxazocin and finasteride reduced the risk of overall clinical progression of BPH more than did treatment with either drug alone.)

AUA Practice Guidelines Committee: AUA Guideline on management of benign prostatic hyperplasia (2003). Diagnosis and treatment recommendations. J Urol 2003;170:530. (Reviews evaluation and treatment of BPH based on current evidence.)

Thompson IM et al: The influence of finasteride on the devleopment of prostate cancer. N Engl J Med 2003;349:215. [PMID:12824459] (This randomized trial suggested that finasteride prevents the appearance of prostate cancer, but increases risk of high grade prostate cancer. Men taking finasteride had fewer urinary problems but higher rates of sexual side effects than the placebo group.)

Principles of Rehabilitation

Laura Mosqueda, MD, & Chinh D. Le, MD

Rehabilitation is one of the most basic components of comprehensive care for the elderly. It is more than a process: it is a philosophical approach that emphasizes function, autonomy, and quality of life. Rehabilitation is defined as restoration of the ill or injured to an optimal functional level in the home or community in relation to physical, psychosocial, vocational, and recreational activity. The American Geriatrics Society defines rehabilitation as the maintenance and restoration of physical and psychological health necessary for independent living and functional independence.

In general, rehabilitation is concerned with lessening the impact of disabling conditions on individuals and their family members. This is especially important in the elderly, who often have multiple comorbid conditions. Although it is possible that a single event such as a stroke leads to the need for rehabilitation, this may be complicated by coexisting morbidity (eg, Alzheimer's disease). In other cases, there may be multiple concomitant conditions that lead to the need for rehabilitation, such as occurs in a person who has severe osteoarthritis, emphysema, depression, and diabetic neuropathy.

As the population ages, the prevalence of chronic diseases increases as does the rate of disability, defined as an inability to perform 1 or more activity of daily living (ADL) or instrumental ADL (IADL). Although there are reports of a decline in disability in the over-65 population, the prevalence of disability among people older than 65 remains quite high (~20%) and significantly increases with age (Figure 37–1).

DISEASE, IMPAIRMENT, DISABILITY, HANDICAP

In 1980, the World Health Organization (WHO) International Classification of Impairments, Disabilities, and Handicaps (ICIDH) used a model of disease, impairment, disabilities, and handicaps to characterize the disablement process. *Disease* is the underlying diagnosis or pathological process, noticeable at a microscopic level. It may progress to a point at which an organ system is unable to function normally, causing an *impairment*. An impairment of an organ system that causes a restriction or lack of ability to perform ADLs is a *disability*. A person with a disability who is unable to fulfill social roles is said to be *handicapped*. A person

is not handicapped by virtue of a disability; rather, it is society that handicaps an individual by not providing adequate accommodations. In May 2001, the WHO released a revision of ICIDH, known as International Classification of Functioning, Disability, and Health (ICF), which introduced the concepts of body functions and structures, activities and participation, and environmental and personal factors to replace the concepts of impairments, disabilities, and handicap. In this model, the function of an individual in a specific domain is an interaction of the complex relationship between the health condition and contextual factors (Figure 37–2).

REHABILITATION SITES

In theory, rehabilitation can and should be given in all care settings. Although a rehabilitative philosophy may be used in all settings, medical reimbursement and the patient's overall condition usually decide the site of rehabilitation practice. Rehabilitation should be started as soon as a patient is able to tolerate the exercises to prevent secondary functional loss and promote early restoration of function. Each setting has its own advantages and disadvantages (Table 37–1).

Acute Inpatient Rehabilitation

Acute inpatient rehabilitation is usually provided for the patient who needs at least 2 different therapies (ie, physical therapy, occupational therapy, speech therapy), is able to tolerate therapy at least 3 h/day 6 days/week, and is likely to show significant improvement. The patient is usually monitored by an interdisciplinary team that includes a physician who is experienced in rehabilitation. Weekly team meetings allow for review, discussion, and planning of the rehabilitation process. The duration of inpatient rehabilitation varies from days to months depending on many factors (eg, clinical diagnoses, potential for functional gain, rate of recovery, family support, and insurance issues).

Subacute Rehabilitation

Patients who are not appropriate candidates for acute inpatient rehabilitation may benefit from subacute rehabilitation in a skilled nursing facility. Medicare and

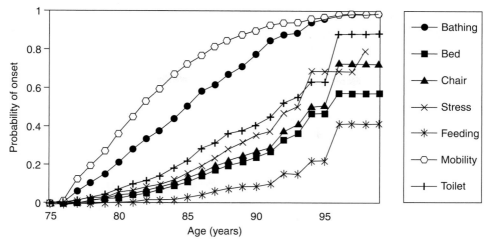

Figure 37–1. Age at onset of activity of daily living disability for all persons (N = 1244). From Jagger C et al: Patterns of onset of disability in activities of daily living with age. J Am Geriatr Soc 2001;49:406. Used with permission.

fee-for-service insurance cover physical therapy, occupational therapy, and speech therapy in the nursing home as long as the patient has been recently hospitalized for at least 3 consecutive days and the patient's condition is expected to improve with therapy. Many managed-care plans do not require a qualifying 3-day hospital stay. The patient is also eligible for rehabilitation in the skilled nursing facility if he or she has been

home < 30 days after a 3-day hospitalization. The patient must be able to tolerate two 30-min sessions of therapy per day and must require at least 1 skilled nursing need. Medicare gives a 100-day benefit for each qualified skilled nursing home admission. When this period ends, the patient must be reevaluated to determine whether he or she qualifies for another 100-day benefit period.

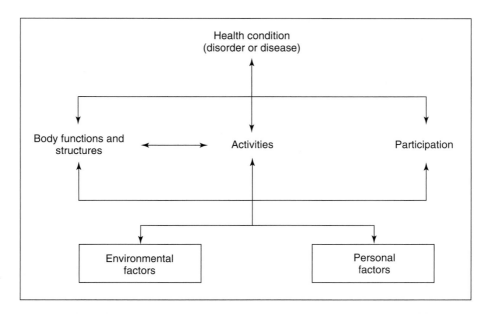

Figure 37–2. Interactions between the components of ICF. From World Health Organization.

Table 37–1. Advantages & disadvantages of rehabilitation setting.

Setting	Advantage	Disadvantage
Acute inpatient	Early start	Not all patients are eligible (must be able to tolerate therapy ≥ 3 h day 6 days/week)
	Therapy can be bedside or in the gym	High cost
	Interdisciplinary team approach	Uses acute Medicare days
Skilled nursing facility	No requirement for 3 h of therapy/day	Eligibility criteria required (3-day hospitalization, need of ≥ 1 nursing skill, able to tolerate two 30-min sessions of therapy per day)
	Does not use acute Medicare days	
	Length of stay longer than acute inpatient	Length of therapy somewhat limited by Medicare
Home	Usually preferred by patient	Usually not well equipped
	Therapist is able to evaluate home environment and need	May be burden on family
	Covered by Medicare	Only a certain number of visits allowed
	No transportation required	No peer group
Outpatient	Access to equipment	Transportation required
	Covered by Medicare and most insurance	
	Peer interaction and support	

Home Rehabilitation

Home is often the best site for the rehabilitation process. A home evaluation by the therapist helps to determine how the physical environment can be adapted to meet the needs of the patient. Home rehabilitation is covered under Medicare and requires ongoing supervision by a physician, who certifies continuing benefit and continuing need.

Outpatient Rehabilitation

For some patients, outpatient rehabilitation is the best option. Outpatient rehabilitation is suited for those who can be at home, have adequate resources for transportation to appointments, and benefit from the equipment in an outpatient rehabilitation department. Another, somewhat hidden, advantage to outpatient rehabilitation is peer interaction. Peers may encourage each other to achieve more.

PROCESS OF REHABILITATION

A comprehensive geriatric assessment is often helpful before the initiation of a rehabilitation program to assist with setting realistic goals with each patient. The assessment should include measures of a person's ability to perform tasks necessary to daily living, leisure activities, and social interactions. Several standardized assessment scales have been developed to facilitate and standardize the assessment process. The functional assessment scale selected should be multifaceted; ideally, it measures the

disability of concern, monitors progress, enhances communication between team members, including patient and family, and measures the effectiveness of rehabilitation interventions. Regardless of whether a standardized instrument is used, a thorough multidisciplinary assessment is essential at a very early stage of the process.

The ultimate goal of a rehabilitation process is to attain optimal function at home and in the community, as defined by the patient. A patient's autonomy must be taken seriously, and time and effort should be spent to ascertain the patient's true wishes. Two people with the same impairment and resulting disability may have very different goals. One may want to return to a very active lifestyle involving exercise, volunteer activities, and baby-sitting grandchildren. The other may wish to return to a sedentary lifestyle that involves staying at home and watching television. The patient and the team will become very frustrated if the patient and team goals are not aligned.

Another important aspect in geriatric rehabilitation is understanding the availability and capability of family caregivers if assistance will be needed after discharge. Many families are willing to provide both emotional and practical support to their loved ones. To minimize caregiver burden and maximize the likelihood of a successful transition to home, the team needs to determine what level of functional recovery is necessary in order for the caregiver to assume care.

The outcome of the rehabilitation process and effectiveness of the rehabilitative intervention can be measured by assessing the patient's function at appropriate intervals and comparing the changes over periods of time. Therefore, it is important to select the functional assessment instruments that are valid and reliable for this purpose. The Functional Independence Measure (FIM; Figure 37–3) was designed as a comprehensive functional assessment instrument, usable by any trained health care professional regardless of discipline. It is short, practical, and easy to use and measures physical function as well as areas of communication and social cognition. It has been proven to have high validity and reliability. However, the FIM does have some limitations. Although it is designed to be scored by any rehabilitation team member, some disciplines may have more difficulty than others in assessing particular items in FIM. In addition, it may not be sensitive enough to measure change in disability among some patient populations (eg, patients with high-level spinal cord injury [C4-5 and C5-6], chronic pain, and traumatic brain dysfunction).

Geriatric rehabilitation (particularly in the inpatient setting) is ideally delivered via an interdisciplinary team, typically including a physician, nurse, physical and occupational therapists, speech and language pathologist, psychologist, social worker, dietitian, and recreational therapist (Table 37–2). Usually the physician is the team leader. In many rehabilitation programs, the physician team leader is a specialist in physical medicine and rehabilitation. In many geriatric programs, it is the geriatrician who leads the interdisciplinary team.

Nursing staff play a key role in the rehabilitation process, especially in inpatient rehabilitation. The nurse provides nursing care, ensures that all orders from all disciplines are performed, and trains family members to assist the patient on discharge. The nurse interacts most frequently with the patient and thus is able to reinforce and apply therapy interventions during daily activities on the ward.

The physical therapist focuses on promoting mobility (eg, ambulation and transfer), whereas the occupational therapist helps with performance in other ADLs and IADLs. The speech and language therapist evaluates and treats communication problems (such as aphasia), cognitive problems, and dysphagia, and the recreational therapist helps modify the treating environment according to patient preferences and prepares the patient to return to leisure activities. Because the intensive therapy sessions typically occupy only 3 h/day, it is important that the techniques, exercises, and approaches learned during these sessions be reinforced when the patient returns to the ward.

EQUIPMENT

Equipment in geriatric rehabilitation should be used appropriately to provide the best benefits and safety. Patients' and caregivers' preferences are also important.

Some types of equipment are very basic but often overlooked, such as eyeglasses, hearing aids, dentures, and appropriate footwear.

For patients with gait problems, canes, crutches, or walkers may be appropriate (Table 37–3). The function of a cane is to widen the base of support and improve balance. Cane height should reach approximately to the level of the greater trochanter and permit elbow flexion to ~20–30°. For relieving weight-bearing pain, it should be placed in the hand opposite the painful lower extremity. The broad-based quad cane provides more stability. Walkers offer bilateral support for balance and stability while walking. Standard walkers have no wheels and must be picked up. Front-wheel walkers require less coordination between upper and lower extremities and, therefore, are often prescribed for patients with ataxic gait and those who are unable to lift and move the standard walker (eg, frail elderly). However, they are less stable than a standard walker and harder to use on thick carpet. Wheelchairs and scooters are other assistive devices for mobility. ADL adaptive devices such as reachers, built-up feeding utensils, swivel spoons, rocker knives, walker baskets, sock aids, and specially designed clothing and shoes may be useful depending on each situation.

Environmental adaptations are usually focused on modification of bathrooms and entryways. Raised toilet seats and associated grab bars or frames make it safer and easier to use the toilet. Tub and shower seats, nonstick tub surfaces, and grab bars are useful bathing aids. The home entrance may be modified with railings, grab bars, and ramps. Wheelchair ramps should rise about 1 in. for every 12 in. in length.

DISCHARGE PLANNING

Discharge planning should begin as soon as the patient's condition is stabilized and probable functional outcome can be predicted. If the patient is a candidate for nursing home living, rehabilitation should be focused on adjusting to disability and on basic functions that will improve quality of life in the nursing home (ie, swallowing, positioning, seating). The patient will often continue to have functional improvement with rehabilitation at a nursing home. If the patient plans to return home, complete detailed information on home structure and support should be provided by the family or through a home visit. Clear, well-informed communication about care needs and rehabilitation goals among the patient, rehabilitation team, and family/caregivers is essential before any discharge and ideally should be discussed throughout the rehabilitation process.

FIM™ instrument

L E V E L S	7 Complete Independence (Timely, Safely) 6 Modified Independence (Device)	**NO HELPER**
	Modified Dependence 5 Supervision (Subject = 100%+) 4 Minimal Assist (Subject = 75%+) 3 Moderate Assist (Subject = 50%+) Complete Dependence 2 Maximal Assist (Subject = 25%+) 1 Total Assist (Subject = less than 25%)	**HELPER**

	ADMISSION	DISCHARGE	FOLLOW-UP
Self-Care A. Eating B. Grooming C. Bathing D. Dressing-Upper Body E. Dressing-Lower Body F. Toileting			
Sphincter Control G. Bladder Management H. Bowel Management			
Transfers I. Bed, Chair, Wheelchair J. Toilet K. Tub, Shower			
Locomotion L. Walk/Wheelchair M. Stairs	W Walk C Wheelchair B Both	W Walk C Wheelchair B Both	W Walk C Wheelchair B Both
Motor Subtotal Score			
Communication N. Comprehension O. Expression	A Auditory V Visual B Both V Vocal N Nonvocal B Both	A Auditory V Visual B Both V Vocal N Nonvocal B Both	A Auditory V Visual B Both V Vocal N Nonvocal B Both
Social Cognition P. Social Interaction Q. Problem Solving R. Memory			
Cognitive Subtotal Score			
TOTAL FIM Score			

NOTE: Leave no blanks. Enter 1 if patient not testable due to risk

Figure 37–3. FIM Instrument. Uniform Data System for Medical Rehabilitation, State University of New York at Buffalo. Used with permission.

Table 37–2. Geriatric rehabilitation team.

Team member	Role
Patient and family	Participate in setting goals, long-term disability management
Rehabilitation nurse	Patient care, case management, patient and family interaction and teaching
Social worker	Case management, assessment of family and community resources, discharge planning
Physician	Provides medical care for disability and comorbid conditions, usually team leader
Occupational therapy	Helps to improve ADLs and IADLs, assesses and applies splints and assistive device
Physical therapy	Assesses and treats mobility problems: strength, flexibility, balance, endurance, coordination, mobility aids
Speech & language pathology	Assesses and manages communication and swallowing problems
Psychologist	Assesses and manages cognitive, behavioral, and affective status
Dietitian	Evaluates nutrition status and therapeutic diets
Recreational therapy	Assesses and manages leisure preferences, adaptations and integration into therapeutic plan

ADLs, activities of daily living; IADLs, instrumental ADLs.

REHABILITATION FOR COMMON GERIATRIC PROBLEMS

Stroke

General Considerations

Stroke is the third leading cause of death in the United States and the leading cause of serious, long-term disability. Each year ~700,000 people experience a new or recurrent stroke. Stroke was the cause of 167,661 deaths (~1 of every 14 deaths) in the United States in 2000; 50% of stroke deaths occurred outside the hospital. There are ~4.5 million stroke survivors alive today.

Treatment

Poststroke care may be divided into 3 phases: acute care, intensive rehabilitation, and long-term care. A rehabilitative approach should be a continuing process

Table 37–3. Common assistive devices for mobility.

Assistive Device	Indications	Advantages	Disadvantages
Single-point cane	To widen the base of stability and improve balance	Low cost; fits easily on stairs or other surfaces where space is limited	Point of support is anterior to the hand, not directly beneath it
Quadruped cane	As above	Provides broad-based support	Some may not be practical for use on stairs; prevents walking quickly
Walk cane (hemiwalker)	As above	Provides very broad-based support; especially useful for patients with hemiplegia	May not allow pressure to be centered over the cane; cannot be used on most stairs
Crutches	To improve balance and lateral stability and relieve weight bearing	Improves balance and lateral stability; relieves weight bearing	Requires good arm strength; awkward in small or crowded area; may damage nerve or vessel in axilliary area
Walker (pick up/standard, four-wheel, front-wheel)	To improve balance and relieve weight bearing	Affords greatest stability; improves anterior and lateral stability. Provides sense of security Several styles are available, depending on need	Tends to be cumbersome in confined area; eliminates normal arm swing; cannot be used safely on stairs; walkers with wheels difficult on carpeting and uneven surfaces
Wheelchair	To maximize mobility in people who cannot ambulate safely	Does not require leg strength Able to move fast outdoors	Cumbersome in confined area; difficult to take in and out of vehicles

started as soon as life-threatening problems are under control during acute hospitalization.

Candidates for intensive rehabilitation are those who are medically stable but have residual disabilities and need help with at least 2 ADLs, are able to sit up (with or without support) for 1 h, and are able to learn and participate in active rehabilitation treatments. Patients who meet these criteria and require moderate to total assistance in mobility or performing ADLs are candidates for an intense inpatient program if they are able to tolerate $\geq$ 3 h of therapy each day. Patients who meet these criteria but require only supervision or minimal assistance in mobility or ADLs are usually candidates for home or outpatient rehabilitation if the home environment and support are adequate or for rehabilitation in a skilled nursing facility if environment and support are not adequate at home.

Individual rehabilitation needs and goals vary greatly. There should be a comprehensive assessment using standardized assessment tools. It is important that a care plan be developed by an interdisciplinary team based on goals that have been discussed with the patient and family.

Factors determining appropriate placement include medical stability, mobility, incontinence, cognitive function, mental health issues, presence of pain, swallowing abilities, communication abilities, evidence of neglect, ability to learn, level of assistance needed for mobility and ADLs, endurance, ability to manage IADLs, amount of medical care needed, and adequacy of family support. Figure 37–4 provides an algorithm to help decision making in rehabilitation placement

Interdisciplinary rehabilitation improves functional outcome, but it is not clear which component of this approach is most important. With rehabilitation, ~10% of stroke patients recover full physical function, 40% have some mild to moderate loss of function, and another 40% have significant functional losses; 10% are likely to need institutional care. Table 37–4 lists factors affecting functional outcome after stroke.

Increasing age is strongly associated with worse functional outcome at hospital discharge and follow-up. However, age is not a significant predictor of change in FIM score, implying that age should not be a factor that influences access to intensive stroke rehabilitation. An elderly person may have more disabilities after a stroke than a younger person but will have the same degree of functional improvement after the stroke. Other factors that are weakly associated with poor functional outcome include lower educational level, poor social supports, single marital status, unemployment, history of stroke, history of coronary artery disease, and presence of diabetes mellitus. Factors that are not associated with stroke outcome include financial resources and history of hypertension, congestive heart failure, or peripheral vascular disease. The presence of the following in the

first 1–4 weeks after a stroke are strongly associated with worse functional outcome at discharge: bowel and bladder incontinence, aphasia, global functional deficits, and sensory, motor, balance, visual, perceptual, and cognitive deficits. Unilateral neglect is also a negative predictor for recovery of function.

Rehabilitation interventions strongly associated with improved functional outcome are early initiation of rehabilitation services (within 72 h poststroke) and rehabilitation provided in an interdisciplinary inpatient setting.

Most of the functional recovery occurs in the first 6 mo after a stroke; some patients continue to gain functional abilities with physical therapy and exercise after 6 mo. Treadmill aerobic exercise training may improve exercise capacity and physical function after stroke. Treadmill training improves physiological reserve by increasing the peak volume of oxygen extraction while lowering the energy cost of a hemiparetic gait and increasing the peak ambulatory workload capacity. These improvements may enhance functional mobility in chronic stroke patients. Anecdoctal evidence supports the use of speech and language pathologists for cognitive rehabilitation of selected patients. In patients who are initially aphasic, ~50% of recovery of speech occurs in the first month and then recovery continues at a slower pace for ~6 mo.

Alternative therapies such as acupuncture have been tested as adjunctive treatment in stroke patients. The effectiveness of acupuncture, however, has not been proven.

Complications

A. Depression

Poststroke depression occurs in 12–27% of patients (Table 37–5), interfering with the ability to perform ADLs. Depression is an underrecognized but treatable condition that improves with medication or psychotherapy or a combination. Thus, this diagnosis should be actively sought and treated in patients after stroke.

B. Falling

Stroke patients are susceptible to falling. Fall incidence can be reduced significantly with appropriate evaluation and intervention (see Chapter 12).

C. Spasticity & Contractures

Spasticity and contractures, both common after a stroke, may greatly interfere with task performance. Treatment includes aggressive and consistent range-of-motion (ROM) exercises, proper positioning, and splinting. Oral medications are generally unsuccessful, although dantrolene sodium may have some beneficial effect. Injection of neurolytic agents such as phenol has variable success. The selective local intramuscular injec-

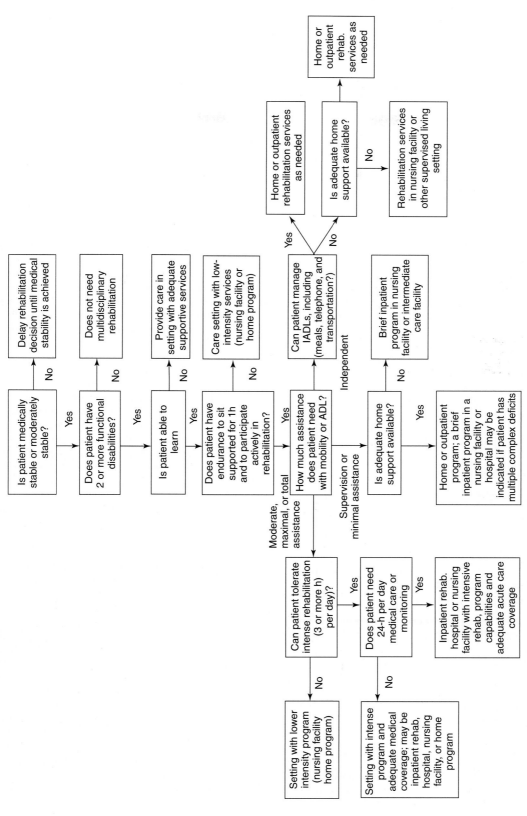

Figure 37–4. Core algorithm for rehabilitative placement of the poststroke patient. From Johnston MV: Rehabilitative placement of poststroke patients: reliability of the clinical practice guidelines of the Agency for Health Care Policy and Research. Arch Phys Med Rehabil 2000;81:541. Used with permission.

Table 37–4. Poststroke negative outcome predictors.

Age > 65
Lower education level
Poor social supports
Nonmarried
Unemployment
History of stroke
Presence of coronary artery disease
Presence of diabetes mellitus
Bowel/bladder incontinence
Cognitive deficits
Global functional deficits

tion of extremely low doses of botulinum toxin A has been found effective in reducing local muscle tone for 3–6 mo, resulting in improved function in selected patients.

D. Poor Caregiver Health

Early hospital discharge with home-based rehabilitation shortens the hospital stay without compromising functional outcome compared with conventional treatment. However, caregivers of the early discharge group may have worse general mental health. Support services for families have been shown to increase social activities significantly and improve quality of life for caregivers.

Osteoarthritis

General Considerations

Osteoarthritis is the most common disabling condition in older people. The first step in evaluating the rehabili-

Table 37–5. Rehabilitation medical complications.

Complication or condition	n	%
Urinary tract infection	569	30
Joint or soft tissue pain	300	16
Depression	235	12
Hypertension	200	10
Electrolyte abnormalities	141	7
Acute urinary retention	95	5
Pneumonia	91	5
No complications	473	25

N = 1903.
From Roth, EJ: Comorbidities in stroke: issues in clinical trials. Paper presented at the National Center for Rehabilitation Research Workshop, August 2001. Used with permission.

tation potential of a person with osteoarthritis is a physical examination with special attention paid to ROM (active and passive), condition of joints (inflamed, deformed, swollen, or unstable), manual muscle testing, postural or gait instability, cardiovascular fitness, and subclinical conditions that could be exacerbated by exercise. Joint pain may affect the accuracy of muscle strength testing; thus, the examiner should document whether the patient has pain during muscle contraction and should estimate strength when pain interferes with an accurate examination of strength.

Treatment

A variety of therapeutic modalities may be of benefit in patients with osteoarthritis. Figure 37–5 provides steps in managing osteoarthritis. Superficial heat (hot packs, heating pads, paraffin baths, fluidotherapy, whirlpool baths, and radiant heat) is more commonly used than deep heat (ultrasonography, short wave, microwave) for osteoarthritic joints. Many patients prefer cold to heat. Trial and patient preference should direct the prescription of heat or cold for symptom relief. Heat application at least temporarily reduces pain and increases the ability to move and exercise inflamed joints. Therefore, superficial heat should be applied before exercising and early in the morning to help relieve morning stiffness. Topical ointments like capsaicin and trolamine salicylate may give symptomatic relief in osteoarthritic joints but are often poorly tolerated by elderly patients. Transcutaneous electronic nerve stimulation may be helpful for hand, wrist, and knee pain. Acupuncture has not been shown to be of benefit.

There is consistent evidence that exercise training does not exacerbate pain or disease progression and is effective in decreasing pain and improving function. Promoting physical exercise should be an integral component in the management of osteoarthritis. Absolute contraindications to exercise are uncontrolled arrhythmias, third-degree heart block, recent electrocardiographic changes, unstable angina, acute myocardial infarction, and acute congestive heart failure. Relative contraindications are cardiomyopathy, valvular heart disease, poorly controlled blood pressure, and uncontrolled metabolic disease. Exercise stress testing should be considered in patients with significant cardiovascular risk factors and may help to establish an individual's initial aerobic exercise program.

To develop the best program for each patient, the physician must understand which functional problems are most important to the patient, help prioritize them, and then work with the patient to set specific short- and long-term goals. This will determine which exercise program to prescribe and will increase the likelihood of patient compliance.

Flexibility exercises decrease stiffness, increase joint mobility, and prevent soft tissue contractures. These are often done during a warm-up period or in conjunction with resistance or aerobic activities. Patients should begin with 1 stretching exercise per muscle group at least 3 times/week, and then the number of repetitions per muscle group can be gradually increased to 4–10 repetitions. Table 37–7 shows general recommendations for static stretching exercises.

Strength training is an essential part of rehabilitation for people with osteoarthritis. Resistance training can reverse many age-related physiological changes and can enhance function by improving the strength of muscles that support the affected joints. Table 37–8 shows general principles for strength training in patients with osteoarthritis.

Isometric exercise is a better option if the joint is inflamed or unstable. This exercise can improve muscle strength and static endurance. Patients should contract the muscles targeted for strengthening, initially at ~30% of maximal effort and gradually increasing to 75% of the maximal voluntary contraction. The contraction should be held for no longer than 6 s. Initially, 1 contraction per muscle group should be performed, and the number of repetitions should be gradually increased to 8–10 as tolerated. At first, contractions should be performed at muscle lengths tolerable to the patient. As joint instability and pain decrease, the patient should gradually shift to dynamic (isotonic) training.

When joint damage is severe enough to cause contractures, more aggressive treatments may be beneficial, including arthroplasty, serial casting, serial casting combined with traction, and manipulation under anesthesia.

The main indication for arthroplasty is pain relief. Conservative (ie, nonsurgical) treatment should be exhausted before considering arthroplasty because joint replacement has limited longevity (~10–20 years).

After an uneventful hip or knee arthroplasty, patients are usually encouraged to sit up in a chair on postoperative day 1 and begin walking on day 2. By day 3, patients are usually switched to oral analgesics and started on intensive physiotherapy. By day 5, patients generally can be discharged from the hospital to either home or a rehabilitation facility depending on their condition. Six weeks after surgery, patients are usually ambulatory without the use of an assistive device. After 3 mo, most patients are able to return to their previous activities (eg, golfing, walking, swimming, cycling). One of the greatest challenges after knee arthroplasty is ensuring the return of flexion and extension of the knee. Vigorous passive exercises should be started immediately postoperatively. Most knee prostheses are now cemented, allowing full weight bearing in the immediate postoperative period. Therefore, partial weight bearing is necessary only when there is grafting or repair of tendon or muscle. The use of continuous passive motion machines immediately after surgery is controversial. ROM exercises, followed by muscle strengthening, are required for 6 weeks to 3 mo after total knee arthroplasty.

Two important issues in rehabilitation after arthroplasty are adequate pain control and prevention of deep vein thrombosis (DVT). Good pain control facilitates early mobilization and rehabilitation, resulting in a shorter convalescence period. Without prophylaxis, prevalence of DVT at 7–14 days after total hip or knee replacement is ~50–60%, with proximal DVT rates of ~15–25%. In 2001, the American College of Chest Physicians recommended either low-molecular-weight heparin (LMWH) or adjusted-dose warfarin as a first-line therapy for prevention of venous thromboembolism in hip and knee replacement surgery. Elastic stockings or intermittent pneumatic compression can be used as an adjuvant prophylaxis for hip replacement surgery; and intermittent pneumatic compression can be used as an alternative prophylaxis option for knee replacement surgery (Table 37–6).

Table 37–6. DVT prophylaxis in arthroplasty.

1. Hip replacement
   Primary: SC LMWH or adjusted-dose warfarin (1A)
   Alternative: adjusted-dose heparin therapy (2A)
   Adjuvant: elastic stocking or intermittent pneumatic compression (2C)
2. Knee replacement
   Primary: SC LMWH or adjusted-dose warfarin (1A)
   Alternative: intermittent pneumatic compression (1B)
3. Hip fracture surgery
   Primary: SC LMWH or adjusted-dose warfarin (1B)
   Alternative: low-dose unfractionated heparin (2B)
Note: a. Optimal duration is uncertain but at least 7–10 days is recommended.
   b. Extended out-of-hospital LMWH prophylaxis (beyond 7–10 days) is recommended for at least high-risk patients (2A)

1A, clear risk vs. benefit, randomized trials without important limitations; strong recommendation, can apply to most patients in most circumstances without reservation; 1B, clear risk vs. benefit, randomized trials with important limitations, strong recommendation, likely to apply to most patients; 2A, unclear risk vs. benefit, randomized trials without important limitations, intermediate-strength recommendation; 2B, unclear risk vs. benefit, randomized trials with important limitation, weak recommendation; 2C, unclear risk vs. benefit, observation studies, very weak recommendation.
Adapted from the Sixth ACCP Consensus Conference on Antithrombotic Therapy: DVT prophylaxis in arthroplasty. Chest 2001;119:132S. Used with permission.

Table 37–7. Static stretching exercise: general recommendations.

Exercise daily when pain and stiffness are minimal (ie, before bedtime).
Exercises can be preceded by a warm shower or by application of superficial moist heat.
Relax before beginning stretching exercise.
Perform movements slowly and extend the range of motion that is both comfortable and produces a slight subjective sensation of resistance. Breathe during each stretch.
Hold this terminal stretch position for 10–30 s before slowly returning the joint or muscle group to the resting length.
Modify the stretching exercises to avoid pain or when the joint is inflamed (decrease the extent if joint range of motion or duration of holding the static position).

Adapted from Exercise Prescription for Older Adult With Osteoarthritis Pain: Consensus Practice Recommendations. J Am Geriatr Soc 2001;49:808. Used with permission.

ISOTONIC TRAINING

Isotonic muscle contractions are used to perform ADLs. Isotonic training has positive effects on energy metabolism, insulin action, bone density, and functional status. Osteoarthritic patients without instability or acute symptoms in the affected joint tolerate this form of exercise very well. It should include 8–10 exercises involving major muscle groups, starting at a low level so that the patient learns the exercises and does not get injured and gradually increasing both the intensity and number of repetitions. Patients should begin at 1 set of 4–6 repetitions and should avoid muscle fatigue. The training should be a maximum of 2

Table 37–8. Principles of strength training in osteoarthritic patients.

Specific exercises should be selected on the basis of the patient's joint stability and degree of pain and inflammation.
Muscles should not be exercised to fatigue.
Exercise resistance must be submaximal.
Inflamed joints should be isometrically strengthened and involved in only a few repetitions; movements should not be resisted.
Joint pain lasting 1 h after exercise and joint swelling indicate excessive activity.

Adapted from Exercise Prescription for Older Adult with Osteoarthritis Pain: Consensus Practice Recommendations. J Am Geriatr Soc 2001;49:808. Used with permission.

days/week. The amount of resistance used for training is increased 5–10%/week.

Hip Fracture

General Considerations

Hip fractures are a major cause of disability in older adults. Rehabilitation may help to reduce the disability of hip fracture.

Treatment

The typical postoperative course of hip fracture is as follows:

- By 1 week postsurgery: ROM exercises, weight-bearing locomotion as tolerated, pivot transfers, isotonic ankle exercises, and isotonic gluteal exercises.

- By 4–6 weeks postsurgery (endosteal and bridging calluses have formed): active ROM exercise around hip and knee, and active resistive exercise as tolerated.

- By 8–12 weeks postsurgery: weight-bearing transfers and ambulation and weaning from assistive devices. Generally, skilled rehabilitation therapy is no longer needed.

A common pattern of functional recovery occurs after hip fracture. That is, recuperation occurs at different rates and plateaus at different times (eg, independence with upper extremity-related ADLs plateaus at 4.3 mo; recovery of cognitive function plateaus at 4.4 mo; and walking speed plateaus at 10.8 mo). Table 37–9 summarizes predictors of a poor rehabilitation outcome.

Although people with dementia have more problems in the immediate postoperative period, those with mild to moderate dementia (eg, Mini-Mental State Exam score 12–17) are often able to return to a community-living situation after an acute rehabilitation program.

Physicians can help facilitate a better outcome by being familiar with the principles guiding choice of operation and prosthesis and the main complications associated with each as well as with appropriate instruction for early weight bearing and movement precautions to prevent dislocation. Appropriate use of opioid analgesics, DVT prevention, good bowel and bladder care, and early recognition of delirium are essential for optimal results.

Deconditioning

Deconditioning is generally a result of prolonged limited mobility. The reason for the limitation of mobility can be physical (eg, pain, imbalance, reduced ROM),

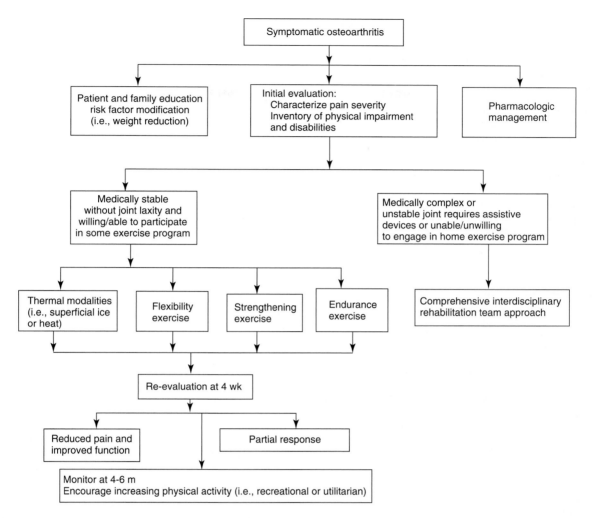

Figure 37–5. Steps in managing osteoarthritis in the older patient. From American Geriatrics Society Panel on Exercise and Osteoarthritis: Exercise prescription for older adults with osteoarthritis pain: consensus practice recommendations. J Am Geriatr Soc 2001;49:808. Used with permission

psychological (eg, fear of falls, depression), or environmental (restraint, neglect) or a result of lifestyle choices. Normal age-related changes, such as sarcopenia, make older adults more vulnerable to a deconditioned state and prolong the recovery process. Those with a high baseline level of function take longer to become deconditioned. However, significant deconditioning may occur in as few as 3 days of immobilization. The primary manifestations of deconditioning are reduced muscle strength, especially in the antigravity and large muscles, reduced joint flexibility, contracture, fatigue,

resting tachycardia or abnormally high heart rate with submaximal exercise, and orthostatic intolerance.

The treatment of deconditioning includes providing adequate sensory and intellectual stimulation, regaining an upright posture, improving joint ROM with active or passive exercise, and increasing strength and coordination with a combination of isometric, isotonic, and functional activities. Four to 8 weeks of resistance exercise can increase strength and improve functional activity in debilitated elderly who need help with 1 or more ADLs. As a generalization, for every day of bed rest,

Table 37–9. Post-hip fracture surgery: negative outcome predictors.

Poor mobility on day 2 postsurgery (requires maximal
    assistance to transfer or moderate assistance to ambulate
    or ambulates < 2 m)
Old age (> 75)
Use of gait aid before fracture
Poor mental status (modified Pfeiffer SPMSQ score < 4)
Nursing home residence
Poor grip and ankle dorsiflexion strength
Significant number of comorbidities
Limited number of leisure activities, poor coping skills, and
    unmarried status
Hip pain, poor self-rated health, and previous employment in
    a prestigious occupation

SPMSQ, Short Portable Mental Status Questionnaire.

2–3 days are needed for recovery. To prevent deconditioning, bed rest is generally avoided.

Falls & Instability

Each year ~30% of community-dwelling people older than 65 and 50% of those older than 80 fall. Falls are the leading cause of accidental death in the elderly. Those who survive a fall may have significant morbidity. Although the majority of falls do not result in injury, falls are associated with significant expense and health care use. Besides physical injury, falls also cause psychological and social consequences, such as fear of falling, anxiety, and admission to long-term care institutions.

The most common risk factors for falls are muscle weakness, history of falls, gait deficit, use of an assistive device, visual deficit, arthritis, depression, cognitive impairment, and age > 80. (The evaluation of falls is reviewed in Chapter 12.)

Because a fall is usually the result of many interacting factors, interventions must address each factor. Interventions are usually a combination of gait training and appropriate use of assistive devices; review and modification of medications; exercise and balance training; treatment of postural hypotension; modification of environmental hazards; and treatment of cardiovascular disorders, including arrhythmias. An interdisciplinary approach has proven most effective in fall rehabilitation and prevention. Although exercise has proven benefits for patients with falls, questions still remain regarding optimal type, duration, and intensity. Exercise programs may be more effective in frail elderly people than younger, more fit people. Tai chi ch'uan has been shown to be helpful in some studies. Home assessment, to ensure elimination of environmental risk factors, should also be considered for patients at high risk for falls.

Amputation

General Considerations

There are > 100,000 new amputees yearly in the United States, many of whom are elderly people with peripheral vascular diseases. Because of advances in vascular surgery and technology, the number of above-knee amputations has decreased; more people now have below-knee amputations. This is important because below-knee amputations greatly reduce energy cost for ambulation and reduce psychological morbidity, both of which are important to successful rehabilitation.

Treatment

If possible, the patient should be evaluated preoperatively to outline the likely rehabilitation plan and to start measures to improve muscle strength (especially in hip extensors and the upper body) and prevent contractures. Because the emotional effect of limb loss is significant, patients and families need a supportive environment where they can acknowledge and express their feelings.

Bed exercise should be started on the first postoperative day. The patient should get out of bed and begin balance training within 3–4 days. A temporary prosthesis or walking aid can be used by the end of the first week. The permanent prosthesis is usually fitted ~6–8 weeks after surgery when the limb stump has resolved and healed. Patients are taught how to take care of the stump with massage and wrapping to reduce edema and how to inspect it for evidence of infection and pressure. The quality of interface between the limb remnant and the prosthesis is the single most critical factor for successful use of the prosthesis. The prosthesis socket (the portion that fits snugly over the limb remnant) determines the patient's comfort and ability to control the artificial limb. Advances in prosthetic technology have led to prostheses that are comfortable and easy to use. Some have dynamic response, shock-absorbing mechanisms, and micro-processor-controlled movement, which allow the person to perform most of the usual ADLs. Factors associated with poor success include increased age, cerebrovascular disease, and dementia. Patient factors that predict a good rehabilitation outcome are independence before amputation, ability to bear weight on the contralateral side, medical stability, and ability to follow instructions.

Phantom sensations in the amputated limb are often felt by amputees, but pain occurs only in a minority.

Sometimes neuromas at the amputation sites are problematic and require injection with a steroid-anesthetic mixture or excision. Socket fit may change with weight alterations. Falls and fear of falling are pervasive among amputees and need to be addressed adequately.

REFERENCES

General Principles

American Geriatrics Society: Geriatric Rehabilitation. American Geriatrics Society, 1993.

Dittmar SS, Gresham GE: Functional Assessment and Outcome Measures for the Rehabilitation Health Professional. Aspen, 1997.

Manton KG, Gu X: Change in the prevalence of chronic disability in the United States black and nonblack population above age 65 from 1982 to 1999. Proc Natl Acad Sci USA 2001;98:6354. [PMID: 11344275]

Schoeni RF et al: Persistent, consistent, widespread, and robust? Another look at recent trends in old-age disability. J Gerontol 2001;56B:S206. [PMID: 11445613]

Waidmann TA, Liu K: Disability trends among elderly persons and implications for the future. J Gerontol 2000;55B:S298. [PMID: 10985301]

Stroke Rehabilitation

Anderson C et al: Home or hospital for stroke rehabilitation? Results of a randomized controlled trial: I. Health outcomes at 6 months. Stroke 2000;31:1024. [PMID: 10797161]

Bagg S et al: Effect of age on functional outcomes after stroke rehabilitation. Stroke 2002;33:179. [PMID: 11779908]

Cherney LR et al: Recovery of functional status after right hemisphere stroke: relationship with unilateral neglect. Arch Phys Med Rehabil 2001;82:322. [PMID: 11245753]

Cifu DX, Flax HJ: Factors affecting functional outcome after stroke. Paper presented at the National Center for Medical Rehabilitation Research Workshop, August 2001.

Cifu DX, Stewart DG: Factors affecting functional outcome after stroke: a critical review of rehabilitation interventions. Arch Phys Med Rehabil 1999;80:S35. [PMID: 10326901]

Mant J et al: Family support for stroke: a randomized controlled trial. Lancet 2000;356:808. [PMID: 11022928]

Silver KH: Chronic stroke: therapeutic intervention. Paper presented at the National Center for Medical Rehabilitation Research Workshop, August 2001.

Teasell R et al: The incidence and consequences of falls in stroke patients during inpatient rehabilitation: factors associated with high risk. Arch Phys Med Rehabil 2002;83:329. [PMID: 11887112]

Arthoplasty Rehabilitation

Brady OH et al: Rheumatology: 10. Joint replacement of the hip and knee—when to refer and what to expect. Can Med Assoc J 2000;63:1285. [PMID: 11107466]

Chen B et al: Continuous passive motion after total knee arthroplasty: a prospective study. Am J Phys Med Rehabil 2000;79:421. [PMID: 11157647]

Geerts WH et al: Prevention of venous thromboembolism. Chest 2001;119:132S. [PMID: 11157647]

Hip Fracture Rehabilitation

Fox KM et al: Intertrochanteric versus femoral neck hip fractures: differential characteristics, treatment, and sequelae. J Gerontol 1999;54A:M635. [PMID: 10647970]

Haentjens P et al: The economic cost of hip fractures among elderly women. A one-year, prospective, observational cohort study with matched-pair analysis. Belgian Hip Fracture Study Group. J Bone Joint Surg Am 2001;83:493. [PMID: 11315777]

Magaziner J et al: Recovery from hip fracture in eight areas of function. J Gerontol 2000;55A:M498. [PMID: 10995047]

Overend TJ et al: Determination of prefracture physical function in community-dwelling people who fracture their hip. J Gerontol 2000;55A:M698. [PMID: 11078101]

Osteoarthritis Rehabilitation

American Geriatrics Society Panel on Exercise and Osteoarthritis: Exercise prescription for older adults with osteoarthritis pain: consensus practice recommendation. A supplement to the AGS clinical practice guidelines on the management of chronic pain in older adult. J Am Geriatr Soc 2001;49:808. [PMID: 11480416]

Gill TM et al: Role of exercise stress testing and safety monitoring for older person starting an exercise program. JAMA 2000;284:342. [PMID: 10891966]

Prevalence of arthritis—United States, 1997. MMWR Morb Mortal Wkly Rep 2001;50:334. [PMID: 11465902]

Deconditioning Rehabilitation

Meuleman JR et al: Exercise training in the debilitated aged: strength and functional outcome. Arch Phys Med Rehabil 2000;81:312. [PMID: 10724076]

Falls Rehabilitation

American Geriatrics Society, British Geriatrics Society, and American Academy of Orthopedic Surgeons Panel on Fall Prevention: Guideline for the prevention of falls in older persons. J Am Geriatr Soc 2001;49:664. [PMID: 11380764]

Close J et al: Prevention of falls in the elderly trial (PROFET): a randomized controlled trial. Lancet 1999;353:93. [PMID: 10023893]

Cumming RG et al: Prospective study of the impact of fear of falling on activities of daily living, SF-36 scores, and nursing home admission. J Gerontol 2000;55A:M299. [PMID: 10819321]

Robertson MC et al: Effectiveness and economic evaluation of a nurse delivered home exercise programme to prevent falls: 1. Randomised controlled trial. Br Med J 2001;322:1. [PMID: 11264206]

Rubenstein LZ et al: Effects of a group exercise program on strength, mobility, and falls among fall-prone elderly men. J Gerontol 2000;55A:M317. [PMID: 10843351]

Wong AM et al: Coordination exercise and postural stability in elderly people: effect of Tai Chi Chuan. Arch Phys Med Rehabil 2001;82:608. [PMID: 11346836]

Amputee Rehabilitation

Fletcher DD et al: Rehabilitation of the geriatric vascular amputee patient: a population-based study. Arch Phys Med Rehabil 2001;82:776. [PMID: 11387582]

Marks LJ, Michael JW: Science, medicine, and the future: Artificial limbs. BMJ 2001;323:732. [PMID: 11576982]

Miller WC et al: The prevalence and risk factors of falling and fear of falling among lower extremity amputees. Arch Phys Med Rehabil 2001;82:1031. [PMID: 11494181]

RELEVANT WORLD WIDE WEB SITE

World Health Organization/International Classification of Functioning, Disability and Health: www.who.int/icf/icftemplate.cfm

Nutrition & Failure to Thrive

Larry E. Johnson, MD, PhD, & Dennis H. Sullivan, MD

CHANGES IN BODY COMPOSITION & ENERGY REQUIREMENTS WITH AGING

The human body is made of lean mass (skeletal muscle, viscera, cells of blood and immune system; 35–50% of body weight); fat (20–30%); extracellular fluid (20%); and bone and connective tissue (10–15%). Body weight in men tends to increase from age 30–60, plateaus for 10–15 years, and then slowly declines. In women, the pattern of weight change is similar, except the changes occur ~10 years later in life. Lean body weight (primarily skeletal muscle) begins to decline by middle age as a result of many factors, including decreasing exercise and age-related declines in hormones (eg, testosterone, estrogen, and growth factors), metabolism, alpha motor units in the spinal column, and muscle protein synthesis. It should be noted also that muscle mass in older adults can rapidly decline with even brief periods of bed rest. Fat mass increases until 60–70 years of age before gradually declining. Even when there is no change in total body weight, total fat mass tends to increase as lean body mass declines. Much of this fat gain occurs within the abdomen (visceral fat) and in the subcutaneous tissue of the torso, and this process accelerates after age 65. Bone mass declines in both older men and women. However, there is an accelerated loss of bone in women in the years after menopause.

Daily energy requirements decline with age, even during healthy aging. The primary reason for this decrease is the loss of muscle mass, which is much more metabolically active than fat tissue. Another cause is a decrease in physical activity.

Older adults have a reduced ability to regulate food intake. They are much less likely, compared with younger persons, to normalize their nutrient intake after either over- or undereating. Thus, appetite can remain poor for an extended period after illness-caused low food intake.

In some settings, such as the intensive care unit, indirect calorimetry is probably the optimal method of determining caloric requirements. In most cases, however, any one of several formulas (Table 38–1) can be used to estimate resting caloric needs. A "middle of the night" quick estimate is 30 kcal (126 kJ)/kg/day. All of these estimations require adjustment for activity level and illness severity; further adjustments depend on change in body weight and clinical response. It is important to not overfeed (see discussion of overfeeding syndrome).

MACRONUTRIENT REQUIREMENTS

Water

Water is often overlooked as a nutrient. Most adults need a maintenance water intake of 30 mL/kg body weight, with a minimum total daily intake of 1.5–2 L. Persons with excessive losses (eg, fever, diarrhea, hot weather) will need more. A decrease in thirst perception, decreased fluid intake in response to elevated serum osmolality, and decreased ability to concentrate urine after fluid deprivation occur in normal aging and increase the risk for dehydration. Cognitive decline, chronic disease, and decreased mobility may also impair fluid intake. Some persons deliberately restrict fluid intake in an effort to control urinary incontinence. Hospitals and nursing homes can easily become "water deserts" because of impaired access to water. The occurrence of an acute febrile illness or inadequate shelter during a heat wave can quickly lead to life-threatening dehydration. It is often necessary to actively encourage and directly observe fluid intake in bed-bound and institutionalized elderly persons. Intake and output measures are notoriously inaccurate in many clinical settings. Giving precise volume goals to caregivers and nurses, including writing fluid intake as a prescription or a formal medication order requiring documentation, is often more effective than simply asking family or staff to "push fluids." Except in the presence of severe protein undernutrition or gastrointestinal bleeding, blood urea nitrogen levels can be used as a guide to detect dehydration and subsequent response to rehydration. "Tenting" of skin is not a specific or sensitive sign of dehydration in older adults.

To treat or prevent dehydration, cooperative adults with an acute illness should be encouraged to drink fluids until their urine is nearly colorless. If a patient is not able to consume adequate amounts of fluid orally, hypodermoclysis (clysis) is a useful alternative to intravenous (IV) hydration or hospitalization for frail older

Table 38–1. Estimation of daily resting caloric (kcal) requirements.

Harris-Benedict equations
Males
$66 + 13.7W + 5H - 6.8A$
Females
$655 + 9.6W + 1.7H - 4.7A$
World Health Organization equations
Males
$13.5\,W + 487$
Females
$10.5W + 596$

A, age in years; H, height in centimeters; W, weight in kilograms.

adults, especially in a nursing home. Insertion of a clysis needle into the subcutaneous space of the back or abdomen requires minimal training and is not as difficult to perform or maintain as an IV. Although not an acceptable route to supply medications or antibiotics, clysis is often adequate to meet fluid needs. In a frail nursing home resident who has stopped drinking because of an acute reversible event such as an infection, clysis may prevent the need for hospitalization during the period before antibiotics or other therapies take effect. Table 38–2 lists tips for improving hydration in older adults.

Dasgupta M et al: Subcutaneous fluid infusion in a long-term care setting. J Am Geriatr Soc 2000;48:795. [PMID: 10894319]

Protein

Protein requirements for older adults are 1.00–1.25 g/kg/day, a bit higher than for younger adults. Protein requirements are influenced by age, activity level, medications, nonprotein content of the diet, and health status. Caloric intake is particularly important because protein requirements to maintain nitrogen balance increase as

Table 38–2. Ways to improve hydration in older adults.

Round with beverage cart offering a variety of liquids.
Offer a midafternoon social snack time.
Provide alternatives, such as Jello, popsicles, health shakes, ice cream, etc.
Try inventive thickening agents like yogurt or pudding mix.
Increase the amount of fluid given with medications.
Remind the patient throughout the day to drink.

total energy intake decreases. Protein requirements also increase with higher levels of physical activity. Corticosteroids, bed rest, injury, infection, and inflammation increase the risk of negative nitrogen balance, which can lead to rapid loss of lean body mass, primarily skeletal muscle. Older hospitalized persons who are very ill or recovering from trauma or major surgery may require ≥ 1.5 g/kg/day of protein to maintain nitrogen balance. Adequate protein intake becomes more challenging in medical conditions requiring protein restriction, such as liver or renal disease. In these situations, patients and families have to work closely with dietitians to avoid undernutrition. Increasing muscular resistance exercise when a lower intake of protein is medically required may improve nitrogen balance.

Campbell WW et al: Increased protein requirements in elderly people: new data and retrospective reassessments. Am J Clin Nutr 1994;60:501. [PMID: 8092084]

Fat

Serum lipid levels remain as strong a predictor of risk for coronary heart disease in older adults as in middle-aged adults. Very low-fat (< 10% of total calories) vegetarian diets have been shown to reverse narrowing within coronary arteries in persons with preexisting coronary artery disease. The dietary restriction required to adhere to this type of diet, however, makes it impractical for most people. Most current recommendations for a healthy diet suggest a diet of 25–30% of total calories coming from fat (American diets frequently have ≥ 40%) and < 300 mg/day of cholesterol). Studies of diet and cardiovascular disease show a small reduction in cardiovascular events and cardiovascular mortality (with little effect on total mortality) when dietary fat intake is reduced or modified. However, this effect was only seen in trials of at least 2 years' duration. It is not clear whether a modified fat diet adds further vascular protection when older adults attain adequate lipid lowering with medications.

Fat in the diet is required for the absorption of fat-soluble vitamins (A, D, E, K). In addition, essential fatty acids must be consumed because they cannot be synthesized in the body. There 2 general categories of essential fatty acids. The omega-6 type, which are generally plentiful in the American diet, have proinflammatory properties and are the substrate for arachidonic acid, prostaglandins, thromboxanes, and leukotrienes. The omega-3 type, including eicosapentaenoic acid (EPA), docosahexaenoic acid (DHA), and prostacyclin, decrease platelet aggregation and vasoconstriction and have anti-inflammatory properties. Per gram, fat has more than twice the calories (9 kcal) than protein or carbohydrates (4 kcal).

Current consensus is that some fats can be particularly cardioprotective, whereas high intakes of others may be harmful. Vegetable oils (particularly flaxseed/linseed, olive, and canola) and nuts (almonds, cashews, hazelnuts, macadamia nuts, pecans, pistachios, walnuts, and legume peanuts) are rich in polyunsaturated and monounsaturated fats (flaxseed/linseed is especially high in omega-3 essential fatty acids) and appear to have particularly healthful properties. Another important source of omega-3 fat is from fatty fish, particularly salmon, mackerel, and albacore tuna. Omega-3 oils can decrease cytokine-mediated inflammation and may play a role in the management of chronic inflammatory diseases such as rheumatoid arthritis. Consuming nuts more than 5 times a week (1 oz = 1 serving) has been shown to reduce coronary heart disease risk by 25–39%, even in very elderly persons and individuals with coronary disease. Saturated fat and partially hydrogenated fats (also called trans fatty acids) can increase total cholesterol and low-density lipoprotein (LDL) cholesterol levels and may even lower HDL cholesterol levels. Intake of these types of fat should be minimized.

Based on current data, in nonfrail adults of all ages, fat intake should not exceed 30% of total calories consumed, polyunsaturated and monounsaturated fats should predominate, and saturated fat and partially hydrogenated fat intake should be reduced. In contrast, in the frail older adult at high risk for weight loss, fat intake of all types can be encouraged to increase total calorie intake before transitioning to the healthier fats.

Harper CR, Jacobson TA: The fats of life: the role of omega-3 fatty acids in the prevention of coronary heart disease. Arch Intern Med 2001;161:2185. [PMID: 11575974]

Carbohydrate

Carbohydrate requirements are generally calculated by default after determining total caloric, fat, and protein requirements. Thus, carbohydrates generally make up about 55% of total caloric intake. On very low-calorie diets, energy requirements are met by the incomplete oxidation of fatty acids, which leads to ketosis and anorexia. To prevent ketosis, at least 50–100 g of carbohydrates should be consumed daily. Unrefined, whole-grain products should be emphasized, with decreased intake of simple sugars. Eating foods with a lower glycemic index (ie, foods that are more slowly digested and absorbed and thus cause a slower rise in blood sugar and lower insulin response) may also be beneficial. Fiber is also a beneficial property of unrefined carbohydrates (see Fiber section).

Ludwig DS: The glycemic index: physiological mechanisms relating to obesity, diabetes, and cardiovascular disease. JAMA 2002;287:2414. [PMID: 11988062]

Sodium

Whether sodium intake plays a clinically significant role in causing diseases of older adults, like hypertension, remains controversial. Most Americans, however, consume far more sodium (3.5 g/day on average) than needed for optimum health. However, many older adults find low-salt diets unpalatable. Indiscriminately recommending that all older adults be on a low-salt diet may cause more undernutrition than benefit.

Among healthy middle-aged adults (with and without hypertension), a diet rich in fruits and vegetables and low fat dairy products has been shown to significantly reduce blood pressure compared with a typical Western diet, and additional sodium restriction further reduces blood pressure in a dose–response manner. It is not known whether these results can be extrapolated to older adults. However, as long as food intake remains good, moderating sodium intake may be beneficial for both hypertensive and nonhypertensive older adults, especially those who are overweight or with a family history of hypertension. Persons with poorly controlled congestive heart failure also may require moderation of sodium consumption. Increased potassium and calcium intake may reduce blood pressure, but no specific recommendations are available.

Sodium chloride (table salt) is the most common source of sodium in the diet. One level teaspoon of table salt contains ~2.3 g of sodium. Therefore, it does not take much salt or salty foods to exceed the restrictions imposed by a low-salt (eg, 2 g sodium) diet. Most canned foods (eg, meats, soups, vegetables) and commercial snack foods contain added salt; elders are advised to read food labels carefully, particularly the number of servings per container.

Fiber

Dietary fiber (including, eg, nonstarch polysaccharides, oligosaccharides, lignin, gum, pectin) is the portion of edible material, most commonly from plants, that is poorly digested in and absorbed from the small intestine but which may undergo bacterial fermentation in the large intestine. Although it is generally recommended that people consume a diet containing 25–35 g of fiber each day, the average American diet contains only 10–15 g. A higher intake of fiber is associated with improved bowel function and is associated epidemiologically with a decreased risk for cardiovascular disease, diverticular disease, and diabetes mellitus type 2. It is unclear whether it is fiber itself or other phytochemicals and minerals associated with fiber-rich foods that may be most important. The purported beneficial effect in preventing colon cancer has been seriously questioned by studies that have shown no effect of either a wheat-bran-fiber supplement or a low-fat, high-fruit, high-vegetable, and high-fiber diet in reducing the recurrence of adenomatous polyps.

Insoluble fiber (eg, fruits, vegetables, and legumes) is incompletely or poorly fermented and improves colonic health by increasing fecal weight, reducing transit time, and improving laxation. Accompanying reduction in intracolonic pressure may lower the risk for diverticular disease. Soluble fiber (eg, oat and rice bran, barley, psyllium, legumes and vegetables, and modified celluloses such as carboxymethylcellulose) decreases total serum cholesterol and LDL–high-density lipoprotein (HDL) cholesterol ratios, reducing cardiovascular disease risk. It also slows stomach emptying and intestinal absorption, which can decrease blood glucose concentrations and insulin levels. Fermentation of fiber in the colon leads to gas production but also produces short-chain fatty acids that provide local nutrition to bowel mucosa, maintaining bowel wall integrity and decreasing bacterial translocation. High fiber intakes can decrease absorption of minerals like calcium, zinc, iron, and copper primarily because of the phytic content of cereals and fruits, but it still appears that the beneficial effects of fiber far outweigh potential side effects.

A diet rich in fruits, vegetables, and whole-grain foods is recommended to increase fiber intake. Most fruits and vegetables contain < 2 g fiber/serving; thus, the U.S. Department of Agriculture (USDA) food guide pyramid recommends 2–3 servings of fruit, 3–4 vegetables, and ≥ 6 servings of grains each day. In considering commercial foods, purchasers are advised to look for whole grain as the first ingredient. If the first ingredient is enriched flour, it is not whole grain and contains very little natural fiber. Supplementing the diet with commercially available concentrated fiber sources may be necessary when fiber intake from natural sources is inadequate. Fiber intake should be increased gradually to avoid bloating, excess flatus, and general discomfort. Adequate fluid intake is also needed, particularly with bed-bound or inactive persons, because constipation may actually worsen.

FAILURE TO THRIVE & UNDERNUTRITION

Failure to thrive (FTT) is a commonly used but vague term that describes a deteriorating state characterized by weight loss (usually with muscle loss, or sarcopenia) and an associated loss of functional and psychological independence. Another commonly used term, cachexia (meaning "poor condition" in Greek), has been defined as the accelerated loss of skeletal muscle in the presence of a chronic inflammatory response; cachexia may occur without anorexia. As with many geriatric syndromes, causes of FTT are likely to be multifactorial. It may be precipitated following a sentinel event (such as an acute illness or hip fracture) superimposed on a background of comorbid illness and age-associated changes, or it may occur more gradually. Some of the possible contributing factors include hormonal changes in estrogen, androgens, and growth hormone; cytokines with known catabolic properties (such as interleukin-1 and tumor necrosis factor [TNF]); changes in trophic signals from the brain to muscle; decreased alpha motor neurons and changes in the neuromuscular junction; and decreased ability of muscle to protect itself from free radical stressors. Extrinsic factors include the interaction between physical activity and muscle and weight loss. Many diverse diseases, like cancer, AIDS, congestive heart failure, rheumatoid arthritis, tuberculosis, chronic obstructive pulmonary disease, and Crohn's disease, can lead to FTT, sarcopenia, and weight loss. Animal studies have shown that loss of skeletal muscle in cachexia exceeds the muscle loss as a result of simple starvation alone. As might be expected, increased nutritional support by itself has little effect on the course of FTT as long as the underlying causes persist.

Depression and dementia can lead to FTT by several pathways. They can cause both decreased appetite and increased disability, each independently resulting in malnutrition. Certain antidepressants are more likely associated with anorexia than others. Tricyclic antidepressants and mirtazapine are more likely to cause weight gain, whereas the selective serotonergic reuptake inhibitors (SSRIs), particularly fluoxetine, and bupropion have an increased association with weight loss (see Chapter 14: Depression & Other Mental Health Issues). The acetylcholinesterase inhibitors for dementia may be associated with gastrointestinal discomfort or diarrhea in some patients (see Chapter 11: Cognitive Impairment & Dementia). Because each patient's particular response to these medications is different, it is wise to monitor appetite and weight closely whenever any new medication is started, so that malnutrition can be quickly recognized and the drug stopped or changed.

Caregiving and care receiving can be associated with adverse emotional and physical effects that increase risk for FTT. Functional disability is more strongly associated with depression than age. As dependency on others escalates, the individual's sense of control diminishes. Elders living in the homes of children or grandchildren have lower satisfaction and morale than those in other living arrangements. Female caregivers rate their levels of caregiver stress and physical health as poorer than similar women not providing care, and daughters providing care are at higher risk of stress and burnout than are sons. The emotional impact on caregivers may include anger, disruption of family relationships, guilt, no time for family or self, frustration, and despair. In-home assessments may lead to recommendations that increase independence and reduce caregiving burden. Failing elders are associated with overstressed caregivers.

Chronic inflammation often plays an important role in FTT and cachexia. Effects include hepatic synthesis of many types of proteins, including opsonins, protease inhibitors, complement factors, C-reactive protein, and fibrinogen. The large quantities of proteins required as liver feedstock for synthesis come from skeletal muscle catabolism. Synthesis of other proteins, like albumin and prealbumin (transthyretin), is greatly reduced. Negative nitrogen balance occurs and weight loss commonly results. Fat metabolism is also affected in this inflammatory process: Lipolysis increases and lipogenesis decreases; triglyceride levels and very low-density lipoproteins increase; and lipoprotein lipase, high-density lipoprotein, and total cholesterol decrease. There is an increase in release of free fatty acids from adipose stores. Changes in carbohydrate metabolism include hyperinsulinemia, peripheral insulin resistance (redirecting glucose to the liver and away from skeletal muscle), and glucose intolerance. Hypermetabolism with an increased resting energy expenditure (REE) occurs in cachexia, unlike uncomplicated starvation. The apathy, malaise, and fatigue associated with cachexia cause a decrease in voluntary energy expenditure but do not balance the increased REE and decreased caloric intake.

Cytokines are protein mediators that regulate the acute-phase response and cachexia. The best studied of the proinflammatory cytokines are TNF-α (also called cachectin), interleukin (IL)-1, and IL-6. Some of the nutritional effects of various cytokines include anorexia, altered gastric emptying, decreased intestinal blood flow, and changes in small bowel motility. The presence of inflammatory markers in the blood of even high-functioning older adults has been found to correlate with subsequent morbidity and mortality. Table 38–3 summarizes common causes of weight loss in older adults.

Kotler DP: Cachexia. Ann Intern Med 2000;133:622. [PMID: 11033592]

Roubenoff R, Harris TB: Failure to thrive, sarcopenia, and functional decline in the elderly. Clin Geriatr Med 1997;13:613. [PMID: 9354744]

PROTEIN-ENERGY MALNUTRITION

Protein-energy malnutrition (PEM; the inadequate intake of protein and calories) or undernutrition is common. Unintentional weight loss is found in up to 13% of elderly outpatients and in 30-80% of nursing home residents. Usual aging is commonly associated with increasing risk for acute illness, chronic illness, and subse-

Table 38–3. Causes of poor food intake & failure to thrive in older adults.[a]

Social/psychological
  Isolation, loss of social meal setting, emotional isolation
  Depression, bereavement, grief
  Unable to drive or walk to the market
  Alcohol abuse (often hidden)
  "Instant bachelors" who have never learned to buy, store, or prepare food
  Finicky eaters
  Elder abuse and neglect
  Inadequate assistance with eating
  Poverty
Physical
  Cancer
  Medications (prescription and nonprescription): digoxin, selective serotonin reuptake inhibitor antidepressants, antacids, laxative abuse, diuretics, NSAIDs, chemotherapy, anticonvulsants, antibiotics, any drug causing delirium
  Decreased sensory pleasure (decreased olfaction and taste)
  Dentures, painful, poorly fitting, absent
  Poor dental health
  Xerostomia
  Physical handicaps and decreased mobility
  Neurological impairments of chewing and swallowing (eg, stroke, dementia, Parkinson's disease)
  Memory and attention disorders (eg, dementia, psychosis)
  Chronic disease interfering with eating: chronic obstructive pulmonary disease, congestive heart failure, renal failure)
  Infections (eg, TB, AIDS, chronic low-grade aspiration)
  Metabolic disorders (eg, diabetes mellitus, hyper- or hypothroidism)
  Atrophic gastritis with decreased stomach acid
  Peptic ulcer disease
  Inflammatory bowel disease
  Intestinal motility disorders (eg, gastroparesis, constipation)
  Negative reinforcers of food intake: hiatal hernia, esophageal reflux, lactose intolerance, exertional hypoxia, intestinal angina (mesenteric ischemia)

[a]Often more than one cause is present.
NSAIDs, nonsteroidal anti-inflammatory drugs; TB, tuberculosis.

quent medication use, all of which can contribute to anorexia. Other mediators of anorexia include cytokines (see Failure to Thrive & Undernutrition section), humoral factors (bombesin-like substances, cholecystokinin), and possible anorectic agents like corticotropin-releasing factor. Common causes for weight loss in older adults are listed in Table 38–3.

In response to energy deprivation, the body reduces its metabolic rate in individual tissues and catabolizes skeletal muscle, while relatively sparing viscera (liver, kidneys, gastrointestinal tract) and blood and immune tissue. This allows the body to compensate for the reduced energy intake. The cost is reduced muscle mass (including heart and respiratory muscle mass) and a decline in functional capacity, resulting in weakness and disability. Factors that prevent successful adaptation to uncomplicated PEM include severe prolonged starvation, micronutrient deficiencies, and onset of catabolic, cytokine-mediated stress (such as infection).

PEM is poorly recognized for many reasons. Early signs and symptoms are nonspecific, mimic usual aging, and often progress slowly. Appetite may decline so slowly that it is not recognized. There is no single gold standard for diagnosing PEM, although weight loss may be the most obvious characteristic to identify. The most common definition of weight loss that cannot be ignored and that must be recognized and addressed is weight loss of 5% in 1 mo, 7% in 3 mo, or 10% over 6 mo. However, more gradual weight loss, especially involuntary weight loss, such as 5% over 6–12 mo is also associated with higher morbidity and mortality. Weight fluctuations associated with fluid changes, such as during treatment for and exacerbations of congestive heart failure, may hide real weight loss. It may be necessary to measure weight more frequently to detect trends, but weighing accuracy in many health care settings is notoriously bad. Workers who weigh frail older adults should be trained and positively reinforced to weigh patients correctly and consistently (using the same amount of clothing, at about the same time of day and relation to meals, and noting the presence or absence of casts, braces, and so on) using calibrated scales. It is very helpful to have a system in place to automatically reweigh a patient if variation of > 5 lbs (2.3 kg) from the previous weight is found. Patients whose weights are most critical to know, unfortunately, are frequently the most problematic to weigh; wheelchair, bed, or lift scales are available for nonambulatory persons.

ASSESSMENT OF NUTRITIONAL STATUS

Anthropometrics

Body weight is the most important anthropometric measurement of nutritional status. Body mass index (BMI) (Table 38–4) is a way of describing weight in re-

Table 38–4. Body mass index (BMI).

BMI = (weight in kg)/(height in m)^2 = (weight in lbs) x 706/ (height in inches)^2

lationship to height; that is, taller persons should weigh more than shorter persons. In persons who are not unusually muscular, an elevated BMI correlates fairly well with obesity. However, BMI does not identify persons who have replaced muscle mass with adipose tissue, nor does it distinguish persons with central obesity. As a general guide, healthier weights in younger adults are between BMIs of 20–25 kg/m^2. A BMI of 25–30 is considered overweight and > 30 is obese (see Obesity in Older Adults section). A BMI < 20 is not necessarily harmful, but many Americans with a BMI < 20 are smokers or have chronic illness or cancer that lowers life expectancy, and older persons with low BMIs have poorer outcomes when they have a serious illness than average-weight or heavier persons.

A variety of other anthropometrics have limited clinical applicability. These have been proposed because adiposity in certain body sites may be more harmful than in others. It has been suggested that central obesity (ie, fat within and around the abdomen) is metabolized differently and has more harmful health consequences than fat located more peripherally (ie, around the hips). It has been proposed that waist circumferences may help identify persons at higher risk (see Obesity in Older Adults section). Skinfold measurements using calipers are prone to many measurement errors and remain primarily a research tool. Bioelectric impedance may prove a better way to assess body composition.

Laboratory Assessment

The initial laboratory assessment of weight loss should include a complete blood count, glucose, electrolytes, renal and liver function, thyroid-stimulating hormone level, urinalysis, and chest x-ray film.

Although serum albumin is commonly ordered to assess protein nutrition or status, serum albumin levels have poor sensitivity and specificity as a measure of nutritional health. Albumin concentration may increase in response to corticosteroids, insulin, and dehydration; levels decrease with hydration, liver and renal disease, malabsorption, and change from an upright to a supine position and in response to inflammatory cytokines. The patient who is undergoing slow, uncomplicated starvation may maintain a near-normal serum albumin until near death by catabolizing muscle stores, reducing metabolic activity, and decreasing protein synthesis and degradation; one can die of starvation with a normal albumin. In contrast, acute and severe injury, even in a well-nourished person, often quickly causes a drop in albumin. The half-life of albumin is ~3 weeks. Levels respond slowly to renutrition alone and may never normalize if inflammation is ongoing. Raising the serum albumin with intravenous albumin replacement does not improve prognosis. However, measurement of serum albumin does have clinical value: A low serum albumin, although not a good indicator of nutritional status, may be a powerful predictor of illness severity and mortality.

Other serum proteins have been used as nutritional markers. There are drawbacks to using serum transferrin as a nutritional marker because levels are also affected by many nonnutritional factors. Serum cholesterol < 160 mg/dL is a marker for increased risk of morbidity and mortality but not a good measure of nutrition. Prealbumin (transthyretin) has a short half-life of 2–3 days and is, like albumin, a negative acute-phase reactant. A low level can be used to confirm the clinical impression of poor nutritional status in the absence of inflammation. A progressively rising prealbumin level may help to confirm improving nutritional status; however, the clinical exam remains the best indicator (eg, the patient is getting stronger, wounds are healing, appetite is improving). Failure of prealbumin to rise when one is assured that the patient is receiving calculated

amounts of nutrition (remember that patients often do not receive the nutritional intake that is medically ordered because of, eg, delirium, anorexia, delayed initiation of feedings, procedures that require feedings to be held, accidental enteral tube removal, or feeding intolerance) should prompt a clinical workup for an occult catabolic or inflammatory process.

Fuhrman MP: The albumin-nutrition connection: separating myth from fact. Nutrition 2002;18:199. [PMID: 11844655]

Sullivan DH: What do the serum proteins tell us about our elderly patients? J Gerontol Med Sci 2001;56:M71. [PMID: 11213278]

Clinical Assessment

A comprehensive clinical assessment of nutritional status is the most useful way to identify undernutrition, and several assessment instruments exist. One tool is the Subjective Global Assessment (Figure 38–1). Another

---

Instructions: Select appropriate category with a checkmark, or enter numerical value where indicated by "#."
A. History
  1. Weight change
    Overall loss in 6 months: amount = #_____kg; % loss = #_____
    Change in past 2 weeks:_____increase,
        _____no change,
        _____decrease.
  2. Dietary intake change (relative to normal)
    _____No change
    _____Change_____duration = #_____weeks.
              _____type:_____suboptimal solid diet,_____full liquid diet
              _____hypocaloric liquids,_____starvation.
  3. Gastrointestinal symptoms (that persisted for > 2 weeks
    _____none,_____nausea,_____vomiting,_____diarrhea,_____anorexia.
  4. Functional capacity
    _____No dysfunction (e.g., full capacity),
    _____Dysfunction_____duration=#_____weeks.
              _____type:_____working suboptimally,
              _____ambulatory,_____bedridden.
  5. Disease and its relation to nutritional requirements
    Primary diagnosis (specify)_____
    Metabolic demand (stress):_____no stress,_____low stress,_____moderate stress,_____high stress.
B. Physical (for each trait specify: 0 = normal, 1+ = mild, 2+ = moderate, 3+ = severe).
  #_____loss of subcutanous fat (triceps, chest)
  #_____muscle wasting (quadriceps, deltoids)
  #_____ankle edema
  #_____sacral edema
  #_____ascites
C. SGA rating (select one)
  _____A = well nourished
  _____B = moderately (or suspected of being) malnourished
  _____C = severe malnourished

Figure 38–1. Subjective Global Assessment (SGA).

tool is the Mini-Nutritional Assessment (Figure 38–2). These tools show promise but have not been rigorously studied in large and varied geriatric populations.

Dietary Assessment

How much is the patient eating and drinking? What seems an easy question is frequently difficult to determine accurately. Accurate calorie counts can be invaluable but are frequently very difficult to obtain. At home, over several days patients or their family can fill out a food diary, which a dietitian can then interpret. There are many barriers to constructing an accurate diary, among them dementia, delirium, psychiatric illness, benign forgetfulness, and illiteracy. Calorie counts in inpatient settings are also frequently inaccurate. Some reasons for this include inaccurate estimations of food consumption by nursing or dietary personnel, misplacement of written estimates, food on meal trays being eaten by other patients or family members, food brought in from the outside that is not recorded, and tube feedings that are stopped and restarted sporadically. Nursing aides can be a valuable resource when asked about global food intake or aversive behaviors in their patients.

Vellas B et al: Nutrition assessment in the elderly. Curr Opin Clin Nutr Metab Care 2001;4:5. [PMID: 11122552]

TREATING UNDERNUTRITION

Once treatment is begun, an organized strategy for periodic reassessment is mandatory to ensure that the patient's nutritional status is improving. If the patient is not improving, appropriate reevaluations must be been done and alternative interventions attempted.

Bouras EP et al: Rational approach to patients with unintentional weight loss. Mayo Clin Proc 2001;76:923. [PMID: 11560304]

Behavioral Interventions for Poor Food Intake

Table 38–5 lists some approaches for improving dietary intake in older adults. Eating is the most social of the activities of daily living, the first one mastered as a child and often the last lost in old age. Patients often eat better, and more, when fed by family members. One reason for this is the length of time the family member dedicates to unhurriedly feeding and encouraging the patient. Successfully motivating anorexic persons to eat requires a multidimensional approach, including treating pain, increasing social supports, identifying realistic goals (eg, being able to care for oneself or being able to return home), encouraging the hope of getting stronger, and adapting to individual food preferences

and meal times. Exercise as simple as daily walking may improve appetite in some patients. Refusal to eat or swallow should not be attributed to a voluntary "death wish" until the patient has undergone a detailed psychiatric assessment and been given appropriate treatment for possible depression.

Oral Supplements

A variety of commercial liquid and powder supplements can be used when patients are unable or unwilling to consume enough regular food. Nutritional supplements are most effective when consumed between meals so patients do not substitute supplement intake for regular meals. However, because of the necessary staff and time demands, between-meal consumption is rarely accomplished. It is common to see unopened canned supplements stacked on patients' bedside tables. Some patients consume these readily and eventually transition back to a regular diet; others, however, find them unpalatable. Powder formulations allow the supplement to be masked by mixing it with other food. A major barrier to the canned supplements is cost, even with generic brands. For patients with no history of lactose intolerance, instant breakfast powders mixed in milk are a satisfactory and less expensive alternative. When calculating water intake, canned protein supplements contain ~70% water. The role for nutritional supplements in healing pressure sores remains uncertain. Supplements targeted to specific patient populations (eg, renal failure, posttrauma, or ventilator dependent) may be useful, though at increased cost.

Potter JM: Oral supplements in the elderly. Curr Opin Clin Nutr Metab Care 2001;4:21. [PMID: 11122555]

Agents to Stimulate Appetite & Promote Weight Gain

A variety of medications have been promoted as helping to improve appetite and increase weight; however, none has proven satisfactory among the elderly. The progestational agent megestrol acetate has been shown to increase appetite and weight in AIDS patients and was found to improve morbidity in frail older adults after it was discontinued. Recent studies of the drug have shown that gained weight tends to be in adipose tissue, whereas skeletal muscle mass actually decreases. Most older adults do not tolerate the dysphoria associated with dronabinol use. Cyproheptadine has not been shown to be effective in older adults. The anabolic agents growth hormone and insulin-like growth factor are extremely expensive and associated with frequent side effects. Androgen therapy with testosterone or its analogues also has many side effects; its use for weight

NESTLÉ NUTRITION SERVICES

Nestlé

Mini Nutritional Assessment
MNA®

Last name:	First name:	Sex:	Date:
Age:	Weight, kg:	Height, cm:	I.D. Number:

Complete the screen by filling in the boxes with the appropriate numbers.
Add the numbers for the screen. If score is 11 or less, continue with the assessment to gain a Malnutrition Indicator Score.

Screening

A Has food intake declined over the past 3 months due to loss of appetite, digestive problems, chewing or swallowing difficulties?
0 = severe loss of appetite
1 = moderate loss of appetite
2 = no loss of appetite

B Weight loss during last months
0 = weight loss greater than 3 kg (6.6 lbs)
1 = does not know
2 = weight loss between 1 and 3 kg (2.2 and 6.6 lbs)
3 = no weight loss

C Mobility
0 = bed or chair bound
1 = able to get out of bed/chair but does not go out
2 = goes out

D Has suffered psychological stress or acute disease in the past 3 months
0 = yes   2 = no

E Neuropsychological problems
0 = severe dementia or depression
1 = mild dementia
2 = no psychological problems

F Body Mass Index (BMI) (weight in kg) / (height in m)²
0 = BMI less than 19
1 = BMI 19 to less than 21
2 = BMI 21 to less than 23
3 = BMI 23 or greater

Screening score (subtotal max. 14 points)
12 points or greater Normal – not at risk – no need to complete assessment
11 points or below   Possible malnutrition – continue assessment

Assessment

G Lives independently (not in a nursing home or hospital)
0 = no   1 = yes

H Takes more than 3 prescription drugs per day
0 = yes   1 = no

I Pressure sores or skin ulcers
0 = yes   1 = no

J How many full meals does the patient eat daily?
0 = 1 meal
1 = 2 meals
2 = 3 meals

K Selected consumption markers for protein intake
• At least one serving of dairy products (milk, cheese, yogurt) per day?   yes ☐   no ☐
• Two or more servings of legumes or eggs per week?   yes ☐   no ☐
• Meat, fish or poultry every day   yes ☐   no ☐
0.0 = if 0 or 1 yes
0.5 = if 2 yes
1.0 = if 3 yes

L Consumes two or more servings of fruits or vegetables per day?
0 = no   1 = yes

M How much fluid (water, juice, coffee, tea, milk…) is consumed per day?
0.0 = less than 3 cups
0.5 = 3 to 5 cups
1.0 = more than 5 cups

N Mode of feeding
0 = unable to eat without assistance
1 = self-fed with some difficulty
2 = self-fed without any problem

O Self view of nutritional status
0 = view self as being malnourished
1 = is uncertain of nutritional state
2 = views self as having no nutritional problem

P In comparison with other people of the same age, how does the patient consider his/her health status?
0.0 = not as good
0.5 = does not know
1.0 = as good
2.0 = better

Q Mid-arm circumference (MAC) in cm
0.0 = MAC less than 21
0.5 = MAC 21 to 22
1.0 = MAC 22 or greater

R Calf circumference (CC) in cm
0 = CC less than 31   1 = CC 31 or greater

Assessment (max. 16 points)

Screening score

Total Assessment (max. 30 points)

Malnutrition Indicator Score
17 to 23.5 points   at risk of malnutrition
Less than 17 points   malnourished

Ref.: Guigoz Y, Vellas B and Garry PJ. 1994. Mini Nutritional Assessment: A practical assessment tool for grading the nutritional state of elderly patients. *Facts and Research in Gerontology.* Supplement #2:15-59.
Rubenstein LZ, Harker J, Guigoz Y and Vellas B. Comprehensive Geriatric Assessment (CGA) and the MNA: An Overview of CGA, Nutritional Assessment, and Development of a Shortened Version of the MNA. In: "Mini Nutritional Assessment (MNA): Research and Practice in the Elderly". Vellas B, Garry PJ and Guigoz Y, editors. Nestlé Nutrition Workshop Series. Clinical & Performance Programme, vol. 1. Karger, Bâle, in press.

Figure 38–2. The Mini Nutritional Assessment tool evaluates the risk of malnutrition in older adults. On the basis of the score, patients are divided into 3 categories: well nourished, at risk for malnutrition, and at risk for undernutrition. Several body measurements must be made, which may be difficult or may require training. From Vellas BJ et al: The Mini Nutritional Assessment: MNA. Serdi Publishing, 1994. Used with permission

Alternative Height Calculations Using Knee to Heel Measurements: With knee at a 90° angle (foot flexed or flat on floor or bed board), measure from bottom of heel to top of knee.

Men = (2.02 x knee height, cm) - (0.04 x age) + 64.19
Women = (1.83 x knee height, cm) - (0.24 x age) + 84.88

Body Weight Calculations in Amputees: For amputations, increase weight by the percentage below for contribution of individual body parts to obtain the weight to use to determine Body Mass Index.

Single below knee	6%
Single at knee	9%
Single above knee	15%
Single arm	6.5%
Single arm below elbow	3.6%

Body Mass Index Table

BMI→ Height	19	20	21	22	23	24	25	26	27	28	29	30	35	40
							Weight (in pounds)							
4'10"	91	96	100	105	110	115	119	124	129	134	138	143	167	191
4'11"	94	99	104	109	114	119	124	128	133	138	143	148	173	198
5'	97	102	107	112	118	123	128	133	138	143	148	153	179	204
5'1"	100	106	111	116	122	127	132	137	143	148	153	158	185	211
5'2"	104	109	115	120	126	131	136	142	147	153	158	164	191	218
5'3"	107	113	118	124	130	135	141	146	152	158	163	169	197	225
5'4"	110	116	122	128	134	140	145	151	157	163	169	174	204	232
5'5"	114	120	126	132	138	144	150	156	162	168	174	180	210	240
5'6"	118	124	130	136	142	148	155	161	167	173	179	186	216	247
5'7"	121	127	134	140	146	153	159	166	172	178	185	191	223	255
5'8"	125	131	138	144	151	158	164	171	177	184	190	197	230	262
5'9"	128	135	142	149	155	162	169	176	182	189	196	203	236	270
5'10"	132	139	146	153	160	167	174	181	188	195	202	209	243	278
5'11"	136	143	150	157	165	172	179	186	193	200	208	215	250	286
6'	140	147	154	162	169	177	184	191	199	206	213	221	258	294
6'1"	144	151	159	166	174	182	189	197	204	212	219	227	265	302
6'2"	148	155	163	171	179	186	194	202	210	218	225	233	272	311
6'3"	152	160	168	176	184	192	200	208	216	224	232	240	279	319
6'4"	156	164	172	180	189	197	205	213	221	230	238	246	287	328

Locate height, then on the same line, locate the closest weight in pounds. Use the lower weight, if midpoint. Do not round up. Read to top of the weight column to obtain the BMI value.

Figure 38–2. **(Continued)**

Table 38–5. Methods to increase food intake in older adults.

Offer comfort foods: chicken soup, tea, ice cream, poached egg on toast.

Offer a happy hour beverage, visually appealing and nutrient dense (shakes, smoothies, coolers, etc.) in social milieu (festive tea cart, staff member's wear chef hats and aprons, beverage in punch bowl, etc.).

Encourage companionship during meal preparation and feeding.

Maximize caloric intake at favorite meal of the day.

Take medications with meals to minimize anorexia and nausea.

Increase physical activity.

Avoid constipation and diarrhea.

Reduce distractions and noise; turn off the television and radio.

Use finger food, including while walking; keep these foods visible during the day.

Give one food item at a time; clear away unnecessary items.

Offer several small meals throughout the day.

gain remains experimental. Anti-inflammatory therapies that affect arachidonic acid metabolism and cytokine release, including the omega-3 fatty acids, are also being studied. Anticatabolic agents, such as those with anticytokine activity, are still investigational.

Persons with persistent anorexia may benefit from a trial of antidepressant therapy.

Artificial (Tube) Feeding

Anorexic patients will often eat more if enough time is taken to hand-feed them. If such a patient is still unable to consume adequate nutrition, the provider should discuss the risks and benefits of other nutritional interventions. If the gastrointestinal tract is functioning, it is strongly preferred to use it for nutritional delivery rather than parenteral routes. Although each state has different laws, it is not clinically mandatory to use artificial feeding when physicians, patients, and their families believe the risks and side effects outweigh the benefits (see Chapter 44: Palliative Care & Pain Management). Some clinicians initiate artificial feeding in a therapeutic trial for a limited and predetermined duration with the understanding that if certain goals (eg, the person will begin to voluntarily consume sufficient calories for survival) are not achieved, the intervention can be withdrawn. A 2- to 4-week trial is reasonable.

Diarrhea is common in tube-fed patients. This is frequently due to medication side effects, because sorbitol is often used as a drug solvent. The use of fiber-enriched supplements or simple antidiarrheal agents may help once it is ensured that the patient does not have liquid stool running around an impaction. When beginning tube feedings, it is useful to periodically assess stomach residuals; high residuals are associated with increased aspiration risk. Bowel motility is commonly impaired in frail bed-bound persons and after surgery. Early initiation of postoperative oral feedings does not invariably improve bowel function. Mobilization of the patient also does not, by itself, improve gastrointestinal function after surgery. Opioid medications almost always cause significant constipation. Metoclopramide may be tried to improve motility but frequently has side effects and should be used at low doses and stopped as soon as possible. Erythromycin cannot be routinely recommended to spur bowel motility.

A common reason to consider tube feeding is because of dysphagia and recurrent aspiration. When counseling patients and families about alternative feeding strategies, it is important to inform them that all tube feeding (both nasogastric and percutaneous) is associated with a significant risk for aspiration and pneumonia. Keeping the head of the bed elevated to 30° during feeding is only somewhat helpful. Maintaining a nasogastric tube in the confused patient may necessitate physical restraints and thus lead to injury and decreased quality of life. Nasogastric tubes are often accidentally pulled out and feedings disrupted. They have to be taped to the face and can cause nasal irritation or erosion. Replacing tubes requires confirmation of placement in the correct location, usually by radiography. Endoscopically placed abdominal (percutaneous endoscopic gastrostomy; PEG) tubes are usually easily maintained, but placement has some risk; these can also be pulled out by patients. If a PEG tube is dislodged, it should be replaced immediately or a catheter inserted because the tract can close quickly, requiring complicated reinsertion.

Continuous tube feeding is usually better than bolus feedings in the bed-bound patient. Nighttime tube feedings can be given if the patient does not meet a defined caloric intake during the day.

Parenteral Nutrition

Nutritional intervention is often delayed in the hopes that a patient will soon begin voluntary eating or because of barriers to artificial feeding. Peripheral parenteral hyperalimentation is easier to initiate and maintain than central hyperalimentation. It is a useful intervention when begun promptly after anticipating that oral intake is likely to be poor for several days. It continues to be underused. Maintaining some enteral nutrition, however, decreases gut mucosal atrophy and the risk of bacterial translocation and peritonitis. In general, delaying nutritional support increases morbidity.

Complication: Refeeding Syndrome

There is danger in rapidly providing large quantities of nourishment, particularly to a slowly starved but stable patient. Overfeeding a debilitated person can cause a potentially fatal refeeding syndrome. If the patient's liver and kidneys are functioning, protein intake should initially not exceed 1.5 g/kg of the patient's normal weight. The Harris-Benedict or World Health Organization (WHO) equations (see Table 38–1) can estimate initial caloric needs if indirect calorimetry is not available. The hyperglycemia associated with overfeeding leads to hyperinsulinemia, with its deleterious effects on blood vessels, and to antinatriuresis, causing fluid retention. Because the patient's heart muscle is also likely to be atrophic, with impaired ability to respond appropriately when overloaded, patients are at high risk of sudden pulmonary edema. Thus, it is important to initiate feeding at intakes of 100% to not more than 120% of the Harris-Benedict/WHO-calculated requirements and to meticulously monitor mineral and electrolyte measures (potassium, phosphate, magnesium) and cardiac status. A rising heart rate may be a subtle indicator of fluid overload. Weight gain > 1 kg/week should be considered fluid retention and avoided.

Crook MA et al: The importance of the refeeding syndrome. Nutrition 2001;17:632. [PMID: 11448586]

OBESITY IN OLDER ADULTS

Aging in the United States is commonly associated with a decrease in lean body mass and a progressive increase in fat stores. This adipose tissue tends to be distributed to the abdomen, even in healthy older adults and those with no change in weight. In the United States, ~42% of men and women between the ages of 60 and 69 and 37% between the ages of 70 and 79 are overweight (BMI > 25 kg/ m²). Among persons older than 80, 18% of men and 26% of women are overweight. Controversy exists as to the definition of healthy weight for adults older than 70. Obesity is associated with highest mortality in young adults; it appears to have less prognostic significance in old age. Obesity in frail older adults may be protective against injury from falls or may provide a nutritional buffer during acute illness. On the other hand, obesity is associated with increased risk of knee and hip arthritis and decreased physical function. Elevated BMI strongly predicts risk for symptomatic knee osteoarthritis in elderly women, and weight loss significantly lowers the osteoarthritis rate in women whose BMI exceeds 25 kg/m^2. Central obesity is associated with increased cardiovascular disease, diabetes mellitus, and hypertension in whites and, perhaps, black men. It has been suggested that a waist circumference > 94 cm (37 in.) in men and 80 cm (31.5 in.) in women is associated with increased cardiovascular risk. However, neither BMI nor fat location seems to predict mortality in black women, except in the case of extreme obesity. Much remains to be learned about racial differences in fat patterning and its health consequences.

Aggressive weight loss should not be attempted or encouraged in most older adults. Those who are obese and have poorly controlled hypertension, diabetes mellitus, functional impairment, or lower extremity arthritis may benefit from gradual weight reduction (under close supervision to prevent malnutrition). Sustained weight loss generally requires a combination of healthy diet and exercise. Exercise does not have to be strenuous; simple walking can be extremely successful, if done regularly.

A relatively small amount of weight loss, perhaps as little as 5–10%, may significantly improve hypertensive or diabetic management. Nevertheless, involuntary weight loss in any older adult, including obese older persons, is associated with high morbidity and mortality and should not be ignored.

Micronutrients

The Recommended Dietary Allowance (RDA) is defined as the average daily intake of a vitamin or mineral that is sufficient to meet the nutrient requirements of most (98%) healthy individuals. Table 38–6 lists RDAs for selected vitamins and minerals. Persons who have medical disorders may need more or less than the RDA for healthy persons. Tolerable upper intake levels (ULs) have also been estimated for certain micronutrients. This is the upper intake that is likely to pose little risk for adverse side effects in most people. The UL allows patients and health care workers to consider possible risks if large amounts of vitamin and mineral supplements are consumed. The ideal intake of vitamins and minerals needed for optimum health may be higher than the RDAs and remains under active study.

Risks for Micronutrient Deficiency

Most persons who have macronutrient undernutrition have multiple micronutrient (vitamin and mineral) de-

Table 38–6. Recommended dietary allowances (RDA) and tolerable upper limits (ULs) for selected vitamins & minerals.[a]

Vitamin/mineral	RDA	UL
Vitamin A (retinol)	Men: 900 µg Women: 700 µg	3000 µg
Vitamin D	Adults < 50: 200 IU Adults 51–70: 400 IU Adults > 70: 600 IU	2000 IU
Vitamin E	15 mg 22 IU natural vitamin E 33 IU synthetic vitamin E	1500 IU
Vitamin K	Men: 80 µg Women: 65 µg	[b]
Vitamin B$_1$ (thiamin)	Men: 1.2 mg Women: 1.1 mg	[b]
Vitamin B$_2$ (riboflavin)	Men: 1.3 mg Women: 1.1 mg	[b]
Niacin (nicotinamide)	Men: 16 mg Women: 14 mg	[b]
Vitamin B$_6$ (pyridoxine)	Men: 1.7 mg Women: 1.3 mg	100 mg
Vitamin B$_{12}$ (cobalamin)	2.4 µg	[b]
Folic acid (folate)	400 µg	1000 mg
Vitamin C (ascorbic acid)	Men: 90 mg Women: 75 mg (increase by 35 mg if a smoker)	2000 mg
Calcium	1200 mg	2500 mg
Selenium	55 µg	400 µg

[a]The RDA is the recommended average daily intake that will fulfill the nutritional needs of most healthy adults. The UL is the highest level of daily nutrient intake that is likely to pose no adverse health risk in most people. As intake above the UL occurs, there is an increasing risk of adverse effects.
[b]Tolerable upper limit not yet determined.

ficiencies as well. In addition, isolated micronutrient deficiencies can occur, particularly as the result of drug–nutrient interactions (Table 38–7). It is difficult to quickly and inexpensively determine micronutrient status for many vitamins and minerals. Moreover, blood micronutrient concentrations, especially those of fat-soluble vitamins and many minerals, may not accurately estimate tissue and storage pools. Micronutrients bound to plasma proteins will be affected by hypoproteinemia; in the presence of PEM or hypoalbuminemic states, ionized fractions may be more useful for assessing status for some micronutrients, such as calcium. Except for vitamin B$_{12}$ and folic acid, water-soluble vitamin nutrition or status is not commonly measured, and specific vitamins are supplemented based on individual risk factors.

Table 38–7. Potential drug–nutrient interactions.

Vitamin A: mineral oil, cholestyramine
Vitamin D: mineral oil, phenytoin, primidone, corticosteroids, cholestyramine
Vitamin E: warfarin (Coumadin)
Vitamin K: antibiotics
Thiamin (vitamin B_1): thiamin antagonists in coffee, tea, raw fish, red cabbage, chronic alcohol abuse
Riboflavin (vitamin B_2): phenothiazines
Pyridoxine (vitamin B_6): levodopa, isoniazid, hydralazine, penicillamine, cycloserine
Niacin: aspirin
Folic acid: sulfasalazine, trimethoprim, phenytoin, primidone, phenobarbital, alcohol, methotrexate, triamterene, metformin, 5-fluorouracil
Vitamin B_{12}: antacids, nitrous oxide, metformin

Bates CJ: Diagnosis and detection of vitamin deficiencies. Br Med Bull 1999;55:643. [PMID: 10746353]

NUTRITION & IMMUNITY

Malnutrition, particularly PEM, is known to impair immune status in older adults, particularly specific B and T cell-mediated functions and nonspecific immunity (polymorphonuclear cells and monocytes). Certain vitamins also appear to have a role in immune function. Vitamin B_6 supplementation causes more robust lymphocyte proliferative responses to T and B cell mitogens and increased IL-2 production in older adults. Supplementation of healthy older adults with vitamin E and beta carotene has been found to increase delayed-type hypersensitivity (DTH) responses and lymphocyte proliferation in some but not all studies. Cell-mediated immunity may also decline in folate deficiency. The evidence that ascorbic acid (vitamin C) deficiency plays a significant role in immune function or that high-dose supplementation reduces viral infections or duration of illness is weak and remains unproven. Studies examining the effect of multivitamin supplementation on immune status have produced mixed results.

Trace minerals play a role in immune function. Zinc, for example, can affect immune function, but readily available measures of tissue zinc status are not available. Serum zinc is not a good marker of tissue status; low serum zinc usually reflects an acute-phase response with hepatic sequestration and wound tissue uptake. Older adults commonly have low zinc intake, which is correlated with poor immune function and tissue healing. Supplementation with the RDA of zinc is recommended. However, high intakes (> 100–150 mg/day) will depress immune status and copper absorption and should not be continued for more than several weeks. Improved wound healing with high-dose zinc supplementation is not seen in zinc-sufficient patients. High zinc intake can cause abdominal discomfort and anorexia.

NUTRITION & COGNITION

The investigation of reversible causes for dementia traditionally includes the assessment of folic acid and vitamin B_{12} status, although the evidence to support this practice remains weak. Persons with low vitamin B_{12} or folic acid levels have been found to be at higher risk for Alzheimer's disease. However, although deficiency of these vitamins is common in frail older adults, vitamin B_{12} and folic acid supplementation rarely changes the course of slowly progressive cognitive decline. At present, any direct relationship between vitamin intake and risk of dementia remains unclear.

One of the hypotheses concerning the cause of Alzheimer's disease is that it is due to oxidative stress. Studies have suggested a potential role for antioxidants, like vitamin E, in modifying the course of Alzheimer's disease; further research will be needed before any convincing protective effect is proven. Cross-sectional data have also implicated a role for carotenoid intake in protecting against cognitive impairment, perhaps by decreasing small vessel disease in the brain.

Foley DJ, White LR: Dietary intake of antioxidants and risk of Alzheimer disease. JAMA 2002;287:3261. [PMID: 12076225]
Seshadri S et al: Plasma homocysteine as a risk factor for dementia and Alzheimer's disease. N Engl J Med 2002;346:476. [PMID: 11844848]

Vitamin B_{12} (Cobalamin)

Recent population studies suggest a prevalence of about 10–15% for vitamin B_{12} deficiency in older adults. Table 38–8 lists the most common causes of vitamin B_{12} deficiency. Pernicious anemia, an autoimmune disorder causing decreased gastric intrinsic factor production, is not a common cause of deficiency among elders. Cobalamin deficiency in older adults is more likely due to malabsorption of cobalamin bound within foods, often the result of atrophic gastritis and hypochlorhydria. Stomach acid helps to remove the vitamin from food and make it bioavailable. Disorders that interfere with enterohepatic absorption (such as small bowel disease or surgery) will lead to deficiency more rapidly than low intake because enterohepatic vitamin B_{12} recycling will be impaired, with the vitamin lost in the stool.

Vitamin B_{12} deficiency can present clinically with 2 relatively independent disorders. One is a hematological disorder characterized by megaloblastosis, macrocy-

Table 38–8. Causes of vitamin B_{12} deficiency.

Atrophic gastritis and hypochlorhydria
Chronic antacid use (H2 blockers, proton pump inhibitors)
Gastric surgery
Ileal surgery
Diseases of the small intestine and terminal ileum: Crohn's disease, sprue, malabsorption syndromes
Helicobacter pylori infection
Pancreatic insufficiency
Parasitic infections of small bowel (eg, fish tapeworm)
Bacterial overgrowth syndromes
Strict vegetarianism
AIDS and AIDS treatment (eg, zidovudine)
Pernicious anemia
Metformin

tosis, and anemia. A separate neurological disorder can cause peripheral neuropathy, with paresthesias and numbness; spinal column lesions, causing loss of vibration and position sense, sensory ataxia, limb weakness, orthostatic hypotension, and plantar extensor responses; and neuropsychiatric symptoms, including delirium, cognitive impairment, and depressive symptoms. Signs and symptoms of vitamin B_{12} deficiency are nonspecific and common in many older adults with multiple medical problems. Many patients with low vitamin B_{12} serum levels are asymptomatic. Current laboratory norms for vitamin B_{12} status are too low and do not identify patients with early deficiency. Many patients with low-normal vitamin B_{12} serum levels (200–350 pg/mL; 150–260 pmol/L) have measurable biochemical indicators of deficiency, including elevated methylmalonic acid (MMA) (> 270 nmol/L) levels, which normalize with supplementation. These apparently asymptomatic cases likely represent an early preclinical deficiency state. Renal insufficiency can also elevate MMA. Homocysteine (Hcy) elevations are less specific and are also affected by folate and vitamin B_6 status; Hcy measurements are not recommended for detecting early vitamin B_{12} deficiency.

Table 38–9 provides an approach to screening for vitamin B_{12} deficiency and treatment guidelines. Intramuscular or oral replacement is most common; alternative formulations (such as nasal gels) are generally more costly and have not been rigorously tested. The practice of prescribing vitamin B_{12} supplementation as a general tonic is not recommended.

Neurological symptoms of B_{12} deficiency may not improve unless therapy is begun very early. Only rarely does a progressive dementia improve in this setting. Older patients and those with more severe or long-standing symptoms appear to have worse odds of recovery.

Table 38–9. Recommendations for screening for & treating vitamin B_{12} deficiency in older adults.

1. Screen with a serum vitamin B_{12} level any older adult who is frail, has macrocytosis or neutrophil hypersegmentation with or without anemia, has peripheral neuropathy or gait disorder, or has otherwise unexplained neuropsychiatric symptoms.
2. Any patient with a vitamin B_{12} serum level < 200 pg/mL (150 pmol/L) can be considered deficient. A serum level between 200–350 pg/mL (150–260 pmol/L) is borderline deficient.
3. Most older adults who are deficient can be treated with supplementation without further investigation. It usually is not essential to prove that the older patient has pernicious anemia or intrinsic factor deficiency by testing for antibodies to intrinsic factor or performing a Schilling test.
4. Most older adults who are borderline deficient should also be treated. If it is necessary to obtain further biochemical evidence that a borderline serum vitamin level represents significant deficiency, an MMA level (serum or urine) can be obtained before and after treatment (an elevated MMA level should fall to normal with correct treatment).
5. All patients with possible symptoms of vitamin B_{12} deficiency should be supplemented parenterally. This can be accomplished by giving several intramuscular injections (1000 µg) within several days to weeks and then continuing supplementation indefinitely with monthly injections.
6. Any healthy patient whose deficiency was found incidentally and is otherwise asymptomatic can be given a trial of oral supplementation (1 mg daily). These patients should have a serum vitamin B_{12} level reassessed within the first month to confirm absorption and periodic (once or twice yearly) screening thereafter.

MMA, methylmalonic acid.

Folate (Folic Acid)

Folate deficiency is associated with general malnutrition and alcohol abuse and with use of folate antagonists, such as methotrexate, phenytoin, sulfasalazine, primidone, phenobarbital, and triamterene. Like vitamin B_{12} deficiency, it can present as a megaloblastic macrocytic anemia. Folate supplementation may improve the hematological picture in combined vitamin B_{12}–folate deficiency states, without correcting the ongoing neurological disorder of vitamin B_{12} deficiency. Clinicians commonly assess both vitamin B_{12} and folate status in any patient with macrocytosis. However, low folate intake is a very unusual cause for macrocytosis. Fortification of grains with folic acid began in the United States in 1998 in a program to reduce neural tube defects. The concern that grain fortification would mask vitamin B_{12} deficiency has not been proven.

Folate deficiency appears to be associated with, and may cause, cognitive impairment. Some studies have found slowed mental processing (including poorer performance on mental status testing) and depressive symptoms in patients with folic acid deficiency. Other research has found associations between low serum folate and cerebral cortical atrophy. Epidemiological investigations point to a connection between hyperhomocysteinemia (which can result from folate deficiency) and Alzheimer's disease or vascular dementia. Ongoing studies are exploring whether vitamin supplementation can reverse or prevent cognitive decline.

Folate status may be assessed by measuring (1) serum folate if dietary intake (diet or vitamin supplementation) has not recently changed or (2) erythrocyte (red blood cell) folate if there has been a recent change in diet (as after hospital admission).

NUTRITION & VASCULAR DISEASE

Elevated levels of Hcy are associated with thrombogenicity and vascular disease throughout the body. Folic acid (and, to a lesser extent, vitamins B_{12} and B_6) supplementation can lower Hcy levels. After fortification of grains in the United States in 1998, Hcy levels have declined in the general population. A combination of folic acid (1 mg), vitamin B_{12} (400 μg), and pyridoxine (10 mg) given for 6 mo to patients averaging 61 years of age after coronary angioplasty significantly reduced Hcy levels and arterial restenosis. Studies are currently underway to determine whether specific vitamin therapy will reduce clinical end points of heart attack and stroke. Consumption of a diet rich in fruits and vegetables continues to be recommended as the best source for folic acid, but folate supplements of 400–1000 μg may additionally be taken.

Antioxidants have been promoted as protective against cardiovascular disease for many years. Many epidemiological observational studies have shown a lower rate of cardiac death in people who consume a diet rich in the antioxidant vitamins E and C and carotenoids. The carotenoids in general, and beta carotene in particular, have antioxidant properties in some model systems but not in others. High levels of serum carotenoids are associated with a lower risk of periventricular white matter lesions on magnetic resonance imaging, particularly in smokers. These findings are difficult to interpret because diets rich in antioxidants are also higher in fiber and lower in cholesterol and saturated fat, and people who consume large amounts of fruits and vegetables or who take vitamin supplements often have healthier lifestyles. Randomized clinical studies for primary prevention of cardiovascular disease have not found that any single vitamin is consistently beneficial. In fact, some studies have

found increased mortality with the use of beta carotene and vitamin E. Vitamin E may increase risk for hemorrhagic stroke.

Overall, the evidence to date is insufficient to conclude that antioxidant vitamin supplementation reduces clinically significant oxidative damage in humans, although large randomized in the United States and Europe are continuing.

Brown BG et al: Simvastatin and niacin, antioxidant vitamins, or the combination for the prevention of coronary disease. N Engl J Med 2001;345:1583. [PMID: 11757504]

Yusuf S et al: Vitamin E supplementation and cardiovascular events in high-risk patients: the Heart Outcomes Prevention Evaluation Study Investigators. N Engl J Med 2000;342:154. [PMID: 10639540]

Hooper L et al: Dietary fat intake and prevention of cardiovascular disease: systematic review. BMJ 2001;322:757. [PMID: 11282859]

Tice JA et al: Cost-effectiveness of vitamin therapy to lower plasma homocysteine levels for the prevention of coronary heart disease. JAMA 2001;286:936. [PMID: 11509058]

NUTRITION & CANCER

In observational studies, populations who consume foods highest in antioxidants (fruits and vegetables) have lower cancer rates. It is difficult to determine whether these findings are due to the antioxidant nutrients themselves or to other healthy behaviors. Some clinical prevention trials using micronutrients have shown promising effects: selenium in lung, prostate, and colorectal cancer; beta carotene, vitamin E, and selenium in stomach cancer; and vitamin E in prostate and colon cancer. Other studies, however, have found an increased risk of cancer in some patients taking beta carotene supplements, and vitamins may impair the effectiveness of cancer therapy by protecting cancer cells during radiation therapy. Fiber intake remains unproven as a protective agent against colon polyps or cancer, but it has other benefits. Any protective role for other nutrients (vitamin D analogues; calcium; phytonutrients such as green tea, lycopene, and soy isoflavones) and general diets (eg, the Mediterranean diet) remain under investigation.

Scheppach W et al: WHO consensus statement on the role of nutrition in colorectal cancer. Eur J Cancer Prev 1999;8:57. [PMID: 10091044]

NUTRITION & AGE-RELATED EYE DISEASES

Evidence to support a protective effect of individual antioxidant vitamins on age-related eye diseases is conflicting. Zinc may have a role in preventing age-related macular degeneration or in slowing its progression. Critical assessment of related studies support a diet rich in antioxidants rather than vitamin supplements to possibly prevent age-related cataract. Smoking has been shown to be the strongest environmental risk factor for age-related macular disorders.

Age-Related Eye Disease Study Research Group: A randomized, placebo-controlled clinical trial of high-dose supplementation with vitamins C and E, beta carotene, and zinc for age-related macular degeneration and vision loss. Arch Ophthalmol 2001;119:1417. [PMID: 11594942]

Age-Related Eye Disease Study Research Group: A randomized, placebo-controlled clinical trial of high-dose supplementation with vitamins C and E and beta carotene for age-related cataract and vision loss. Arch Ophthalmol 2001;119:1439. [PMID: 11594943]

NUTRITION & BONE HEALTH

Low bone density is common in older adults and is associated with hip and vertebral fractures. One common cause is osteoporosis, a multifactorial disease that causes brittle bones (see Chapter 27: Osteoporosis & Hip Fractures). Another cause is osteomalacia, resulting from vitamin D deficiency. In older adults, osteoporosis and osteomalacia frequently coexist.

Daily intake of elemental calcium should be ~1200–1500 mg in most persons after adolescence. There are a variety of calcium sources. A cup of milk or yogurt contains ~300 mg of calcium. Green vegetables contain some calcium, but they also contain other phytochemicals that interfere with calcium absorption. Therefore, calcium bioavailability from vegetables may be limited. Many persons will be unable to consistently obtain the recommended intake of calcium from natural sources and will need to take calcium supplements. Some brands of orange juice, candy, and other foods now contain added calcium. In pill form, calcium carbonate is the least expensive; absorption improves when consumed with food (although high-fiber foods may reduce absorption somewhat). Some formulations, like calcium citrate, are better absorbed but cost more. Calcium supplements can increase constipation in some individuals. Perhaps paradoxically, persons who develop calcium oxalate kidney stones should not be on a low-calcium diet because dietary calcium can bind with and reduce food oxalate absorption and thereby decrease risk of stone formation.

Vitamin D is required for calcium absorption, and vitamin D receptor density in the intestine decreases with age. The capability of the skin to manufacture vitamin D when exposed to sunlight also decreases with age and with use of sunscreens. In addition, in the winter in many parts of the United States, low sun exposure prevents significant cutaneous production of the vitamin. Thus, for various reasons, supplementation of vitamin D is often necessary for many older adults. A combined vitamin D–calcium supplement is recommended because most older adults will benefit from both. Persons taking glucocorticoids also need supplementation of calcium and vitamin D to reduce bone loss. Because of the toxicity of vitamin D, it is important not to exceed the UL of 2000 IU.

Very high intakes of vitamin A are associated with an increased incidence of hip fractures in postmenopausal women who are not taking estrogen. It is recommended that the UL for vitamin A (3000 μg) not be exceeded.

Janssen HCJP et al: Vitamin D deficiency, muscle function, and falls in elderly people. Am J Clin Nutr 2002;75:611. [PMID: 11916748]

VITAMIN & MINERAL SUPPLEMENTATION

Many older adults, including those who are healthy and living independently as well as those who are frail, ill, or institutionalized, are at risk for subtle micronutrient deficiencies. Most adults do not consistently consume recommended amounts of fruits and vegetables. As aging progresses, risk factors for poor intake, adverse drug–nutrient interactions, and nutrition-related diseases increase. Many persons in the United States (currently ~40% of adults) consume supplemental vitamins. Current evidence suggests that daily intake of a vitamin–mineral supplement, supplying the RDA, can be recommended for all older adults and is associated with no significant adverse effects. It remains unclear whether intakes above the RDA are associated with significant health benefits, and high intake of some micronutrients (particularly vitamins A, D, and pyridoxine) and many minerals is well known to cause toxicity. Certain subgroups (eg, smokers, persons at risk for hemorrhagic stroke) may be at higher risk for side effects from vitamin supplementation.

Patients should be counseled not to exceed the UL (see Table 38–6), except under medical guidance, and should be reminded that improved health is directly related to modifying more clearly associated cancer and cardiovascular risk factors, such as smoking, hypertension, diabetes mellitus, saturated fat intake, and exercise. Vitamin and mineral supplementation does not substitute for healthy nutrition. Clinicians should ask about vitamin and mineral supplement use when reviewing their patients' medications lists.

Willett WC, Stampfer MJ: What vitamins should I be taking, doctor? N Engl J Med 2001;345:1819. [PMID: 11752359]

Use of Alcohol, Tobacco, & Nonprescribed Drugs

39

James W. Campbell, MD, MS

ESSENTIALS OF DIAGNOSIS

- Definition of harmful use of any substance: "Use resulting in a negative consequence followed by repeated use."
- Negative consequences occur in the medical, legal, family, occupational, social, psychological, and/or economic arenas.
- Questions of quantity and frequency of use can be misleading, especially in older persons.
- Alcohol abuse in older persons can exacerbate or cause congestive heart failure, dementia, depression, delirium, falls, fractures, hypertension, incontinence, insomnia, malnutrition, osteoporosis, sexual dysfunction, and gastrointestinal complaints.
- Treatment for alcoholism is more likely to be successful in older persons.
- Screening and intervention for tobacco abuse should be part of primary care for all older adults because tobacco use is still prevalent and health benefits of smoking cessation are substantial.

SMOKING

General Considerations

Studies from the Center for Medicare and Medicaid report that smoking is the single most preventable cause of illness. Over 10% of the population 65 years and older are smokers; specifically, 12.9% of persons aged 65–74 smoke and 6.1% of persons older than 75 smoke. Smokers older than 65 are identified as the most likely to benefit from smoking cessation.

Prevention

Tobacco abuse reduction is one of the most well-developed areas of prevention. Strategies include public education, office interventions, formal cessation programs, and pharmacological assistance. In 2002, Medicare began a limited program to address smoking cessation specifically in the older population, but no large-scale prevention programs target seniors.

Complications

Smoking is debated in terms of its effect on cognition. Recent studies have not shown a relationship between smoking and measures of general cognitive ability, executive function, and memory when corrected for age, education, and other health conditions. These studies need to be examined closely; when one controls for other tobacco-use related health conditions (ie, cerebrovascular accidents, coronary artery disease, and hypertension), the mechanisms by which tobacco places a person at greater risk of cognitive decline may be eliminated and create a false protective effect. An association with osteoporosis is found for smokers and former smokers with chronic obstructive pulmonary disease independent of their use of corticosteroids.

Treatment

The pharmacological options in smoking cessation are well substantiated. Nicotine substitution by patch improves success rates in smoking cessation. Adjunctive pharmacotherapy is also beneficial. The use of bupropion assists with smoking cessation. Smoking cessation highlights another important aspect of behavior change; despite common assumptions to the contrary, repeated attempts to quit improve success. This suggests the value of educating those who have quit and relapsed that their chance for success in the future is significant. Each attempt to quit provides the quitter with a new set of skills and knowledge. Interest in quitting appears to be rising among older persons. Medicare Stop Smoking Programs funded by Medicare are underway in Alabama, Missouri, Ohio, Oklahoma, Nebraska, and Wyoming.

Arday DR et al: Smoking patterns among seniors and the Medicare stop smoking program. J Am Geriatr Soc 2002;50:1689. [PMID: 12366623]

Neafsey PJ, Shellman J: Misconceptions of older adults with hypertension concerning OTC medications and alcohol. Home Health Nurse 2002;20:300. [PMID: 12045697]

Schinka JA et al: Effects of the use of alcohol and cigarettes on cognition in elderly adults. J Int Neuropsychol Soc 2002;8:811. [PMID: 12240745]

Yeh SS et al: Risk factors for osteoporosis in a subgroup of elderly men in a Veterans Administration nursing home. J Invest Med 2002;50:452. [PMID: 12425432]

ALCOHOL ABUSE

General Considerations

Alcoholism is the third most common psychiatric disorder among older persons. Up to 16% of men and 8% of women have alcohol use disorders. Alcohol use significant enough to impair health is present in up to 20% of patients hospitalized on medical-surgical units. Too often the diagnosis is missed as a result of not screening. Simple screening tools with good sensitivity are available, and excellent tools for diagnostic confirmation with high specificity are validated in older populations. Treatment for substance abuse disorders through brief intervention and more classical treatments have been found to be effective in older patients.

Alcoholism, alcohol dependence, and alcohol addiction are used synonymously in this chapter. Many classify alcoholism as chronic or late onset depending on the presentation of first symptoms before or after age 65. Although of interest, these 2 groups do not perform significantly differently in treatment. Alcoholism can be considered to be active or in remission, and activities such as relapse prevention groups act as mechanisms to prolong a remission.

Pathogenesis

Although alcoholism is at its core a heritable disease, much of the inherent medical risk in the elderly patient's consumption of various substances lies in the altered pharmacokinetics present in older individuals (see Chapter 41: Principles of Drug Therapy). All ingested agents have a decrease in volume of distribution. The volume of distribution of water-soluble agents is particularly altered as the body fat–body water ratio changes with age. Alcohol, a classic water-soluble drug, produces a much higher blood alcohol concentration in an older person than in a younger person of the same weight. Genetic predisposition to alcoholism is estimated to account for 40–60% of alcoholism cases.

Prevention

Alcohol abuse prevention is predominantly aimed at younger persons. However, there are significant programs now specifically designed to address alcoholism prevention in elders. In Virginia, a statewide program to detect and prevent geriatric alcoholism has included a 7-year follow-up; this follow-up documented the program's ability to enhance detection and increase assistance to identified persons with alcoholism risks.

Clinical Findings

A. SYMPTOMS & SIGNS

Alcoholism in elders is often missed. Many of the classical clues are mistakenly attributed to age-related changes or diseases common in old age (Table 39–1). Many of the consequences that drive a younger person into treatment—job loss, divorce, or legal pressures—are less likely to occur in older persons. One of the best clinical clues is the use of other substances, particularly nicotine. Seventy percent of alcoholics smoke > 20 cigarettes/day compared with 10% of the general population. Alcohol abuse should be investigated in patients with anxiety and mood disorders. Even such common conditions as hip fractures should trigger screening for alcoholism because research has shown a 2.6-times increased risk of hip fracture over 5 years in patients with a history of admission for alcohol-related disorders. Physical stigmata of alcoholism do occur but are a late

Table 39–1. Clinical clues to the diagnosis of alcoholism misattributed to diseases common in old age.

Clue	Disease	Alcohol
Fracture	Osteoporosis	Alcohol directly induces falls and osteoporosis.
Sleep disturbance	Insomnia of old age	Alcohol impairs the normal sleep cycle.
Elevated blood pressure	Essential hypertension	Alcohol is a direct cause of secondary blood pressure elevation.
Cognitive impairment	Alzheimer's-type dementia	Alcohol is a direct cause of dementia, Wernicke-Korsakoff syndrome, and delirium.
Incontinence	Urge incontinence	Alcohol-induced diuresis.
Congestive heart failure	Ischemic heart disease	Alcohol-induced cardiomyopathy.
Sexual dysfunction	Peripheral vascular disease	Alcohol-induced hormonal dysfunction.

finding in alcoholism, and screening is best aimed at an earlier stage of the disease.

Confusion, dizziness, drowsiness, and dryness of mouth are among the common side effects of alcohol use.

B. LABORATORY FINDINGS

Many attempts have been made to find a useful screening laboratory test for detecting early alcoholism. To date, no test with reasonable sensitivity and specificity exists. Elevations in MCV and γ-glutamyltransferase are reasonably sensitive but nonspecific. Alterations in AST and ALT most often represent advanced disease.

Carbohydrate-deficient transferrin (currently available at specialized centers) is a possibly useful test to measure intake over time. However, the test shows more promise as a monitor of treatment than as a tool for screening patients for alcoholism.

C. IMAGING STUDIES

Currently, no imaging studies are useful in the detection of early-stage disease.

D. SPECIAL TESTS

Standardized questionnaires are the current gold standard for diagnosis. The Geriatric version of the Michigan Alcoholism Screening Test is still one of the best tools available (Figure 39–1). The short version is a brief test with a sensitivity of 52% and a specificity of 96%. The AUDIT tool also has very high specificity. The CAGE assessment has been well studied and exhibits excellent sensitivity. This tool is composed of 4 simple questions based on the CAGE mnemonic:

1. Have you ever felt you should *C*ut down on your drinking?
2. Have people *A*nnoyed you by criticizing your drinking?
3. Have you ever felt bad or *G*uilty about your drinking?
4. Have you ever had a drink first thing in the morning to steady your nerves or get rid of a hang-over (ie, as an *E*ye opener)?

The CAGE is 91% sensitive and 48% specific.

Interview technique is important because the order of questions has been shown to affect the screening tools. The CAGE becomes less sensitive if preceded by questions on quantity and frequency. The CAGE, well delivered, can enable the diagnosis of alcoholism even in a patient with significant denial. The patient may offer as evidence of control the ability to cut down on drinking. The simple fact that the patient is working to limit intake helps make the diagnosis of alcoholism. Another more recently developed tool, the Alcohol-Re-lated Problems Survey (short version), also has a sensitivity of 92% and a specificity of 51%.

E. SPECIAL EXAMINATIONS

There are a large number of prolonged standardized diagnostic tools (eg, the Substance Abuse Disorders Diagnostic Schedule). These tools are valuable in research settings and are used as entry points to intensive treatment but are not appropriate for primary care settings. The most important goal in primary care is to perform some form of screen on all persons.

It is noteworthy that older women are often omitted from clinical studies even though 12% of older women regularly drink in excess and older women have a swifter progression to alcohol-related illnesses. Older women represent the most underscreened and underdiagnosed population. Older women who are moderate to heavy drinkers have been found to have many misconceptions about alcohol and drug use. They are also less likely to be assessed for nonprescribed drug use despite the fact that OTC drug use is higher in women than in men.

Differential Diagnosis

Alcoholism is in the differential diagnosis, either as a cause or exacerbating factor, in almost all geriatric syndromes. Likewise, alcohol abuse, heavy alcohol use, or alcoholism can be a direct etiological factor or a clear cause of worsening of many of the diseases prevalent in old age. One important consideration is the differentiation of aging from substance use abuse disorders. Table 39–2 lists some examples of presentations often incorrectly attributed to aging that may actually be symptomatic of pathological alcohol use.

Complications

As many as 10% of demented individuals suffer from an alcohol-induced dementia. This dementia often goes unrecognized despite being one of the most responsive to treatment. Differentiating alcohol-induced dementia from Alzheimer's disease or multi-infarct dementia is critical since alcohol-induced dementia improved dramatically with sobriety. Alcohol abuse often coexists with depression, dysthymia, or anxiety. An estimated 10–15% of depressed persons use alcohol to self-medicate. Alcohol has been associated with an increased risk of falls, osteoporosis, and fractures.

There is continued great debate regarding the beneficial effects of low-dose drinking. In younger persons, this may well represent a chance to influence cardiovascular risk factors. However, no clear evidence exists of benefits from drinking for elders. On the contrary, many diseases and medications used by the elderly have contraindications to alcohol use.

		YES	NO
1.	After drinking have you ever noticed an increase in your heart rate or beating in your chest?	☐	☐
2.	When talking with others, do you ever underestimate how much you actually drink?	☐	☐
3.	Does alcohol make you sleepy so that you often fall asleep in your chair?	☐	☐
4.	After a few drinks, have you sometimes not eaten or been able to skip a meal because you don't feel hungry?	☐	☐
5.	Does having a few drinks help decrease your shakiness or tremors?	☐	☐
6.	Does alcohol sometimes make it hard for you to remember parts of the day or night?	☐	☐
7.	Do you have rules for yourself that you won't drink before a certain time of day?	☐	☐
8.	Have you lost interest in hobbies or activities you used to enjoy?	☐	☐
9.	When you wake up in the morning do you have trouble remembering part of the night before?	☐	☐
10.	Does having a drink help you sleep?	☐	☐
11.	Do you hide your alcohol bottles from family members?	☐	☐
12.	After a social gathering, have you ever felt embarrassed because you drank too much?	☐	☐
13.	Have you ever been concerned that drinking might be harmful to your health?	☐	☐
14.	Do you like to end an evening with a night cap?	☐	☐
15.	Did you find your drinking increased after someone close to you died?	☐	☐
16.	In general, would you prefer to have a few drinks at home rather than go out to social events?	☐	☐
17.	Are you drinking more than in the past?	☐	☐
18.	Do you usually take a drink to relax or calm your nerves?	☐	☐
19.	Do you drink to take your mind off your problems?	☐	☐
20.	Have you ever increased your drinking after experiencing a loss in your life?	☐	☐
21.	Do you sometimes drive when you have had too much to drink?	☐	☐
22.	Has a doctor or nurse ever said they were worried or concerned about your drinking?	☐	☐
23.	Have you ever made rules to manage your drinking?	☐	☐
24.	When you feel lonely does having a drink help?	☐	☐

Scoring 5 or more "yes" responses is indicative of an alcohol problem. For further information, contact Frederic Blow, PhD, at University of Michican Alcohol Research Center, 400 E. Eisenhower Parkway, Suite A, Ann Arbor, MI 48104, 313/988-7952.

Figure 39–1. Geriatric version of the Michigan Alcoholism Screening Test. Courtesy F. Blow. Used with permission.

Treatment

A. TWELVE-STEP PROGRAMS

An organized approach to screening, diagnosis, and treatment of substance abuse in elders is summarized in Figure 39–2. The treatment of all substance abuse disorders is based on the model of Alcoholics Anonymous (AA) and similar 12-step programs. Brief counseling in a primary care setting is often effective to initiate recovery. Family involvement is key to success in the treatment of substance abuse. Paradoxically, a patient co-erced into treatment has nearly as good a chance of long-term success as a patient who initially self-referred. The standard prescription includes discontinuation of all substance use, attendance at 90 meetings in the first 90 days, and regular involvement in the program and meetings.

AA is the most readily available program, and its tenets can be adapted for any substance. Although formal research on the principles of AA is by definition difficult, studies have shown that patient attendance at 90 meetings in the first 90 days to be the most powerful predic-

Table 39–2. Clinical clues to the diagnosis of alcoholism misattributed to normal aging.

Decreased socialization
Forgetfulness
Functional decline
Gait instability
Impaired driving
Increased use of analgesics
Increased use of over-the-counter drugs
Peripheral neuropathy
Poor dentition
Poor nutrition
Sexual dysfunction
Self-neglect
Sleep impairment
Slow postsurgical recovery

tor of long-term sobriety. AA is geriatric friendly, and 33% of all calls to AA are from persons older than 55. A nonjudgmental approach without "labeling" appears to be more effective in older persons, who are still strongly averse to accepting the label "alcoholic." A less threatening approach such as "you may be drinking more than is healthy" or "your drinking appears to be having a negative impact on your life" gives better results. Presenting treatment in the framework of hope is a far more successful strategy for behavior change than fear.

B. DETOXIFICATION

Detoxification needs to be closely medically monitored because the older person is more susceptible to medical complications. Aversive drugs such as disulfiram are of limited utility in older persons because a disulfiram reaction may have major medical consequences. Newer

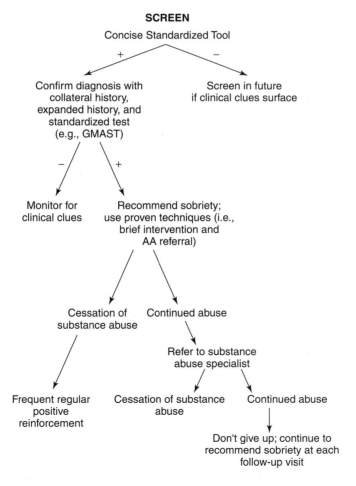

Figure 39–2. Organized approach to screening, diagnosis, and treatment of substance abuse in elders.

drugs such as naltrexone, although well grounded in appropriate physiology, are substantially limited by cost.

C. PHARMACOLOGY

Pharmacological adjuncts to treatment still require a solid primary treatment program.

Prognosis

Problem drinking can be successfully treated by brief intervention by primary care physicians. This technique is time and cost efficient with surprisingly good results. Simple physician education of patients regarding risks and benefits of continued use combined with 1 follow-up resulted in a significant success rate on the order of 10–15%. Although this rate is low in absolute terms, it is high compared with the success of treatment of other chronic diseases in 2 visits. At the end of intensive treatment, older patients showed significant change in most areas targeted for treatment; motivation, cognition, and interpersonal support improved more than expected. Older alcoholics in general have a better prognosis than younger alcoholics, which may be because the older cohort is more likely to have monosubstance abuse.

Arndt S et al: Screening for alcoholism in the primary care setting: are we talking to the right people? J Fam Pract 2002;51:41. [PMID: 11927063]

Blow FC: Treatment of older women with alcohol problems: meeting the challenge for a special population. Alcohol Clin Exp Res 2000;24:1257. [PMID: 10968666]

Coogie CL et al: Follow-up to the statewide model detection and prevention program for geriatric alcoholism and alcohol abuse. Community Ment Health J 2001;37:381. [PMID: 11419516]

Eliason MJ, Skinsted AH: Drug & alcohol intervention for older women: a pilot study. J Gerontol Nurs 2001;27:18. [PMID: 11820530]

Enoch M, Goldman D: Problem drinking and alcoholism: diagnosis and treatment. Am Fam Physician 2002;65:441. [PMID: 11858627]

Hanlon JT et al: Epidemiology of over-the-counter drug use in community dwelling elderly: United States perspective. Drugs Aging 2001;18:123. [PMID: 11346126]

Hinkin CH et al: Screening for drug and alcohol abuse among older adults using a modified version of the CAGE. Am J Addict 2001;10:319. [PMID: 11783746]

Lemke S, Moos RH: Prognosis of older patients in mixed-age alcoholism treatment programs. J Subst Abuse Treat 2002;22:2. [PMID: 1189905]

Menninger JA: Assessment and treatment of alcoholism and substance related disorders in the elderly. Bull Menninger Clin 2002;66:166. [PMID: 1214183]

Moore AA et al: Beyond alcoholism: identifying older, at risk drinkers in primary care. J Stud Alcohol 2002;63:316. [PMID: 12086132]

Yuan Z et al: Effects of alcohol related disease on hip fracture and mortality: a retrospective cohort study of hospitalized Medi-

care beneficiaries. Am J Public Health 2001;91:1089. [PMID: 11441736]

OTHER DRUGS

General Considerations

The rates of use of nonprescribed illicit drugs are thought to be low among the elderly, although rigorous studies are not currently available. The national comorbidity study suggests that illicit drug use declines with age. Screening based on consequences and treatment based on brief intervention and 12-step programs are effective for all substance abuse disorders.

Elders tend to use nonprescribed over-the-counter (OTC) drugs frequently. However, only 11% of physicians routinely ask about OTC use during primary care encounters.

Complications

Interactions among alcohol, illicit drugs, and prescription and over-the-counter medications are potentially serious problems in the elderly. Two thirds of older people use OTC and two thirds of OTC use is analgesics; arthritis pain accounts for ~75% of analgesic use. These analgesics include aspirin, nonsteroidal anti-inflammatory drugs, and acetaminophen products. Acetaminophen specifically interacts with alcohol and can form a dangerous drug–drug interaction. Acetaminophen is found in many OTC and prescription combination agents and, therefore, can easily be ingested in toxic doses. Older patients are also taking significant amounts of prescription drugs. These prescribed drugs can interact with the OTC agents. Special caution must be exercised because many drugs are now available both OTC and by prescription. This creates the potential for error as a patient may be getting excessive doses of a class of drugs by combining OTC drugs with prescribed medications.

Hinkin CH et al: Screening for drug and alcohol abuse among older adults using a modified version of the CAGE. Am J Addict 2001;10:319. [PMID: 11783746]

Sleath B et al: Physician-patient communication about over-the-counter medications. Soc Sci Med 2001;53:357. [PMID: 11439819]

Rigler SK: Alcoholism in the elderly. Am Fam Physician 2000;61:1710, 1883, 1887. [PMID: 10750878]

 EVIDENCE-BASED POINTS

- *Pharmacokinetic changes make alcohol more potent in older persons.*

- *Quantity and frequency inquiries perform poorly as screening for alcohol problems; consequence-based questionnaires are the best screening tools.*
- *No laboratory tests or physical exam findings perform as well as screening tools.*
- *Heavy alcohol use and alcohol abuse are associated with osteoporosis and hip fracture.*
- *Alcohol-induced dementia, which is often mistaken for progressive degenerative dementia of the Alzheimer's disease type, improves significantly with sobriety.*
- *Cigarette smoking is still prevalent in the young–old population, and cessation is beneficial.*

Barnett NL et al: Over-the-counter medicines and the elderly. J R Coll Physicians Lond 2000;24:445. [PMID: 11077655]

RELEVANT WORLD WIDE WEB SITES

Centers for Medicare and Medicaid Services: www.cms.hhs.gov/healthyaging/1b.asp (Issues related to tobacco use.)

National Institutes of Health, National Institute on Alcohol Abuse and Alcoholism: www.niaaa.nih.gov (Many government reports on alcoholism.)

U.S. Public Health Service: www.surgeongeneral.gov/library/mentalhealth/chapter4/sec5.html#service_substance (Contains the Surgeon General's 1999 mental health report.)

National Institute on Aging: www.niaaa.nih.gov/ (Report on age and alcohol abuse.)

Elder Mistreatment: Abuse, Neglect, & Exploitation

40

Carmel Bitondo Dyer, MD, & Lucia Kim, MD

ESSENTIALS OF DIAGNOSIS

- Elder mistreatment may be broadly defined as any action or lack of action that leads to harm or threatened harm to the health or welfare of the elderly person.
- Elder mistreatment includes physical or psychological abuse, caregiver or self-neglect, and financial exploitation.
- Elder mistreatment can be committed by another person, such as a caregiver, or by self and can be intentional or unintentional.
- The common denominator in any form of elder mistreatment is that the needs of the elderly person are unmet or have been violated.
- The definition of elder mistreatment varies from state to state.

General Considerations

Elder mistreatment is a complex phenomenon and a major public health issue. It comprises neglect, abuse, and financial exploitation. Epidemiological studies reveal prevalence rates of 1.3–5.4%. However, many of these studies were based on self-reporting and, therefore, may underrepresent the actual prevalence rate. The National Elder Abuse Incidence Study estimated that at least one-half million community-dwelling elders were abused or neglected or experienced self-neglect during 1996. This study revealed that almost 80% of cases of elder abuse, neglect, and self-neglect were unreported. Lack of awareness (especially among health care professionals), social isolation, and the elderly person's fear of threatening the relationship with the caregiver and feeling that there is nowhere else to go, that nothing can be done to help, or of shame in admitting abuse by one's own family are some barriers to reporting elder mistreatment. Two or more types of mistreat-

ment often coexist, and evidence of mistreatment is not always clear-cut. Regardless of the type of mistreatment, family members comprise a large portion of the mistreaters.

Nursing home residents have all the same risk factors for mistreatment as community-dwelling elders and are often so cognitively impaired that they cannot report abuse. They are also frequently physically impaired and cannot defend themselves. Multiple reports describe nursing home abuse. The 1998 compilation of complaints received by the State Long-Term Care Ombudsman program (whose aim is to "identify, investigate, and resolve individual and systems level complaints" that affect residents in nursing homes and residential care facilities) and its parent agency, the Administration on Aging, found that, nationwide, physical abuse was 1 of the 5 most frequent complaints in nursing homes. Ten percent, or ~20,000, of the complaints received by ombudsmen during fiscal year 1998 were about abuse, gross neglect, or exploitation, whereas another 5% related to financial abuse and misappropriation of property. Ombudsmen reported > 1700 cases of sexual abuse of nursing home residents during a 2-year period. Because the number of people in nursing homes is increasing, the number of abuse cases in nursing homes will undoubtedly increase as well.

Huber R et al: Data from long-term care ombudsman programs in six states: the implications of collecting resident demographics. Gerontologist 2001;41:61. [PMID: 11220816]

Administration on Aging: Long-Term Care Ombudsmen Report for Fiscal Year 1998: www.aoa.dhhs.gov/ltcombudsman/98report/98finalreport.html

A. NEGLECT

Neglect is the failure of a caregiver to provide adequately for the needs of the elder. Neglect is the most common form of elder mistreatment, representing almost 70% of all cases of mistreatment in the United States. Neglect can be committed by a caregiver and can be unintentional, if the caregiver is unaware of the needs of the elder, or intentional, if the caregiver willfully fails to provide care. Self-neglect occurs when the older person is unable to perform basic daily tasks of self-care as a result of mental or physical impairment. Diogenes syndrome is a term used to describe situations in which an elderly person lives in squalor and isolation, refusing help from the outside world.

B. ABUSE

Abuse can be physical, psychological, or sexual. Physical abuse includes hitting, pinching, kicking, and inappropriate use of restraints. Psychological abuse includes verbal aggression or making threats, which lead to emotional distress. Physical, sexual, and psychological abuse can be a part of intimate partner violence or spousal abuse.

C. FINANCIAL EXPLOITATION

Exploitation occurs when resources of an elderly person are used illegally or improperly for monetary or personal gain. The clinician must determine whether there is an explicit agreement between the patient and caregiver when money or property is being exchanged. Many elders who are lonely or who have functional but not mental limitations may knowingly enter into agreements in which personal care or friendship is traded for money, goods, or property. In other circumstances, perpetrators use undue influence by gaining a victim's confidence and then systematically isolating the victim from family and friends. These perpetrators then have the elder transfer assets into their possession. Financial exploitation when the patient has the capacity to understand the consequences of his or her actions is theft.

Comijs HC et al: Elder abuse in the community: prevalence and consequences. J Am Geriatr Soc 1998;46:885. [PMID: 9670877]

Pavlik VN et al: Quantifying the problem of abuse and neglect in adults-analysis of a statewide database. J Am Geriatr Soc 2001;49:45. [PMID: 11207841]

Pillemer K, Finkelhor D: The prevalence of elder abuse: A random survey. Gerontologist 1998;28:51. [PMID: 3342992]

Department of Health and Human Services, Administration on Aging: ww.aoa.gov/eldfam/elder_rights/elder_abuse/elder_abuse.asp

Clinical Findings

A. SYMPTOMS & SIGNS

If the presence of elder mistreatment seems likely based on screening, the clinician should look for specific clinical findings. Although seemingly obvious, these findings can be missed if the clinician is not mindful of the possible diagnosis. Red flags for possible elder mistreatment are presented in Table 41–1.

The clinician should observe the patient–caregiver interaction. A mistreated elder may display behavioral

Table 40–1. Red flags for possible elder mistreatment.

Delay in presentation for medical care after an onset of illness or injury
Frequent emergency room visits
Conflicting stories between the caregiver and the elder
Repeated injuries ("accident prone")
Missed appointments or "doctor shopping"
Medication noncompliance

problems. The caregiver may be outwardly hostile toward the patient or the health care provider.

A unifying feature of abuse, neglect, and exploitation is a state of vulnerability. This vulnerability appears to be largely due to neuropsychiatric disease, which is seen in a significant percentage of mistreated elders. The most common neuropsychiatric diagnoses include dementia, depression, psychosis, and alcohol abuse. These disorders limit the patient's ability to care for self and can lead to a failure to fulfill major role or societal obligations. Abuse of substances such as prescription medication or illegal drugs may produce similar consequences. The associated behavior patterns and loss of decision-making capacity resulting in self-neglect place older persons at risk of becoming victims of crime.

1. Physical abuse—Patients who are physically abused may have lacerations or bruises in multiple sites, fractures in unusual locations such as distal fractures of the femur, burns from cigarettes or hot liquids, or evidence of restraints on the wrist, waist, neck, or legs. Physically abused patients may display behavioral problems, such as agitation or fear of strangers.

2. Sexual abuse—Victims of sexual abuse may present with oral venereal lesions. Bruising of the uvula, the palate, and the junction of the hard palate may indicate forced oral copulation. In addition, the clinician may note bleeding and bruising of the anogenital area as well as bruising on other areas of the body, especially the abdomen. New diagnoses of sexually transmitted disease in nursing home residents or other elders may indicate abuse. Urinary tract infections in unusual clusters have been described in nursing home residents who have been victims of sexual abuse. Difficulty sitting and walking may indicate sexual abuse in elderly women. Behavioral signs indicating potential sexual abuse may include withdrawal, fear, depression, anger, insomnia, increased interest in sexual matters, or increased sexual or aggressive behavior.

3. Neglect—The diagnosis of neglect can be much less obvious than physical or sexual abuse. Therefore, potential signs and symptoms of neglect must be considered in conjunction with the patient's overall health, comorbid conditions, and functional and nutritional status. Pressure ulcers, malnutrition, and dehydration are often signs of caregiver neglect. They can also occur in the absence of neglect as a result of immobility and illness. However, multiple deep pressure ulcers or malnutrition and dehydration, arising in situations in which care should be provided, can be considered clinical findings of neglect.

Patients who neglect themselves often fail to seek medical care. When they do consult a physician, findings include poor hygiene and advanced medical disease. Self-neglecting patients often dress in dirty clothes, bathe infrequently, and have ungroomed, matted hair. Skin infestations from lice, fleas, and scabies are common, as are multiple skin excoriations from scratching.

4. Financial exploitation—Clinicians may detect clues to exploitation during the interview. Exploited elders may report being evicted from multiple dwellings. Poor nutritional status or medical noncompliance may occur because of lack of funds despite adequate income. The patients may fail to pay bills or maintain their health insurance. A new caregiver can appear on the scene to handle financial matters.

B. Physical Exam

Comprehensive physical examination should include a thorough skin, oral, and musculoskeletal evaluation. Nutrition and volume status should be assessed through physical examination and laboratory tests.

C. Assessment of Home Environment

Evaluation of the home environment is important to assess fully the patient's functional capabilities. Visiting nurses, adult protective services (APS) specialists, and medical teams that make house calls can perform in-home assessments. These professionals can make observations about patient–caregiver interaction, food supplies, and the upkeep and cleanliness of the home. In-home assessments reveal information about the ability of the patient to perform activities of daily living beyond what can be learned during an office visit.

Dyer CB et al: The high prevalence of depression and dementia in elder abuse and neglect. J Am Geriatr Soc 2000;48:205. [PMID: 10682951]

D. Assessment of Risk Factors

Potential risk factors that pertain to the elderly victim include advanced age, female gender, poverty, cognitive or functional impairment (especially recent decline), minority ethnic or racial group, and depression. Risk factors pertaining to caregivers include depression, external stress such as sudden change in economic status,

alcohol and other substance abuse, history of violence, and dependency on the elder for finances or housing. Although some elders are at higher risk for mistreatment, it is important to note that elder mistreatment can happen to any elder regardless of age, gender, and race or socioeconomic status.

E. Screening

Screening for elder mistreatment is essential, particularly in older persons who are cognitively impaired or unwilling to file a report. Elders are often reluctant to reveal abusive situations because they may feel humiliated or responsible. They may be afraid of threatening their relationship with the caregiver. They may be averse to pressing charges against their own family members. One study noted that 72% of elder abuse victims did not complain of the abuse at the time of presentation to an emergency center. The American Medical Association (AMA) recommends screening of geriatric patients if physical signs are present regardless of whether they complain of abuse. Screening for elder mistreatment should be a part of the routine health assessment for all older persons and part of comprehensive geriatric assessment.

Ideally, the health care provider has developed good rapport and is trusted by the elderly patient before addressing the issue of mistreatment. Patients and caregivers must be interviewed separately. One may start with general statements regarding safety in the house and with caregiving concerns. Direct questions must then be asked regarding abuse, neglect, and exploitation, using plain language in an unintimidating, nonconfrontational, and nonjudgmental manner (Table 40–2). If injury or harm has occurred, one must determine the frequency, severity, and location. A detailed social history must be obtained, including living arrangement, family composition, nonfamily member support, and socioeconomic status. This information will be helpful in formulating the management options.

Table 40–2. Direct questions about mistreatment.

Do you have frequent disagreements with your son or daughter?
When you disagree, what happens? Are you yelled at?
Are you made to wait long periods of time for food or medicine?
Are you made to stay in your room?
Are you ever slapped, punched, or kicked?
Has anyone ever threatened you or made you feel afraid?
Has anyone ever made you sign a document that you did not understand?

Numerous types of screening tools relevant to elder abuse and neglect exist, but most professionals collect information on the observations of others and assess risk factors. If the screening test suggests abuse, tools for performing a more comprehensive assessment for victims of elder mistreatment are available.

In some settings, such as the emergency room, comprehensive screening procedures cannot be performed because of time limitations. Instead, a single question or a 3-question screen can be used:

1. Single-question screen. When time is limited, simply asking the patient whether he or she is being abused or neglected can be helpful.
2. Three-question screen. Three important questions to ask when screening for elder mistreatment are as follows:

- Do you feel safe where you live?
- Who prepares your meals?
- Who takes care of your checkbook?

Fulmer T et al: Abuse of the elderly: screening and detection. J Emerg Nurs 1984;10:131. [PMID: 6374226]

Jones J et al: Emergency department protocol for the diagnosis and evaluation of geriatric abuse. Ann Emerg Med 1988;17:1006. [PMID: 3177986]

Differential Diagnosis

Many of the clinical features of elder mistreatment can be confused with the physical examination changes seen with normal aging.

A. Skin Tears

Skin tears are lacerations seen commonly in nonabused elderly persons and occur most frequently on the forearms and occasionally on the legs. Persons usually have no more than 1–2 skin tears at a time, and skin tears often heal completely without scarring.

B. Bruises

Ecchymoses often occur more frequently and resolve much more slowly in older persons than in younger persons and can last for months instead of the usual 1–2 weeks.

C. Spontaneous Fractures

The bones of older persons are thinner and less dense, making them more susceptible to fractures as the result of bone disease or injury. Metabolic bone disease, osteoporosis and all its causes, such as chronic steroid use, osteomalacia, and Paget's disease, and cancer that invades bone make the bones more brittle. The 2 types of bone fractures known to occur spontaneously are vertebral fractures in osteoporotic older women and hip fractures.

D. Malnutrition

Both smell and taste decline with age, resulting in decreased appetite. Many patients with cancer will lose weight regardless of efforts to maintain nutritional status. Poor health, including poor dentition, depression, dementia, and malabsorption syndromes, also may contribute to weight loss and undernutrition. Numerous other disorders can lead to malnutrition, including stroke, Parkinson's disease, amyotrophic lateral sclerosis, and disorders of the esophagus.

E. Dehydration

The elderly are much more prone to dehydration with minimal provocation than younger people. Dehydration is a common reason for emergency department visits by older persons. The elderly have decreased body water reserves and thirst drive; their thirst drive may remain depressed even after 12–24 h of water deprivation. The central nervous system regulation of water is altered; although antidiuretic hormone (ADH) is secreted properly in response to volume depletion, the older kidney responds less well to changes in ADH and continues to excrete water in the face of dehydration. Hydration is particularly difficult to monitor in older persons, who can experience very rapid changes in their fluid status without much in the way of symptomatology.

F. Pressure Ulcers

Pressure ulcers most often occur in medically ill or cognitively impaired individuals. Intrinsic causes such as acute illness, neurological disease, peripheral vascular disease, incontinence, and poor nutritional status place individuals at higher risk. Although poor nutrition is a risk factor, improving nutritional status does not always reverse or prevent the process despite good care. Pressure ulcers may take weeks to months to heal depending on the underlying comorbidities and the extent of the lesions.

Finucane TE et al: Tube feeding in patients with advanced dementia: a review of the evidence. JAMA 1999;282:1365. [PMID: 10527184]

Complications

In situations of physical abuse, any of the sequelae of blunt trauma can be seen, such as broken bones, peritoneal bleeding, and organ injury as well as subdural hematomas or intracranial bleeding with head injury. Acute illnesses such as delirium, diabetic ketoacidosis, and sepsis are commonly seen in neglected elders. Because of a lack of usual medical care, neglected patients often suffer from untreated chronic illness, such as uncontrolled diabetes or hypertension, which can lead to stroke and extensive functional limitations. Neglected patients who have insect infestations may have superinfected areas of skin excoriation. Pressure ulcers, malnutrition, and burns are other clinical findings that can be complications of neglect.

Treatment

Elder mistreatment is a complex medical problem that involves the domains of health, function, and social support and thus requires intervention on multiple levels.

There are no data regarding interventions in nursing home abuse. Clinicians need to understand the principles of good geriatric medical care, recognize mistreatment when it occurs, report it in accordance with the laws of each jurisdiction, and work with the facility staff to help correct problems.

A. MEDICAL INTERVENTION

1. History & physical—The medical approach first involves recognition of the mistreatment through the use of screening tools and comprehensive history and physical examination to look for the clinical findings. Delirium should be excluded. If the clinician suspects elder mistreatment, radiological examinations and blood tests should be ordered. Radiographs may show unsuspected fractures, often in various stages of healing. Laboratory data such as serum chemistries may reflect dehydration or electrolyte imbalance. Anemia may be present, suggesting malnutrition. Serum levels of prescribed medications may be low or undetectable, indicating that a caregiver may not be administering them. There may be high levels of sedating drugs noted on a toxicology screen.

2. Documentation—Documentation of the abuse or neglect should be complete regardless of the health care setting. The AMA recommends specific documentation. The physician should record the chief complaint in the patient's own words if possible. Proper documentation should include a complete medical and social history. If appointments are repeatedly canceled, the name of the caller should be noted. If injuries are present, the type, number, size, location, and color as well as the patient's overall state of health, the resolution of the problems, and possible causes should be included. The physician should render an opinion on whether injuries are adequately explained by the history. All laboratory or radiological and imaging studies should be recorded. If it is possible, obtaining color photographs can be very helpful. If the police are called, the name of the officer, actions taken, and police incident number should be documented as well as the date and time the report was made to the APS and the name of the person taking the report. The diagnosis of elder

mistreatment should be included in the medical problem list.

3. Reporting—Cases of elder mistreatment are reported to the APS or a similar agency depending on the jurisdiction. Reporting requirements for physicians vary from state to state; presently all but 6 states have mandatory reporting laws. Failure to report in many instances is a misdemeanor and is punishable by law. The reporting statutes specifically state that persons whose professional communications are generally considered confidential, such as physicians, attorneys, and mental health professionals, have a duty to report and that persons filing reports of mistreatment or otherwise participating in judicial proceedings resulting from the report are immune from criminal or civil liability unless they acted in bad faith or with a malicious purpose. Even in states without mandatory reporting, a report should be filed because it can trigger social service support or legal help for the patient.

When reporting, physicians need only to provide basic demographic data, information about the nature of the mistreatment, and the demographics and names of other parties, including the alleged perpetrator, if applicable. Mistreatment that occurs in facilities such as nursing homes is handled separately in some states, and physicians should know the laws and responsible agencies in their states. The National Center on Elder Abuse web site has a complete listing of reporting laws and the telephone numbers to call for each state.

4. Discharge or care planning—The clinician must be sure that the elder's medical and safety needs have been met. If the patient does not meet the criteria for admission to the hospital after the clinician has documented the findings and filed a report, the clinician must be sure that the home environment is safe and that there is assistance at home for functionally impaired patients. A social work consultation or consultation with an APS specialist may be necessary before discharge in order to develop a safety plan.

Elder mistreatment is often a chronic problem, and the patient should be referred to a physician or medical team with whom he or she can have an ongoing relationship. Elder mistreatment presents special difficulties for the patient in terms of function, decision-making capacity, and health and social support. These interrelated problems are best handled by a team of professionals from medicine, law, and social services. Geriatricians are skilled in the recognition of geriatric syndromes and are often very familiar with local agencies that could provide service to the mistreated elderly patient. Comprehensive geriatric assessment and intervention may be the ideal intervention for vulnerable abused or neglected elders.

If geriatric consultation is not available, developing a relationship with other health professionals and local agencies will be necessary to make the appropriate referrals for elder mistreatment patients. It is often helpful to discharge the patient to home with as many services as possible. Home health agencies can provide in-home assessments by social workers or nurses. Other referral sources include drug and alcohol rehabilitation services, homemaker services, and legal assistance or advocacy groups.

5. Assessment of decision-making capacity—In many instances, the mistreated elder is vulnerable because he or she lacks the capacity to participate fully in decision making. Additionally, acute illness can reduce an older person's ability to make rational and informed decisions. Diminished decision-making capacity can have serious medical consequences when a patient with diminished capacity decides against necessary surgery or hospital transport, resulting in inadequate medical care, worsening suffering, exacerbation of an illness or injury, or even death. A competent individual has the right to be a fully informed participant in all aspects of decision making and, of course, has the right to refuse. However, those patients who lack decision-making capacity and whose expressed choices may lead to harm or even death need protection and assistance.

The determination of neglect versus poor choices hinges on an elder's capacity to participate in his or her own care. There are no easily administered standard tools that assess capacity. The gold standard is psychiatric interview, which is a process that takes time and requires a specialist, rendering it impractical in more urgent circumstances. If geriatric or psychiatric consultation is not available, the clinician should be sure that the patient understands the risks and benefits of any decisions that impact his or her health or living situation.

B. SOCIAL SERVICE INTERVENTION

APS or some similar entity provides social intervention in almost every jurisdiction in the United States. APS specialists usually receive reports, conduct investigations, and coordinate social interventions. They elicit input from collateral sources such as friends and family members of the patient and consult with other social workers, physicians, and nurses. After the APS specialists complete the investigation and comprehensive in-home assessment of the patient's situation, they develop service plans to resolve mistreatment issues and other problems they have identified. They work closely with victims, families, and other involved parties. Their goal is to ensure that service is the least restrictive alternative, reflects the patient's preferences, and maximizes independence. When a patient has the capacity to make informed decisions, the APS specialists advocate for the right to refuse services if the individual does not want intervention. As advocates of a legal jurisdiction, APS specialists are bound by statutory limitation and may not impose services such as medical care if the patient is capable of making decisions.

C. LEGAL INTERVENTIONS

Laws differ from state to state, but in general law enforcement is involved in cases in which crimes are committed against the elderly, such as physical abuse, neglect with malicious intent, and financial exploitation. Police officers investigate cases, looking for evidence to help prosecutors pursue perpetrators. Officers of the court and judges participate in guardianship hearings when appropriate. Members of law enforcement and the legal profession help link older persons with agencies and other resources available to victims of crime. Forensic pathologists work closely with law enforcement officers to determine the cause of death in cases of suspected homicide resulting from abuse or neglect.

Dyer CB et al: Elder neglect: a collaboration between a geriatrics assessment team and adult protective services. South Med J 1999;92:242. [PMID: 10071677]

Prognosis

Little is known about the natural history of mistreated elders. However, studies have shown that there is an increased mortality associated with physical abuse, caregiver neglect, and self-neglect; each is an independent risk factor. Elderly victims of mistreatment and self-neglect have significantly higher mortality than nonmistreated elders.

Lachs MS et al: The mortality of elder mistreatment. JAMA 1998;280:428. [PMID: 9701077]

 EVIDENCE-BASED POINTS

- *The risk factors for elder mistreatment include age, dependency, poverty, minority race or ethnicity, and cognitive impairment.*
- *The prevalence of elder abuse ranges from 1.3–5.4%.*
- *Dementia and depression are more prevalent in persons reported as abused, especially those reported for self-neglect.*

- *Persons with elder mistreatment reported to the APS have nearly triple the mortality rate of older persons never reported as mistreated.*

REFERENCES

American Medical Association: Diagnostic and treatment guidelines on elder abuse and neglect. American Medical Association, 1992.

Aravanis SC et al: Diagnostic and treatment guidelines on elder abuse and neglect. Arch Fam Med 1993;2:371. [PMID: 8130916]

Elder Justice Roundtable Report: Medical forensic issues concerning abuse and neglect. The U.S. Department of Justice medical forensic roundtable discussion: www.ojp.usdoj.gov/nij/elderjust

National Center on Elder Abuse: http://www.elderabusecenter.org

Principles of Drug Therapy: Changes With Aging, Polypharmacy, & Drug Interaction

Rebecca Boxer, MD, & Ronald Shorr, MD

More than 80% of older adults take at least 1 medication daily. As the American population ages, more patients will be treated for acute and chronic diseases, including hypertension, arthritis, stroke, cancer, dementia, and diabetes. A larger proportion of older patients will be exposed to and consuming drug therapies. However, we have limited knowledge of age-related risks of many medications. Patients older than 75 infrequently participate in clinical trials, and if they do it is in relatively small numbers and they are often healthy.

Useful information on various medications used to treat the frail elderly has been gleaned from pharmacoepidemiological studies. For example, invaluable data on nonsteroidal anti-inflammatory drugs (NSAIDs), benzodiazepines, hypoglycemics, and gastric motility agents have come from pharmacoepidemiological data. Because it is unlikely that large trials involving frail elderly will occur, these studies will continue to grow in value to guide therapeutic decisions for the geriatric patient.

PRINCIPLES OF PHARMACOKINETICS

Pharmacokinetics refers to the processes of absorption, distribution, metabolism, and elimination of a medication. These processes depend on the individual taking the medication and the properties of the medication. These processes can change with age but also can vary greatly between individuals. The impact is difficult to determine. The pharmacokinetic processes are also influenced by various diseases, environment, and use of other medications. In general, the impact of the individual patient's physiological status (eg, hydration, nutrition, and cardiac output) and health status on the pharmacology of a particular drug is just as important as age-related changes.

Absorption

The absorptive process includes appropriate absorptive surface, gastric pH, splanchnic blood flow, and gastrointestinal (GI) tract motility. However, the absorption of drugs seems to be relatively unaffected by age, although it can be affected by other medications, diseases, and environment.

Distribution

Drugs distribute into both intracellular and interstitial spaces. Multiple physiological changes in the elderly can affect the distribution of drugs. The rate of drug distribution will be affected by cardiac output, blood flow to various tissues, and tissue volume. Older patients have an increased fat–lean body mass ratio, decreased total body water, and often somewhat decreased serum albumin. These changes can affect the distribution of some drugs in various ways depending on the properties of the drug. Drugs that distribute in fat (eg, diazepam) will have a larger volume of distribution. Hydrophilic medications (eg, digoxin) will have a decreased volume of distribution. Drugs that bind to serum proteins reach an equilibrium between bound (inactive) and free (active) drug. Levels of serum albumin can fluctuate and often decrease during periods of illness. The amounts of free to bound drug can increase with illness, and patients can develop toxicity (eg, with warfarin). This toxicity can be compounded if the processes of metabolism and elimination are also affected by the illness. Adding a new drug that competes for protein binding (eg, thyroid hormone, digoxin, warfarin, phenytoin) with drugs the patient is already taking can also result in higher levels of free drug. When high-protein drugs are used together, drug levels and effects must be monitored.

Metabolism

The metabolism of drugs varies between individuals and with aging. Hepatic enzyme activity, mass, and blood flow can decrease with age but are highly variable. In some patients, these changes are important in metabolizing drugs that have a high first-pass metabolism (eg, propranolol) where small reductions in metabolizing ability can have a greater impact.

There are 2 main metabolizing pathways in the liver. Phase I is catalyzed by cytochrome P450 through the process of oxidation and reduction. Phase II conjugates drugs through acetylation, glucuronidation, sulfation, and glycine conjugation. Phase II metabolism is not affected by age. The CYP groups of enzymes are predominately in the liver but also exist in the brain, kidney, and intestine. Enzyme activity varies greatly among individuals, but there also may be an age-related decline in cytochrome P450 activity. There is no way to predict which patients are affected. Metabolism is also influenced by other medications that either up- or downregulate various enzyme substrates, which can greatly change concentration of drugs. In addition, alcohol intake, smoking, diet, and illness can affect drug metabolism. Older adults tend to be on more medications, each with the potential to influence metabolism of another.

Excretion

Renal function often decreases with age, by much as 50% by age 85 compared with younger patients. Glomerular filtration rate and tubular function both decline. This can greatly affect elimination of various drugs that are renally excreted. The serum creatinine is not an accurate predictor of renal function in older adults because of their decreased muscle mass. Decreased creatinine clearance results in higher serum levels of the drug as well as a longer drug half-life. This is increasingly important for drugs with a narrow therapeutic index (eg, digoxin, aminoglycosides). To adjust the doses of these medications, the patient's creatinine clearance should be estimated using a formula such as:

$$\text{Creatinine clearance} = \frac{(140 - \text{age}) \times \text{weight (kg)}}{\text{Serum creatinine} \times 72}$$

(multiply by 0.85 for women to allow for 15% less muscle mass).

Although this formula is generally helpful, it is unclear whether it accurately estimates creatinine clearance in frail elderly patients, such as those living in nursing homes.

The half-life of various medications can be prolonged in older adults because of changes in drug distribution or clearance. The half-life of a drug depends on both the volume of distribution and the clearance of the drug.

$$\text{Half-life} = \frac{\text{Volume of distribution}}{\text{Clearance}}$$

Changes in volume of distribution resulting from increased body fat and decreased body water alter the expected volume of distribution of various drugs. This, in combination with changes in creatinine clearance, will produce a concentration difference of a drug greater than that seen in a younger person.

PRINCIPLES OF PHARMACODYNAMICS

The pharmacodynamics of a drug refers to the effect the drug has on an individual at the organ site. Pharmacodynamics has not been as carefully studied in older adults as pharmacokinetics, and much information is derived from observational data. Many drugs in older adults can have an exaggerated or paradoxical effect. Older adults are more sensitive to medications that depress the central nervous system (CNS; eg, benzodiazepines), which can result in adverse effects of delirium, confusion, and agitation. Patients taking psychoactive medications need close monitoring of doses and effects. Increased sensitivity (greater response at a given concentration of drug at the organ site) to drugs can have effects such as hemorrhage with anticoagulants (especially in combination with NSAIDs, acetylsalicylic acid [ASA]); orthostatic hypotension with various blood pressure medications and α-blockers; and delirium with various psychotropics and medications with anticholinergic properties.

GERIATRIC THERAPEUTICS
Adverse Drug Reactions

Adverse drug reactions occur about twice as often in older than younger patients. Hospital admissions as a result of drug-related illness range from 2.3–27.3%. Risk of an adverse drug reaction increases with greater severity of illness, multiple comorbidities, smaller body size, changes in hepatic and renal metabolism and excretion, and prior drug reactions. The increased number of adverse drug reactions tends to correlate with age, but, when controlled for other factors such as environment and disease, age is not as important as number of medication and number of disease conditions. Patients with multiple comorbidities tend to take more medications and are at increased risk for adverse drug reactions. Medications with a narrow therapeutic index and prolonged half-life cause the most trouble for the elderly patient.

The incidence of adverse drug reactions increases sharply when the older patient uses 5 or more medications daily. The risk of adverse reactions is increased by prescribing errors and the prescribing of drugs that interfere with normal hepatic metabolism or protein binding. The symptoms of an adverse drug reaction are often nonspecific and can mimic other illnesses. Adverse reactions such as fatigue, memory loss, confusion, incontinence, gait instability, and parkinsonism are common and can mistakenly be attributed to age rather than medication. Adverse drug reactions misinterpreted as disease-related symptoms can result in treatment with another medication rather than discontinuation of the offending medication. Medication reactions should always be considered when evaluating an older adult with new symptoms. The physician also needs to pay close attention to drug–drug interactions when prescribing a new medication.

Polypharmacy

Polypharmacy, the use of multiple medications, correlates strongly with the incidence of adverse drug reactions. To lessen the risks of adverse reactions resulting from polypharmacy, a carefully detailed medication history is important. Patients often have to be prompted to report medications such as eyedrops, herbal medications, and vitamins. Patients who visit multiple physicians or who have been hospitalized recently are at greater risk for polypharmacy. In addition, white patients who are sicker and older also are at increased risk for polypharmacy. For example, a patient being treated for benign prostatic hypertrophy with an α-blocker, hypertension with a β-blocker, and pain or depression with a tricyclic antidepressant (TCA) is at increased risk of orthostatic hypertension and falls. Polypharmacy can be reduced by eliminating unnecessary, suboptimally effective, or ineffective medications as well as medications with duplicate effects.

Inappropriate Medications

Inappropriate prescribing occurs when the risks of the medication outweigh the benefits. The prevalence of inappropriate drug use in the elderly population ranges from 12–40%. Medications are deemed inappropriate by either their side effects or by the potential for disease-medication interactions. Expert consensus panels generated lists of inappropriate medications in the treatment of nursing home patients. These lists are now widely used in other settings but have not been evaluated in controlled clinical trials. Medications considered inappropriate for use in elderly patients include disopyramide, anticholinergic drugs (including antihistamines such as diphenhydramine for sleep), benzodiazepines with long elimination half-lives, methyldopa, chlorpropamide, and meperidine, among others. However, many other medications that are considered appropriate can cause adverse effects in vulnerable older adults. For example, antidepressants increase the risk for falls even at therapeutic doses, emphasizing the need to carefully monitor patients and inform them of potential problems arising from medications adverse effects.

Prescribing Hazards

A patient's response to a drug can be affected by multiple illnesses, hepatic and renal impairment, as well as drug–drug interactions. In general, lower doses of medications are advised compared with the usual doses used in young adults. Protocols or guidelines for drug dosaging are typically based on studies of younger and healthy older patients. For many commonly used medications, pharmacokinetic data with patients older than 75 are not available. It is prudent to consider initiating therapy at lower than published doses for many medications and slowly increasing the dosage as needed for therapeutic effect.

Discontinuing medications can also result in adverse events as a result of alterations in drug metabolism. Some medications will induce the CYP-450 enzyme system (ie, barbiturates, carbamazepine, phenytoin, primidone, rifampin, and rifabutin). Through the CYP-450 enzyme system, these drugs can increase the metabolism of other medications. For example, patients on anticonvulsants were found to have a much lower concentration of felodipine than those not on anticonvulsants. When the anticonvulsant is discontinued, the enzyme activity decreases and the level of the affected drug can become dangerously elevated. Also, a drug level may never reach a therapeutic range while a patient is on an enzyme-inducing medication. This may require prescribing very high doses of a drug to reach a therapeutic effect. For example, patients taking rifampin will usually need large doses of warfarin to achieve a therapeutic prothrombin time. When the enzyme-inducing agent is stopped, the dose of other medications will need to be adjusted to prevent excessive effects. Medication with a narrow therapeutic index should be closely monitored with all medication changes.

New Medications

Physicians should be especially aware of potential and unexpected adverse effects and disease–drug or drug–drug interactions. Physicians should be wary of using new medications without reviewing data on their use in vulnerable older adults.

Underuse of Medications

Clinicians may be overcautious in using medications that have limited data on use in older adults. Underuse of medications can increase morbidity and mortality. For example, β-blockers are underused in older patients after myocardial infarction. Other conditions that are typically undertreated are hyperlipidemia, depression, isolated systolic hypertension, iron deficiency anemia, chronic obstructive pulmonary disease (COPD) (bronchodilators), pain, and constipation. Elderly heart failure patients are undertreated with angiotensin-converting enzyme (ACE) inhibitors. Anticoagulants (eg, warfarin for atrial fibrillation) are still underused.

Adherence

Adherence is more difficult for patients as the drug regimen becomes more complicated. Older adults often have complicated drug regimens. Patients may not fill their prescriptions or may use them for a different use than was intended. It can be difficult to determine adequate adherence if the patient is a poor historian or has no reliable informant. Patients can have a poor understanding of disease processes and the relevance of prescribed treatment. Patient and family goals may not be expressed, and physician's goals may not be the same. Patient barriers to adherence, such as cognitive decline, illiteracy, and negative attitudes toward taking medications, need to be considered. Nonadherence could also be related to inability to open safety closure bottles or the patient's inability to afford the medication.

Risk of complications increase when a physician is unaware of nonadherence. Medications may appear to be ineffective, and dosages may be increased or a more powerful medication prescribed. Complications also arise when a patient becomes hospitalized or when supervision is increased. Patients then receive the prescribed medication and can have serious complications (eg, thyroxine dose is increased and atrial fibrillation develops). Changes in diet can have profound effects, especially for patients taking hypoglycemics, diuretics, or anticoagulants. Medications prescribed in a hospital setting may work well in the controlled environment, but outside the hospital a patient can rapidly get into trouble. Typical conditions for this scenario are congestive heart failure (CHF) with changes in salt intake and diabetes with changes in carbohydrate intake.

Adherence can improve with careful explanation of the purpose of the medication. A good patient–physician relationship and open communication can help one to realize why a patient may have trouble adhering to recommendations. Formulating a reminder system for when medication should be taken, such as setting an alarm or a receiving a reminder telephone call from a friend or family member, may be helpful. Medications can be organized in pillboxes for day and time. Medication regimens and dosing schedules should be simple with clear written and verbal instructions.

COMMON MEDICATIONS

Many valuable medications are commonly used but can cause adverse effects. Cardiovascular and psychotropic drugs are the most often associated with adverse reactions. CNS side effects of commonly used medications—α-blockers, hypnotics, and drugs with histaminic and anticholinergic effects—can result in decreased ability to perform activities of daily living, increased risk of falls, and incontinence.

Nonsteroidal Anti-Inflammatory Drugs

NSAIDs are widely used for treating arthritis and chronic pain. NSAIDs provide fast and effective pain relief. However, adverse effects occur more frequently in older adults. Both age and age-related changes in NSAID pharmacokinetics increase the risk of adverse effects.

NSAIDs inhibit cyclo-oxygenase (COX) enzymes, which catalyze the conversion of prostaglandins from arachidonic acid. Prostaglandins have many roles throughout multiple organ systems and are a primary cause of pain, swelling, and inflammation. Their inhibition can also result in increased blood pressure and other adverse effects, most notably in the kidney and GI tract. Prostaglandins are vasodilators and help maintain blood flow and glomerular filtration through the kidneys, especially when blood volume is decreased. Inhibition by NSAIDs can result in decrease renal blood flow. Patients on NSAIDs who have low absolute or effective blood volume are at increased risk for renal insufficiency and renal failure. Both COX-1 and COX-2 enzymes are produced in the kidney. Inhibition of either can result in adverse renal effects, cause fluid retention, and affect sodium homeostasis. Patients who are most affected already have fluid-related morbidity (eg, CHF, liver disease, renal insufficiency). Concomitant diuretic therapy can increase risk of adverse effects. Patients with comorbidities, especially renal insufficiency and hypertension, who are given NSAIDs should be closely monitored. Preferably the lowest dose to control symptoms and intermittent shorter acting medications (eg, ibuprofen) should be used.

Infrequently, NSAIDs can also cause hyperkalemia. This is mediated though prostacyclin inhibition, resulting in decreased renin and aldosterone production, which affects potassium excretion. Patients at increased risk are those taking potassium supplements, ACE inhibitors, or potassium-sparing diuretics and those with renal insufficiency. Hyperkalemia resolves when NSAID therapy is stopped.

In the GI tract, prostaglandins have a protective effect on gastric mucosa by decreasing gastric acid production, increasing mucus production, and increasing bicarbonate production in the duodenum. COX-1 is the enzyme that catalyzes production of prostaglandin in the GI tract. Inhibition of COX-1 by nonselective NSAIDs can result in peptic ulcers and injury to the gastric mucosa. Older adults may produce less gastric prostaglandin at baseline, placing them at increased risk of gastropathy. In addition, comorbidity, use of multiple medications (steroids, diuretics, anticoagulants), and amount of NSAIDs consumed increase the risk. The specific COX-2 inhibitors (celecoxib, rofecoxib) have decreased toxicity of the GI tract while still providing anti-inflammatory effect.

Prostaglandins through COX-1 also play a role in platelet aggregation, which may also be a factor in GI bleeding. NSAIDs lack cardiovascular protection, unlike aspirin. NSAIDs do not replace aspirin in treating cardiovascular diseases. Patients with higher risk of adverse events from NSAIDs as a result of comorbidity (liver disease may affect hepatic metabolism, renal insufficiency CHF/edematous states, peptic ulcer disease) and multiple medication use should be monitored closely, or a different class of medication should be used to control symptoms. If an NSAID is necessary for prolonged use, COX-2 selective inhibitors should be considered. Misoprostol or proton pump inhibitors can be added to COX-1 NSAIDs to protect the gastric mucosa when costs restrict the use of the COX-2 agents.

Anticoagulants

Warfarin has been shown to decrease the risk of stroke in patients with atrial fibrillation (AF). Despite this, older adults (age 80 and older) with AF who are at the highest risk are more likely not to be receiving anticoagulation therapy. Physicians are often hesitant to start their patients on anticoagulation because of concerns of hemorrhage and difficulties controlling the therapy in an appropriate range. Regardless of age, dose response to warfarin varies among patients. Some studies have shown that effective dosing decreases with age.

The decision to start a patient on warfarin needs to be individualized. The risks and benefits of taking warfarin depend on the clinical situation and the goals of therapy. Anticoagulation will lower the risk of thromboembolic events, but older adults are at increased risk for bleeding complications. Risk of hemorrhage increases with history of hemorrhage, alcohol bingeing, use of aspirin and NSAIDs, cancer, liver disease, and renal insufficiency. Advanced age, thrombocytopenia, previous stroke, uncontrolled hypertension, and non-white ethnicity may also increase risk of hemorrhage.

Hemorrhagic complications are more frequent when the international normalized ratio (INR) is > 4; the therapeutic index ranges from 2.0–3.0. Older adults with acute or chronic illness taking multiple medications tend to be at the highest risk for INR fluctuations and should be closely monitored to avoid adverse events. Factors that can influence the therapeutic dose of warfarin, often requiring lower doses, include mutations in cytochrome P450, other medications (espe-

cially if highly albumin bound), low body weight, low serum albumin level, CHF, liver disease, and hyperthyroidism. In addition, warfarin can become sub- or supertherapeutic when patients experience a mild illness or changes in diet, placing them at risk for stroke or hemorrhage and necessitating close monitoring of the INR. Patients are vulnerable to complications of anticoagulation when they change settings (eg, when going from hospital to home, nursing home) and should be monitored more closely. Doses may need to be reduced in patients with CHF, COPD, liver disease, malignancy, prolonged diarrhea, or enteral feedings/poor nutritional status.

Many medications can affect the anticoagulation of warfarin by elevating or lowering the therapeutic effect. Some drugs will increase the metabolism of warfarin by induction of hepatic enzymes. This results in a lowering of the INR. Other medications will potentiate the anticoagulation effect by competing for degrading enzymes. Medications can also compete for protein-binding sites and result in more unbound warfarin. (Medication interactions with warfarin are listed in Table 41–2.) Patients must be educated about the use of warfarin and warned about use of over-the-counter (OTC) medications (no NSAIDs or ASA) and herbal remedies. Vitamin K intake should be maintained at the same level because fluctuations in intake can result in supra- or subtherapeutic INR levels (Table 41–1). The body

Table 41–1. Vitamin K-containing foods.

Green leafy vegetables
Spinach
Kale
Lettuce
Collard greens
Turnip greens
Cabbage
Watercress
Oils
Soybean
Olive
Canola
Cottonseed
Vegetables
Avocado
Brussel sprouts
Chickpeas
Broccoli
Cauliflower
Asparagus
Green beans
Meat
Beef liver

Table 41–2. Drugs that affect warfarin.

Drugs that potentiate effect	Drugs that diminish effect
Antibiotics/antifungals	Antibiotics/antifungals
Cephalosporins (cefamandole, cefoperazone, cefotetan, ceftriaxone)	Griseofulvin
Tetracyclines	Rifampin
Macolides	
Quinolones	
Sulfonamides (Bactrim has marked potentiating effect)	
Isoniazid	
Metronidazole	
Fluconazole	
Itraconazole	
Ketoconazole	
Anti-inflammatories	Benzodiazepines
Celecoxib	
Rofecoxib	
Piroxicam	
Fenprofen?	
Diflunisal?	
Tramadol	
Anticonvulsants	Anticonvulsants
Phenytoin	Barbiturates
Valproic acid	Carbamazepine
Antidepressansts	
Selective serotonin reuptake inhibitors	
Antiarrythmics	
Amiodarone (has a marked potentiating effect)	
Propafenone	
Propranolol	
Quinidine	
Diruretics	
Ethacrynic acid	
Gastrointestinal	Gastrointestinal
Cimetidine	Sulcralfate
Omeprazole	
Lipid-lowering agents	Lipid-lowering agents
Clofibrate	Cholestyramine
Gemfibrozil	
Lovastatin	
Simvastatin	
Pulmonary	
Zafilukast	
Zileuton	
Other	Other
Allopurinol Alcohol	Vitamin K
Danazol Disulfiram	
Flutamide	
Methylphenidate	
Pentoxlfylline	
Endocrine	Endocrine
Levothyroxine	Oral contraceptives
Tamoxifen	
Anabolic steroids	
Sulfonylureas	

Adapted from Honig PK, Gillespie BK: Clinical significance of pharmacokinetic drug interactions with over-the-counter (OTC) drugs. Clin Pharmacokinet 1998;35:167. Used with permission.

stores only small amounts of vitamin K and is dependent on oral intake and gut flora to synthesize it. Impaired absorption of vitamin K or antibiotic therapy can affect gut bacterial flora and disrupt vitamin K absorption. Intracranial bleeding is the most feared adverse effect from anticoagulation; its incidence ranges from 0.3–2% per year. Risk factors of intracerebral hemorrhage are similar to those of ischemic stroke: age, prior stroke, and hypertension. A concern regarding hemorrhage from falls is often the deterrent to anticoagulation therapy. Patients and caregivers should be made aware of signs and symptoms of bleeding so they may receive prompt medical attention.

The decision to use anticoagulation is made in agreement with the patient and caregivers, weighing the benefits against the risks.

Oral Hypoglycemics

The prevalence of diabetes mellitus type 2 is increasing in the United States. Control of diabetes helps to avoid complications and maintain quality of life. However, elderly patients are believed to be at increased risk for hypoglycemia and hypoglycemic-related events while on oral hypoglycemics. Symptoms of hypoglycemia can be blunted in elderly diabetics, raising concern about optimal treatment. One must pay careful attention to various comorbidities when choosing a medication to treat diabetes.

A. SULFONYLUREAS

Sulfonylureas act on the beta cells in the pancreas to increase insulin secretion. The second-generation sulfonylureas (glipizide, glyburide, glimeperide) are equal in efficacy, safer, and more potent than first-generation drugs (chlorpropamide, tolbutamide, tolazamide). Chlorpropamide should not be used in elderly patients because of its increased risk of hypoglycemia related to its long half-life (renal excretion). Of the second-generation medications, glyburide is the longest acting and has an increased risk of hypoglycemia compared with other agents. These drugs are metabolized by the liver and cleared by the kidney. Caution should be used in patients with renal or liver disease. Drugs should be started at the lowest dose and carefully monitored because elderly patients are at increased risk for hypoglycemia at onset of therapy and with increased dosing. Weight gain is not an uncommon side effect of this class of medication.

B. BIGUANIDES

Biguanides (metformin) act as insulin sensitizers and decrease hepatic glucose production. They also have the added benefits of promoting weight loss and lowering low-density lipoprotein (LDL) cholesterol and triglycerides. In addition, metformin has been shown to decrease macrovascular complications, including myocardial infarction. Compared with sulfonylureas, metformin causes much less hypoglycemia.

With initiation of metformin therapy, ~50% of patients will experience GI side effects, including abdominal pain, diarrhea, and nausea. These side effects tend to decrease and resolve as patients continue therapy. To keep side effects to a minimum, dosages should be started low and slowly increased for therapeutic effect. The risk of lactic acidosis with metformin is low, but this medication should not be used in patients with renal insufficiency, heart failure, liver disease, dehydration, or alcoholism. It should be discontinued when patients become acutely ill, have major surgery, or receive radiocontrast dye.

C. THIAZOLIDINEDIONES

Thiazolidinediones (rosiglitazone, pioglitazone) enhance insulin sensitivity by increasing skeletal muscle uptake of glucose, decreasing hepatic glucose production in the liver, and decreasing lipolysis. These drugs stimulate production of adipocytes and can cause weight gain while decreasing serum free fatty acid levels. This class of drugs can cause edema and increase plasma volume, so they should be used cautiously in patients with mild CHF and avoided in patients with class III or IV heart failure. Anemia is a rare complication. Liver enzymes should be checked periodically. Patients with liver disease should not receive this agent.

D. α-GLUCOSIDASE INHIBITORS

α-Glucosidase inhibitors (acarbose and miglitol) inhibit the enzyme α-glucosidase in the small intestine, which decreases the breakdown of complex carbohydrates and delays absorption. These drugs work best after meals and lower glucose less than other hypoglycemic drugs. These agents are not absorbed systemically and will not cause hypoglycemia or weight loss. Side effects are mostly GI and include flatulence, bloating, loose stools, and abdominal discomfort; these tend to decrease with continued therapy. If these drugs are used in combination with other oral hypoglycemics, glucose needs to be used to reverse a hypoglycemic episode because complex carbohydrates will not be absorbed.

Nonsulfonylurea Secretagogues

Nonsulfonylurea secretagogues (repaglinide, nateglinide) are short-acting drugs that stimulate insulin secretion. These drugs are taken with meals and require the presence of glucose for action. They decrease postprandial hyperglycemia and, because of their short duration of action, have less risk of hypoglycemia compared with sulfonylureas. Nateglinide has less effect on insulin secretion in the fasting state than postprandially. Repaglinide has an efficacy equal to metformin and the sulfonylureas. Side effects include weight gain and hypoglycemia. They should be used cautiously in patients with renal or liver disease.

Psychoactive

The aging brain is much more susceptible to oversedation and delirium with psychoactive agents. Drugs such as neuroleptics, antidepressants, sedatives, and hypnotics are a common cause of adverse reactions and paradoxical effects. Barbiturates should be completely avoided if possible because they are very sedating and addictive, and they interact with other medications. In general, the most common adverse effects from all psychoactive drugs are oversedation, delirium, falls, and confusion. Patients on these medications need to be closely monitored.

Neuroleptic medications are often used to control behavioral problems in demented patients. Extrapyramidal side effects (EPSs), including dystonia, parkinsonism, and akathesia, are of concern. Akathesia, which can be mistaken for agitation or psychosis, is less common with the newer neuroleptics (atypical), but when it develops it often requires discontinuation of the medication. EPSs often do not manifest themselves until 1–2 weeks after initiation of therapy. The adverse affects can then appear anytime during therapy, especially with dosage increases. Patients taking these drugs should be monitored periodically for EPSs. If they are present, dosage decreases can be attempted. Changing the neuroleptic to a low potency or changing to an atypical neuroleptic are options.

Tardive dyskinesia (TD) develops with longer term use of neuroleptic drugs, and older adults are at increased risk, as much as 5–10 times that of a younger person. The risk of TD is lower with atypical drugs, clozapine, risperidone, olanzapine, and quetiapine fumarate.

A. CLOZAPINE

Clozapine is the oldest atypical agent and is often used as a last resort when patients are not controlled on other medications. It has not been studied in patients with dementia. Clozapine has anticholinergic properties but does not cause EPSs. It can cause agranulocytosis. White blood cell count must be checked weekly for the first 6 mo and then every 2 weeks. Clozapine can also cause marked sedation, ataxia, falls, fever, delirium, and sialorrhea, weight gain, and diabetes.

B. RISPERIDONE

Risperidone has been carefully studied in patients with Alzheimer's dementia. It is effective against both psychosis and aggression, and EPSs are less common compared with haloperidol use. The higher the dosage, the greater is the risk for extrapyramidal and other side effects. A recent black box warning was added because of a slight increased risk of stroke while on this medication.

C. OLANZAPINE

Olanzapine has some anticholinergic and antihistaminic side effects and minimal risk of EPSs at low doses. This drug has a long half-life, and sedation is common. Sedation may not occur until 10 days after the drug has been initiated. Slow titration is advised to avoid oversedation, and it should not be used on an as-needed basis. Weight gain and an increase in triglyceride level are common.

D. QUETIAPINE FUMARATE

Quetiapine fumarate is used to control agitation in dementia, but studies of its effectiveness are limited. EPSs are uncommon, but it has marked antihistaminic effects. Sedation, dizziness, and orthostatic hypotension are the common side effects. Patients may be at increased risk of diabetes.

E. BENZODIAZEPINES

Benzodiazepines are used to treat anxiety and insomnia. These drugs have a high rate of adverse effects and can often result in dependency. Side effects include confusion, falls, gait impairment (ataxia), anterograde amnesia, sedation, and dizziness. Patients do build up a tolerance to these drugs over time, and a withdrawal syndrome may occur if therapy is stopped suddenly. These agents are best used on an as-needed basis for acute behavioral difficulties as a result of anxiety or drug withdrawal in order to avoid side effects. Long-acting agents should be avoided (flurazepam, diazepam), and chronic use is discouraged.

F. ANTIDEPRESSANTS

The best tolerated antidepressants are the serotonin reuptake inhibitors (SSRIs). Unlike TCAs, there is less risk of anticholinergic side effects, orthostatic hypotension, adverse cardiac effects, or seizures. Side effects include GI disturbances, either insomnia or sedation, sexual dysfunction, and agitation (movement disorder). TCAs are, for the most part, avoided in older adults because of high rates of adverse effects. Desipramine and nortriptyline are the only recommended agents for elderly patients. Venlafaxine, a combination serotonin and norepinephrine reuptake inhibitor, tends to be activating. It can elevate blood pressure, especially in patients with hypertension. Mirtazapine has a postsynaptic serotonin effect and some serotonin and norepinephrine reuptake effect. Its effects can range from calming to sedating. Higher doses can be activating. Mirtazapine can also stimulate appetite. Doses for all antidepressants should be started low and increased slowly (weeks to months) to monitor adverse effects.

Opioid Analgesics

Underprescribing for pain is common in older adults. Concern regarding side effects (eg, oversedation, constipation, delirium) is justified but should not prohibit use of options. Addiction/dependence can be a concern of both the physician and the patient. Elderly patients tend to clear opioids more slowly. For example, absorption from fentanyl patches can be slower and take longer to reach maximum plasma concentrations. Long-acting drugs also need to be titrated slowly to avoid accumulation. Patients should be closely monitored when this therapy is initiated and with dosage titration. Meperidine is avoided as an opioid analgesic because it has a metabolite that can cause delirium. All opioids can potentially cause delirium, and patients taking these medications should be frequently assessed. Constipation is common. A bowel regimen is usually required to avoid constipation and impaction.

Anticholinergics

Various medications have anticholinergic properties (Table 41–3). Older adults are particularly susceptible to anticholinergic side effects. The side effects for these medications can be mistaken as normal signs of aging (eg, dry mouth, constipation, tachycardia, confusion). Treatment of side effects with other medications leads to polypharmacy. Other adverse effects of anticholinergic drugs include delirium, urinary retention, orthostatic hypotension, tachycardia, seizure, constipation, exacerbation of glaucoma, and blurred vision. Patients and caregivers should be aware of potential side effects. The physician should also note whether the patient is taking multiple medications that have anticholinergic effects because the side effects are additive.

Diuretics

Concomitant use of other medications with diuretics, notably NSAIDs, can increase adverse effects on renal function. Both loop and thiazide diuretics place a patient at risk for hypokalemia, which can lead to ventricular arrhythmias. Physicians may choose to supplement potassium or change the medication to avoid hypokalemia. Potassium-sparing diuretics (eg, triamterene, spironolactone) can cause hyperkalemia. Potassium levels should be monitored periodically. Care should be taken to instruct patients on the most appropriate time of day to take diuretics to minimize disruption of daily activities (eg, because of incontinence) and to enhance compliance. Loop diuretics can cause postural hypotension or postprandial hypotension.

ACE Inhibitors

ACE inhibitors have beneficial effects on cardiac and renal function. Patients with heart failure and left ventricular systolic dysfunction benefit from ACE inhibitor therapy. Older adults may be at increased risk for re-

Table 41–3. Common medications with anticholinergic properties.

Antibiotics	Ampicillin, cefalothin, cefamandole, cefoxitin, clindamycin, cycloserine, gentamicin, pipercillin, tobramycin, vancomycin
Antidepressants	All tricyclic antidepressants, especially amitriptyline, desiprimine, clomipramine, imipramine, and doxepin
Antipsychotics	All have some, but the strongest anticholinergics are chlorpromazine, thioridazine, and clozapine; resperidone has the least, if any, anticholinergic effects
Antihistamines	Chlorpheniramine, diphenhydramine, hydroxyzine, cryoheptadine promethazine, dexchlorpheniramine
Benzodiazepines	Alprazolam, chlordiazepoxide, flurazepam, oxazepam
Cardiovascular agents	Captopril, chlorthalidone, digoxin, diltiazem, dipyridamole, furosemide, hydrochlorothiazide, hydralazine, isosorbide mononitrate, methyldopa, nifedipine, triamterene, warfarin
Corticosteroids	Cortisone, dexamethasone, hydrocortisone, prednisolone
Gastrointestinal agents	Atropine, cimetidine, dicyclomine, hysoscyamine, propantheline, belladonna, clidinium, ranitidine chlordiazepoxide
Immunosuppressive agents	Azathioprine, cyclosporine
Muscle relaxants	Carisoprodol, methocarbamol, cyclobenzaprine, chlorzoxazone, metaxalone, orphenadrine
Respiratory	Theophylline
Opiates	Codeine, oxycodone
Urinary agents	Oxybutynin, tolterodine

Adapted from Temple RJ, Himmel MH: Safety of newly approved drugs: implications for prescribing. JAMA 2002;287:2273. Used with permission.

lated renal dysfunction and hypotension. Low doses are used to initiate therapy, and dose titration proceeds cautiously. Excessive diuresis at initiation or when increasing the dose of therapy may place the patient at increased risk for renal insufficiency.

ACE inhibitors render older adults at increased risk for hyperkalemia and renal insufficiency. Patients should have their renal function and potassium level monitored shortly after starting an ACE inhibitor. ACE inhibitor therapy may need to be stopped for cough, hypotension, persistent hyperkalemia, and renal dysfunction. NSAIDs used with ACE inhibitors can worsen adverse effects of renal dysfunction and hyperkalemia. Cough and angioedema can occur with any of the ACE inhibitors.

Angiotensin II Receptor Blockers

These drugs are often an option when ACE inhibitors are not tolerated. There is still a risk of renal dysfunction and hyperkalemia similar to that of ACE inhibitors. Lower doses may decrease this risk. There is no risk of cough.

β-Blockers

β-Blockers are clearly beneficial in postmyocardial infarction (MI) patients as well as in those with mild to moderate heart failure. Nonselective β-blockers (carvedilol) may have increased benefit over β_1-selective β-blockers (metoprolol). Older adults may have comorbid conditions that limit their tolerance of β-blockers (eg, COPD). Older adults are at higher risk for bradycardia. However, β-blockers may have cardioprotective effects, even for patients with risk factors for complications such as pulmonary disease, heart failure, depression, and diabetes.

Topical β-blockers are used to treat glaucoma. Topical agents are readily absorbed through the lacrimal system and the nasopharyngeal mucosa. Patients on ophthalmic β-blockers should be monitored for side effects (most notably respiratory and cardiovascular effects and decreased exercise tolerance).

Digoxin

This drug has not been shown to decrease mortality, but it has been shown to reduce hospitalizations and symptoms in heart failure patients of all ages. Digoxin has a narrow therapeutic index, and older adults are at increased risk of toxicity. Decreased renal function and lean body mass are contributing factors. Digoxin interacts with many other medications, and many disease states can cause the level of the drug to become toxic (Table 41–4). Toxicity is a clinical diagnosis, and the

Table 41–4. Digoxin interactions.

Drugs that increase digoxin levels	Disease states that increase toxicity
Quinidine, amiodarone	Hypoxia
Cyclosporine	Acidosis
Itraconazole, triamterene, tetracycline, erythromycin	Hypokalemia
Calcium	Hypomagnesemia
Verapamil, diltiazem	Hypercalcemia
Spironolactone	Lung disease
Propafenone	Hypothyroidism
Propantheline	Myocardial ischemia

serum digoxin level does not always predict toxicity. Digoxin is protein bound, and the level of free digoxin can fluctuate. Older adults should be monitored carefully and maintained at lower doses than might be used in younger patients (0.5 ng/mL–0.8 ng/mL). Patients should be reassessed when adding new medications, with electrolyte abnormalities, or when illness occurs.

Hepatic Hydroxymethylglutaryl Coenzyme A Reductase Inhibitors (Statins)

Lowering LDL and increasing high-density lipoprotein (HDL) cholesterol reduces the risk of cardiovascular diseases. Statins inhibit the enzyme hepatic hydroxymethylglutaryl coenzyme A (HMG-Co) reductase in the liver. This action decreases the production of cholesterol and upregulates the LDL receptors in the liver, resulting in increased removal of LDL from the circulation. Decreasing LDL and increasing HDL decreases the risk of cardiovascular disease.

Statins should be taken at night. The risks of statin medication are the same in old and young patients alike. Older adults should start at the lowest dose, or perhaps even half of the starting dose, and be monitored for effect in 4–6 weeks. Liver transaminases should be evaluated at initiation of therapy and then again in 6–12 weeks (and every 6 mo thereafter). The drug should be discontinued when transaminases are 3 times the upper limit of normal. Patients with persistent unexplained elevations in transaminases or with chronic liver disease should not receive statin medication. The physician should carefully monitor patients who use alcohol and may choose to not prescribe a statin medication to these patients. Rhabdomyolysis is an infrequent complication of statin therapy, but the creatine kinase should be checked if muscle pain or weakness develops. Statins combined with gemfibrozil, niacin, erythromycin, or cyclosporine will increase the risk of rhabdomyolysis.

Iron

Iron supplements can interact with many other medications. Most notably, iron can form complexes with medications in the GI tract, rendering them less effective. Drugs that most commonly interact with iron are levodopa, methyldopa, penicillamine, quinolones, tetracyclines, and L-thyroxine. Interactions can result in a 50% decrease in the concentration of these drugs. There should be at least a 2-h difference in dosing times between iron and these medications.

Herbal Medications

Herbal medications are used for a multitude of medical and psychiatric problems. Patients often erroneously assume that herbal medications can be taken without risk of adverse effects, drug interactions, or perioperative complications (Table 41–5). However, patients are often unaware that labeling of herbals can be faulty, dosing and potency can vary among manufacturers, and additives can be omitted or misidentified. The product can be tainted with pesticides, herbicides, or heavy metals.

A. ECHINACEA

Echinacea, a member of the daisy family, has multiple uses but is best known for prophylaxis of upper respiratory tract infections. It is thought to have short-term immunostimulatory effects and can be used for various other infections as well. Evidence regarding its therapeutic effects is inconclusive. Echinacea should be avoided in patients taking immunosuppressive drugs. Prolonged use (> 8 weeks) may result in immunosuppression. Adverse effects are primarily allergic. Because of hepatotoxicity concerns, patients with liver disease should avoid using this herbal remedy.

B. EPHEDRA

Ephedra (ma huang) has been used for a multitude of purposes, including weight loss, fatigue, treatment of asthma, and bronchitis. The active compound is ephedrine, a noncatecholamine sympathomimetic agent with activity at the α_1-, β_1-, and β_2-receptors. Adverse events include hypertension, tachycardia/palpitations, stroke, and seizure. Multiple problems can occur perioperatively with use of this herbal (see Table 41–5) and should be discontinued before surgery. This herbal is contraindicated with use of monoamine oxidase inhibitors, causing hypertension, hyperpyrexia, and coma. This herbal should not be used with theophylline, TCAs, pseudoephedrine, cardiac glycosides, or any other drugs that may have cardiac effects. This herbal should likely be avoided in older adults. Herbal medications should be discontinued 24 h preoperatively.

C. GARLIC

Garlic is used to decrease the risk of atherosclerosis. It has the potential to mildly lower cholesterol and blood pressure and decrease thrombus formation and platelet aggregation. Garlic may potentiate the effect of other platelet inhibitors. Use of this herbal is considered relatively safe, but it is recommended that patients discontinue use 1 week preoperatively to decrease the risk of bleeding.

D. GINKGO BILOBA

Ginkgo biloba has been used historically for a variety of problems, most notably cognitive difficulties. It also is used for vertigo, tinnitus, headache, asthma, peripheral vascular disease, macular degeneration, erectile dysfunction, and altitude sickness. Ginkgo is believed to have multiple effects: to act as an antioxidant, free radical scavenger, vasodilator, neurotransmitter, and receptor modulator; to enhance cell use of oxygen and glucose; and to inhibit platelet aggregation. Some data indicate that its use will mildly improve memory, but there is no evidence that it improves normal cognitive function. It is unclear whether use of this herbal will improve tinnitus. The common side effects are GI upset and headache. There is concern regarding increased risk of bleeding; some studies have reported spontaneous intracranial bleeding. This herbal medication should probably be avoided in patients receiving anticoagulant therapy. Presurgical patients should stop using this herb 36 h before surgery.

E. GINSENG

Ginseng has multiple varieties and has been used in Chinese medicine for centuries. It is thought to help maintain a sense of well-being, decrease stress, prolong life, have diuretic effects, and improve sexual functioning. This herb may also have an effect on platelet function and increase the risk of bleeding, which could be irreversible in humans. In addition, it has the potential to lower postprandial glucose by increasing glycogen storage and lipogenesis in both diabetic and nondiabetic patients. This could increase risk of hypoglycemia. It is recommended that this herb be discontinued 7 days before surgery. There are case reports of interactions with warfarin and digoxin. When used in high doses, ginseng may cause elevations in blood pressure, insomnia, diarrhea, headache, anxiety, schizophrenia, and Stevens-Johnson syndrome. It should be avoided in patients with high blood pressure. Evidence regarding its therapeutic effects is inconclusive.

F. KAVA

Kava is used as an anxiolytic and hypnotic. Kava has multiple CNS effects, including a weak effect on the benzodiazepine-binding sites and anticonvulsant, neu-

Table 41–5. Medicines & perioperative care: Clinically important effects & perioperative concerns of 8 herbal medicines & recommendations for discontinuation of use

Common names	Relevant pharmacological effect	Perioperative concern	Preoperative discontinuation
Echinacea, purple coneflower root	Activation of cell-mediated immunity	Allergic reactions; decreased effectiveness of immunosuppressants, potential for immunosuppression with long-term use	No data
Ephedra, ma huang	Increased heart rate and blood pressure through direct and indirect sympathomimetic effects	Risk of myocardial ischemia and stroke from tachycardia and hypertension; ventricular arrhythmias with halothane; long-term use depletes endogenous catecholamines and may cause intraoperative hemodynamic instability; life-threatening interaction with monoamine oxidase inhibitors	At least 24 h
Garlic, ajo	Inhibition of platelet aggregation (may be reversible); increased fibrinolysis; equivocal antihypertensive activity	Potential to increase risk of bleeding, especially when combined with other medications that inhibit platelet aggregation	At least 7 days before surgery
Ginkgo, duck foot tree, maidenhair tree, silver apricot	Inhibition of platelet-activating factor	Potential to increase risk of bleeding, especially when combined with other medications that inhibit platelet aggregation	At least 36 h before surgery
Ginseng, American ginseng, Asian ginseng, Chinese ginseng, Korean ginseng	Lowers blood glucose; inhibition of platelet aggregation (may be irreversible); increased PT, PTT in animals; many other diverse effects	Hypoglycemia; potential to increase risk of bleeding; potential to decrease anticoagulation effect of warfarin	At least 7 days before surgery
Kava, awa, intoxicating pepper, kawa	Sedation, anxiolysis	Potential to increase sedative effect of anesthetics; potential for addiction, tolerance, and withdrawal after abstinence unstudied	At least 24 h before surgery
St. John's wort, amber, goat weed, hardhay, hypericum, klamatheweed	Inhibition of neurotransmitter reuptake; monoamine oxidase inhibition is unlikely	Induction of cytochrome P450 enzymes, affecting cyclosporine, warfarin, steroids, protease inhibitors, and possibly benzodiazepines, calcium channel blockers, and many other drugs; decreased serum digoxin levels	At least 5 days before surgery
Valerian, all heal, garden heliotrope, vandal root	Sedation	Potential to increase sedative effect of anesthetics; benzodiazepine-like acute withdrawal; potential to increase anesthetic requirements with long-term use	No data

PT, prothrombin time; PTT, partial thromboplastin time.
From Ang-Lee MK et al: Herbal Medicines and perioperative care. JAMA 2001;286:208. Used with permission.

roprotective, and anesthetic properties. Concomitant benzodiazepine use may increase effects. It potentially could have effects on any substances acting on the CNS, and concomitant use with alcohol should be avoided. Kava does have the potential for abuse and a withdrawal syndrome after long-term use, but this concern is not well established. Kava dermopathy can occur with heavy use and manifests itself as a yellow scaly eruption, which resolves when it is discontinued. It can also cause ataxia, hair loss, hearing problems, decreased appetite, and weight loss. High doses can also lead to elevation in liver enzymes or liver damage and may result in elevated cholesterol. Kava should be discontinued 24 h before surgery.

G. Saw Palmetto

Saw palmetto is effective for treating benign prostatic hypertrophy, but the mechanism is not completely understood. It has been shown to inhibit 5α-reductase as well as prostate estrogen receptors. Prostate size has not been proven to decrease with use of saw palmetto, but there have been beneficial effects on nocturia and peak urine flow. It is less effective than α-blocking agents but has fewer side effects. GI side effects, dizziness, headache, and increase in blood pressure are most common but still infrequent. There have been no reports on interactions with other drugs.

H. St. John's Wort

St. John's wort is currently used to treat mild to moderate depression but is not indicated for major depression. Its effect is due to inhibition of serotonin, norepinephrine, and dopamine uptake. It is considered to be safe overall. Adverse effects include insomnia, diarrhea, rare photosensitivity, and potential to unmask mania. Use with SSRIs may cause the syndrome of serotonin excess, especially in older adults. In addition, St. John's wort can induce or reduce various cytochrome P450 isoenzymes and affect levels of many drugs. Effects of warfarin can be reduced and cyclosporine levels decreased. The use of St. John's wort may affect multiple drugs used during surgery and, because of its long half-life, should be discontinued 5 days before surgery.

I. Valerian Root

Valerian root is used as a treatment for insomnia and anxiety and is included in most herbal insomnia remedies. Side effects include morning drowsiness and headache. Effects are dose dependent. Benzodiazepines may amplify effects. Patients on long-standing doses could potentially have related withdrawal if it is stopped abruptly, justifying tapering before surgery.

OTC Medications

It is important to discuss nonprescription medication use with older adult patients because it can interfere with the effectiveness of prescription drugs and potentiate harmful effects. Many patients do not consider these therapies as part of their medication regimen, and the physician needs to ask specifically about such medications.

A. Gastrointestinal Agents

Antacids (eg, aluminum/magnesium hydroxide) can interfere with medication absorption, especially when absorption is pH dependent. The bioavailability of some antibiotics, notably the quinolones, and some beta-lactams as well as tetracycline can be affected.

The H_2 receptor agonist cimetidine at its OTC dosage can interact with prescription medication. It affects pH-related absorption of ketoconazole, theophylline levels can be increased, and it can affect various benzodiazepines, either increasing or decreasing levels. Cimetidine and ranitidine can prolong prothrombin time during therapy with warfarin by decreasing its clearance. It also decreases the clearance of flecainide, ethmozine, procainamide, quinidine, lidocaine, propranolol, and phenytoin.

B. NSAIDs

The physician needs to specifically inquire about the use of NSAIDs to alert patients to potential adverse effects. Aspirin can affect serum concentrations of phenytoin and valproic acid. Both ibuprofen and naproxen can increase lithium concentrations. They can reduce renal excretion of digoxin, especially in patients with renal insufficiency.

 EVIDENCE-BASED POINTS

- *Drugs that are prescribed should have a clear and documented indication.*
- *Patient and caregivers should be educated regarding each drug's indication and side effects so that the therapeutic effect can be monitored.*
- *Medications are started at low doses and increased cautiously.*
- *Changes in pharmacokinetics can occur when stopping medications.*
- *Patient adherence with the medication is ensured before increasing the dose or adding a new medication.*
- *New medications should be added cautiously; the medication list should be checked for potential drug–drug and drug–disease interactions.*
- *Medication side effects are considered a potential cause of new symptoms.*
- *Drugs that are not having the desired effect or are having adverse effects are discontinued in a timely fashion.*
- *Medication lists are kept up to date and available if the patient is hospitalized or needs consultation.*
- *Medications are periodically reviewed with the patient and caregiver, allowing for drugs to be stopped and drug oversights corrected.*

- *Inquiry is made about OTC and herbal medications.*
- *Medications with strong anticholinergic properties are avoided, or patients and caregivers are made aware of common side effects.*
- *Primum non nocere (first do no harm).*

REFERENCES

Ang-Lee MK et al: Herbal medicines and perioperative care. JAMA 2001;286:208. [PMID: 11448284]

Aronow WS: Cholesterol 2001. Rationale for lipid-lowering in older patients with or without CAD. Geriatrics 2001;56:22. [PMID: 11582971]

Astin JA et al: Complementary and alternative medicine use among elderly persons: one-year analysis of a Blue Shield Medicare supplement. J Gerontol A Biol Sci Med Sci 2000;55:M4. [PMID: 10719766]

Avorn J: Improving drug use in elderly patients: getting to the next level. JAMA 2001;286:2866. [PMID: 11735764]

Bandyopadhyay S et al: Age and gender bias in statin trials. Q J Med 2001;94:127. [PMID: 11259687]

Beers MH: Explicit criteria for determining potentially inappropriate medication use by the elderly. An update. Arch Intern Med 1997;157:1531. [PMID: 9236554]

Bell GM, Schnitzer TJL: Cox-2 inhibitors and other nonsteroidal anti-inflammatory drugs in the treatment of pain in the elderly. Clin Geriatr Med 2001;17:489. [PMID: 11459717]

Beyth RJ: Hemorrhagic complications of oral anticoagulant therapy. Clin Geriatr Med 2001;17:49. [PMID: 11270133]

Beyth RJ, Shorr RI: Epidemiology of adverse drug reactions in the elderly by drug class. Drugs Aging 1999;14:231. [PMID: 10220106]

Capewell S et al: Reduced felodipine bioavailability in patients taking anticonvulsants. Lancet 1988;2:480. [PMID: 2900404]

Cohen JS: Avoiding adverse reactions. Effective lower-dose drug therapies for older patients. Geriatrics 2000;55:54. [PMID: 10711307]

Demirkan K et al: Response to warfarin and other oral anticoagulants: effects of disease states. South Med J 2000;93:448. [PMID: 10832939]

Ernst E: The risk-benefit profile of commonly used herbal therapies: ginkgo, St. John's wort, ginseng, echinacea, saw palmetto, and kava. Ann Intern Med 2002;136:42. [PMID: 11777363]

Fine PG: Opioid analgesic drugs in older people. Clin Geriatr Med 2001;17:479. [PMID: 11459716]

Foster DF et al: Alternative medicine use in older Americans. J Am Geriatr Soc 2000;48:1560. [PMID: 11129743]

Gage BF et al: Warfarin therapy for an octogenarian who has atrial fibrillation. Ann Intern Med 2001;134:465. [PMID: 11255522]

Gloth FM III: Geriatric pain. Factors that limit pain relief and increase complications. Geriatrics 2000;55:46. [PMID: 11054950]

Gurwitz JH: Using pharmacoepidemiological findings to guide clinical practice: sulfonylureas and hypoglycemia in older adults. J Am Geriatr Soc 1996;44:871. [PMID: 8675941]

Haller CA, Benowitz NL: Adverse cardiovascular and central nervous system events associated with dietary supplements containing ephedra alkaloids. N Engl J Med 2000;343:1833. [PMID: 11117974]

Hanlon JT et al: Recent advances in geriatrics: drug-related problems in the elderly. Ann Pharmacother 2000;34:360. [PMID: 10917384]

Hanlon JT et al: Suboptimal prescribing in older inpatients and outpatients. J Am Geriatr Soc 2001;49:200. [PMID: 11207875]

Holmboe ES: Oral antihyperglycemic therapy for type 2 diabetes: clinical applications. JAMA 2002;287:373. [PMID: 11790217]

Honig PK, Gillespie BK: Clinical significance of pharmacokinetic drug interactions with over-the-counter (OTC) drugs. Clin Pharmacokinet 1998;35:167. [PMID: 9784931]

Hylek EM: Oral anticoagulants. Pharmacologic issues for use in the elderly. Clin Geriatr Med 2001;17:1. [PMID: 11270124]

Inzucchi SE: Oral antihyperglycemic therapy for type 2 diabetes: scientific review. JAMA 2002;287:360. [PMID: 11790216]

Izzo AA, Ernst E: Interactions between herbal medicines and prescribed drugs: a systematic review. Drugs 2001;61:2163. [PMID: 11772128]

Kagansky N et al: Cholesterol lowering in the older population: time for reassessment? Q J Med 2001;94:457. [PMID: 11528008]

Knight EL, Avorn J: Quality indicators for appropriate medication use in vulnerable elders. Ann Intern Med 2001;135:703. [PMID: 11601953]

Lasser KE et al: Timing of new black box warnings and withdrawals for prescription medications. JAMA 2002;287:2215. [PMID: 11980521]

McLeod PJ et al: Defining inappropriate practices in prescribing for elderly people: a national consensus panel. CMAJ 1997;156:385. [PMID: 9033421]

Mintzer J, Burns A: Anticholinergic side-effects of drugs in elderly people. J R Soc Med 2000;93:457. [PMID: 11089480]

O'Brien JT, Ballard CG: Drugs for Alzheimer's disease. BMJ 2001;323:123. [PMID: 11463665]

Rochon PA, Gurwitz JH: Prescribing for seniors: neither too much nor too little. JAMA 1999;282:113. [PMID: 10411177]

Schneider LS: Treatment of Alzheimer's disease with cholinesterase inhibitors. Clin Geriatr Med 2001;17:337. [PMID: 11375139]

Shorr RI et al: Incidence and risk factors for serious hypoglycemia in older persons using insulin or sulfonylureas. Arch Intern Med 1997;157:1681. [PMID: 9250229]

Sweitzer NK et al: Drug therapy of heart failure caused by systolic dysfunction in the elderly. Clin Geriatr Med 2000;16:513. [PMID: 10918645]

Tariot PN et al: Pharmacologic therapy for behavioral symptoms of Alzheimer's disease. Clin Geriatr Med 2001;17:359. [PMID: 11375140]

Temple RJ, Himmel MH: Safety of newly approved drugs: implications for prescribing. JAMA 2002;287:2273. [PMID: 11980528]

Tune LE: Anticholinergic effects of medication in elderly patients. J Clin Psychiatry 2001;62:11. [PMID: 11584981]

Vander Zanden JA et al: Systemic adverse effects of ophthalmic beta-blockers. Ann Pharmacother 2001;35:1633. [PMID: 11793633]

Wirshing DA: Adverse effects of atypical antipsychotics. J Clin Psychiatry 2001;62:7. [PMID: 11584988]

Wirshing WC: Movement disorders associated with neuroleptic treatment. J Clin Psychiatry 2001;62:15. [PMID: 11584982]

Zhan C et al: Potentially inappropriate medication use in the community-dwelling elderly: findings from the 1996 Medical Expenditure Panel Survey. JAMA 2001;286:2823. [PMID: 11735757]

Exercise

Stephanie Studenski, MD, MPH

General Considerations

Although physical exercise has clear benefit to health and function, most older adults do not engage in any regular exercise activity. The challenge for the clinician is to promote exercise that is appropriate and feasible for the individual needs of the patient.

A. Types of Exercise & Exercise Settings

Exercise can promote cardiopulmonary fitness, musculoskeletal power, balance, flexibility, and a general increase in capacity to expend metabolic energy. All types of exercise require a minimum intensity, frequency, and duration to achieve gain by inducing moderate physiological stress. Thus, exercise must include a plan for progression of duration and intensity over time. Exercise can be performed in the community, within the health care system, or at home. It can be self-managed or supervised, in groups or one on one. It can involve much or little equipment and cost.

B. Fitness Levels in Older Adults

The exercise capacity and needs of older adults depend on their initial health and functional status and history of physical activity and exercise. Many older adults, especially the young–old (< 75), are in good health and have no functional limitations. These healthy elders include both usual healthy elders with no symptoms and fit elders. The usual can be differentiated from the fit by their capacity to perform demanding physical work or exercise. For healthy elders, standard exercise recommendations and precautions are appropriate. Some older adults who are independent in activities of daily living (ADLs) have subclinical disability, demonstrated by reduced physical performance. These persons require some adaptations to the exercise program. Those with frank disability benefit from therapeutic exercise for recovery of function. If the change in functional status is recent, exercise is offered as a part of a rehabilitation program. If the disability is chronic, exercise is more often part of a self-care program. Older adults with conditions involving the heart, lungs, bones, and joints or other organ systems need exercise targeted at certain physiological and functional parameters and require activity modifications for the condition.

Prior experience, knowledge, and beliefs about exercise will influence attitudes and expectations. Individuals who have personally experienced improved physical function with exercise in the past may be more receptive, whereas those who have had no experience or who have had prior injury with exercise may be less interested.

C. Types of Goals for Exercise

Exercise can be preventive or therapeutic. Preventive goals for exercise aim to reduce adverse events in the future. In healthy adults, exercise can be a form of primary prevention, delaying disability and disease. Exercise in persons with subclinical disability or disease is a form of secondary prevention, like the treatment of hypertension, in which a detectable abnormality (high blood pressure, reduced physical performance, decreased bone density) is treated before it causes overt disease and disability (Table 42–1). Exercise for tertiary prevention has the goal of reducing recurrence or complications. Therapeutic exercise has immediate goals to improve symptoms and functions.

General Guidelines for Exercise

The health care provider should be able to assess medical safety for exercise and recommend medically indicated exercise modifications. The provider should also be able to give the independent older adult key recommendations for safe unsupervised exercise and should be involved in improving patient adherence to exercise programs.

A. Medical Evaluation

Even though a medical evaluation is recommended before exercise for nearly all older adults, there are no clear guidelines for the medical assessment of exercise safety. Most guidelines tend to focus on cardiac screening and contraindications. Many other conditions also require specific exercise modification (Table 42–2).

There are long-standing misconceptions about the need for bed rest. Absolute bed rest is almost never a good thing; almost everyone benefits from some degree of physical activity. The very few contraindications to physical activity include recent myocardial infarction, unstable angina or uncompensated congestive heart failure, critical aortic stenosis, and significant abdominal aortic aneurysm. Some acute conditions such as major bone fracture, nonhealing lesion on a weight-

Table 42–1. Benefits of physical activity & exercise for older patients with chronic health conditions.

Condition	Benefits
Obesity	Reduces total abdominal adiposity
Diabetes mellitus type 2	Increases insulin sensitivity and glucose tolerance
Atherosclerosis	Increases luminal diameter of coronary arteries
Hypertension	Reduces resting blood pressure
Vascular disease	Increases resting and exercise stroke volumes and lowers resting and exercising heart rates
Cardiovascular disease: coronary diseases, congestive heart failure	Lowers risk of death after myocardial infarction; improves endothelial function and skeletal muscle aerobic metabolism and reduces afterload
Cerebrovascular disease	Reduces risk of total and ischemic stroke in women
Peripheral vascular disease	Increases maximal treadmill walking distance
Chronic obstructive pulmonary disease	Improves dyspnea
Obstructive sleep apnea	Weight loss
Sarcopenia	Resistance training improves muscle strength and size and improves mobility
Physical frailty	Postpones disability
Osteopenia/osteoporosis	Delays the decrease of bone mineral density
Low back pain	Improves performance of daily activities
Alzheimer's disease	Women with higher levels of physical activity are less likely to develop cognitive decline
Recovery from surgery, immobilization, debilitating illness	Decreases morbidity, morality, rehospitalization; improves quality of life, depression scores, and physical functioning
Depression	Improves symptoms of depression and anxiety

From Chakravarthy MV et al: An obligation for primary care physicians to prescribe physical activity to sedentary patients to reduce the risk of chronic health conditions. Mayo Clin Proc 2002;77:170. Used with permission.

Table 42–2. Modifications of exercise prescription for selected conditions.

Condition	Modification
Degenerative joint disease	Non-weight-bearing activities: stationary cycling, water exercises, chair exercises; low resistance–low repetition strength training
Coronary artery disease	Symptom-limited activities: moderate endurance activities (eg, walking, cycling); more vigorous activities at physician's discretion: lower resistance, higher repetition strength training
Diabetes mellitus	Daily, moderate endurance activities; low resistance, higher repetition strength training; flexibility exercises
Dizziness, ataxia	Chair exercises, low-resistance and low-repetition strength training; moderate flexibility activities with minimal movement from supine or prone to standing positions
Back syndrome	Moderate endurance activities and flexibility exercises; low-resistance, low-repetition strength training; modified abdominal strengthening activities; water activities
Osteoporosis	Weight-bearing activities with intermittent bouts of activity spaced throughout the day; low-resistance, low-repetition strength training and chair-level flexibility activities
Chronic obstructive lung disease	Moderate endurance activities using interval or intermittent approach; low-resistance, low-repetition strength training; modified flexibility and stretching exercises
Orthostatic hypotension	Minimize movements from standing to supine and supine to standing; sustained moderate endurance activities with short rest intervals
Hypertension	Dynamic large-muscle endurance activities; minimize isometric work and focus on low-resistance, low-repetition isotonic strength training

From American College of Sports Medicine: ACSM position stand on exercise and physical activity for older adults. Med Sci Sports Exer 1998;30:992. Used with permission.

bearing extremity, or febrile illness transiently limit activity. Those who are recovering from acute illness benefit from early mobilization (see Chapter 7: Hospital Care).

Some medical conditions must be identified to modify the exercise program, to implement special safety procedures, or to prepare to adapt therapy to the condition itself. Most commonly, the screening focuses on risk of major cardiac events during exercise such as silent ischemia and exercise-induced arrhythmias. This is a controversial area in the literature. Cardiac screening recommendations are not consistent among official organizations. Exercise stress testing is expensive, is difficult to perform for many older adults, and uncovers a huge reservoir of silent cardiac disease of unclear clinical significance. Many older adults do not plan to undertake a vigorous exercise program, and moderate activity may be associated with negligible accumulated cardiac risk because there are also cardiac risk reductions associated with moderate exercise. Ideally, exercise should occur in a monitored environment after standard cardiac evaluation for persons at higher risk for cardiac events during exercise. This category includes persons with myocardial infarction within 6 mo, angina, symptoms or signs of congestive heart failure, resting systolic blood pressure > 200 mm Hg or resting diastolic blood pressure > 110 mm Hg, chest pain or shortness of breath during observed exercise, such as climbing a flight of stairs or cycling in the air while lying on the exam table, or a resting electrocardiogram with new Q waves, ST-segment depression, or T-wave inversions. Systolic blood pressure that drops with exercise is also a danger sign. There is no consensus about how to evaluate cardiac risk of exercise in asymptomatic persons with risk factors such as old myocardial infarction, other vascular diseases, pulmonary conditions, diabetes, hyperlipidemia, smoking, and hypertension. For individuals who do not have these risk factors, the provider may consider 2 options. Cardiac stress testing could be ordered in all cases, in accordance with the American Heart Association and American College of Sports Medicine guidelines, or a moderate activity program can be prescribed with cautious initiation and progression. Cardiac stress testing is indicated before a vigorous exercise program is implemented. The patient and family may wish to be involved in this choice.

Noncardiac conditions influence exercise plans. For example, exercise increases insulin sensitivity and reduces insulin requirements in the diabetic patient. These patients should monitor glucose levels and adjust hypoglycemic regimens when increasing activity. Because exercise can transiently increase blood pressure in persons with hypertension, it is ideal to check blood pressure before, during, and after exercise at least during exercise initiation. The proposed exercise plan can be adapted for chronic conditions both to benefit specific needs and to avoid problems (see Table 42–2).

B. Patient Guidelines

The health care provider should offer general safety guidelines to the older adult who plans to exercise in an unsupervised setting (Table 42–3). Many web sites offer extensive advice about safety. Some of the key recommendations are to start low and go slow, to increase duration before increasing intensity, to stay well hydrated, to monitor exertion, and to discontinue if serious symptoms develop.

C. Exercise Adherence

Convincing an older sedentary person to exercise can be a formidable challenge. Modern civilization has created a living environment that, although immeasurably beneficial, reduces the need for physical activity in daily life. Modern transportation and labor-saving devices mean many people can go years without needing to walk further than a block or performing any physically demanding activity. The reduced demands for physical capacity in modern society have 2 negative effects on physical function. First, a great deal of capacity can be lost without detectable symptoms or limitations. Second, interventions are difficult to build into daily routines. One can get through the day with little physical demand and must intentionally add "nonessential" obligations to build up physical capacity.

Preventive interventions can be difficult to implement. Preventive actions such as taking a pill for blood

Table 42–3. General patient instructions for exercise.

1. Start slowly and increase gradually.
2. Avoid holding your breath.
3. If you are on a medication or have a heart condition that changes your natural heart rate, do not use your pulse rate to judge how hard you should exercise.
4. Use safety equipment as recommended for the activity.
5. Drink plenty of fluids if doing activities that make you sweat unless your doctor has asked you to limit fluids.
6. Bend from the hips, not the waist, when bending forward.
7. Warm up muscles before stretching.
8. No exercise should be painful.
9. You can find the right amount of effort using the guideline "If you can talk without any trouble at all, your activity is probably too easy. If you cannot talk at all, it is too hard."
10. Always include a warm-up and cool-down with an activity that moves your body but doesn't tire you.

Adapted from National Institute on Aging: Exercise for older adults: www.nihseniorhealth.gov/exercise/toc.html.

pressure reduction may demand less of the individual than undertaking an exercise program. Preventive aims such as weight reduction, quitting smoking, or increasing exercise require the individual to make a significant behavior and lifestyle change. Although many behavior change strategies have been proposed, and a few tested, most have only a modest effect on the target behavior. The new behavior is frequently short lived, and benefits are not sustained. Given all the challenges of inducing behavior change and the constraints on time and resources available to the clinician, many proposals for the clinician's role in promoting exercise behavior seem daunting and not feasible. Although there are no simple answers, useful suggestions and guidelines are provided in Table 42–4. Adherence is improved when an individual commits to personally meaningful and measurable goals, decides on and uses a self monitoring plan such as a calendar or record of exercise, receives specific feedback such as objective increase in performance, and has access to support as desired from others. A physician's formal recommendation to exercise, delivered as a prescription based on individualized risks and needs, increases motivation and adherence.

Older adults need a choice of sites and schedules. Some may prefer group activities with supervisors in community settings, whereas others may prefer to exercise alone at home. For many older adults, a socialization opportunity is a key to continued motivation. Cost and access are important considerations. Many older adults prefer modest rather than high-intensity exercise and may have strong personal preferences about public changing facilities and privacy.

For the clinician, adherence-promoting concepts can be translated into actions. A health risk appraisal presents the individual with a personal profile of health risks and potential benefits of exercise. For example, a patient with mild hypertension and osteopenia could undergo blood pressure and bone density assessments; office testing of endurance, strength, and balance using a 6-min walk test; and performance tests such as timed repeated chair rises and tandem stands. The patient could respond to a questionnaire about activity practices and preferences. The results can be presented as a personalized summary of health status and future health risk, linked to specific exercise recommendations.

The next step is to determine individual goals, interests, and barriers to exercise. The exercise recommendations should be derived from the individual's target accomplishments and preferences. Early success is a key to a positive outcome. Decide on modest initial goals, write them down as a prescription, and follow up in a few weeks to help motivate the patient. For example, a person with subclinical disability may wish to become less dyspneic when carrying groceries or laundry. She may prefer to exercise at home because she is a caregiver. An initial goal might be to start neighborhood walks or slow stair climbing for 5 min at a time a few times a day 4–5 days/week. The patient might keep a calendar or diary of exercise distance and time. The exercise is to be done at a pace that can be sustained but feels moderately tiring as demonstrated by increased work of breathing or gradual muscle fatigue. A return visit in a few weeks offers an opportunity to discuss initial challenges and successes. Repeated measures of symptoms and physical performance can be used as a feedback measure of progress. Reimbursable encounter time focused on exercise prescription can be linked to many cardiopulmonary or neuromusculoskeletal conditions in which exercise is medically recommended.

General Physical Activity

A. Principles & Benefits

General physical activity is a measure of overall energy consumption. Higher levels of physical activity have been repeatedly linked to reduced morbidity and mortality in epidemiological studies. Physical activity has been linked to reduced problems with heart disease, diabetes, and osteoporosis and improved mental well-being. Because many older adults have asymptomatic deconditioning, they have very little reserve if faced with any event or process that exacerbates the problem. In this sense, physical activity can increase physiological reserve and tolerance to stress. General physical activity differs from exercise in that the latter is more formally defined. Exercise is characterized by specific activities with expected physiological responses. Exercise is structured, scheduled, and repeated, whereas physical activity represents accumulated energy expenditure over time in all activities. General physical activity may not

Table 42–4. Strategies to promote physical activity in older adults.

A. Personal and interpersonal
  1. Goal setting
  2. Self-monitoring
  3. Feedback
  4. Support from family, friends, staff
  5. Physician advice
B. Environmental and societal
  1. Easy access to safe and low-cost exercise site
  2. Opportunity for social interaction
C. Program factors
  1. Choice of sites and schedules
  2. Choice of activities and intensity

achieve the increased fitness levels that can be expected with formal endurance training. Physical activity can be expected to reduce the risks and complications of many chronic conditions and to increase well-being.

Using the framework described in Table 42–5, the older adult can be clinically "staged" by the kind of activity that causes fatigue or dyspnea and by the frequency and duration of energy-consuming activity. Energy demands are often compared in units called metabolic equivalents, or METS. Energy demands are based on oxygen or calorie consumption. The MET is a ratio comparing the energy consumption of an activity to energy consumption at rest. Oxygen consumption is often presented in milliliters per kilogram per minute. Oxygen consumption at rest (the resting metabolic rate) is ~3.5 mL/kg/min. A 3-MET activity consumes 3 times the oxygen per kilogram per minute, or ~10.5 mL/kg/min. Energy consumption can also be assessed in terms of caloric expenditure. The resting metabolic rate is about 1 kcal/kg/h. A 3-MET activity that is performed for 30 min (0.5 h) by a 50-kg person consumes 3 METs × 50 kg × 0.5 h, or 75 calories. Estimates of the metabolic demands of various activities are based on averages from several sources and are summarized by the American College of Sports Medicine in the *Compendium of Physical Activities*. These estimates are based on studies of healthy adults. Many conditions such as neurological or musculoskeletal problems decrease the metabolic efficiency of movement and increase the metabolic demands of activity.

There are no studies of the energy demands of activities done by healthy or frail older adults. Because energy use may be more inefficient in many older adults, metabolic demands of activities may be somewhat higher than listed in Table 42–5. For this reason, the best use of the METs and activity table is to create a hierarchy of activities. The hierarchy can be used to gauge relative energy capacity between older adults and to select gradually increasing energy demanding activities for exercise prescription.

It is possible to link MET estimates to performance measures that can be done in the clinic or other health care settings. Table 42–6 relates walking speed in miles per hour and METS to walking speed, 6-min walk distance, 400-m walk time, and typical history. Walking speed test procedures are not yet standardized; distances and instructions vary. Table 42–6 lists walking speeds in meters per second over a 4-m course at a usual pace. If the timing of the walk starts from a standing position, then a period of acceleration is included, and walking speed calculations will underestimate actual walking speed. If the timing starts after the patient has started walking (a rolling start), then gait speeds are fairly consistent over various distances from 8 ft to 50 m. The 6-min walk distance or 400-m walk time can be used to estimate walking time in miles per hour and then METs. Many people who walk slowly (especially < 2.5 mph) may be unable to walk for the whole 6 min without rests and may have walk distances that are lower than those listed in Table 42–6.

Table 42–5. Physical energy demands of common activities.

MET	Representative activities
1.0	Sitting quietly, sleeping, watching television
1.5	Eating, sitting and talking, playing cards
2.0	Bathing while sitting, making the bed, driving a car, slow walking on level ground at < 2 mph
2.5	Dressing, shaving, sweeping or vacuuming floors, cooking, filling gas tank, riding lawn mower, walking on level ground at 2 mph
3.0	Walking on level ground at 2.5 mph, descending stairs, very light stationary bicycling (50 watts), very light weight lifting, slow dancing, bowling
3.5	Walking and carrying 15-lb load, food shopping with cart, golfing with cart, walking level ground at 3 mph
4	Showering while standing, toweling off, leisure bicycling, treading water, fishing, sweeping floors, raking lawn, playing with children, walking at 3.5 mph
4.5	Washing windows, washing car, mopping floors, weeding, mowing lawn with power mower, doing home calisthenics
5	Walking upstairs with light load, digging in garden
5.5	Square or folk dancing, scrubbing floors, house painting, stationary bicycling at 100 watts
6	Walking up hill at 3.5 mph, walking up stairs with moderate load (16–30 lbs), moving furniture, tilling garden, mowing with push mower, shoveling snow, light swimming
7	Playing tennis, backpacking, walking up hill with light load, stationary bicycling at 150 watts (moderate effort)
8	Carrying up to 50 lbs up stairs, slow lap swimming, race walking or slow running at 5 mph, walking up hill with moderate load

Adapted from American College of Sports Medicine: ACSM Resource Manual, 3rd edition. Williams & Wilkins, 1998. Used with permission.

Table 42–6. Translating walking speed: clinical assessment of energy capacity.

Functional status	Miles per hour	Meters per second: 4-m walk		6-min walk distance		400-m walk time	METs	Typical history of fatigue with activity
		Stand	Roll	Meters	Feet			
Overt disability	1.0	0.41	0.46	165	541	14 min 24 s	< 2	Self-care, walking very short distances
	1.5	0.57	0.69	248	813	9 min 36 s	< 2	
Sub clinical disability	2.0	0.75	0.93	335	1098	7 min 12 s	2.5	Household activities, walking .25 mile
	2.5	0.88	1.15	414	1358	5 min 45 s	3.0	Carrying groceries or light yard work
Usual healthy elders	3.0	1.0	1.38	497	1630	4 min 48 s	3.5	Moderate housework, climbing several flights of stairs
	3.5	1.1	1.60	576	1889	4 min 7 s	4.0	Carrying loads up stairs or up hills, heavy household or yard work
Fit elders	4.0	1.25	1.84	662	2171	3 min 36 s	> 4	Heavy work or sports

METs, metabolic equivalents.

The ability to sustain a given MET level is an important part of endurance. Many sedentary older adults are able to sustain a moderate MET level for only a few minutes. For this reason, the exercise program often must begin with a gradual increase in duration of exercise before any effort to increase the MET intensity is even considered.

B. Activities & Prescription

A medical assessment evaluates the medical safety for exercise and modifications for specific conditions. The practitioner is often expected to approve a proposed exercise program, including appropriate types of activity and related patient safety instructions. The physical activity prescription is based on the individual's current health and physical activity level. The current public health recommendation for older adults is to accumulate 30 min of moderate physical activity on most days of the week. This averages out to about 100 calories/day expended in moderate exercise. For every activity level, the prescription includes frequency, duration, intensity, warm-up and cool-down, stretching and other precautions, and progression. All activity should begin with a warm-up of somewhat easy activities that slightly increase energy demands. After the warm-up, the individual should stretch all major muscle groups using slow stretches that last ~30 s. Stretching helps reduce risk of injury in older adults and is safer and more effective after a warm-up. The cool-down after exercise is also important. This is the transition phase for heart rate and oxygen consumption to return to resting level. Slower walking or biking are appropriate activities. The intensity of physical activity that will have a training ef-

fect but be tolerable can be estimated from a person's predicted MET level. The predicted MET level can be based on history and clinical assessment. The proposed activities should be in the upper range of energy expenditure for the individual (Table 42–7). The recommended duration of activity, often 30 min or more in younger people, may be intolerable for more deconditioned older adults. Brief episodes of activity lasting 5–10 min several times per day can help build toward more sustained activity. All programs should progress over time. In the more frail, duration is progressed toward bouts of activity that last 20–30 min, before intensity is increased. It can take weeks or even months to reach this goal. The rate of progression can be gauged by perceived difficulty using the Borg Scale, ranging from 1 (very, very light) to 20 (very, very hard). The target is "somewhat hard," or in the 12–13 range. This degree of difficulty can be described as "not hard enough if it is easy to talk but too hard if one can't talk while doing it." Physiological effects of training take days to weeks to emerge. Progression based on physiological response in healthy adults is based on an increase in METs no more than every few weeks.

Aerobic Exercise

A. Principles & Benefits

Formal aerobic exercise is designed to increase fitness or aerobic capacity. Higher levels of fitness have been associated with reduced mortality and can increase reserve and resistance to deconditioning. Structured aerobic exercise is more targeted than general physical activity toward increasing cardiopulmonary fitness. Specific aero-

Table 42–7. Physical activity prescription by patient type.[a]

Patient type	Intensity (METs)	Duration (minutes)	Frequency	Examples of exercise
Overt disability				
Recently bed bound	1.5	5–10	Several times per day	Sitting ADL, passive and active range of motion, progress to standing and walking
Nonambulatory	2	5–10	Several times per day	Self-propel wheelchair, seated self-care, upper extremity games and activities individually and in groups
Subclinical disability				
Very sedentary	3	5–10	Several times per day	Slow walking program, group recreation
Inactive	4	20 or more	Most days of the week	Walking, gardening, housework, bicycle
Usual aging	4–5	30	Most days of the week	Brisk walking, stair climbing, moderate endurance recreation
Fit	5 +	30 or more	Most days	Moderate to high intensity: very brisk walks on uneven surfaces and hills, brisk stair climbing, moderate to vigorous sports

METs, metabolic equivalents; ADL, activity of daily living.
[a]Prescribing exercise: (1) Let the patient select the preferred mode of activity; (2) start with an intensity and duration that is well tolerated; (3) initial exercise sessions should be observed if there has been no recent moderate activity; (4) initial sessions of moderate activity should include assessment of blood pressure and heart rate; (5) increase duration to a target training level (20–30 min or a set of 10 reps) before increasing intensity; (6) teach about self-monitoring of effort.

bic training can probably achieve greater gains in cardiopulmonary fitness than can physical activity alone.

Cardiopulmonary fitness is generally assessed as maximal exercise capacity, measured as maximum oxygen consumption or VO_2max. Maximal exercise capacity is influenced by heart rate, cardiac stroke volume, and peripheral oxygen extraction. Older adults who undergo training have been shown to have demonstrable improvements in VO_2max attributable to improvements in cardiac stroke volume and oxygen extraction. Aging itself limits peak performance but not the ability to benefit from training.

B. Prescription & Activities

Unsupervised physical activity rather than unsupervised formal aerobic training is appropriate for persons who have clinical or subclinical (difficulty performing self-care activities) disability and cannot exercise continuously at a moderate intensity. Supervised aerobic training may be appropriate as part of a structured and supervised restorative program. Unsupervised formal aerobic training is appropriate for healthy older adults who are able to walk steadily at a brisk pace. Healthy older adults may desire greater gains from exercise than they can achieve with a general physical activity program, in large part because vigorous activity is more effective at increasing aerobic capacity than is moderate activity.

The training program is likely to include more vigorous activity, justifying stress testing for sedentary and untrained adults. The same processes of warm-up, stretch, exercise, and cool-down should be followed. For structuring training, heart rate or perceived exertion can be used. Maximum predicted heart rate is traditionally estimated as 220 − age. The training range is considered to be 60–90% of maximum heart rate. Moderate training is at a heart rate of 50–70% of predicted maximum. A higher percentage of predicted maximum is for vigorous exercise. Heart rate estimates are not useful in the presence of any condition that alters heart rate response to exercise, such as the use of β-blockers, some pacemakers, and many atrial arrhythmias.

The Borg Scale of perceived exertion can also be used to target intensity. Another way of describing vigorous intensity is that it should induce sweating over time but be sustainable without exhaustion. Training should start with a moderate intensity pace and duration. Intensity can be increased with interval training, in which the individual establishes a tolerable MET level and adds brief periods of increased intensity every 5–10 min. The goal is to gradually increase the duration of the higher intensity intervals. Cross-training promotes variability in the program. Activities such as swimming and use of exercise equipment that requires upper extremity effort can complement lower extremity training and reduce boredom. Upper extremity exercise induces a higher heart rate response per MET level than does lower extremity training. Many people have more deconditioned arms than legs. The Borg Scale perceived exertion should be used to estimate intensity of upper extremity exercise. Initial durations may be much briefer than with lower extremity exercise.

Strength Training

A. Principles & Benefits

Aging is associated with loss of muscle mass and power. Loss of muscle mass is *sarcopenia,* similar to the loss of bone mass, or *osteopenia.* The loss of muscle mass with age has been attributed to both smaller and fewer muscle cells. Muscle power is affected by both muscle mass and nervous system factors involving every level from the brain to the neuromuscular junction. Thus, muscular performance can improve faster and to a greater extent than can be attributed to increased muscle mass alone. Both muscle mass and power are responsive to exercise in older adults. The increase in muscle mass with exercise not only improves strength but also contributes to improved carbohydrate and lipid metabolism.

Muscle strength can be measured in many ways. The numerous and variable strength assessment techniques make it difficult to interpret and compare training programs and relative strength gains. Some measures of strength are reported in kilograms or pounds, as in 1-repetition maximum or isometric strength. The 1-repetition maximum (1-rep max) is the maximum mass that can be moved in a given maneuver, such as knee extension. Peak isometric force is the maximum force that can applied without moving (a single muscle length) using a dynamometer. Isokinetic strength measures the peak or average force applied by a muscle group through the range of motion at a given distance and speed of contraction. Isokinetic strength is reported in foot-pounds or Newton-meters. Power is often measured across multiple muscle groups in the lower extremity. This measure incorporates the rate of force development and is measured in Newton-meters per second. Functional strength is affected not only by the absolute ability to generate force but also by the ability to generate force across the varying lengths of the muscle during movement. The relationship between gains in force production and power are not linear and are not well understood. The muscle must perform at speeds that are useful for functions such as stopping a fall. Muscles need to work both when they are getting shorter (a concentric contraction) and to control the rate of lengthening, as in sitting down (an eccentric contraction). Isokinetic strength assessments can mea-

sure either concentric or eccentric contractions. Muscle endurance is a marker of the ability to sustain contractions. Some dynamometers can be used to assess the ability to sustain an isometric contraction.

The evidence linking strength to function is variable. Some of this variability is attributable to the diversity of strength measurement techniques. In addition, the relationship between strength and function may not be linear. There may be thresholds that define strength requirements for usual functions. Persons who are very weak could increase strength without reaching the minimal threshold for an activity. For example, a bed-bound person could increase leg strength without achieving the minimal strength requirements needed for climbing stairs. Healthy persons may already be capable of many functions, and further strength gain could increase reserve without a detectable effect on usual function.

B. Prescription & Activities

Strength gain is important for almost all older adults, from the most disabled to the most fit. Programs can be offered at intensity levels from light to vigorous. Medical concerns relate primarily to acute energy demands on the cardiovascular system and the need to avoid injury. Strength training is appropriate for persons with many chronic conditions.

The main safety rules for strength training are to breathe properly and to move in a smooth and controlled fashion. The most important breathing guideline is to avoid holding one's breath, which induces increased internal body pressure (the Valsalva maneuver). Other breathing guidelines are to start with taking a breath before lifting, exhaling during lifting, and inhaling during controlled release. Smooth movement means that the muscle moves against resistance at a steady rate without shaking or jerking.

Strength training can incorporate body weight for resistance or low-tech items such as elastic bands, wrist, and ankle weights, free weights, or household items like milk jugs and tin cans. Strength equipment can offer safer ways to lift heavier weights and can provide complex systems to control the rate of muscle contraction. For most older persons with clinical or subclinical disability, simpler weight training equipment is probably sufficient.

For all types of older adults, the program should start with a baseline assessment of intensity. Intensity is determined as a level of resistance for each major muscle group in the upper extremity, lower extremity, and trunk. A proper level of resistance is one in which a set of 8–15 repetitions feels somewhat hard but can be completed using smooth control. Intensity can be prescribed as a percentage of the 1-rep max as well. For each level of intensity, sessions are repeated 2 or 3 times per week until 1 or 2 sets of repetitions can be done in a smooth manner. Resistance can then be increased. There is no clear evidence that training more frequently or increasing the number of sets accelerates gains in frail persons. More rapid increases in intensity and more frequent training can increase the risk of injury. Healthy elders may be interested in a more aggressive program and can participate in most community-based programs. For the very frail, body weight offers sufficient resistance for initial training. Using body segment weight alone for training is similar to active range of motion. Bearing the weight of the whole body in standing, transfers, and walking is a strength training activity for many frail elders.

Balance Training

A. Principles & Benefits

Balance exercise training can improve markers of stability and reduce fall rates. Balance can be described in biomechanical or in physiological terms. From a biomechanical perspective, balance is the ability to control the displacement and recovery of the moving mass of the body over the base of support. The base of support is the contact surface of the body with the support surface, as in the feet with the ground or the buttocks with a chair. Static balance is the ability to remain upright when controlling the mass of the body over a fixed base of support, as in standing. Better balance involves remaining upright on a smaller base of support and being able to move the mass of the body further toward the margins of the base of support. Dynamic balance is the ability to control the mass of the body over a moving base of support, as in walking. Mobility requires dynamic balance. Improved dynamic balance involves more rapid and accurate corrections of the moving base of support as the body mass moves.

A physiological approach to balance incorporates the detection, planning, and execution of the movements required to remain upright. Balance reactions can be corrective, as in responding to a push, or anticipatory, as in planning to step over an obstacle. Although most balance assessment has been static and corrective, the balance requirements for mobility are mostly dynamic and anticipatory. The physiological subsystems of balance include sensory, central processing, and effector factors. There are 3 sensory systems: vision, vestibular, and somatosensory. Central processing requires alertness, attention, integration of sensory information, and response planning. Effector subsystems important for balance include strength and range of motion. Most balance training programs are based on biomechanical principles. Balance tasks are ordered in difficulty according to the size of the base of support and the speed and size of displacements of the body. For example, in static balance, standing with feet together is harder that standing with feet apart, and standing on 1 foot is even harder. Some balance training involves awareness of the shifting of weight within the base of support from 1 foot to the other. Stepping over obstacles requires planning and executing displacements while moving. Some balance training is specific to a physiological deficit such as vestibular dysfunction.

B. Prescription & Activities

A global assessment of balance capacity can be obtained clinically with simple measures such as the Tinetti Performance Oriented Mobility Assessment, timed stands, or tandem walking. Persons who need assistive devices such as walkers for standing and walking by definition require a larger base of support and have limited balance. Balance training requires progression in difficulty, making it inherently somewhat more dangerous than other forms of exercise because there is an increased risk of falling.

Balance training for everyone but the healthy elder requires supervision. Balance training for the very frail person involves movement practice in a seated position that requires displacement of the trunk and arms. For the person who needs an assistive device, balance training often involves experience maneuvering around the home or while holding to a support surface. Persons with subclinical disability can practice maintaining static balance with a progressively smaller base of support while standing, walking with a narrow base of support, and controlling weight shift and lower extremity movement, as in playing catch with a ball or swinging a golf club. Healthy elders can improve balance through many recreational activities that require displacement and recovery, such as dancing or tennis.

Some forms of balance training target specific issues and opportunities. Tai chi ch'uan requires slow, controlled motions that involve displacement and recovery. There is a focus on body awareness. Balance training in water allows patients to explore the margins of their ability to displace and recover without fear of injury, because falls are cushioned by the water. Balance training with visual feedback involves force plates under the feet and a video monitor to show the location of the center of pressure. As weight is shifted forward, backward, and from side to side, a point on the screen moves, allowing patients to increase awareness of body position and control. They also get feedback that they are able to move closer and closer to the margins of the base of support, a sign of progress.

Flexibility

A. Principles & Benefits

Flexibility decreases with age and can become significantly restricted with disuse or disease. Loss of range of motion affects mobility and function. In the worst case, contractures occur, limiting walking, standing, and reaching. Flexibility is rarely an isolated deficit, because loss of mobility and movement also affect strength and fitness.

B. Prescription & Activities

There are few contraindications to flexibility exercise. Even the bed-bound person with an injury or illness benefits from range of motion of uninjured body segments. Specific contraindications include acutely inflamed joints, joints that are therapeutically fused, and recent fracture. General light to moderate activity helps warm up the muscle before stretching for flexibility. Stretches should last 10–30 s and involve all the major joints of the upper and lower extremity and trunk. The stretch should cause a sensation of pulling but not acute pain.

Combined Programs

A. Principles & Benefits

Most older adults benefit from exercises that improve fitness, strength, balance, and flexibility. All components are needed to improved mobility and function. Many people who have frank or subclinical disability are so deconditioned and weak that almost all exercise stresses their limits and has a training effect.

B. Prescription & Activities

The medical approval process for combined programs is based on the specific issues already described. Major constraints on combined programs are time and fatigue. It is usually unrealistic for a frail older adult to undertake a program that demands hours of exercise each day. This limited exercise capacity can be a barrier to formal rehabilitation programs that require 3 h/day of active therapy.

For healthy elders and those with subclinical disability, the challenge is to make the most of available time and energy. Some programs are based on alternating activities on different days. For example, one could walk ≥ 3 days/week and perform strength training 2–3 times/week on the "off" days. Some programs combine a mix of aerobic, strength, and balance activities into an hour-long session 3 days/week. Some activities can combine several goals. Stair climbing increases both muscle power and fitness.

EVIDENCE-BASED POINTS

- *Aging is associated with losses of peak fitness, strength, and flexibility, but training prevents or reverses some of these losses.*

- *Exercise is safe and effective for most older adults, from the most frail to the most fit.*

- *Exercise testing before moderate aerobic exercise in the asymptomatic older adult is controversial.*

- *Regular exercise involves a behavior change that is hard to initiate and maintain.*

- *The formal prescription of exercise by a health care provider increases patient exercise behavior.*

REFERENCES

American College of Sports Medicine: ACSM position stand on exercise and physical activity for older adults. Med Sci Sports Exer 1998;30:992. [PMID: 9624662] (Primary source for current recommendations and evidence-based justification for exercise in older adults.)

American College of Sports Medicine: ACSM Resource Manual, 3rd edition. Williams & Wilkins, 1998. (Core reference for exercise physiology, prescription, and management.)

Chakravarthy MV et al: An obligation for primary care physicians to prescribe physical activity to sedentary patients to reduce the risk of chronic health conditions. Mayo Clin Proc 2002;77:165. [PMID: 11838650] (Summary of the physiological effects of exercise on chronic health conditions.)

Chandler JM, Hadley EC: Exercise to improve physiologic and functional performance in old age. Clin Geriatr Med 1996; 12:761. [PMID: 8890115] (Review of the exercise evidence in the literature.)

Christmas C, Anderson RA: Exercise and older patients: guidelines for the clinician. J Am Geriatr Soc 2000;48:318. [PMID: 10733061] (Overview of the evidence for the benefits of exercise in older adults.)

Gill TM et al: Role of exercise stress testing and safety monitoring for older persons starting an exercise program. JAMA 2000; 284:342. [PMID: 1089166] (Summary of the evidence and discussion of the issues related to stress testing before exercise in older adults.)

Judge JO: Physical activity. Clin Geriatr 2001;9:19. (Practical guideline to promoting physical activity.) (PMID: not available)

Keysore JJ, Jette AM: Have we oversold the benefits of late-life exercise? J Gerontol MS 2001;56A:M412. [PMID: 11445600] (Thoughtful summary of exercise intervention trials.)

King AC: Interventions to promote physical activity by older adults. J Gerontol MS 2001;56A:M36. [PMID: 11730236] (Summary of behavioral principles, strategies, and future issues to promote exercise in older adults.)

Mazzeo RS, Tanaka H: Exercise prescription for the elderly: current recommendations. Sports Med 2001;31:809. [PMID: 11583105] (Overview of key aspects of exercise prescription, especially for endurance and strength.)

O'Grady M et al: Therapeutic and physical fitness exercise prescription for older adults with joint disease: an evidence based approach. Rheum Dis Clin North Am 2000;26:617. [PMID: 10989515] (Thoughtful discussion of exercise benefits and recommendations for exercise adaptation for older persons with arthritis.)

Van der Bij AK et al: Effectiveness of physical activity interventions for older adults. Am J Prev Med 2002;22:120. [PMID: 11818183] (Overview and summary of the evidence on interventions designed to promote exercise adherence in older adults.)

Vincent KR et al: Resistance exercise and physical performance in adults aged 60 to 83. J Am Geriatr Soc 2002;50:1100. [PMID: not available] (Report of a randomized controlled trial in healthy elders of 2 levels of resistance training.)

Wu G: Evaluation of the effectiveness of Tai Chi for improving balance and preventing falls in the older population–a review. J Am Geriatr Soc 2002;50:746. [PMID: 11982679] (Review of the various forms of Tai Chi Ch'uan and a summary of the evidence to date of its effectiveness on maintaining balance.)

RELEVANT WORLD WIDE WEB SITES

American College of Sports Medicine: ACSM position stand on exercise and physical activity for older adults: www.acsm-msse.org

Extendedcare.com: www.extendedcare.com/library/informedliving.asp (Practical guide to exercise for older adults.)

National Institute on Aging: www.nihseniorhealth.gov/exercise/toc.html (Focuses on exercise for older adults with guidelines and suggested exercise programs.)

National Institute on Aging: Exercise: a guide from the National Institute on Aging: www.nia.nih.gov/exercisebook (Recommendations and examples of exercise for older adults; includes examples of diaries an self monitoring of progress.)

National Institute on Aging and National Aeronautics and Space Administration: http://weboflife.ksc.nasa.gov/exerciseandaging/home.html
(Guidelines and examples for exercise for older adults.)

President's Council on Physical Fitness: www.fitness.gov/activelife/activelife.html (Provides recommendations for older adults.)

Common Pain Syndromes & Management of Pain

43

Jerry O. Ciocon, MD, Diana J. Galindo, MD, & Daisy G. Ciocon, PhD, ARNP

Patients with pain often seek immediate relief and alleviation of discomfort. Success of treatment depends on the accuracy of the diagnosis and provision of the most appropriate medications. Prescription drugs (eg, analgesics, anti-inflammatory agents, and muscle relaxants) may be helpful, but appropriate trigger point injections might provide more effective treatment.

In many instances in this chapter, we recommend injections as a therapeutic modality. The amount of corticosteroid (Depo-Medrol) used should be ~40 mg for small areas and 80 mg for larger areas. Long-acting local anesthetics (eg, bupivacaine) are preferred and are mixed with the corticosteroid before injection. Complicated pain syndromes may benefit from evaluation and treatment by a physiatrist or anesthetist who specializes in pain management.

■ TEMPOROMANDIBULAR JOINT PAIN

ESSENTIALS OF DIAGNOSIS

- Myofascial pain of the mastication muscles, pain in the temporomandibular joint radiating to the mandible, ear, neck, and tonsillar pillars.
- Point tenderness in the external and internal portions of the joint.

General Considerations

Whiplash injury, head, neck, and facial trauma (direct and indirect) are common preceding events.

Pathogenesis

External stress, including dental malocclusion and external head and neck injuries, causes internal derangement of the synovial articular disk of the temporomandibular joint (TMJ), resulting in pain and joint dysfunction. The muscles of mastication, namely, the temporalis, masseter, pterygoids, trapezius, and sternocleidomastoids, tighten into spasm during joint injury, causing facial pain.

Prevention

Regular dental maintenance, immediate medical attention after head and neck trauma, especially after a vehicular accident with whiplash injury, might help prevent muscle spasm that leads to myofascial pain.

Clinical Findings

A. SYMPTOMS & SIGNS

Headache with pain in the ear and neck, with point tenderness in the internal and external portions of the TMJ, are the common findings.

B. LABORATORY FINDINGS

Sedimentation rate may reflect inflammation of the joint (a nonspecific finding).

C. IMAGING STUDIES

Radiographic imaging of the TMJ may not show any abnormalities, except perhaps for malalignment. Magnetic resonance imaging (MRI) may show irregularities of the synovial disk.

D. SPECIAL TESTS

Injection of the joint with a small amount of anesthetic may serve as a diagnostic test to determine whether the TMJ is the source of pain.

E. SPECIAL EXAMINATIONS

The internal portion of the TMJ must be palpated, and the pain should be reproduced to give a definite diagnosis.

Differential Diagnosis

Cervicalgia, cervical degenerative disk disease, tooth abscess, otitis media, otitis externa, and temporal arteritis must be differentiated from TMJ disease. Nocturnal bruxism can also cause pain in the TMJ area.

Complications

Chronic headache, depression, weight loss as a result of trouble chewing, insomnia, tinnitus, dizziness, altered taste, and decline in function may result from untreated TMJ pain.

Treatment

Timely correction of dental occlusion with acrylic bite appliances will prevent worsening of malocclusion. Myofascial massage of the tender muscles of mastication may alleviate the pain. Trigger point injection (Table 43–1) with long-acting anesthetics around the joint may also relieve discomfort. The joint space between the mandibular condyle and the glenoid fossa of the zygoma may be injected with a small amount of local anesthetic and steroid. Narcotic analgesics and benzodiazepines should be avoided.

Kropmans TJ et al: Repeated assessment of temporomandibular joint pain: reasoned decision-making with use of unidimensional and multidimensional pain scales. Clin J Pain 2002; 18:107. [PMID: 11882774]

Greene CS: The etiology of temporomandibular disorders: implications for treatment. J Orofacial Pain 2001;15:93. [PMID: 11443830]

RELEVANT WORLD WIDE WEB SITES

American Academy of Orofacial Pain: www.aaop.org/TMD/info_factors.htm

Table 43–1. Suggested dosage of corticosteroids (methylprednisolone) & local anesthetic agent (bupivacaine 0.5%).

Site	Methylprednisolone (mg)	Bupivacaine 0.5% (mL)
TMJ	10	1
Trapezius	40	1
Shoulder pain syndrome	80	2
Elbow pain syndrome	80	1
Wrist pain syndrome	40	1
Chest pain syndrome	40	1
Abdominal wall pain	40	2
Groin pain syndrome	40	2
Lumbar related pain	80	2
Knee pain syndrome	80	2
Ankle/foot pain	40	1

TMJ, temporomandibular joint.

American Academy of Orofacial Pain: www.aaop.org/guidelines.htm

■ TRAPEZIUS MYOFASCIAL PAIN SYNDROME

ESSENTIALS OF DIAGNOSIS

- *Discomfort in the neck, mastoid region, angle of the jaw, and upper extremity and localized trigger point tenderness in these areas.*
- *Mechanical stimulation of the trigger point by palpation or stretching produces intense local pain and referred pain.*
- *An involuntary withdrawal of the stimulated muscle, or a "jump sign," is often observed.*

General Considerations

This common condition may not be clinically recognized, and pain is often thought to be due to cervical spine arthritis or even angina pectoris. Poor posture while doing desk work, computer work, watching television, and engaging in unaccustomed physical activity are predisposing factors.

Pathogenesis

Flexion and extension injuries to the neck area secondary to pressure from the straps of purses, backpacks, or laptop computer cases may result in trapezius myofascial pain syndrome. Taut bands of muscle fibers resulting from repeated muscular contractions lead to microtrauma of the affected muscle, causing still more muscle deformity and pain. This often leads to chronic deconditioning of the agonist and antagonist muscle unit. The trapezius muscle is also very vulnerable to stress-induced tension, leading to muscle spasm and pain.

Prevention

Patients should be advised to balance the weight distribution of purses, golf bags, and other items when carried on the shoulders. Regular exercise with proper stretching before and after any activity will condition the trapezius muscle and prevent taut bands from forming.

Clinical Findings

A. SYMPTOMS & SIGNS

Pain in the neck, mastoid region, angle of the jaw, and upper extremity and neck stiffness are the common manifestations. Patients may believe the symptoms are of cardiac origin. Point tenderness in these areas and the jump test (involuntary withdrawal of the stimulated muscle) are characteristic clinical findings.

B. LABORATORY FINDINGS

Blood tests are typically not helpful.

C. IMAGING STUDIES

Computed tomography (CT) or MRI may reveal other causes of neck pain (eg, cervical spondylosis, cervical disk herniation) that may mimic this syndrome.

D. SPECIAL TESTS

Liquid crystal contact thermography may demonstrate a higher than normal temperature in the trapezius muscles. Electromyographic (EMG) increases in electrical activity of the trapezius can provide objective evidence for this disorder; when pain is relieved, EMG activity decreases.

E. SPECIAL EXAMINATIONS

Localizing a defined trigger point and a positive jump test support the diagnosis of trapezius myofascial syndrome.

Differential Diagnosis

Angina pectoris, cervical spondylosis, cervical radiculopathy, occipital neuralgia, and tension headache can mimic the symptoms of trapezius myofascial syndrome.

Complications

Chronic and unrecognized conditions may lead to chronic pain, fatigue, anxiety and depression, and functional decline caused by pain with simple motions such as hair combing, fastening of brassieres, or reaching overhead. Inactivity caused by pain may result in muscle wasting and frozen shoulder.

Treatment

Heat and cold compress therapy accompanied by proper trapezius muscle stretching may help prevent repeated muscle spasm. Anti-inflammatory medications may relieve some discomfort. Injections (see Table 43–1) directed at the primary trigger point with long-acting anesthetics and methylprednisolone may provide

benefit, although multiple administrations may be necessary.

Carlson CR et al: Reduction of pain and EMG activity in the masseter region by trapezius trigger point injection. Pain 1993;55:397. [PMID: 8121703]

RELEVANT WORLD WIDE WEB SITES

www.drshankland.com/myofascial.html

■ SHOULDER PAIN SYNDROMES

ACROMIOCLAVICULAR JOINT PAIN; SUPRASPINATUS, INFRASPINATUS, SUBSCAPULARIS TENDINITIS; BICIPITAL TENDINITIS, & ROTATOR CUFF TEAR

 ESSENTIALS OF DIAGNOSIS

- *Pain at the shoulder that is made worse by stretching the affected arm across the chest (as in removing a coat or long-sleeved shirt); pain that disturbs sleep when lying on the involved shoulder.*
- *Point tenderness of the acromioclavicular joint or the rotator cuff areas.*

General Considerations

Shoulder pain may be mistakenly attributed to osteoarthritis when insufficient historical information is obtained and inadequate examination is performed. Acromioclavicular (AC) joint pain is aggravated by stretching the affected arm across the chest. With subdeltoid bursitis and supraspinatus, infraspinatus, subscapularis (SIS) tendinitis, shoulder pain is exacerbated by abduction.

Pathogenesis

The AC joint is vulnerable to injury from both acute trauma and repeated microtrauma. Falls, breaking a fall with the arm outstretched, repeated strain from throwing injuries, or working with the arm raised across the body may result in injury to the AC joint, causing inflammation and pain. Overuse or misuse of the shoulder, such as carrying heavy loads in front of and away from the body, and vigorous exercise without adequate stretching may also precipitate injury. When not treated, calcium deposits may form and cause permanent changes in the lining of the joint, leading to the development of chronic arthritis. This may further limit movement of the shoulder.

Prevention

Recognition of the disorder may prevent further injury. Patients can avoid carrying heavy objects with an outstretched arm, avoid heavy handbags, maintain improved posture, and implement fall prevention strategies (see Chapter 12: Falls & Mobility Disorders).

Clinical Findings

A. SYMPTOMS & SIGNS

Pain is experienced in the shoulder with specific movements. Point tenderness may be appreciated over the acromion (AC bursitis), rotator cuff area (SIS), and subdeltoid areas. Pain may be reproduced with resisted abduction and lateral rotation of the shoulder joint. Sudden release of resistance during this maneuver will markedly increase the pain.

A. LABORATORY FINDINGS

Complete blood count, sedimentation rate, and antinuclear antibody may be indicated if an inflammatory or infectious cause is suspected.

B. IMAGING STUDIES

Plain radiographs of the shoulder may reveal calcification of the bursa and associated structures consistent with chronic inflammation. In acute conditions, the radiograph will be normal. MRI may reveal tendinitis, partial disruption of the ligaments, or rotator cuff tear. Radionucleotide bone scan is indicated if metastatic diseases or primary bone tumor is suspected.

C. SPECIAL TESTS

EMG studies (ordered rarely) in patients with shoulder bursitis may reveal decreases in electrical activity of the deltoid muscle compared with the supraspinatus muscle. This reflects inhibition of the deltoid as a compensatory mechanism for inflamed rotator cuff ligaments.

D. SPECIAL EXAMINATIONS

Trigger point tenderness at a specific site in the shoulder and reproduction of pain with shoulder passive and active maneuvers will often define the specific site of shoulder inflammation. In rotator cuff tear, there is weakness on external rotation of the shoulder if the infraspinatus is involved and weakness in abduction above the level of the shoulder if supraspinatus is involved. A positive drop-arm test (inability to hold the arm abducted at the level of the shoulder after the supported arm is released) is often present with complete rotator cuff tears. Moseley's test is performed by having the patient actively abduct the arm to 80° and then adding gentle resistance, which will force the arm to drop if complete rotator cuff tear is present. A positive Yergason's sign, or production of pain on active supination of the forearm against resistance with the elbow flexed at a right angle, is characteristic of bicipital tendinitis.

Differential Diagnosis

Polymyalgia rheumatica, rheumatoid arthritis, rotator cuff tear, osteoarthritis of the shoulder, and Lyme disease may mimic symptoms of this disorder. Rotator cuff tear is often the result of ongoing tendinitis of the shoulder.

Complications

Frozen shoulder, chronic pain, handicap resulting from limitations of upper extremity function, and interrupted sleep are common complications.

Treatment

Range of motion (ROM) and stretching exercises may be beneficial after acute flares subside. Trigger point injections (see Table 43–1) at the specific site (AC, supraspinatus, infraspinatus, bicipital, or subscapularis tendon) may alleviate the pain.

Short-term (2–4 weeks) immobilization of shoulder with sling and swath is recommended when there is significant trauma to the shoulder joint.

Glockner SM: Shoulder pain: a diagnostic dilemma. Am Fam Physician 1995;51:1677. [PMID: 7754927]

Turnbull JR: Acromioclavicular joint disorders. Med Sci Sports Exerc 1998;30(suppl):S26. [PMID: 9565953]

RELEVANT WORLD WIDE WEB SITES

www.hopkinsmedicine.org/orthopedicsurgery/sports/acjoint.html

E-Medicine: Acromioclavicular Injury: www.emedicine.com/emerg/topic14.htm

North Wales Sports Physiotherapy Clinic: www.north-wales-sports-physiotherapy-clinic.co.uk/shoulder2.htm

E-Medicine: Rotator Cuff Injury: www.emedicine.com/aaem/byname/rotator-cuff-injury.htm

■ ELBOW PAIN SYNDROMES

ARTHRITIS OF THE ELBOW, TENNIS ELBOW, GOLFER'S ELBOW, OLECRANON BURSITIS

ESSENTIALS OF DIAGNOSIS

- *Pain in the elbow and around the forearm area with everyday tasks such as using a computer keyboard, holding a glass of water, turning a door knob, or driving.*
- *Presence of tenderness around the elbow.*
- *Cause depends on location of the elbow pain and physical examination findings.*

General Considerations

True elbow arthritis is uncommon. Frequently, tendinitis and bursitis will coexist with arthritis pain of the elbow. The olecranon bursa lies in the posterior aspect of the elbow joint and may become inflamed as a result of direct trauma or overuse of the joint.

Pathogenesis

Recurrent microtrauma to the extensor tendons of the forearm with microtearing at the origin of the extensor carpi radialis and extensor carpi ulnaris leads to lateral epicondylitis (tennis elbow). Secondary inflammation from continued overuse or misuse of the extensors of the forearm can become chronic. Coexistent bursitis, arthritis, and gout may also perpetuate the pain and disability of tennis elbow. Similarly, microtrauma of the flexor tendons of the forearm and microtearing at the origin of the pronator teres, flexor carpi radialis and flexor carpi ulnaris, and palmaris longus leads to medial epicondylitis (golfer's elbow). Repeated irritation, acute trauma, and infection of the olecranon bursa lead to bursitis.

Prevention

Proper stretching of the elbow before and after any sports or regular activity that subjects the elbow to repeated trauma (eg, golf, tennis, hockey, repeated hand shaking, scooping of ice cream) may prevent microtrauma to tendons. Proper positioning of the arm when engaged in sports activities and use of elbow support may also prevent unnecessary trauma and irritation.

Clinical Findings

A. SYMPTOMS & SIGNS

Pain in the elbow worsened by movement and relieved by rest and heat are characteristic of elbow pain syndrome. Pain may interfere with sleep. Specific symptoms depend on the location of the inflammation. In elbow arthritis, the pain is felt deep inside the joint, and crepitus may be present. In tennis elbow, elbow pain in the lateral epicondyle is constant and made worse with active contraction of the wrist, leading to diminished grip strength, difficulty holding items such as a coffee cup or a hammer, and sleep disturbance. On physical examination, there will be tenderness along the extensor tendons or just below the lateral epicondyle. Forcing the clenched fist into flexion further aggravates the elbow pain.

In golfer's elbow, pain is constant in the medial epicondyle and is made worse with active contraction of the wrist. Forcing the clenched fist into extension aggravates the elbow pain. In olecranon bursitis, pain and swelling of the olecranon bursa occur.

B. LABORATORY FINDINGS

In infectious olecranon bursitis, leukocytosis may be found, and Gram's stain and culture of aspirates from the bursa may reveal an infectious cause. Sedimentation rate, antinuclear antibody testing, and examination of joint fluid for uric acid crystals are indicated if collagen vascular disease or gout is suspected.

C. IMAGING STUDIES

Plain radiographs of the elbow may reveal calcification of the tendons, bursa, or elbow joint. MRI is indicated if there is joint instability or failure to respond to conservative treatment and surgical procedure is contemplated.

D. SPECIAL TESTS

If ulnar nerve entrapment of the elbow is suspected, electromyography and nerve conduction velocity studies (EMG/NCS) may be used; these tests are extremely sensitive. EMG/NCS can sort out other causes of pain that may mimic ulnar nerve entrapment at the elbow, including cervical radiculopathy and plexopathy.

E. SPECIAL EXAMINATIONS

A diagnostic trial with trigger point injection using a local anesthetic and corticosteroid may prove revealing.

Differential Diagnosis

Septic arthritis, collagen vascular disease, gout, and pseudogout are common disorders that may present with elbow pain and may have similar clinical findings to the elbow pain syndrome. Ulnar nerve entrapment at the elbow is one of the most common entrapment neuropathies encountered in clinical practice. Nerve irritation may mimic elbow pain syndrome.

Complications

Flexion contractures, chronic pain, upper extremity disability, sleep disturbance, and depression may complicate elbow pain syndrome if it is not treated aggressively.

Treatment

Trigger point injection (see Table 43–1) with anesthetic or corticosteroids, acupuncture, shock wave therapy, use of orthotic devices, physiotherapy, and antibiotics (if infection is identified) are common treatment modalities for elbow pain syndrome.

Buchbinder R et al: Shock wave therapy for lateral elbow pain. Cochrane Database Syst Rev 2002;1:CD003524. [PMID: 11869669]

Fink M et al: Acupuncture in chronic epicondylitis: a randomized controlled trial. Rheumatology 2002;41:205. [PMID: 11886971]

Pienimaki TT et al: Chronic medial and lateral epicondylitis: a comparison of pain, disability and function. Arch Phys Med Rehabil 2002;83:317. [PMID: 11887110]

Sevier TL, Wilson JK: Treating lateral epicondylitis. Sports Med 1999;28:375. [PMID: 10593647]

RELEVANT WORLD WIDE WEB SITES

Sports Injury Clinic: www.sportsinjuryclinic.net/cybertherapist/front/elbow/tenniselbow.htm

■ WRIST PAIN SYNDROMES

ARTHRITIS, CARPAL TUNNEL SYNDROME, DE QUERVAIN'S TENOSYNOVITIS, DUPUYTREN'S CONTRACTURE, TRIGGER FINGER OR THUMB

ESSENTIALS OF DIAGNOSIS

- Pain, swelling, decrease in function of the wrist and hands with or without trauma and point tenderness to specific site.

General Considerations

The hands and wrists are vulnerable to trauma or inflammation because of the presence of multiple joints and the repeated motion with activities of daily living (ADLs) or work. Pain is often aggravated by motion and relieved by rest or heat therapy.

Pathogenesis

Recurrent and frequent repetitive movement of the joints in the hands and wrists leads to wear and tear, resulting in inflammation and possible arthritis. Rheumatoid arthritis may affect the wrists and hands even in the absence of trauma. Posttraumatic arthritis is commonly observed in athletes, in those who fall, and in those who perform strenuous manual work or operate heavy equipment.

Compression of the median nerve is commonly due to flexor tenosynovitis, rheumatoid arthritis, myxedema, amyloidosis, and other space-occupying lesions. This leads to carpal tunnel syndrome. Repeated twisting motions of the hands (eg, using a screwdriver, frequent hand shaking) and high-torque wrist turning (eg, scooping ice cream) may lead to inflammation and swelling of the abductor pollicis longus and extensor pollicis brevis at the level of the radial styloid process, resulting in de Quervain's tenosynovitis. Compression and repeated trauma to the tendon of the flexor pollicis longus lead to trigger thumb, and repeated trauma to the tendons of the flexor digitorum superficialis resulting from compression against the heads of the metacarpal bones lead to trigger finger.

Prevention

Use of protective gloves, proper hand positioning with use of computers and keyboards, and frequent rest from strenuous and repetitive hand and wrist movements reduce risk of wrist injury.

Clinical Findings

A. SYMPTOMS & SIGNS

Wrist and hand pain made worse by activities and relieved by rest and heat are characteristic of wrist and hand pain syndromes. When severe, sleep interruption is common. Grating and popping sensation with use of the joint and crepitus may be present on physical examination. Rheumatoid arthritis commonly causes swelling and tenderness of the metacarpophalangeal joints with deformities. With continued disuse, muscle wasting may occur and joint stiffness will be observed.

B. LABORATORY FINDINGS

Rheumatoid factor, sedimentation rate, and antinuclear antibody are useful if inflammatory rheumatological disease is suspected. Complete blood count, Gram's stain, and culture of aspirated synovial fluid may reveal an infectious cause of inflammation and pain.

C. IMAGING STUDIES

Plain radiography may reveal bony displacement, joint instability, and occult bony disease. MRI may reveal joint deformity, space-occupying lesion, and inflammation of the tendons involved, although clinical examination with proper anatomic correlation may obviate the need for such studies.

D. SPECIAL TESTS

EMG/NCS may reveal objective evidence of nerve irritation in carpal tunnel syndrome.

E. SPECIAL EXAMINATIONS

The injection of anesthetics to the site of pain may serve as a diagnostic maneuver to identify the cause of the pain. In suspected carpal tunnel syndrome, Tinel's or Phalen's signs and the application of pressure over the median nerve (by inflating a sphygmomanometer over the wrist) support the diagnosis. Tinel's sign is the induction of paresthesias by tapping over the site of the median nerve at the wrist. Phalen's sign is positive if symptoms are reproduced by maximum flexion of the wrist for 60 s.

Differential Diagnosis

Rheumatoid arthritis, septic arthritis, Lyme disease, and posttraumatic arthritis may mimic the symptoms of hand and wrist pain syndromes.

Complications

Muscular atrophy of the thenars and hypothenars, decreased joint ROM, chronic pain, insomnia, depression, and a decrease in functional level, including work-related disabilities, are common complications.

Treatment

Use of specific splints to reduce compression and irritation of the tendons and nerves, trigger point injections (see Table 43–1) with corticosteroids and anesthetics, and surgical release or removal of structures that cause mechanical compression are common treatment modalities. Infection requires aggressive treatment with appropriate antibiotics. If carpal tunnel syndrome is diag-

nosed (positive Tinel's or Phalen's signs) or significant osteoarthritis is noted, referral to a hand surgeon for operative treatment may be warranted, if symptoms are severe and the patient is a surgical candidate.

D'Arcy CA, McGee S: The rational clinical examination. Does this patient have carpal tunnel syndrome? JAMA 2000;283:3110. [PMID: 10865306]

Hayward AC et al: Primary care referral protocol for carpal tunnel syndrome. Postgrad Med J 2002;78:149. [PMID: 11884696]

■ CHEST PAIN SYNDROMES

COSTOSTERNAL SYNDROME, INTERCOSTAL NEURALGIA, DIABETIC TRUNCAL NEUROPATHY, TIETZE'S SYNDROME, FRACTURED RIBS, POSTTHORACOTOMY PAIN, ACUTE HERPES ZOSTER OF THE THORACIC DERMATOME, XIPHODYNIA SYNDROME, SLIPPING RIB SYNDROME, THORACIC VERTEBRAL COMPRESSION FRACTURE

 ESSENTIALS OF DIAGNOSIS

- Chest pains with physical examination findings of point tenderness or reproducible pain.
- Normal electrocardiogram and normal screening blood test for myocardial injury.

General Considerations

Because of concerns about potentially life-threatening thoracic disease, chest pain is a serious matter and one of the most common reasons for urgent medical attention. A clear history of trauma may clarify the diagnosis, especially when specific clinical findings (eg, point tenderness that reproduces the pain) are present.

Pathogenesis

Inflammation of chest wall structures is caused by overuse or misuse or trauma secondary to acceleration or deceleration injuries or blunt impact. Costal joints are susceptible to the development of arthritis, spondylitis,

Reiter's syndrome, and psoriatic arthritis, even without any history of trauma. With severe trauma, chest wall joints may sublux or dislocate. The chest wall joints are also subject to tumor invasion from malignancies, including thymoma and metastatic disease.

Prevention

Use of seat belts when driving, attention to fall prevention, conscious effort to avoid excessive and repeated use of chest wall muscles, and stretching before strenuous sports or physical activities may prevent these injuries.

Clinical Findings

A. SYMPTOMS & SIGNS

Patients suffering from either costosternal syndrome or Tietze's syndrome (second or third costochondral joint inflammation) show vigorous splinting by keeping the shoulders stiffly in neutral position. Pain is reproduced with active protraction or retraction of the shoulder, deep inspiration, and full elevation of the shoulder. Coughing and shrugging of the shoulder also reproduce the pain. Patients may also complain of a clicking sensation with movement of the costal joints or ribs (slipping rib syndrome). Physical examination findings in intercostal neuralgia are minimal unless there is a history of thoracic or subcostal surgery or cutaneous findings of herpes zoster involving the thoracic dermatomes. Motor involvement of the subcostal nerve (eg, from diabetic neuropathy) leads to weakening and bulging of the abdominal muscles.

B. LABORATORY FINDINGS

Complete blood count, sedimentation rate, antinuclear antibody, and prostate-specific antigen laboratory tests may provide further information about the degree of inflammation, presence of infection, and metastatic bone deposits from prostate carcinoma.

C. IMAGING STUDIES

Plain radiographs of the ribs and sternocostal region are indicated for chest wall pain resulting from trauma and to rule out suspected bony disease, including tumors.

MRI of the costosternal joints is indicated if joint instability or occult mass is suspected. Radionuclide bone scanning may also confirm the presence of fractures of the ribs or sternum and detect inflammatory disease.

D. SPECIAL EXAMINATIONS

Direct trigger point injection of local anesthetics with subsequent alleviation of pain may identify a specific cause of the chest wall pain syndrome. The hooking maneuver is performed by having the patient lie in the supine position with the abdominal muscles relaxed while the examiner hooks the fingers under the lower rib cage and pulls gently outward. The presence of clicking, or a snapping sensation, of the affected ribs and cartilage indicates the slipping rib syndrome.

Differential Diagnosis

The costochondral and sternocostal joints are susceptible to trauma, osteoarthritis, ankylosing spondylitis, rheumatoid arthritis, Reiter's syndrome, and psoriatic arthritis. These joints are also subject to invasion by tumor either from direct extension of primary malignancies (eg, thymoma) or from metastatic disease. Infectious agents (eg, herpes zoster, *Candida albicans,* and bacterial infection in the case of open chest wall injuries) or surgical trauma may also cause chest wall pain syndromes.

Complications

Chronic pain may develop with insufficient therapy and inadequate preventive measures for recurrent injuries. Subsequently, patients may experience functional decline, sleep disturbance, or depression. Pneumothorax may result from rib fractures or attempted therapeutic injections.

Treatment

Proper recognition of the specific cause of the chest wall pain syndrome must precede appropriate therapy. Once potentially serious diseases are ruled out, reassurance should be provided. Nonsteroidal anti-inflammatory drugs (NSAIDs), cyclo-oxygenase-2 (COX-2) inhibitors, local application of heat followed by cold packs, elastic rib belt, and localized trigger point injection (see Table 43–1) using local anesthetic and corticosteroids are reasonable therapeutic options. Intercostal nerve block may be beneficial for postthoracotomy syndrome and postherpetic neuralgia. Narcotic analgesics, adjuvant analgesics (such as anticonvulsants), and antidepressants are often used for chronic pain.

Aeschlimann A, Kahn MF: Tietze's syndrome: a critical review. Clin Exp Rheumatol 1990;8:407. [PMID: 1697801]

Wise CM et al: Musculoskeletal chest wall syndromes with noncardiac chest pains: a study of 100 patients. Arch Phys Med Rehab 1992;73:147. [PMID: 1543409]

RELEVANT WORLD WIDE WEB SITES

NetDoctor: www.netdoctor.co.uk/diseases/facts/costochondritis.htm

ABDOMINAL & GROIN PAIN SYNDROMES

ILIOINGUINAL NEURALGIA, GENITOFEMORAL NEURALGIA

ESSENTIALS OF DIAGNOSIS

- *Myofascial abdominal pain may present with severe pain and often significant tenderness on examination.*
- *Groin pain syndromes are characterized by abdominal or pelvic pain aggravated by certain body movements, pain radiating to the thighs, scrotum, or labia, and findings of point tenderness.*

General Considerations

Potentially fatal diseases causing abdominal pain, such as pancreatitis, ruptured viscus, ischemic bowel, sigmoid volvulus, and intra-abdominal abscess, should be ruled out before considering the possibility of myofascial pain or specific neuralgia. Thorough abdominal examination will often reveal deep intra-abdominal disease. With support of laboratory data, these conditions can be ruled out.

Pathogenesis

Ilioinguinal neuralgia is caused by compression of the ilioinguinal nerve as it passes through the transverse abdominis muscle at the level of the anterior superior iliac spine. Genitofemoral neuralgia is caused by compression of the genitofemoral nerve as it arises from L1 and L2 nerve roots and passes the psoas muscles or from either the inguinal or genital branches of the nerve as they pass beneath the inguinal ligament. Direct injury, blunt trauma after inguinal herniorrhaphy, and pelvic surgery are the most common causes of this injury.

Prevention

Stretching of the leg and lower abdominal muscles before anticipated physical activities and early therapy using heat and gentle massage at the inguinal areas after inguinal surgery may prevent irritation and inflammation of nerves.

Clinical Findings

A. SYMPTOMS & SIGNS

In ilioinguinal and genitofemoral neuralgia, paresthesias, burning pain, and numbness over the lower abdomen radiating to the legs, scrotum, or labia and occasionally the inner thigh are common. The patient often assumes a bent-forward "novice skier's position" to relieve pressure on the nerve. Chronic pain leads to bulging of the abdominal muscle wall and may be confused with inguinal hernia.

B. LABORATORY FINDINGS

Sedimentation rate and antinuclear antibody may be helpful for the neuralgias to rule out secondary causes.

C. IMAGING STUDIES

In an evaluation of abdominal pain, a plain radiograph of the abdomen may reveal calcification in the pancreas, calcified gallstones, or evidence of ileus. Plain radiographs of the hip and pelvis help to rule out occult bony disease. MRI of the lumbar plexus is indicated if tumor or hematoma is suspected and may also define inflammation around the specific nerve affected.

D. SPECIAL TESTS

EMG will help distinguish ilioinguinal or genitofemoral neuralgia from lumbar plexopathy, lumbar radiculopathy, and diabetic polyneuropathy.

E. SPECIAL EXAMINATIONS

Tinel's sign elicited by tapping over the ilioinguinal nerve where it pierces the transverse abdominal muscle or the genitofemoral nerve where it passes beneath the inguinal ligament helps identify respective neuralgia syndromes.

Differential Diagnosis

Other causes of abdominal pain (see also Chapter 23: Abdominal Complaints & Gastrointestinal Disorders) include cholecystitis, bowel obstruction, renal calculi, myocardial infarction, diabetic ketoacidosis, pneumonia, perforated bowel, ischemic bowel, and irritable bowel syndrome. Clinical and laboratory information as well as history will often provide clues to the diagnosis. Acute herpes zoster may present with abdominal pain before the appearance of skin rash. Lesions of the lumbar plexus from trauma, hematoma, tumor, diabetic neuropathy, or inflammation can mimic pain, numbness, and weakness of genitofemoral or ilioinguinal neuralgia.

Complications

Ilioinguinal and genitofemoral neuralgia are often missed; when recognized, and if nerve blocks are given, ecchymosis and hematoma formation are common.

Treatment

Initial treatment of the neuralgias consists of treatment with NSAIDs or COX-2 inhibitors and avoidance of repetitive activities that cause pain. Nerve block to the ilioinguinal or genitofemoral area may also alleviate discomfort; when not effective, epidural block may be considered. A home program for sustained stretch of myofascial trigger points has also been shown to reduce pain.

Hanten WP et al: Effectiveness of a home program of ischemic pressure followed by sustained stretch for treatment of myofascial trigger points. Phys Ther 2000;80:997. [PMID: 11002435]

RELEVANT WORLD WIDE WEB SITES

www.physsportsmed.com/issues/1997/02feb/fomby.htm

■ LUMBAR SPINE & RELATED SYNDROMES

LUMBAR RADICULOPATHY, SPINAL STENOSIS, ARACHNOIDITIS, SACROILIAC JOINT PAIN, PIRIFORMIS SYNDROME, ISCHIOGLUTEAL BURSITIS, COCCYDYNIA, TROCHANTERIC BURSITIS

ESSENTIALS OF DIAGNOSIS

- Low back pain with and without leg pain, numbness, loss of reflexes.
- Identifying site of nerve root irritation, trigger point tenderness, and imaging studies can aid in making specific diagnosis.
- Lumbar radiculopathy causes pain in the back or the legs.

General Considerations

Back pain and leg pain are often disabling and may affect daily function, work, and safety with ambulation. Lumbar radiculopathy often affects the lower extremities. Other inflammatory conditions in the hip, pelvic, and lower back area may present with similar symptoms but may be differentiated by specific tender trigger point areas.

Pathogenesis

Lumbar radiculopathy can be due to herniated disk, foraminal stenosis, tumor, osteophyte formation, and, rarely, infection. Most of these processes are due to wear and tear, especially in overweight and underactive persons. Sacroiliac joint pain is often caused by poor posture, but other causes include ankylosing spondylitis, rheumatoid arthritis and other collagen vascular diseases, and overaggressive bone graft.

Prevention

Proper posture and avoidance of excessive bending prevent worsening of the pain and repeat injuries. Professionally guided exercise programs designed to strengthen back and leg muscles may help with pain control and mobility.

Clinical Findings

A. SYMPTOMS & SIGNS

Pain, numbness, tingling, and paresthesias in the distribution of the affected lumbar nerve root or roots and lack of coordination of the affected extremities may cause difficulty with ambulation and even falls. Continuous irritation to the nerve roots may lead to urinary and fecal incontinence. Patients suffering from lumbar stenosis or lumbar radiculopathy often stoop forward to walk or may shift their body weight onto a shopping cart to relieve pressure on the affected nerve root of the lumbar spine. Calf pain with ambulation (pseudoclaudication) is also a common presentation of lumbar stenosis or radiculopathy.

B. LABORATORY FINDINGS

Complete blood count and blood cultures may be indicated if an infectious cause (eg, abscess) is suspected. Sedimentation rate, antinuclear antibody, and human leukocyte B-27 antigen screening help to differentiate other rheumatological diseases.

C. IMAGING STUDIES

MRI of the lumbar spine, sacroiliac area, and other specific areas may help identify abnormalities and provide guidance for further therapy. Computed tomography complemented by myelography is a reasonable second choice to MRI. Radionucleotide bone scanning and plain radiography are indicated when fracture or other bony abnormalities such metastatic disease are suspected.

D. SPECIAL TESTS

EMG/NCS provides the neurophysiological information that can delineate the actual status of individual nerve roots and the lumbar plexus.

E. SPECIAL EXAMINATIONS

Identifying trigger tender points and performing the straight-leg test to document nerve root irritation and the pelvic rock test for sacroiliac joint pain may help in locating the cause of lower back and leg pain. The pelvic rock test is performed by placing the hands on the iliac crests and the thumbs on the anterior superior iliac spines and then forcibly compressing the pelvis toward the midline. A positive test is indicated by the production of pain around the sacroiliac joint.

Differential Diagnosis

Low back strain, lumbar bursitis, lumbar fibromyositis, lumbar disk herniation, and spinal stenosis can mimic lumbar radiculopathy.

Complications

Failure to accurately diagnose lumbar radiculopathy can lead to lumbar myelopathy, which, if untreated, may progress to paraparesis, paraplegia, cauda equina syndrome, and gait disorders, resulting in falls.

Treatment

Physical therapy, heat modalities, deep sedative massage, NSAIDs, and skeletal muscle relaxants are reasonable initial therapeutic options for lumbar radiculopathy and spinal stenosis. Caudal epidural blocks with local anesthetic and corticosteroids may alleviate pain temporarily. Use of an antidepressant (eg, nortriptyline) may help depression and sleep disturbance. Trigger point injections (see Table 43–1) at the specific tender location—sacroiliac joint, ischiogluteal bursa, sacrococcyx junction, trochanteric bursa, and sciatic nerve at the level of the piriformis muscle in piriformis syndrome—may alleviate pain and improve function and gait. Referral to a physiatrist or anesthetist (pain clinic) may be necessary for trigger point injections.

Maigne JY et al: Causes and mechanisms of common coccydynia: role of body mass index and coccygeal trauma. Spine 2002;25:3072. [PMID: 11145819]

RELEVANT WORLD WIDE WEB SITES

E-Medicine: Piriformis Syndrome: www.emedicine.com/sports/topic102.htm

E-Medicine: Coccygodynia: www.emedicine.com/orthoped/topic383.htm

■ KNEE PAIN SYNDROMES

ARTHRITIS OF THE KNEE, MEDIAL COLLATERAL LIGAMENT SYNDROME, SUPRAPATELLAR BURSITIS, PREPATELLAR BURSITIS, BAKER'S CYST

 ESSENTIALS OF DIAGNOSIS

- *Pain, swelling, limited ROM, and imaging of the knee joint make the diagnosis of osteoarthritis.*
- *Bursitis or a ligament syndrome is a more likely diagnosis when there is specific point tenderness, absence of significant intra-articular knee abnormalities on examination, and normal radiographic imaging.*

GENERAL CONSIDERATIONS

Osteoarthritis of the knee is the most common cause of knee pain. Movement of the knee results in more pain; pain may be relieved by rest and application of heat therapy. Coexisting bursitis, tendinitis, and internal derangement of the knee may make the clinical diagnosis of arthritis difficult unless detailed imaging is performed.

Pathogenesis

Excessive weight and repeated movement lead to wear and tear of the lining of the knee, causing inflammation, fluid accumulation, prostaglandin production, and further inflammation. Soft tissues around the knee may also be subjected to strain and become irritated and inflamed, resulting in bursitis or tendinitis. Baker's cyst is due to excess synovial fluid accumulation in the knee.

Prevention

Proper knee support and adequate stretching before and immediately after any strenuous sports or physical activity are important. Use of knee guards may minimize direct irritation of knee structures by a hard floor surface and prevent myofascial inflammation.

Clinical Findings

A. SYMPTOMS & SIGNS

In osteoarthritis of the knee, pain is felt around the knee and distal femur. Pain is constant and achy. Pain may interfere with sleep. Grating and popping sensations and crepitus are often observed. Later, ROM is diminished and ADLs become difficult. Ultimately, muscle wasting and stiff "frozen knee" may develop.

B. LABORATORY FINDINGS

Synovial fluid cell count and culture (along with complete blood count and blood cultures) are essential when septic arthritis is a consideration. In addition, crystal analysis should be performed if gout or pseudogout is suspected.

C. IMAGING STUDIES

Plain radiographs are indicated for most patients who complain of knee pain. MRI of the knee is indicated if aseptic necrosis or occult mass or tumor is suspected.

D. SPECIAL TESTS

EMG will help distinguish patellar bursitis from femoral neuropathy, lumbar radiculopathy, and plexopathy. Sonography of the patellar tendon and adjacent structures may confirm patellar bursitis syndrome.

E. SPECIAL EXAMINATIONS

Knee manipulation is used to assess joint instability or appreciate joint stiffness as in "frozen knee" resulting from adhesive capsulitis. Pain with passive and active resisted extension of the knee will reproduce pain in patellar bursitis, and sudden release during this maneuver will markedly increase the pain. On palpation of the patellar bursa, a boggy sensation, erythematous appearance, and warm skin surface may also be found.

Differential Diagnosis

Lumbar radiculopathy may mimic pain and associated symptoms of knee arthritis. Bursitis and other soft tissue inflammatory processes can cause pain around the knee. Primary and metastatic tumors of the femur and spine may also present with symptoms similar to knee osteoarthritis. Dysfunction of the quadriceps tendon can mimic symptoms of patellar bursitis.

Complications

Failure to identify neoplasm and septic arthritis may result in venous thrombosis, pulmonary embolism, joint destruction, and sepsis. Intra-articular or trigger point injections may lead to infection.

Treatment

Weight reduction, use of NSAIDs, and physical therapy are the initial therapeutic modalities. Aseptic intra-articular injection (see Table 43–1) with corticosteroids and local anesthetic may reduce inflammation and pain. Trigger point injection of corticosteroids at the tender myofascial area or specific knee bursa (suprapatellar or prepatellar), followed by knee muscle strengthening exercise, may alleviate pain. Baker's cysts must be drained.

Dawn B et al: Prepatellar bursitis. J Rheumatol 1997;24:976. [PMID: 9150094]

RELEVANT WORLD WIDE WEB SITES

Clinical Sports Medicine: www.clinicalsportsmedicine.com/chapters/24f.htm

E-Medicine: Myofascial Pain in Athletes: www.emedicine.com/sports/topic158.htm

www.physsportsmed.com/issues/1999/07_99/yu.htm

■ ANKLE & FOOT PAIN SYNDROMES

ARTHRITIS OF THE ANKLE & MIDTARSAL JOINTS, TARSAL TUNNEL SYNDROME, ACHILLES TENDINITIS, MORTON'S NEUROMA, PLANTAR FASCIITIS

 ESSENTIALS OF DIAGNOSIS

- *Pain in the ankle and foot area causes discomfort with pressure and weight bearing and often is relieved by rest. Presence of specific point tenderness and location of pain with activity usually provide the diagnosis.*

- *Arthritis of the ankle presents with pain around the ankle joint proper.*

- *Anterior tarsal tunnel syndrome presents with deep, aching pain in the dorsum of the foot.*

- *Posterior tarsal tunnel syndrome presents with pain, numbness, and paresthesias of the sole of the foot.*

- Plantar fasciitis is characterized by hindfoot pain on awakening, which is worsened by foot pressure.
- Morton's neuroma is the most common cause of pain in the forefoot, usually affecting the second and third toes. It is often associated with wearing tight shoes.

General Consideration

Osteoarthritis and tendinitis of the soft tissue around the ankle and feet may cause disabling discomfort. Detailed history and comprehensive examination of the foot and ankle joints often lead to a specific diagnosis.

Pathogenesis

Excessive strain and frequent use of the ankle joint leads to inflammation and pain. Compression of the tarsal ligaments is commonly due to repeated trauma with daily use of high-heel shoes. Inflammation from rheumatoid arthritis results in a higher incidence of tarsal tunnel syndrome. Repeated trauma to the plantar aspect of the foot leads to plantar fasciitis. Perineural fibrosis of the interdigital nerves is the cause of Morton's neuroma.

Prevention

Use of comfortable shoes when taking long walks and avoidance of sudden ankle and foot motion without proper stretching may prevent trauma to joints and supporting structures.

Clinical Findings

A. SYMPTOMS & SIGNS

Osteoarthritis of the ankle and feet presents with pain localized to the ankle and foot, which is made worse by walking and relieved by rest and heat. Plantar fasciitis is characterized by pain localized to the hindfoot and is most painful on awakening in the morning. Muscle atrophy resulting from disuse and "frozen ankle" may be seen in patients with ankle or foot pain syndromes.

B. LABORATORY FINDINGS

Complete blood count and synovial fluid analysis (cell count, culture) are essential when septic arthritis is a consideration. Crystal analysis of synovial fluid is helpful in suspected gout or pseudogout.

C. IMAGING STUDIES

Plain radiographs are indicated in most patients with ankle pain to rule out fractures, occult mass, and tu-

mors. MRI may show aseptic necrosis, osteomyelitis (a consideration if there is an open wound), and tumors.

D. SPECIAL TESTS

Bone scan may be helpful if an acute inflammation or metastatic bone lesion is suspected. EMG will help distinguish lumbar radiculopathy and diabetic polyneuropathy from tarsal tunnel compression symptoms.

E. SPECIAL EXAMINATIONS

A positive Tinel's sign—an electric shock sensation when the deep peroneal nerve (just medial to the dorsalis pedis artery) is palpated—is often observed in anterior tarsal tunnel syndrome (ATSS). Active plantar flexion will often reproduce the symptoms of ATTS. Weakness of the extensor digitorum brevis may also be observed. Tinel's sign just below and behind the medial malleolus over the posterior tibial nerve is seen in posterior tibial tunnel syndrome (PTTS). In PTTS weakness of the flexor digitorum brevis and the lumbrical muscles may also be present.

Differential Diagnosis

Lumbar radiculopathy, diabetic polyneuropathy, stress fracture of the ankle or feet, and primary bony or metastatic bony tumors present with symptoms similar to other foot and ankle pain syndromes.

Complications

Failure to adequately treat or recognize these disorders may lead to gait disorder, falls, depression, and disability.

Treatment

Weight reduction, proper use of foot orthotics, use of comfortable shoes, NSAIDs therapy, and trigger point injections (see Table 43–1) with corticosteroids and local anesthetics are the treatment modalities for patients with this pain syndrome.

Barrett SJ, O'Malley R: Plantar fasciitis and other causes of heel pain. Am Fam Physician 1999;59:2200. [PMID: 10221305]

Coughlin MJ: Common causes of pain the forefoot in adults. J Bone Joint Surg 2000;82:781. [PMID: 10990297]

Wu KK: Morton neuroma and metatarsalgia. Curr Opin Rheumatol 2000;12:131. [PMID: 10751016]

RELEVANT WORLD WIDE WEB SITES

American Orthopaedic Foot and Ankle Society: www.aofas.org/footpain.asp

E-Medicine: www.emedicine.com/sports/

E-Medicine: Plantar Fasciitis: http://www.emedicine.com/emerg/topic429.htm

Podiatry Online: www.podiatryonline.com/best_practice/tarsal. html

Palliative Care

44

William L. Lyons, MD, & Steven Z. Pantilat, MD

A century ago, Americans commonly died quickly and at young ages as a result of infections or trauma. With improved sanitation, nutrition, and medical technology, most Americans can now expect to live into their later years, often with multiple and interacting chronic illnesses. Death now comes more often at an old age as a result of 1 or more chronic illnesses (eg, heart disease, cancer, emphysema, dementia) after months or years of declining health. This change has created significant challenges. Physicians caring for chronically ill persons need to be able to provide meaningful prognostication about life expectancy, help patients set priorities for their stage in life, ensure that health care actions are consistent with these priorities, and identify and treat suffering.

The various trajectories of decline and death experienced by older Americans have been described in the literature. Cancer prognosis is relatively clear and is the basis for Medicare's hospice benefit. After being diagnosed with cancer, an individual has a variable period of stable function before a steady decline and death. A second trajectory, typified by heart failure or chronic obstructive pulmonary disease, entails slow, steady decline, with superimposed, unpredictable, dramatic exacerbations, one of which leads to death. The third trajectory involves a slow, steady, inexorable decline over years characterized by functional dependence; elderly persons with dementia or profound frailty usually show this pattern. Caring for patients whose trajectories are like the second or third types can be very challenging because predicting such individuals' life expectancy with accuracy is difficult and orchestrating therapies and health services (eg, assistive devices, family respite care) is often complex.

Blanchard J et al: Quality improvement in end-of-life care. Small-scale innovations can make a dramatic difference. Postgrad Med 2002;111:21. [PMID: 11912995]

ADVANCE CARE PLANNING & ADVANCE DIRECTIVES (see also Chapter 46: Common Legal & Ethical Issues)

The ethical principle of autonomy dictates that capable persons have the right to decide what medical treatments they will undergo. It is very common for geriatric patients and their families to be faced with serious decisions toward the end of life, such as whether to allow attempted resuscitation, artificial nutrition and hydration, or transfers from nursing home to hospital. Often the patient is incapable of participating in the necessary discussions at a moment of crisis. Advance care planning allows patients to project their autonomy into the future. The process invites patients to take time, when they have the capacity, to reflect about serious matters and to sketch out their health-related goals and articulate strong feelings about particular medical treatments. Unfortunately, < 25% of older Americans have executed advance directives, and few such documents offer very specific instructions about desired care.

Advance directives can be categorized as either proxy directives, in which the patient designates an individual to make health-related decisions on his or her behalf in the event of decisional incapacity, or instructional directives, in which the patient specifies in advance what kinds of treatment he or she would want under various circumstances. The most useful advance directives accomplish both goals, identifying a surrogate decision maker and spelling out clear health-related treatment goals and preferences. To make advance directives as useful as possible, clinicians should counsel patients who designate a proxy to talk with this individual about goals and preferences, not simply to provide the clinician with that individual's name. Instructional directives will be of limited use if inadequate effort is expended in their preparation. In particular, instructional directives are of limited utility if they state nothing more specific or inclusive than "avoid heroic measures if my condition is terminal."

Outpatient clinicians, in the first few visits with any older patient, should ask whether an advance directive has been previously completed. If so, the document should be obtained, reviewed with the patient, photocopied, and placed in the medical record. If not, the clinician should proactively and deliberately start the advance care planning discussion. In caring for older patients with dementing illnesses (assuming some decisional capacity remains), time is of the essence. Clinicians should succinctly summarize in the medical chart the advance planning discussions held with patients. Further, because such advance directives often appear not to be transferred to, or recognized in, the hospital charts of inpatients, communication about advance directives from the primary provider to other physicians involved in the patient's care in the hospital is crucial. Some clinics use prompts to remind clinicians to review advance directives, analogous to those used for immunizations or cancer screening. Once completed, advance directives should be revisited frequently (eg, yearly) and whenever a significant change in health status occurs. Patients should be instructed to keep copies of advance directives in an accessible location at home and to provide copies to surrogate decision makers.

Although eliciting goals, values, and treatment instructions from patients can be a challenging task, clinicians can improve their skills. Table 44–1 provides suggested open-ended questions that are often fruitful in catalyzing these discussions. The questions place more emphasis on goals and values and less on particular treatment modalities. Given the rapid pace of development in medical technology, it is daunting to attempt to cover every conceivable option that might be considered at some future time in a patient's life. Moreover, asking patients to consider hypothetical burdens and benefits of such treatments is, in many instances, unrealistic. It is often preferable to elicit a patient's general goals and values; when the time comes, the clinician can then work with the surrogate to determine whether the burdens of a particular treatment are justified in an effort to reach those goals.

Kaufman SR: Intensive care, old age, and the problem of death in America. Gerontologist 1998;38:715. [PMID: 9868851]

Table 44–1. Tips for advance care planning.

1. In the first few clinic visits, solicit previously completed advance directives. Obtain them, review with patients, photocopy, and maintain them in the medical record. Clinicians should proactively and deliberately initiate discussions with those who have not already completed a document.
2. Ask patients to designate a proxy decision maker: "Who would you want to make medical decisions for you if you become too sick to make decisions for yourself? The best person is someone who knows you and cares about you and who is able to make difficult decisions."
3. Ask patients to talk about their goals and values: "What's important to you in life?" "What do you fear most about being sick or injured?" "Do you believe that medical treatments should be used to keep you alive as long as possible?" "Can you imagine any situation related to your health that you would consider to be worse than death? For example, are there any circumstances in which you think death would be better than living with severe impairments?" "Do you know of any medical treatments that you would not want to be used under any circumstances?" "Often it is not clear whether a particular treatment is going to help a sick patient. If such a situation arose in caring for you, would you permit your doctors to try the treatment for a limited period and then consult with the surrogate about whether the treatment is helping more than it is hurting?"
4. Urge patients to discuss their answers to Tip 3 with their designated surrogate.
5. Reassure patients: "Advance directives only come into play if you lose the ability to make your own decisions, and you can change them at any time."
6. Revisit advance directives frequently and whenever a significant change in health status occurs.
7. Track completion of advance care planning in a manner analogous to other health care maintenance activities (eg, immunizations or cancer screening).

COMMUNICATION & DECISION MAKING

Ideally, clinicians attend to symptom palliation throughout a patient's life and continuously readjust treatment priorities on the basis of frequent consultation with the patient or other key decision makers. In reality, for a multitude of reasons, curative and life-prolonging care is typically the focus of attention until some clear transition occurs, at which time all parties consider a major shift in goals. Relief of suffering then becomes the major emphasis. Skilled geriatric end-of-life care requires the practitioner to be adept at discussing transitions with patients and families and to be capable of facilitating meetings in which important decisions are made. The following guidelines might serve as a general blueprint for a family meeting.

1. **Recognize a key transition** is taking place. One common trigger or indicator is a major change in prognosis (eg, a new, serious diagnosis has been made or a patient has not recovered from an infection despite use of an appropriate antibiotic). Another indicator may be something articulated by the patient (eg, "I am getting tired of all of this").
2. **Collect important medical information** regarding prognosis, treatment options, benefits and burdens of these options, and probability estimates for various outcomes.
3. With help from the patient, **identify and assemble key** stakeholders.
4. **Elicit all parties' understanding of the patient's diagnosis and prognosis.**
5. **Correct misperceptions.** Use of "I wish" statements can be helpful (eg, "I wish the chemotherapy had eliminated the cancer, but it appears to

have come back"). Avoid numerical predictions (patients mentally mark their calendars when told they "have 6 months to live"); it is better to say, for example, "I think we are talking about weeks to months."

6. **Elicit goals, hopes, and values** that may relate to a treatment's potential benefits and burdens. Does the patient hope to live to see a granddaughter graduate from college? Is she happy to sacrifice some degree of mental clarity to be free of pain? How unpleasant is the prospect of depending on family for matters of personal care? "If your mother were sitting with us now, what do you think she'd tell us to do?"

7. **Discuss treatment options** (eg, dialysis, care in the hospital or intensive care unit, mechanical ventilation, antibiotics) **that are consistent with the patient's goals and values.** If appropriate, **offer a recommendation.** "Based on what you have told me, I think it would be best if I write an order instructing the nursing home not to transfer you to the emergency room if you have another bad emphysema episode. Instead, we will focus on treating you here so that you don't feel so breathless."

8. **Summarize** the results of the discussion (and write a brief synopsis in the medical record).

Lo B et al: Discussing palliative care with patients. Ann Intern Med 1999;130:744. [PMID: 10357694]

Quill TE: Perspectives on care at the close of life. Initiating end-of-life discussions with seriously ill patients: addressing the "elephant in the room." JAMA 2000;284:2502. [PMID: 11074781]

Steinhauser KE et al: Factors considered important at the end of life by patients, family, physicians, and other care providers. JAMA 2000;284:2476. [PMID: 11074777]

SYMPTOM MANAGEMENT

Providing meticulous management of symptoms of terminal illness is important not only for humanitarian reasons but to allow the patient to focus attention on essential considerations like saying goodbye at life's end. Some providers worry about being too generous with symptom-relieving medications, fearing that they may expedite a patient's demise. The ethical **principle of double effect,** however, states that it is acceptable to use a treatment to relieve suffering, even if a known but unintended consequence is that it may hasten a patient's death.

Pain

Nociceptive pain is pain arising from nonneural tissue injury. Most pain resulting from metastatic deposits,

for example, is nociceptive. Although mild nociceptive pain can be treated satisfactorily with acetaminophen, moderate or severe pain should be treated with opioids. In the unusual instance when pain appears only infrequently and sporadically, a simple as-needed regimen may suffice. More commonly, the patient's pain is present at a constant background level, with episodes of exacerbations that may or may not be predictable. This pattern is best treated using a scheduled (basal) dosage of opioid, with additional drug available as needed for breakthrough pain. The basal opioid chosen should be a long-acting preparation to provide continuous pain control for continuous pain. Patients should also have medications available for breakthrough pain at a dose equivalent to 100% of the basal amount given in the same 24-h period. For example, a patient who is taking 30 mg twice daily (60 mg total/24 h) of long-acting morphine could be offered a breakthrough regimen of short-acting morphine, 10 mg orally every 4 h as needed (60 mg/24 h). Table 44–2 lists commonly used opioids, with estimated conversions from one drug to another and one route to another. It often does not make a large difference which drug is chosen in a particular instance; attention to drug cost and ease of administration may be helpful when making a selection. Of note, morphine metabolites accumulate in patients with poor renal function, and meperidine should be avoided because of its short half-life and the significant risk of delirium and seizures in the elderly.

Opioids can cause several adverse effects: somnolence, delirium, nausea, constipation, urinary retention, pruritus, and even myoclonus when used in high doses.

Table 44–2. Opioid drugs & equivalent potency conversions.

Oral dose (mg)	Drug	Parenteral dose (mg)
100	Codeine	60
—	Fentanyl[a]	0.1
15	Hydrocodone	—
4	Hydromorphone	1.5
2	Levorphanol	1
150	Meperidine	50
10	Methadone	5
15	Morphine	5
10	Oxycodone	—

[a]Transdermal fentanyl may be approximately converted to oral morphine as follows: 25 μg/h transdermal fentanyl = 50 mg/day oral morphine.

Adapted from Education for Physicians on End-of-Life Care Project, funded by Robert Wood Johnson Foundation. Used with permission.

Although somnolence may resolve at a stable dose after 2–3 days, constipation tends to persist, even when serum drug levels have stabilized. A bowel regimen (eg, senna, starting at 1 tablet at bedtime) should generally be used in managing any patient started on an opioid regimen. Other side effects of opioids may resolve with lowering of the drug dose. If that is not possible, clinicians may try treating the symptom (eg, diphenhydramine 25 mg orally every 6 h for pruritus) or changing to a new opioid.

Neuropathic pain is the result of injury to nerves, such as can occur with tumor encasement of a nerve trunk. Opioids typically provide only partial relief of neuropathic pain. Gabapentin (beginning 100 mg orally every night and titrating slowly up to 1200 mg 3 times daily) or desipramine or nortriptyline (either beginning 10 mg orally every night and titrating every 2–3 days slowly to 150 mg every night, if needed) are more likely to provide relief.

Nonsteroidal anti-inflammatory drugs (eg, ibuprofen at 400–600 mg orally 3 times/day) may provide relief of bone pain or pain with an inflammatory component and may also allow reduction of opioid dosing. Patients who have gastrointestinal discomfort with nonsteroidal drugs may derive benefit from simultaneous use of a proton-pump inhibitor. Peritumor edema often contributes to cancer pain (eg, metastatic disease in the liver), and prednisone use (10–20 mg orally daily) can be helpful in this context for patients whose life expectancy would reduce concerns about corticosteroid adverse effects.

In many cases, pain from bony metastases is best treated by judicious use of radiotherapy. Patients who are expected to live more than a few days and for whom transportation to a treatment center is feasible may benefit from consultation with a radiation oncologist.

Dyspnea

It is very common for patients with malignancy, end-stage cardiac disease, or end-stage pulmonary disease to experience shortness of breath at end of life. Skillful management of this symptom can substantially reduce suffering. Generally, chronic dyspnea is best treated with opioids, and the principles discussed in connection with pain management apply here as well. Supplemental oxygen may provide relief even for patients whose oxygen saturation levels are not low. Similarly, a bedside fan or open window may be beneficial. Lorazepam (in doses of 0.5–1 mg as needed) may help reduce dyspnea-induced anxiety. Drugs used in management of congestive heart failure (diuretics, digoxin, angiotensin-converting enzyme [ACE] inhibitors) need not necessarily be discontinued when goals of care become purely palliative because such a regimen can provide relief of dyspnea as well.

Nausea & Vomiting

Nausea and vomiting may result from a disease process itself or from medications used to combat the disease or its symptoms. One common cause is constipation (see later discussion), a common problem in terminal, bedbound, dehydrated patients taking opiates. Opioids themselves may cause nausea by stimulation of receptors in the chemoreceptor trigger zone. Other metabolic derangements and medications can cause nausea by the same mechanism. This cause of nausea can be managed by attempting to design a regimen that minimizes blood stream fluctuations in opiate levels (eg, by increasing the ratio of basal to breakthrough dosing). If unsuccessful, haloperidol (starting 0.5 mg orally 3 times/day) may provide relief of opiate-induced nausea. When the cause of nausea cannot be clearly identified, as commonly occurs, prochlorperazine (5–10 mg orally 3 times/day or 25 mg rectally every 12 h) is often helpful as a first agent. If symptoms persist, it is appropriate to add additional agents. Metoclopramide (10 mg orally 4 times/day 30 min before meals and at bedtime) may be beneficial when upper gastrointestinal tract motility is compromised. Finally, dexamethasone (1–4 mg orally or subcutaneously every 6 h) often relieves nausea, particularly if it results from extrinsic compression of the gut by tumor.

Constipation

It is easier to prevent constipation (eg, by instituting a bowel regimen when prescribing opioids) than treat it. Senna (starting at one 8.6-mg tablet at bedtime, with doses ranging up to 3 tablets 2 or 3 times/day if necessary) can be used alone or with sorbitol (30–150 mL of 70% solution) to ensure regularity. Some patients have difficulty titrating sorbitol or are bothered by drug-induced bloating. Bisacodyl suppositories (5–10 mg daily as necessary) can be used to treat constipation if the oral route become unreliable. Docusate is effective as a stool softener but lacks cathartic properties.

Delirium

Elderly patients nearing the end of life commonly experience acute confusional states (see also Chapter 10: Delirium). The extent to which the underlying cause of the episode needs to be determined depends on life expectancy and the likelihood that a reversible cause can be identified and addressed in time. A patient who appears to be suffering from anxiety-inducing delusions, hallucinations, or perceptual distortions should be provided reassurance at the least, and consideration should be given to use of a neuroleptic. Haloperidol (starting 0.5 mg orally 3 times/day) may reduce agitation from psychotic symptoms; chlorpromazine (starting 10 mg orally 2 times/day) may also prove effective and may add a potentially useful sedative effect. However, some patients experience greater confusion as a result of this drug's anticholinergic properties. Benzodiazepines tend to worsen delirium and should be avoided.

Depression

An elderly person coming to terms with the fact that life is drawing to a close is entitled to "feel blue," cry, and think of death. Such symptoms may represent preparatory grief, an expected part of the dying process. These grieving patients may benefit from support from loved ones and their health care providers as well as from counseling. Patients whose mood is characterized by hopelessness or decreased self-esteem or who entertain thoughts of suicide are more likely to be suffering from clinical depression. Although sadness is normal in dying patients, depression is not and should be treated. For depressed dying patients with a life expectancy measured in (many) weeks, a trial of an antidepressant (see Chapter 14: Depression & Other Mental Health Issues) may help. Dextroamphetamine or methylphenidate (for each drug, start 2.5 mg orally each morning and noon) may help those with a shorter life expectancy. Those individuals who benefit from psychostimulants typically report an effect within 1–2 days of starting the drug.

Other Issues

The oral cavity is commonly a site of discomfort in dying patients. In the final few days and hours of life, a patient's oral mucosa may become very dry, which can generate pain, difficulty with speaking and swallowing, and halitosis. Meticulous attention to oral care and use of moistened swabs and artificial saliva can improve symptoms related to dryness. Dentures not only assist with chewing but may provide desired aesthetic structural support to the lower face. They require daily cleaning to avoid painful candidal infections.

Emollients maintain skin moisture in dehydrated patients, and their application can be pleasurable. Management of decubitus ulcers in a patient's last few hours or days of life can be controversial; often the most humane approach is to minimize painful wound care and mandatory repositioning and opt instead for chronic analgesic use.

Chochinov HM: Dignity-conserving care—a new model for palliative care: helping the patient feel valued. JAMA 2002;287: 2253. [PMID: 11980525]

Gloth FM: Pain management in older adults: prevention and treatment. J Am Geriatr Soc 2001;49:188. [PMID: 11207874]

Luce JM, Luce JA: Perspectives on care at the close of life. Management of dyspnea in patients with far-advanced lung disease: "once I lose it, it's kind of hard to catch it...." JAMA 2001;285:1331. [PMID: 11255389]

NUTRITIONAL QUESTIONS IN END-OF-LIFE CARE

Food has great cultural and symbolic significance so that, when a patient's oral intake declines as a result of a life-threatening disease, many questions arise. Is the patient dying from slow starvation? Does reduced intake of food and fluids lead to suffering? Should some kind of measures be taken (up to and including the provision of artificial nutrition and hydration) to ensure adequate nutrition?

In most cases, patients lose appetite and interest in eating as a natural consequence of dying: their declining to eat is a normal part of dying, not the cause of it. Moreover, data show that such patients do not typically experience significant hunger or thirst. Fasting-induced ketones may even provide some measure of natural euphoria.

Although artificial nutrition and hydration may be appropriate for patients with good functional status who lack the ability to eat because of gastrointestinal tract disruptions or obstructions, it has not been demonstrated to prevent aspiration pneumonia, promote comfort, increase weight, improve functional status, or prolong life. Further, providing hydration to patients nearing death runs the risk of generating wet respiratory secretions or pulmonary edema. It is reasonable to offer a diet the patient prefers and suggest gentle spoon feeding by caregivers. Table 44–3 provides rec-

Table 44–3. Recommendations for nutrition and hydration in end-of-life care.

Assess patient and family concerns regarding feeding.
Explain risks and benefits of nutrition (natural and artificial); correct misperceptions.
Describe natural dying.
Empathize with family.
Elicit preferences from patient and family.
Make a recommendation.
Where appropriate, encourage careful spoon feeding of ad lib diet.
Consider artificial nutrition and hydration in patients with good functional status who have mechanical obstructions or disruptions of gastrointestinal tract.
Minimize nutrition and hydration in near-terminal patients to promote comfort.

ommendations for nutritional management in end-of-life care.

PSYCHOLOGICAL, SPIRITUAL, & SOCIAL ISSUES

Dying is less a biomedical event than a psychological, social, and existential one. A person reaching the end of life may question the deepest meaning of identity, the quality of relationships, and even the purpose of existence. Excellent care at the end of life focuses on more than management of physical symptoms.

Kubler-Ross's description of 5 psychological stages experienced by dying individuals (denial, anger, bargaining, depression, and acceptance) captures much emotional truth, but not every patient experiences each stage or traverses such an orderly progression. Beyond these, anxiety and fear of the unknown are commonly voiced emotions. Clinicians can provide emotional support by listening and providing information and reassurance, signaling fidelity and nonabandonment regardless of what may come, and giving reason for hope even if only to feel better tomorrow.

As death approaches, patients may worry about unfinished business in their social or family spheres. A death that is not sudden may be a gift to the patient, allowing for completion of interpersonal relationships. According to hospice leader Ira Byock, a dying person should give voice to 5 statements in order for such relationships to be brought to a healthy close: Forgive me, I forgive you, Thank you, I love you, and Goodbye.

Clinicians can elicit existential or spiritual concerns by asking a few well-phrased and well-timed open-ended questions: "Do you find yourself wondering what is the purpose of all of this? Has spirituality or faith been important to you in the past? Is it now?" A timely referral to a pastor or chaplain can be a great service. Some patients derive spiritual solace by leaving a legacy in the form of shared stories, an audio- or videotape, a scrapbook, or an autobiography.

HOSPICE CARE

Hospice care refers to the provision of services to persons with an incurable illness, using an interdisciplinary team to focus on minimizing physical symptoms, providing spiritual and psychological support, and assisting with family bereavement. In the United States, hospice also refers to the Medicare hospice benefit, through which federal funds provide this type of end-of-life care to eligible patients.

There are 2 fundamental eligibility criteria for the Medicare hospice benefit. First, the patient must have a life expectancy, as certified by a physician, < 6 mo, assuming the disease runs its usual course. Second, the patient's goals of care must be palliative, not curative. Although some hospice agencies may require that a do-not-resuscitate order be in effect, this is not a mandatory criterion of Medicare regulations.

It is typically more difficult for a physician to certify a prognosis of < 6 mo for a patient with a noncancer diagnosis. To assist with prognostication, the National Hospice Organization has published a set of useful guidelines.

Two special populations of terminal geriatric patients deserve special consideration: those with terminal dementia and those dying of old age.

Terminal Dementia

Many dementing illnesses, such as Alzheimer's disease, are terminal afflictions. Nevertheless, the terminal stage can last for a prolonged period, a fact that may make hospice agencies unwilling to admit such patients (if dementia is given as the terminal diagnosis). The following characteristics are typical of demented patients with life expectancy of < 6 mo and should prompt a hospice approach: progressive weight loss, decubitus ulcer formation, recurrent pneumonia, recurrent urinary tract infection, inability to ambulate (even with assistance), inability to track objects with the eyes, and a vocabulary < 6 words.

Dying of Old Age

Some debilitated elderly persons with a combination of illnesses and disabilities show such progressive frailty that it is apparent to all that a terminal process is at work, even if no single terminal diagnosis can be applied. Such individuals typically have poor appetite and ongoing weight loss, are substantially (and increasingly) dependent in activities of daily living, and may have repeated hospitalizations and emergency department visits. The International Classification of Diseases (ninth edition) code 799.3, for "debility, unspecified," has been applied to this population, and hospice agencies will accept this as a terminal diagnosis if adequate supporting evidence is provided. Table 44–4 lists the kinds of information that should be gathered in support of this label.

Table 44–5 summarizes Medicare hospice benefits. Of note, medications are a covered benefit (if used to treat the terminal illness) in contrast to traditional Medicare coverage. Also of interest, although continuous nursing is not available (except for short-term management of a medical crisis), hospice nurses are available by telephone 24 h/day. Hospitalization is discouraged (because it is seldom required to provide purely palliative care) but may be used when medically necessary for acute symptom management.

Table 44–4. Evidence in support of hospice diagnosis "Debility, Unspecified".[a]

Multiple comorbid conditions (particularly affecting central nervous, cardiac, or pulmonary systems)

Clinical progression of disease or disability, with multiple emergency department visits or hospitalizations in recent months

Progressive decline in functional status (dependence in at least 3 activities of daily living or Karnofsky Performance Status worse than 50%) (eg, patient has progressed to spending > 50% of waking hours in bed or chair).

Recent impaired nutritional status (unintended weight loss exceeding 10% over previous 6 mo)

Disrupted skin integrity (eg, decubitus ulceration)

Sepsis

---

[a]International Classification of Diseases code 799.3.

Lynn J: Perspectives on care at the close of life. Serving patients who may die soon and their families: the role of hospice and other services. JAMA 2001;285:925. [PMID: 1180736]

National Hospice Organization: Hospice Care: A Physician's Guide. National Hospice Organization, 1998. (Frequently referenced guide to rudiments of Hospice care, with useful prognostic guidelines for noncancer diagnoses.)

CROSS-CULTURAL ISSUES

Culture is particularly important at times of life transition, such as weddings, births, and deaths. In the context of end-of-life care, culture renders human what is otherwise a biological event. Physicians who are knowledgeable about their patients' cultures are better able to provide compassionate palliative care. Culture includes not only ethnicity, but also religion, educational level, socioeconomic status, generational cohort, and geography. American biomedicine, of course, is also a culture, with its own jargon and intrinsic value system.

One consistent element of American bioethical tradition is the emphasis on patient autonomy. This may be an unfamiliar concept to many patients and their loved ones; often, families wish to spare the patient the perceived burden of decision making at times of serious illness. Some families go further and request that the patient not be informed of an ominous diagnosis. One way to satisfy these cultural requests, while still respecting the tradition of autonomy, is for the physician to offer the patient the opportunity to cede discussions of diagnosis, prognosis, and treatment to someone else.

Culturally competent physicians deliberately learn about the cultural traditions of populations they serve. Such knowledge allows providers to probe individual patients about particular beliefs and practices that may affect care at the end of life. Table 44–6 lists areas of potential inquiry.

A clinician should have a low threshold for involving a translator when a patient's primary language differs from that of the clinician. Family translators may not be ideal because they may feel motivated to sanitize bad news or sidestep taboo subjects. When cultural

Table 44–5. Services covered under Medicare hospice benefit.

Symptom management (including medications for this purpose)

Skilled nursing

Medical supplies

Durable medical equipment

Social services

Respite care (maximum 5-day stay) to give family relief from caregiving

Home health aide services

Psychological counseling

Pastoral care and spiritual support

Volunteers (to help with chores, provide companionship)

Bereavement services for family after death

Table 44–6. Issues to explore in cross-cultural end-of-life care (sample questions).

To patient

"How should we take account of your religious or spiritual beliefs as we provide care for you (eg, involvement of clergy, handling of the body, rituals at time of death)?"

"Are there any traditions that I should be aware of?"

"Do you have any particular concerns related to grief or loss?"

"Would you like to be informed of findings that present during the course of our testing?" or should we discuss all these matters, and any decisions, with your [son/daughter]?"

"In your tradition or culture, are there particularly sensitive or taboo subjects that need delicacy when being addressed?" (eg, can the disease be discussed openly? Can death?)

"How do you and your family feel about hospice or palliative care? I have found, for example, that some people think of it as just giving up."

"Is there anything you want me to keep in mind as we work to treat your symptoms? For example, some people find great meaning in suffering, whereas others want me to do everything I can to eliminate it."

To family at patient's death "Do you have a strong point of view about autopsy?"

---

miscommunication appears likely, it can also be helpful to involve a staff member of the same cultural group as the patient.

Crawley LM et al: Strategies for culturally effective end-of-life care. Ann Intern Med 2002;136:673. [PMID: 11992303]

Kagawa-Singer M, Blackhall LJ: Negotiating cross-cultural issues at the end of life: "you got to go where he lives." JAMA 2001;286:2993. [PMID: 11743841]

AFTER DEATH

At and after death, the clinician is called on to perform a number of important tasks. The pronouncement of death is the first such task. To confirm the patient's physical death is generally not a significant professional challenge. The ritual aspect of this event, however, in which the physician formally declares to loved ones that a life has reached an end, is rich in meaning. In serving this ancient ministerial role, a physician may wish to assure family that the patient died peacefully and that all appropriate care had been given. This may also be the first opportunity to express sympathy for the loss.

An autopsy may help surviving family members, as well as clinicians, to understand the underlying causes of an elderly person's death and can provide a sense of closure. Autopsy rates have fallen over the last several years. Some families report refusing permission out of fear of disfigurement of the body or delay of the funeral. When families are offered autopsy, they should be informed that they may limit the autopsy (eg, to abdomen only) and that the procedure may be performed without interfering with funeral plans or the appearance of the deceased.

A telephone call or letter from the clinician to the family after a death is usually much appreciated. By following up with the family, the provider can express concern and ask about the grieving process. Crying, difficulty sleeping, and even fleeting thoughts of death are probably normal reactions for the recently bereaved. However, persistent blaming of oneself, decline in self care, or suicidal ideations and plans are indicators of complicated grief or depression, and persons demonstrating such signs need prompt (and, in some instances, emergent) referral to a therapist or psychiatrist.

Prigerson HG, Jacobs SC: Perspectives on care at the close of life. Caring for bereaved patients: "all the doctors just suddenly go." JAMA 2001;286:1369. [PMID: 11560543]

Anti-Aging & Complementary Therapies

45

Alfred Fisher, MD, PhD, & John E. Morley, MBBCh

Most older Americans expect to live longer and more independently than previous generations, and many seek increasingly to be involved in their own health through diet, exercise, and participation in health care. Never before has information about health, disease, and treatments been more available through conventional media and the Internet. Ironically, during an era when the number of seniors has grown dramatically, the societal focus on youthfulness has remained strong. The combination of the desire to be involved in health care, the ready access to information which can create consumer demand, the wish to promote health and avoid aging, and interest in new ways to approach problems have created tremendous interest both in therapies designed to prevent or retard aging and in complementary and alternative approaches to health care.

ANTI-AGING THERAPIES

Knowledge about the biological mechanisms involved in aging and the physiological changes associated with aging provides a rational basis for the quest for anti-aging therapies. An anti-aging therapy could act by 1 or more of the following 3 mechanisms:

1. Modify the biochemical and molecular events that cause aging.
2. Correct physiological changes that cause signs or symptoms associated with aging.
3. Lessen the susceptibility of an individual to diseases associated with aging.

Practices that act through the third mechanism (eg, colonoscopy, blood pressure reduction, cholesterol reduction, and other practices that aim to prevent age-associated diseases) are common in medical practice and are dealt with in Chapter 3 and elsewhere in this book.

Antioxidants: Vitamin A, Vitamin C, Vitamin E, Beta Carotene

Aging has long been hypothesized to be due, in part, to oxidative stress. Many cellular processes produce reactive oxygen or reactive nitrogen species, which via a free radical mechanism can chemically modify and hence damage proteins, DNA, and lipids. Aged animals show accumulation of oxidative damage, with markers of oxidative damage being elevated 2- to 3-fold between reproductive maturity and death. Experimental studies in animals have supported a role for oxidative damage in aging. For example, in the worm, *Caenorhabditis elegans,* and in mice, genetic mutations enhance endogenous antioxidant defense pathways and increase life span by 30–100%. Also experimental treatment with antioxidants has increased their life span by 10–50%, maintained mobility in worms, and preserved cognition in mice.

In humans, oxidative damage may contribute to atherosclerosis, cancer, Parkinson's disease, and Alzheimer's disease. The antioxidants most commonly used in people are vitamin A and its precursor beta carotene, vitamin C, and vitamin E. When vitamins are used as anti-aging therapies, they are often used in doses that are higher than the replacement doses that are appropriate for vitamin deficiencies. Although ingestion of vitamin supplements was not associated with increased life span in participants in the U.S. National Health and Nutrition Examination Surveys, it has been hoped that antioxidants might prevent diseases associated with oxidative damage.

A. VITAMIN E

Vitamin E is the safest of the lipid-soluble vitamins and is most commonly given as α-tocopherol in doses ranging from 150 IU/day–2000 IU/day. Side effects include nausea, flatulence, diarrhea, and inhibition of vitamin K.

Vitamin E (800 IU/day) may be used in patients with end-stage renal disease and coronary artery disease to prevent myocardial infarction and other cardiovascular end points. There is no compelling evidence, however, that vitamin E prevents coronary artery disease or its sequelae in other clinical situations. In fact, vitamin E could be harmful in patients with low high-density lipoprotein (HDL) and normal low-density lipoprotein. An antioxidant cocktail including vitamin E blunted the effects of niacin and simvastatin on raising HDL, reducing progression of atherosclerosis and reducing cardiovascular events. With regard to primary prevention, 1 study found no effect of vitamin E during

468

3.6 years of follow-up in patients with cardiovascular risk factors but no history of cardiovascular disease. Similarly, the Alpha-Tocopherol and Beta Carotene Cancer Prevention Study (ATBC) showed no effect of vitamin E on the development of angina or myocardial infarction in patients without coronary artery disease. With regard to secondary prevention, several studies showed no effect of vitamin E supplementation on cardiac outcomes; these findings contrast to a 50% reduction in recurrent myocardial infarction attributed to vitamin E in the smaller Cambridge Heart Antioxidant study. Other studies have found no beneficial effect of vitamin E on progression of carotid atherosclerosis or the development of abdominal aortic aneurysm or peripheral vascular disease.

The effect of vitamin E on the progression of Alzheimer's disease of moderate severity may be promising. In an analysis adjusting for baseline Mini-Mental State Examination, progression was delayed as indicated by longer time to the composite end point of death, institutionalization, loss of ability of 2 of 3 basic activities of daily living, or development of severe dementia (670 days vs. 440 days). However, falls were more frequent in patients treated with vitamin E.

The effect of vitamin E on rates of cancer is not fully defined. Among smokers, the ATBC study found no effect on the development of lung cancer, an increase in the incidence of stomach cancer, and fewer cases of prostate and colorectal cancer. The decrease in prostate cancer seen in the ATBC study has been suggested to be due in part to lowered serum androgen levels because patients receiving vitamin E had significantly lower serum levels of testosterone and androstenedione. Observational studies of vitamin E in the prevention of colorectal cancer have produced mixed results. One study found no effect of vitamin E on the development of breast cancer.

In patients with preexisting age-related macular degeneration, a combination of antioxidants including vitamin E decreased progression to advanced macular degeneration in the Age-Related Eye Disease Study. In contrast, vitamin E for 6 years had no effect on the incidence of age-related macular degeneration in smokers in the ATBC trial. The development of cataracts was not prevented by an antioxidant regiment including vitamin E in another study.

B. Vitamin A

Vitamin A and its precursor, beta carotene, are lipid-soluble vitamins that affect vision, cell growth, and differentiation by interacting with retinoic acid receptors to control gene expression. Both vitamin A and beta carotene have antioxidant properties. The recommended daily allowance of vitamin A is 5000 IU (1.5 mg)/day; intake of 10,000 IU/day is considered safe. Vitamin A is the most toxic of the lipid-soluble vitamins, and both acute toxicity and chronic toxicity are seen. Acute toxicity requires the ingestion of large quantities substantially greater than 200,000 IU. Chronic toxicity occurs with the ingestion of 50,000 IU/day for > 3 mo. Symptoms of chronic toxicity include hair loss, mouth sores, nausea and vomiting, dry skin, hepatomegaly, and increased intracranial pressure, which can result in headaches and altered mental status. Vitamin A consumption in the 10,000 IU/day range may result in an elevated risk of hip fracture in postmenopausal women. This may be due in part to increased production of parathyroid hormone with resultant hypercalcemia. In contrast, the consumption of the provitamin beta carotene is believed to be safe, apart from causing yellowing of the skin, because its conversion to vitamin A is regulated. As a result of these safety issues, most studies use beta carotene instead of vitamin A.

Despite benefits seen in observational studies of vitamin A or beta carotene supplements, experimental studies provide no evidence of benefit for and potential harm in smokers, former smokers, and postmenopausal women. In observational studies, higher intake of fruits and vegetables containing beta carotene was associated with lower risks of cancer and cardiovascular disease. These benefits were not confirmed, however, by randomized trials of beta carotene for preventive effects with respect to cancer and cardiovascular disease. Finnish male smokers treated with beta carotene, as part of the ATBC study, had no decrease in cancer at the major sites and instead had an increase in the incidence of lung, prostate, and stomach cancers. The finding of a possible link to increased risk of lung cancer was supported by the Beta Carotene and Retinol Efficacy trial, which treated smokers, former smokers, and workers exposed to asbestos with vitamin A and beta carotene for 4 years. This study found no change in the incidence of cancer at other sites. The Physician's Health Study found no impact of beta carotene on the incidence of cancer, including lung cancer, during 12 years of treatment. In the Women's Health Study, women treated with beta carotene for ~2 years and then monitored for 2 years had no change in the incidence of cancer. With regard to cardiovascular disease, the ATBC study, Physician's Health Study, the Beta Carotene and Retinol Efficacy trial, and Women's Health Study found no effect of beta carotene on cardiovascular outcomes such as myocardial infarction or stoke. Subgroup analysis of the ATBC trial found no effect of beta carotene in the prevention of myocardial infarction in either primary or secondary prevention. Also, results from the HDL-Atherosclerosis Study suggest that antioxidant cocktails including beta carotene could be harmful to patients with normal LDL and low HDL levels treated with niacin and simvastatin: The use of the antioxidants blunted the effects of niacin and simvastatin on raising HDL, reducing progression of atherosclerosis, and reducing cardiovascular events.

In patients with preexisting age-related macular degeneration, a combination of antioxidants including beta carotene decreased progression to advanced macular degeneration in the Age-Related Eye Disease Study. In contrast, beta carotene for 6 years had no effect on the incidence of age-related macular degeneration over 6 years in the smokers studied in the ATBC trial.

C. Vitamin C

Vitamin C is water-soluble vitamin that is involved in multiple oxidation-reduction reactions in vivo, including the synthesis of collagen. Vitamin C also has antioxidant properties. The recommended daily allowance for vitamin C is 90 mg/day for men and 75 mg/day for women. Supplementation beyond these levels has progressively less effect on the serum levels of vitamin C because both the absorption from the gastrointestinal (GI) tract and excretion via the urine is tightly regulated. Vitamin C has low toxicity, even in large doses. The most common side effects include GI upset, flatulence, and diarrhea. Oxalate kidney stones are also a concern as a result of the metabolism of vitamin C to oxalate. Vitamin C also impairs tests measuring glucose in blood and urine. There is a theoretical concern that supplementation with 500 mg/day of vitamin C could lead to oxidative damage to DNA because levels of 8-oxoadenine, a form of adenine produced by oxidative damage, are increased in patients taking vitamin C daily for 6 weeks.

There is no compelling evidence that vitamin C prevents or retards cardiovascular disease or prevents cancer. However, in patients with precancerous lesions of the stomach, the rate of progression to stomach cancer was lower in those given vitamin C.

Vitamin C may be helpful in preventing progression to advanced macular degeneration and in improving appearance in patients with photodamage. Vitamin C was part of the combination of antioxidants that decreased progression to advanced macular degeneration in the Age-Related Eye Disease Study. Topical vitamin C improved appearance and the synthesis of new collagen in patients with photodamage when applied topically.

D. Alpha-Lipoic Acid

Alpha-lipoic acid is considered to be a potent antioxidant because it can oxidize and regenerate other antioxidants such as vitamin E and glutathione. Studies have suggested that it may be helpful in treating diabetic neuropathy and have a role in retarding the progression of neurodegenerative diseases. Alpha-lipoic acid is not recommended, however, before further studies.

LIMITED EFFICACY OF ANTIOXIDANTS & THE ANTIOXIDANT THEORY OF AGING

How should the largely negative results of randomized studies of the antioxidant vitamins be interpreted? Some have suggested that these findings draw into question the oxidative damage theory of aging, as does the observation that transgenic mice that overproduce CuZn superoxide dismutase do not have any increase in life span. Others have pointed out that the negative results could be due to reasons other than the role of oxidative damage in aging. For example, dose finding studies have not been performed to determine optimal dosages. Also, the antioxidants studied may be unable to reach adequate levels in the proper anatomic or cellular locations. One study using vitamin E found increased serum levels of serum vitamin E in patients taking increasing doses of the vitamin, but the increased serum levels did not translate into changes in measures of lipid peroxidation as a measure of membrane oxidative damage. This study questions both the dosages of vitamin E used in existing studies and the appropriateness of using vitamin E as an antioxidant in patients eating a standard American diet. Finally, it is unclear when during the life course antioxidants would be most effective. Most animal studies treated animals for their entire lives, whereas clinical studies used antioxidants for limited periods of time, generally in adult patients. Interest in newer antioxidants, such as the catalase/superoxide dismutase mimetics, will it is hoped lead to future studies designed to address both clinical concerns as well as these more practical concerns.

Age-Related Eye Disease Study Research Group: A randomized, placebo-controlled, clinic trial of high-dose supplementation with vitamins C and E, beta carotene, and zinc for age-related macular degeneration and vision loss: AREDS report no. 8. Arch Ophthalmol 2001;119:1417. [PMID: 11594942]

Brown BG et al: Simvastatin and niacin, antioxidant vitamins, or the combination for the prevention of coronary disease. N Engl J Med 2001;345:1583. [PMID: 11757504]

Guarente L, Kenyon C: Genetic pathways that regulate ageing in model organisms. Nature 2000;408:255. [PMID: 11089983]

Huang TT et al: Ubiquitous overexpression of CuZn superoxide dismutase does not extend life span in mice. J Gerontol A Biol Med Sci 2000;55:B5. [PMID: 10719757]

Meagher EA et al: Effects of vitamin E on lipid peroxidation in healthy persons. JAMA 2001;285:1178. [PMID: 11752359]

Willett WC, Stampfer MJ: Clinical practice. What vitamins should I be taking, doctor? N Engl J Med 2001;345:1819. [PMID: 11752359]

Yu BP: Approaches to anti-aging intervention: the promises and the uncertainties. Mech Ageing Dev 1999;111:73. [PMID: 10656527]

Growth Hormone

Growth hormone secretion reaches its maximum during the growth spurt accompanying puberty before beginning a steady decline with age in both men and women. Much of this decline is due to a selective reduction in the nocturnal pulsatile secretion of growth hormone. Some of the changes associated with aging are reminiscent of those seen in adult patients with frank growth hormone deficiency, such as reduction in lean body mass, increase in body fat (especially abdominal obesity), decrease in muscular strength, and difficulty with cognitive functioning. As a result, there has been much interest in supplementing growth hormone in the elderly.

Responses to growth hormone or growth hormone secretagogues as measured by serum insulin-like growth factor (IGF-1) levels, which is made by the liver and muscle in response to growth hormone, persist in the elderly. Most studies have titrated the doses of growth hormone or secretagogues to produce IGF levels in the low- to mid-normal range seen in young adults. Treatment with growth hormone increases lean body mass, skin thickness, and vertebral bone mineral density and decreases fat mass. These changes were more pronounced in elderly men than in postmenopausal women. Growth hormone-induced increases in muscle mass were not accompanied by increases in physical strength, stamina, or functional status, however. Effects of exogenous growth hormone on cognition and memory have not been well studied. Short-term use of growth hormone or secretagogues improves sleep.

Side effects of growth hormone include fluid retention, arthralgias, glucose intolerance, headache, and carpal tunnel syndrome. Growth hormone treatment is associated with 2 additional risks. The first is a possible increase in cancer related to the cell growth stimulant properties of IGF-1. The second relates to emerging evidence that growth hormone and IGF-1 signaling shorten life span rather than prolong it. In both worms and fruit flies, increased activity of IGF-1 like signaling pathways shortens life span. Mice deficient in growth hormone live longer than those with normal growth hormone levels, and treatment with supplemental growth hormone in adulthood has led to premature aging. Also, mice treated with caloric restriction not only live longer but also have lower serum IGF-1 levels than normally fed control mice. In a study of Paris policemen, those with physiologically high growth hormone levels died at a higher rate than those with growth hormone in the lower third of the normal range. In summary, the limited benefits of growth hormone, its high cost, and potential long-term risks weigh against the use of growth hormone in the elderly.

Anawalt BD, Merriam GR: Neuroendocrine aging in men andropause and somatopause. Endocrinol Metab Clin North Am 2001;30:647. [PMID: 11571935]

Khorram O: Use of growth hormone and growth hormone secretagogues in aging: help or harm. Clin Obstet Gynecol 2001;44: 893. [PMID: 11600869]

Hormone Replacement

A. TESTOSTERONE

In men, testosterone levels peak during late adolescence then decrease by roughly 0.5–1% per year. Hypogonadism is present in ≤ 10% of men aged 50–69 years and in ≤ 30% of men 70 years of age and older. In parallel with the declines in testosterone levels, aging men experience decreases in muscle mass and strength, bone mass, sexual interest and potency, and cognitive function and increases in fat mass. It is unknown, however, whether these changes can be attributed to declines in testosterone levels.

Several studies have reported on the supplementation of testosterone in men with low testosterone levels via either injections or a scrotal patch (Table 45–1). Most studies have shown increases in lean body mass and bone mineral density and decreases in fat mass and bone mineral density. Accompanying the increase in muscle mass has been an increase in either upper or lower extremity strength. However, only 1 experimental study has shown an increase in functioning with testosterone replacement. Sexual function has shown mixed results with supplementation, and men with lower initial testosterone levels tend to have the most significant improvements. Three studies have suggested small improvements in cognitive function in middle-aged men receiving testosterone.

Concerns have been raised regarding potential effects of supplementation on prostate disease, cardiovascular risk, and erythrocytosis. Testosterone supplementation does not worsen prostatic hypertrophy, and it is unknown whether it increases risk of prostate cancer. Administration of testosterone leads to no change or slight decreases in total cholesterol and LDL cholesterol combined with no change or slight decreases in HDL cholesterol. Testosterone therapy decreases angina, causes coronary artery dilation, and decreases ST depression during exercise stress testing. Erythrocytosis can be seen in up to 25% of patients receiving treatment. This can be easily managed by either decreasing the dose of testosterone given or using phlebotomy.

Hypogonadism can be detected by the Androgen Deficiency in Aging Males Questionnaire followed by direct measurement of a bioavailable testosterone. This questionnaire also identifies patients with depression,

Table 45–1. Hormone replacement & its actions.

Hormone	Actions	Evidence
Testosterone		
Males	Increase lean body mass	++
	Decrease fat mass	++
	Increase bone mineral density	++
	Increase sexual functioning	+
Females	Increase libido	+
	Increase bone mineral density	+/–
	Increase muscle mass	+/–
Hormone replacement therapy with estrogen		
Females	Decrease vasomotor symptoms	++
	Prevent osteoporosis	++
	Prevent coronary artery disease	–
	Prevent dementia	+/–
	Prevent colon cancer	+/–
	Improve mental health	–
Dehydroepiandrosterone		
Females	Increase sense of well-being	+
	Increase bone mineral density	+
	Increase sexual interest (those older than 70)	+
	Decrease skin pigmentation	+
	Decrease skin sebum production	+
Males	Increase sense of well-being	+
	Increase strength	+
	Increase skin thickness	+
	Increase skin hydration	+
Pregnenolone	Increase memory	–
	Improve sleep	+

which should be treated before replacement therapy is considered.

Testosterone levels decline from age 20 to menopause in females. Levels then stay constant through the menopausal transition and then increase after menopause. Estrogen therapy increases sex hormone-binding globulin and, therefore, decreases free testosterone levels. Testosterone replacement therapy in menopausal women improves libido and increases bone mineral density and muscle mass (see Table 45–1). Further studies are required to determine the role of testosterone in women as an anti-aging hormone.

Anawalt BD, Merriam GR: Neuroendocrine aging in men andropause and somatopause. Endocrinol Metab Clin North Am 2001;30:647. [PMID: 11571935]

Hermann M, Berger P: Hormonal changes in aging men: a therapeutic indication? Exp Gerontol 2001;36:1075. [PMID: 11404052]

Morley JE, Perry HM: Androgen deficiency in aging men: role of testosterone replacement therapy. J Lab Clin Med 2000;135:370. [PMID: 10811051]

Morley JE, Unterman TG: Hormonal fountains of youth. J Lab Clin Med 2000;135:364. [PMID: 10811049]

Morley JE et al: Validation of a screening questionnaire for androgen deficiency in aging males. Metabolism 2000;49:1239. [PMID: 11016912]

B. HORMONE REPLACEMENT THERAPY WITH ESTROGEN/PROGESTIN

The changes in estrogen that occur with menopause are well known, and hormone replacement therapy (HRT) to address these changes has been widely used. Large-scale randomized trials demonstrate, however, that HRT leads to increased rates of coronary events, stroke, pulmonary embolism, and breast cancer that are not outweighed by decreased rates of hip fracture and colon cancer. Moreover, HRT did not make asymptomatic or mildly symptomatic women feel better or improve cognition.

Vasomotor symptoms are relieved by HRT, most often with < 1 year of therapy. In women with bothersome vasomotor symptoms, estrogen may be started at a low dose, increased until symptoms are relieved, and tapered every 6 mo until they can be discontinued. In a 50-year-old woman, this strategy will lead to an extra serious adverse event for every 1000 women treated for 1 year. Vasomotor symptoms may also be treated with clonidine, selective serotonin reuptake inhibitors (SSRIs), vitamin E, or phytoestrogens, but these approaches are not as effective as estrogen.

Grady D: Postmenopausal hormones—therapy for symptoms only. N Engl J Med 2003;348:1835. [PMID: 12642636]

Hays J et al: Effects of estrogen plus progestin on health-related quality of life. N Engl J Med 2003;348:1893. [PMID: 12642637]

Hlatky MA et al: Quality-of-life and depressive symptoms in postmenopausal women after receiving hormone therapy: results from the Heart and Estrogen/Progestin Replacement Study (HERS) trial. JAMA 2002;287:591. [PMID: 11829697]

Manson JE, Martin KA: Clinical practice. Postmenopausal hormone-replacement therapy. N Engl J Med 2001;345:34. [PMID: 11439947]

New England Journal of Medicine: http://content.nejm.org/cgi/reprint/NEJMp030038v1.pdf.

New England Journal of Medicine: http://content.nejm.org/cgi/reprint/NEJMoa030311v1.pdf.

C. Dehydroepiandrosterone

Dehydroepiandrosterone (DHEA) and its sulfated derivative, DHEAS, are synthesized by the adrenal cortex and are the most abundant steroid hormones in young adults. After age 30, serum levels of DHEA declines ~2% per year. As a result, in 80-year-olds, DHEA levels are 10–20% of levels in young adults. Low levels of DHEA have been correlated with an increased risk of breast cancer in premenopausal women, an increase in cardiovascular disease and mortality in elderly men, a lower bone mineral density in perimenopausal women, a higher likelihood of depressed mood in elderly women, and a higher likelihood of cognitive decline in both sexes.

Several short-term studies in older persons have supplemented DHEA levels to those seen in young adults with 50–100 mg/day doses (see Table 45–1). In women, DHEA supplementation led to an improved sense of well-being, increased bone mineral density, and, in women older than 70, increased sexual interest and satisfaction. In men, DHEA supplementation has led to improved well-being, increased strength, and decreased fat mass. In both sexes, DHEA supplementation improved skin thickness, hydration, sebum production, and pigmentation. Adverse effects on lipid profile and glycemic control were not seen.

In conclusion, short-term DHEA supplementation appears safe, but the effects have been modest. Routine supplementation is not recommended until long-term studies have demonstrated the safety and benefits of DHEA supplementation.

Gurnell EM, Chatterjee VK: Dehydroepiandrosterone replacement therapy. Eur J Endocrinol 2001;145:103. [PMID: 11454504]

D. Pregnenolone

Pregnenolone is the precursor of all steroid hormones. In the 1940s, pregnenolone was shown to increase attention and decrease arthritic pain. In mice, pregnenolone is the most potent known memory enhancer. However, pregnenolone fails to improve memory in humans, but it does enhance sleep in humans (see Table 45–1). Currently, there is no evidence to support the use of pregnenolone as an anti-aging hormone.

Vallee M et al: Role of pregnenolone, dehydroepiandrosterone and their sulfate esters on learning and memory in cognitive aging. Brain Res Brain Res Rev 2001;37:301. [PMID: 11744095]

COMPLEMENTARY & ALTERNATIVE MEDICINE

General Considerations

Complementary and alternative therapies have been defined as therapies that either fall outside of the conventional thought and approach to a given disease or that are not taught in U.S. medical schools or widely provided by U.S. hospitals. The National Center for Complementary and Alternative Medicine divides these therapies into 5 major domains.

1. Alternative medical systems, which consist of complete systems of theory and practice that are completely independent of a biomedical approach (eg, traditional oriental medicine, homeopathy, naturopathic medicine, and urvedic medicine).

2. Mind–body interventions, which target the potential for the mind to affect the body's basic function and reaction to disease (eg, meditation, prayer and mental healing, hypnosis).

3. Biological therapies, which consist of using herbs, dietary manipulation, supplements, or mixtures prepared from biological sources to enhance health or treat disease (eg, herbal remedies such as ginseng and ginkgo, supplements such as glucosamine or vitamin E, and mixtures such as shark cartilage).

4. Manipulative and body-based systems in which therapies such as massage, chiropractic manipulation, or osteopathic manipulation use a relationship between form and function to treat disease.

5. Energy therapies, which modify internal sources or flow of energy or alternately apply external sources of energy to modify body function or health (eg, use of magnets or electromagnetic fields, which involve external sources of energy, or the practice of Qi Gong or therapeutic touch,

which involve manipulating the internal balance or flow of energy).

Barrett B: Complementary and alternative medicine: what's it all about? West Med J 2001;100:20. [PMID: 11816777]

National Institutes of Health, National Center for Complementary and Alternative Medicine: http://nccam.nih.gov

Prevalence of Use

Among seniors, the most commonly used complementary and alternative therapies are chiropractic therapy, herbal remedies, relaxation techniques, and high dose or megavitamins.

Patients using complementary and alternative therapies often do not report their use to their physicians. Physicians should ask specifically whether patients are using them or seeing practitioners. Some therapies such as herbs may have side effects or may interact with conventional therapies. Asking about interest in and use of complementary and alternative therapies may also strengthen the physician–patient relationship and facilitate exploration of a patient's needs and expectations.

Eisenberg DM et al: Trends in alternative medicine use in the United States, 1990–1997: results of a follow-up national survey. JAMA 1998;280:1569. [PMID: 9820257]

Eisenberg DM et al: Perceptions about complementary therapies relative to conventional therapies among adults who use both: results from a national survey. Ann Intern Med 2001;135:344. [PMID: 11529698]

Foster DF et al: Alternative medicine use in older Americans. J Am Geriatr Soc 2000;48:1560. [PMID: 11129743]

Pappas S, Perlman A: Complementary and alternative medicine. The importance of doctor-patient communication. Med Clin North Am 2002;86:1. [PMID: 11795082]

Wolsko PM et al: Insurance coverage, medical conditions, and visits to alternative medicine providers: results of a national survey. Arch Intern Med 2002;162:281. [PMID: 11822920]

Legal Aspects of Use

Physicians looking to incorporate complementary and alternative therapies into their practice should consider the potential legal and malpractice implications, which may require consultation with legal or risk management experts.

Each state regulates the practice of medicine, allied health professions, and complementary and alternative therapy practitioners differently. Practitioners of complementary and alternative therapies may need to be formally licensed to be able to practice their discipline, may need to be certified not to practice but instead to use a specific title, or may need to register their name and location of practice with the state before opening a practice. Additionally, each state limits the scope of practice for practitioners. Usually, medical doctors are given unlimited authority to diagnose and treat medical illnesses. The scope of practice for complementary and alternative therapy providers is usually more limited. These limits can take the form of prohibitions against the practice of medicine or surgery or against the practice of services granted legally to other disciplines. For example, state statues may bar an acupuncturist from performing massage or providing psychological counseling because these abilities have been granted to licensed massage therapists and psychologists, respectively. Before contacting or referring patients, it is important that physicians learn about relevant state statutes to ensure that providers are appropriately licensed, certified, or registered and adhere to their appropriate scope of practice.

Malpractice consists of care that deviates from the current standard of care, lacks professional skill, and results in harm to a patient. Because all complementary and alternative therapies lie outside widely accepted conventional medical therapies, the integration of these therapies into medical practice could risk malpractice. Physicians can mitigate this risk by choosing therapies that have supporting data presented in peer-reviewed journals, especially mainstream medical journals, using therapies in an adjuvant manner along with traditional treatments for the same condition, initiating therapy only after obtaining informed consent from the patient wherein the patient has chosen to assume the risk of a given treatment, or using therapies only after standard treatments have failed or proved to be intolerable. Referring patients to practitioners of complementary and alternative therapies instead can also expose physicians to malpractice liability in a few specific situations. These situations include referring a patient for a condition for which a conventional therapy would be more appropriate, referring a patient to a provider whose record of lack of skill or judgment deems him or her a "known incompetent," or referring a patient to a practitioner who is connected to the physician within a joint practice, such as working for the same multispecialty practice, clinic, or health maintenance organization.

Cohen MH: Legal issues in complementary and integrative medicine. Med Clin North Am 2002;86:185. [PMID: 11799969]

Massage/Chiropractic

Massage therapy and chiropractic therapy are the most widely used complementary and alternative therapies in the United States. Swedish massage, the Trager method, and reflexology are the most commonly used types of massage. Swedish massage involves using smooth stroking and kneading movements often with the use of a massage oils. The Trager method involves holding the joints of the arms and legs in specific positions and gently rocking the joint. Reflexology is based on an alternate medical system in which parts of the body are represented by points on the feet, hands, and ears. Manipulation of these points transmits energy to the appropriate body part and can affect its function. Often massage therapy involves the use of multiple techniques tailored to a patient's symptoms.

Studies have consistently found benefit for massage therapy in the treatment of pain. Massage has been evaluated for the treatment of back pain, fibromyalgia, and headaches with positive results. Massage has also been found to be of benefit in the palliative care of terminal cancer pain. The improvements include decreases in pain, anxiety, and depression along with improved sleep. Massage has also been found to be a potentially helpful adjunct to conventional therapies for HIV and breast cancer. These studies looked at levels of anxiety and depression as well as markers of physiological stress such as cortisol and catecholamines. These later studies did not address clinical outcomes such as survival, alteration in responses to treatments, rates of hospitalization, or physical functioning. Hence, it is unclear whether these improvements have any impact on patients beyond improvements in psychological well-being.

Chiropractic medicine is a manipulation-based practice, which has spinal manipulation as the core clinical activity. Originally, chiropractic was envisioned to be an alternate medical system based on the tenet that neurological dysfunction at the spine was the cause of most disease and that spinal manipulation could correct the dysfunction. Over time, the field has moved away from this tenet and redefined its practice. Some within chiropractic have sought to incorporate other alternative therapies along with exercise, nutrition, and smoking cessation education to create a primary care practice. Others have viewed chiropractic as a limited medical specialty such as dentistry or podiatry. Most patients seem to view chiropractic in the latter sense as the vast majority of patients seek chiropractic care for back, neck, or head pain. Chiropractic treatment involves a history and physical exam, with the exam focusing on joint, muscle, and soft tissues. Plain x-ray films can also be an important part of the evaluation. On the basis of history, exam, and x-ray findings, the chiropractor determines whether the patient's condition will be amenable to chiropractic treatment and also plans a treatment regimen. Treatment involves spinal manipulation with or without adjunctive treatments such as heat, cold, electricity, and counseling about exercise, fitness, nutrition, weight loss, and relaxation techniques.

Chiropractic treatment has been studied for back and neck pain in > 50 individual studies. Several systematic reviews have found sufficient evidence to sup-port the beneficial use of chiropractic therapy for acute and chronic back pain but not for neck pain or sciatica. Chiropractic treatment has not been shown to be effective treatment of nonmusculoskeletal illnesses such as hypertension, dysmenorrhea, and asthma.

Common side effects of manipulation include localized pain, headache, and fatigue. More serious side effects include cauda equina syndrome from lumbar manipulation or stroke resulting from vertebral artery dissection have been reported. The risk of serious complications from lumbar manipulation have been estimated to be 1 in 100 million manipulations. The risk of stroke from cervical manipulation is low, but higher than lumbar manipulation, estimated at between 1 in 400,000 to 2 million manipulations.

Field T: Massage therapy. Med Clin North Am 2002;86:163. [PMID: 11795087]

Meeker WC, Haldeman S: Chiropractic: a profession at the crossroads of mainstream and alternative medicine. Ann Intern Med 2002;163:216. [PMID: 118277498]

Acupuncture

Acupuncture is a popular alternative therapy that involves the use of needles to stimulate points on the surface of the body. Acupuncture derives from an alternate medical system that holds that a vital energy called Qi circulates through the body along 12 pathways known as meridians. Alterations in the flow of Qi result in illness. Meridians have internal and surface projections, and stimulation of appropriate points on the surface restores the proper flow and restores health. Practitioners assess patients using either a more traditional Chinese medicine approach involving examination of the tongue, pulse, abdomen, and acupuncture points or a more Western approach involving a medical history and exam. From the evaluation, an acupuncture regimen is selected. Treatments consist of weekly to biweekly sessions involving the insertion of up to 15 needles at selected points for times ranging from several seconds to 30 min. The needles are solid disposable stainless steel and are ~37 gauge in size. Once inserted, the needles can be stimulated manually or with electricity, heat, or burning herbs.

Acupuncture has been shown to be efficacious in the treatment of postoperative and dental pain and for the management of nausea and vomiting resulting from a wide variety of causes. Acupuncture has also been used to treat chronic pain, osteoarthritis, headache, and back pain, but its efficacy in treating these conditions has not been established. A systematic review of the use of acupuncture in the treatment of chronic pain found insufficient evidence of benefit, and one randomized trial found acupuncture to have no benefit in the treatment of chronic back pain. Reviews of the evidence supporting the use of acupuncture for back pain have had conflicting results.

The 2 most common adverse effects are pain from needles and bleeding or hematoma. Other minor but common adverse effects are fatigue, nausea, and dizziness. The most serious, but rare, adverse events have been pneumothorax from needle insertion on the thorax and needle fracture requiring surgical removal. Patients should be cautioned to ensure that practitioners count needles before and after a session, use only new needles, and only insert needles to recumbent patients to minimize harm from fainting.

Cherkin DC et al: Randomized trial comparing traditional Chinese medical acupuncture, therapeutic massage, and self-care education for chronic low back pain. Arch Intern Med 2001; 161:1081. [PMID: 11322842]

Ernst E: Complementary therapies in palliative cancer care. Cancer 2001;91:2181. [PMID: 11777363]

Ernst E, White AR: Prospective studies of the safety of acupuncture: a systematic review. Am J Med 2001;110:481. [PMID: 11331060]

Ezzo J et al: Is acupuncture effective for the treatment of chronic pain? A systematic review. Pain 2000;86:217. [PMID: 10812251]

Kotani N et al: Preoperative intradermal acupuncture reduces postoperative pain, nausea and vomiting, analgesic requirement, and sympathoadrenal responses. Anesthesiology 2001;95: 349. [PMID: 11506105]

Herbs/Supplements

Herbs are the second most common complementary or alternative therapy used by older persons. In contrast to pharmaceuticals, the production, marketing, and sale of herbs and supplements is regulated only by the Dietary Supplement Health and Education Act, which does not regulate the purity, quality, or standardization of preparations. As a result, active ingredients can vary among manufacturers and even from lot to lot for a given manufacturer. Patients and physicians should select products made by larger, more reputable companies, which specify the amounts of ingredients and standardization of the active ingredients to an accepted standard.

Ernst E, Pittler MH: Herbal medicine. Med Clin North Am 2002; 86:149. [PMID: 10793599]

Massey PB: Dietary supplements. Med Clin North Am 2002; 86:127.

http://home.mdconsult.com/das/book/17756751/view/862 (Complete German Commission E Monograph on herbal medications.)

A. GINKGO

Ginkgo is the top-selling herbal medicine in the United States. The clinical use of ginkgo can be traced to Chinese medicine more than 2000 years ago. In Germany, a standardized ginkgo extract, Egb 761, has been approved for the treatment of intermittent claudication and cognitive impairment. Gingko extracts are prepared from ginkgo leaves and contain several active constituents, such as ginkgolides, bilobides, and flavone glycosides. Good-quality extracts contain 22–27% flavone glycosides and 5–7% terpin lactones, which include the ginkgolides and bilobides. The daily dosage used in clinical trials ranged from 120–320 mg/day; the most common dose is 40 mg 3 times/day (Table 45–2). Common side effects include headache, GI upset, and nausea, all of which are mild. There are also concerns about antiplatelet and warfarin-like effects, so patients should be cautioned about the potential for bleeding and gingko should be avoided in patients taking anticoagulants.

Ginkgo is clinically used for dementia, memory impairment, tinnitus, and intermittent claudication (see Table 45–2). A qualitative systemic review and a meta-analysis have addressed the effectiveness of ginkgo in the treatment of dementia and found positive results. The pooled effect size on cognitive function is comparable to that of donepezil. The pooled studies did not address whether ginkgo is useful in the treatment of other manifestations of dementia such as global functional status or problem behaviors. Ginkgo has also been studied for the treatment of memory impairment, or cerebral insufficiency. These terms encompass memory impairment associated with aging and probably clinically reflect mild cognitive impairment or age-related declines in memory. The studies of ginkgo for these indications are overall weak with regard to methodology, but a qualitative systemic review and a meta-analysis, including only the better studies, have found evidence of benefit. A qualitative systemic review of the studies examining the effectiveness of ginkgo for tinnitus found that only 1 of 5 studies used sound methodology. This study revealed that ginkgo produced a small but statistically significant reduction in the perception of tinnitus. Finally, a meta-analysis that included 8 randomized controlled trials of gingko for intermittent claudication found a statistically relevant increase in pain-free walking distance of 34 m compared with placebo. The results for gingko are similar to those for pentoxifylline but less than those seen with walking exercises. Hence, there is reasonable evidence to support the use of gingko for dementia or intermittent claudication and weaker evidence to support its use for memory impairment in nondemented patients and for tinnitus.

Ernst E: The risk-benefit profile of commonly used herbal therapies: ginkgo, St. John's wort, ginseng, Echinacea, saw palmetto, and kava. Ann Intern Med 2002;136:42. [PMID: 11777363]

Table 45–2. Herbal medicines: dose & use.

Herb/supplement	Dose	Use	Evidence
Gingko	40 mg tid	Dementia	++
		Cerebral/insufficiency	+
		Tinnitus	+
		Claudication	++
St. John's wort	300 mg tid	Depression	–
Glucosamine	1500–2000 mg qd or divided bid	OA	++
Chondroitin	1000–1500 mg qd or divided bid	OA	++
S-adenosyl methionine	1600 mg bid to qid	Depression	+
		OA	++
Saw palmetto	320 mg divided bid to tid	Benign prostatic hypertrophy	+/–
Shark cartilage	750 mg qd to 1 g/kg tid	Cancer treatment	–
		Cancer prevention	
Valerian root	300–900 mg 30–60 min before bedtime	Insomnia	+/–
Ginseng	200–600 mg qd or divided bid	Physical performance	+/–
		Psychomotor performance	+/–
		Immune system function	+/–
Garlic	600–900 mg qd	Hypercholesterolemia	+
		Hypertension	–
		Cancer prevention	+/–
Ginger	0.5–1.0 g qd	Vertigo	+
		Motion sickness	+
		Postoperative nausea	+/–
		OA	+

tid, 3 times/day; bid, 2 times/day; qd, every day; qid, 4 times/day; OA, osteoarthritis.

Massey PB: Dietary supplements. Med Clin North Am 2002;86: 127. [PMID: 11795085]

B. St. John' Wort

St. John's wort is widely used in Europe to treat depression. Preparations include both hypericin and hyperforin, which are believed to be at least 2 of the active ingredients. Good-quality extracts are usually standardized to a 0.3% hypericin content. St. John's wort is believed to work through selective inhibition of the reuptake of serotonin, dopamine, and norepinephrine in the brain. The dose used in most clinical trials is 900 mg/day (300 mg 3 times/day); effects take at least 2–3 weeks to appear (see Table 45–2). Side effects are mild; nausea, photosensitivity, and headache are most common. Given the role of serotonin, dopamine, and norepinephrine reuptake in the action of St. John's wort, patients should not take tricyclic antidepressants, SSRIs, or monoamine oxidase inhibitors while taking St. John's wort. St. John's wort activates P450 enzymes, so care should be used in treating patients also taking warfarin, digoxin, or other drugs with hepatic metabolism.

Several meta-analyses and qualitative systemic reviews have reported on the use of St. John's wort for either first-time or recurrent depression. These studies have found St. John's wort to be superior to placebo and comparable to tricyclic antidepressants. These studies also included 2 trials that compared St. John's wort with fluoxetine and sertraline and found roughly equal effectiveness. Early studies had substantial methodological flaws, however, and 2 multicenter randomized controlled trials found no effect of St. John's wort in patients with significant depression. Until more data are available, St. John's wort may be used cautiously in the treatment of mild depression but should not be used for moderate to severe depression, which should be treated with pharmacological or cognitive–behavioral interventions of proven efficacy (see Table 45–2).

Ernst E: The risk-benefit profile of commonly used herbal therapies: ginkgo, St. John's wort, ginseng, echinacea, saw palmetto, and kava. Ann Intern Med 2002;136:42. [PMID: 11777363]

Hypericum Depression Trial Study Group: Effect of Hypericum perforatum (St. John's wort) in major depressive disorder: a randomized controlled trial. JAMA 2002;287:1807. [PMID: 11939866]

Massey PB: Dietary supplements. Med Clin North Am 2002; 86:127. [PMID: 11795086]

Shelton RC et al: Effectiveness of St. John's wort in major depression: a randomized controlled trial. JAMA 2001;285:1978. [PMID: 11308434]

C. GLUCOSAMINE/CHONDROITIN

Glucosamine and chondroitin are commonly used for the treatment of osteoarthritis (see Table 45–2). Both glucosamine and chondroitin are components of proteoglycans found in articular cartilage and synovial fluid. How oral glucosamine or chondroitin work physiologically is not clear, and there is little evidence that patients with osteoarthritis are deficient in these substances or that oral glucosamine or chondroitin is selectively taken to joints. Glucosamine is usually taken at dosages of 1500–2000 mg/day every day or divided twice daily (see Table 45–2). Chondroitin sulfate is usually taken at 1000–1500 mg/day every day or divided twice daily. Combination pills containing both glucosamine and chondroitin are also available. Glucosamine alone tends to be most inexpensive of the preparations. Studies have found these substances to be very safe, with no more side effects than placebo.

Meta-analyses of early clinical trials of glucosamine and chondroitin have shown both to be superior to placebo in improving pain and disability (see Table 45–2). A randomized trial provides further evidence of efficacy: Patients with osteoarthritis of the knee who were treated with glucosamine and chondroitin had less pain, disability, and joint space narrowing after 3 years. Small studies have shown that glucosamine and chondroitin may also improve pain resulting from osteoarthritis of the TMJ. It is unknown whether glucosamine and chondroitin improve symptoms of osteoarthritis at other sites such as the hand or hip.

Ernst E: Complementary and alternative medicine for pain management in rheumatic disease. Curr Opin Rheumatol 2002; 14:58. [PMID: 11790998]

Reginster JY et al: Long-term effects of glucosamine sulphate on osteoarthritis progression: a randomised, placebo-controlled clinical trial. Lancet 2001;357:251. [PMID: 11214126]

Thie NM et al: Evaluation of glucosamine sulfate compared to ibuprofen for the treatment of temporomandibular joint osteoarthritis: a randomized double blind controlled 3 month clinical trial. J Rheumatol 2001;28:1347. [PMID: 11409130]

D. S-ADENOSYLMETHIONINE

S-adenosylmethionine (SAMe) is used to treat osteoarthritis and depression. The oral dose of SAMe is 400–1600 mg/day. Most studies use a 1600 mg dose divided 2–4 times daily (see Table 45–2). This dosage costs ≥ $120/mo. Side effects are rare and include mild GI upset, headache, dizziness, insomnia, hypersomnia, and anxiety. Mania has developed in some patients treated for depression.

In studies of patients with depression (see Table 45–2), SAMe consistently leads to significant but modest improvements compared with placebo. Studies

comparing SAMe and tricyclic antidepressants have found both to be roughly equivalent, although the doses of tricyclic antidepressant used or the follow-up period were often inadequate to see effects of the tricyclic agent. No studies compared SAMe with newer antidepressants such as SSRIs. More studies are needed before SAMe can be recommended for the treatment of moderate to severe depression.

In the treatment of osteoarthritis, SAMe is equivalent to NSAIDs in pain relief except that SAMe may require several weeks of treatment for full effect. SAMe has a lower incidence of side effects than NSAIDs, and patients rate its tolerability higher. SAMe has not been compared with acetaminophen in terms of pain control or side effects.

SAMe has also been studied for use in patients with cirrhosis or cholestasis and has proven beneficial. For example, in cirrhosis a significant decrease in death or need for a liver transplant was seen in patients with alcoholic cirrhosis treated for 2 years.

Echols JC et al: SAMe (S-adenosylmethionine). Harv Rev Psychiatry 2000;8:84. [PMID: 10902097]

Massey PB: Dietary supplements. Med Clin North Am 2002;86: 127. [PMID: 11795086]

E. SAW PALMETTO

Saw palmetto is made from the berries of the American dwarf palm and is commonly used to treat symptoms of benign prostatic hypertrophy (BPH). In western Europe, saw palmetto is used much more commonly than finasteride or α-blockers for BPH. Saw palmetto ingredients inhibit the 5α-reductase enzyme that converts testosterone to 5-dehydrotestosterone and may also inhibit prostaglandin synthesis and growth factor actions. Saw palmetto is usually given at a dose of 320 mg divided either 2 or 3 times daily (see Table 45–2). Side effects are infrequent and mild and include headache, diarrhea, constipation, nausea, and decreased libido.

Saw palmetto was superior to placebo in reducing nocturia and increasing peak urinary flow in 2 metaanalyses and was equivalent to finasteride in 1 (see Table 45–2). Its overall effect on BPH symptoms has not been determined, however, and its effects relative to α-blockers are unknown. Until more data are available, saw palmetto is appropriate for patients who prefer it to either α-blockers or finasteride.

Ernst E: The risk-benefit profile of commonly used herbal therapies: ginkgo, St. John's wort, ginseng, echinacea, saw palmetto, and kava. Ann Intern Med 2002;136:42. [PMID: 11777363]

Lowe FC: Phytotherapy in the management of benign prostatic hyperplasia. Urology 2001;58:71. [PMID: 11750257]

F. SHARK CARTILAGE

Shark cartilage is used as an anticancer supplement without compelling supporting evidence. Available preparations often contain capsules with 750 mg of shark cartilage powder with dosing ranging from 750 mg/day to 1 g/kg divided 3 times/day (see Table 45–2). A phase I/II study in patients with advanced cancer found no benefit for shark cartilage (1 g/kg divided 3 times/day) in survival and quality of life. Observed toxicity was low and limited mainly to mild GI upset, nausea, and constipation. Further trials are underway.

Ernst E, Cassileth BR: How useful are unconventional cancer treatments? Eur J Cancer 1999;35:1608. [PMID: 10673970]

Gonzalez RP et al: Shark cartilage as source of antiangiogenic compounds: from basic to clinical research. Biol Pharm Bull 2001;24:1097. [PMID: 11642310]

Hillman JD et al: Treatment of Kaposi sarcoma with oral administration of shark cartilage in a human herpesvirus 8-seropositive, human immunodeficiency virus-seronegative homosexual man. Arch Dermatol 2001;137:1149. [PMID: 11559209]

G. VALERIAN ROOT

Valerian root is often used as a sleep aid. The active ingredient is not known, but extracts bind directly to γ-aminobenzoic acid (GABA) receptors, enhance the release of GABA, and decrease the reuptake and degradation of GABA. Valerian root can either be consumed as a tea from 3–5 g of dried root with straining after 15 min of brewing or taken as commercial supplements that range in dose from 300–900 mg taken 30–60 min before bedtime (see Table 45–2). Side effects are infrequent and consist of dizziness, headache, and "hangover." Valerian root appears to have mild impacts on concentration, reaction time, motor skill, and vigilance 1 h after ingestion and essentially no impact the next day. However, the effect on these parameters in older patients is not known. Addiction to valerian root has not been described, but a case report of possible withdrawal symptoms after termination of chronic use, with successful treatment with midazolam, has been published.

The evidence that valerian root helps patients with insomnia is not compelling (see Table 45–2). Three of 9 studies of prolonged continuous use of valerian root showed a tendency toward benefit, but there were inconsistencies among studies. Maximum benefit may require 2–4 weeks of continued use. The 6 studies of intermittent dosing of valerian root were inconclusive.

Assemi M: Herbs affecting the central nervous system: gingko, kava, St. John's wort, and valerian. Clin Obstet Gynecol 2001;44:824. [PMID: 11600863]

Stevinson C, Ernst E: Valerian for insomnia: a systematic review of randomized clinical trials. Sleep Med 2000;1:91. [PMID: 10767649]

H. GINSENG

Ginseng is among the best selling herbal supplements. It is also one of the herbs with the most reported benefits, including central nervous system effects of increased vigilance, increased concentration, increased sense of well-being, and increased relaxation along with systemic anticancer, antidiabetic, and aphrodisiac effects. There are multiple types of ginseng, and most studies have used Asian ginseng, *Panax ginseng*. Ginseng is made from dried roots, and among the ingredients of ginseng extracts are > 25 different kinds of ginsenosides as well as panaxans. The usual dosage of ginseng is 200–600 mg of standardized extract either given every day or divided 2 times/day (see Table 45–2).

The incidence of side effects is low, but some can be serious, such as vaginal bleeding or Stevens-Johnson syndrome. Most side effects are less serious and include insomnia, diarrhea, euphoria, headache, mastalgia, and nausea. Interactions between ginseng and warfarin have been reported, so caution should be exercised. High doses of ginseng have also been shown to lower blood glucose levels, so patients should take ginseng with meals to minimize the risks of hypoglycemia. Ginseng abuse syndrome is believed to be due to contaminants in the preparation instead of ginseng itself.

There is insufficient evidence that ginseng improves physical performance, psychomotor performance, and immune function. One study attempted to determine the evidence for the multiple health claims made for ginseng (see Table 45–2). The review found significant methodological issues with most studies and possible publication bias.

Ernst E: The risk-benefit profile of commonly used herbal therapies: ginkgo, St. John's wort, ginseng, echinacea, saw palmetto, and kava. Ann Intern Med 2002;136:42. [PMID: 11777363]

Vogler BK et al: The efficacy of ginseng. A systematic review of randomized clinical trials. Eur J Clin Pharmacol 1999;55:567. [PMID: 10541774]

I. GARLIC

Garlic is widely advertised and used in the United States with the aims of lowering cholesterol and blood pressure and preventing cancer. The active ingredient is allicin, and most preparations are standardized to contain 0.6–1.3% allicin. The most widely studied form is the Kwai powder, which contains 1.3% allicin. Studies of this preparation have used doses of 600–900 mg/day (see Table 45–2). Side effects include odor, flatulence, diarrhea, and stomach upset. The most serious, although rare, side effect is increased bleeding, which may be due to reductions in platelet aggregation.

Garlic has been found to be superior to placebo in reducing total cholesterol but not blood pressure (see Table 45–2). The total reduction in cholesterol is 12–25 mg/dL at 3 mo, which is similar to the effect of dietary intervention and less than the effect of statins. None of the underlying studies lasted more than 10 mo, and 1 meta-analysis suggested that the benefit of garlic may not last beyond 6 mo.

Garlic was associated with reduced rates of stomach and colorectal cancer in cohort and case–control studies, but there are no randomized studies of garlic for these indications. The effect of garlic on cancer at other sites has not been studied sufficiently to support any conclusions.

Ackermann RT et al: Garlic shows promise for improving some cardiovascular risk factors. Arch Intern Med 2001;161:813. [PMID: 11268223]

Fleischauer AT, Arab L: Garlic and cancer: a critical review of the epidemiologic literature. J Nutr 2001;131:1032S. [PMID: 11238811]

Stevinson C et al: Garlic for treating hypercholesterolemia. A meta-analysis of randomized clinical trials. Ann Intern Med 2000; 133:420. [PMID: 10975959]

J. GINGER

Ginger has been used in Chinese and Ayurvedic medicine for > 2500 years for the treatment of musculoskeletal pain and GI illnesses. Ginger is prepared from the root of plants in the Zingiberaceae family, which includes the genera *Zingiber* and *Alpinia.* Most studies have used extracts from *Zingiber officinale,* but it is unclear whether extracts from ginger plants in other genera and species would have similar effects. Ginger can be given as powdered root, 0.5–1 g/day (see Table 45–2). Alternately, extracts made from *Zingiber* and *Alpinia* roots are also available, and these have been used 2–3 times/day. Side effects are mild; dyspepsia, heartburn, and nausea are most common.

Ginger has been studied for the prevention of postoperative nausea and motion sickness and the treatment of vertigo and osteoarthritis pain (see Table 45–2). Studies of ginger in the prevention of postoperative nausea have produced mixed results. Small studies found ginger to be effective in reducing vertigo from caloric stimulation and preventing vomiting and sweating from sea sickness. The study of sea sickness found nonstatistically significant reductions in nausea and vertigo as well. Two studies evaluated ginger for the treatment of osteoarthritis pain; the 3-week study found mild to no effect, whereas the 6-week study found significant improvement in pain with more improvement from weeks 2–6 than weeks 0–2. Hence, the effect of ginger on osteoarthritis pain may require several weeks to appear.

Altman RD, Marcussen KC: Effects of a ginger extract on knee pain in patients with osteoarthritis. Arthritis Rheum 2001; 44:2531. [PMID: 11710709]

Bliddal H et al: A randomized, placebo-controlled, cross-over study of ginger extracts and ibuprofen in osteoarthritis. Osteoarthr Cartil 2000;8:9. [PMID: 10607493]

Ernst E, Pittler MH: Efficacy of ginger for nausea and vomiting: a systematic review of randomized clinical trials. Br J Anaesth 2000;84:367. [PMID: 10793599]

Homeopathy

Homeopathy is an alternative medical system based on the vitalistic theory that illness results from imbalances in the patient's vital force. The goal of homeopathy is to use medications to restore the balance and then to rely on the self-healing potential of the body to lead to a cure. The practice relies on 2 tenets: the principle of similars and the principle of dilution. The principle of similars suggests that an effective treatment can come from a diluted form of a substance that causes similar symptoms in a healthy person. The principle of dilution holds that high dilutions of these substances are equally or more effective than more concentrated solutions. Although this latter principle draws most skepticism, it is important to note that most homeopathic remedies are not infinite dilutions but instead contain small but measurable amounts of the active ingredients. A practitioner selects a remedy, after a thorough history and physical exam, by matching symptoms and findings to remedies.

Homeopathic remedies have been shown to be effective. However, studies have been limited by methodological flaws and publication bias. In particular, the studies of better methodological quality were more likely to report negative results. Until rigorous studies have validated the use of specific remedies, it would be prudent to approach their use with caution.

Cucherat M et al: Evidence of clinical efficacy of homeopathy. A meta-analysis of clinical trials. Eur J Clin Pharmacol 2000; 56:27. [PMID: 10853874]

Merrel WC, Shalts E: Homeopathy. Med Clin North Am 2002; 86:47. [PMID: 11795090]

Aromatherapy

The practice of aromatherapy consists of using volatile essential oils extracted from plants for therapeutic benefit. Essential oils can be topically applied, aerosolized, or used in massage.

Aromatherapy partially relieves anxiety, and the favorable side effect profile makes aromatherapy a useful adjunctive therapy. The aerosolized and massage use of essential oils has been best studied with respect to calming and anxiolytic effects. A systematic review found evidence to support a mild anxiolytic effect of essential oils when combined with massage. Essential oils combined with massage have been tried in terminal cancer patients receiving palliative care and hospitalized dementia patients. In cancer patients, aromatherapy massage using Roman chamomile resulted in decreased anxiety and improvements in physical and psychological symptoms as well as quality of life. Topical use of essential oils can also be directed at the treatment of a given skin condition, and tea tree oil has been shown to have benefits in the treatment of acne and onychomycosis. A study of dementia patients found essentially no benefit of massage with essential oils. The side effects related to aromatherapy are low and are almost exclusively limited to either topical or massage use. These side effects include allergic reactions and photosensitivity.

Cooke B, Ernst E: Aromatherapy: a systematic review. Br J Gen Pract 2000;50:493. [PMID: 10962794]

Smallwood J et al: Aromatherapy and behaviour disturbances in dementia: a randomized controlled trial. Int J Geriatr Psychiatry 2001;16:1010. [PMID: 11607948]

Common Legal & Ethical Issues

46

Marshall B. Kapp, JD, MPH, FCLM

Many aspects of the medical care of patients throughout the age spectrum raise important legal and ethical issues. However, a variety of legal and ethical questions are either uniquely relevant to geriatric practice or take on added significance and special nuances when applied to the treatment of older individuals. Legally and ethically pertinent characteristics of older individuals include their greater likelihood to have impaired cognitive capacity, closer chronological proximity to critical illness and death, higher prevalence of serious and multiple chronic diseases and disabilities requiring long-term care, particular family dynamics, a more urgent need to engage in various aspects of life planning, and extensive reliance on public financing for their medical care.

INFORMED MEDICAL DECISION MAKING

Diagnostic & Treatment Interventions: Informed Consent

Under the ethical principle of autonomy or self-determination, every adult patient (with no upper age limit) has the right to make personal decisions regarding medical care, including decisions about which diagnostic and treatment interventions to undergo. This ethical principle has been translated into the legal doctrine of informed consent.

Although the patient has the right to decline a particular suggested diagnostic or therapeutic intervention, the principle of autonomy does not establish a right to demand tests or treatments that the physician believes would be worthless or even harmful to the patient. The clash between patient desires for aggressive medical intervention and medical skepticism about the value of such intervention has arisen most vividly in the context of futile life-sustaining medical treatments. There is broad consensus that physicians are under no ethical or legal obligation to provide, and indeed should not provide, futile or nonbeneficial treatment to a patient. However, enormous controversy continues about how one can reliably and fairly determine whether a particular intervention would be futile—physiologically, quantitatively, or qualitatively—for a specific patient.

In order for a patient's choice about any specific medical intervention to be considered an ethically and legally valid exercise of informed consent, 3 elements must be present. First, the patient's participation in the decision-making process and the ultimate decision must be voluntary (ie, free of force, fraud, duress, intimidation, or any other form of undue constraint or coercion).

Second, the patient's choice must be adequately knowing or informed. The physician must communicate in understandable lay terms material information about the patient's situation (ie, information that might make a difference in how an ordinary, reasonable patient would think about the choices involved). Particular pieces of data that should be shared with the patient include the diagnosis, nature, and purpose of the proposed interventions; reasonably foreseeable risks; probability of success; viable alternatives and their anticipated benefits and risks; the result expected without the intervention; and advice (ie, the physician's recommendation).

Third, valid decisions require a capable decision maker. A patient must be cognitively and emotionally able to weigh alternatives rationally. Our culture starts with a legal and ethical presumption that every adult is sufficiently capable of making his or her own medical decisions. For some geriatric patients, however, this aspect of medical decision making may be problematic. When a patient lacks adequate capacity, someone else must act as decision maker on the patient's behalf; the subject of surrogate decision making is discussed later.

A determination of one's mental competence technically is a legal matter resolvable only by a court and carrying clear legal consequences. As a practical matter, however, formal judicial proceedings for this purpose are rare. Most of the time, the attending physician, in collaboration with other members of the health care team, makes clinical, working, de facto judgments about a patient's present decisional capacity.

There exists no single, uniform, scientific standard of legal competence/decisional capacity. Questions that should be included in the physician's inquiry about a patient's capacity are as follows:

1. Can the person make and communicate (verbally or otherwise) any choices regarding medical interventions?

2. Can the person express any reasons for the choices made (to indicate that some reasoning process is taking place)?

3. Are the stated or apparent reasons underlying the person's choices rational in the sense that the person starts with a factually accurate understanding of the medical situation and can reason logically to a conclusion?

4. Does the person understand or appreciate the implications, including the likely personal risks and benefits, of the alternatives presented and choices made?

Several considerations should guide the physician's assessment of a patient's decisional capacity. Foremost, capacity is a matter of whether the patient has a minimal degree of functional ability, regardless of the clinical diagnosis or whether the physician personally agrees with the patient's decision. Capacity needs to be determined on a decision-specific basis. A patient may be capable of rationally making certain kinds of decisions but not others. How much intellectual and emotional capacity is necessary depends on the difficulty and seriousness of the decision being faced. Partial or limited capacity is not synonymous with incapacity. The patient may be capable enough to make the specific decision in question.

Decisional capacity is variable, rather than steady state, in many older patients. It may wax and wane in particular cases depending on environmental factors, such as time of day (eg, sundowning), day of the week, physical setting, presence of acute or transient medical problems, other persons involved in supporting or pressuring the patient's decision, or reactions to medications. Physicians often can affect patients' capacity—for better or worse—through their care (eg, choice and timing of medications). Physicians should try to communicate with patients about their care as much as possible during the patient's windows of lucidity.

Additionally, many older persons may be capable of assisted consent with extra time and effort on the physician's part, especially if a person has supportive family or friends available. For instance, an older patient who cannot process information as swiftly as a younger person may be able to understand the complexities of a proposed test or treatment if afforded enough time and emotional support.

Surrogate Decision Making

When a patient is determined to lack present decisional capacity, decisions must be made for that patient by a surrogate or proxy. One may obtain formal legal authority to act as a surrogate for medical decision-making purposes either through a judicial guardianship order or the patient's having executed in a timely fashion a durable power of attorney (DPOA).

A. GUARDIANSHIP

Creation of a guardianship or conservatorship (precise terminology varies among jurisdictions) is the chief means of transferring decision making to a surrogate without the patient's permission. This entails appointment by a state court (in most jurisdictions, the probate division) of a surrogate (the guardian or conservator), who is empowered to make certain decisions on behalf of an incompetent person (the ward). Ordinarily, this occurs in response to a petition filed by the family, a health care facility, or the local adult protective services (APS) agency. The legal proceeding involves review by the court of the sworn affidavit or live testimony of a physician who has examined the alleged incompetent person. Most courts prefer to appoint a relative of the ward to act as guardian; in the absence of a family member who is willing and able to act in that role, however, a court may appoint someone else (eg, a close friend) or a public guardian or volunteer guardianship program if those options are locally available.

Because creating total, or plenary, guardianship usually entails an extensive deprivation of an individual's basic personal and property rights, the least restrictive/least intrusive alternative doctrine makes limited or partial guardianship preferred. In every jurisdiction, courts possess the statutory authority to limit the surrogate's power in terms of duration and types of decisions covered.

The modern trend in surrogate decision making has been toward the substituted judgment standard. Under this approach, the guardian is required to make the same decisions that the patient would make, according to the patient's own preferences and values to the extent they can be ascertained, if the patient were able to make and express competent decisions. The substituted judgment standard is highly consistent with respect for patient autonomy. When it cannot reasonably be ascertained what the patient would have decided if competent, the guardian is expected to rely on the traditional best interests standard. That test mandates that decisions be made in a manner that, from the guardian's perspective, would confer the most benefit and the least burden on the ward.

B. DURABLE POWER OF ATTORNEY

A person may take steps while still decisionally capable to anticipate and prepare for eventual incapacity by voluntarily delegating or directing future medical decision-making power. The DPOA is a legal document, explicitly authorized by state statute, in which a competent individual (the principal) directs, through the appointment of an agent (the attorney in fact, who need not be an attorney at law), the making of medical decisions in the event of future incapacity. The principal may give the agent general or specific instructions to direct future decision making or may make the grant of authority unrestricted. The DPOA is distinguishable from the regular or ordinary power of attorney, which ordinarily is used to delegate power to make arrangements and take actions regarding financial or property affairs.

DPOAs fall into 2 categories. An immediate DPOA comes into effect immediately on the naming of an agent. In a springing DPOA, the legal authority is transferred ("springs") from the patient to the agent only when some specified future event (such as confirmation of the principal's incapacity by an examining physician) has occurred.

Medical Decision Making for the Critically Ill

Rapidly unfolding advances in medical technology create exciting new opportunities for the successful medical treatment of critically ill patients. However, it frequently is impossible to predict accurately whether a particular intervention will benefit a particular patient at a particular point in time. Complex dilemmas regarding if, when, and for how long various life-sustaining medical treatments (LSMT) ought to be introduced or continued in specific situations carry perplexing ethical and legal ramifications.

Under both common law and constitutional interpretation, *Cruzan v. Director, Missouri Department of Health,* 110 S. Ct. 2841 (1990), a competent adult patient's right to make informed, voluntary medical choices encompasses the right to permit or refuse particular LSMT (including artificial nutrition and hydration). If the patient has been formally adjudicated incompetent, the court-appointed guardian acts as the decision maker regarding the initiation, continuation, withholding, or withdrawal of LSMT. When no guardian has been appointed, LSMT choices for a decisionally incapacitated patient devolve to the agent named in a DPOA instrument, if one was executed while the patient was still capable of doing so.

A. Advance Directives & Oral Statements

When neither a guardianship nor a DPOA exist for a patient who cannot speak autonomously for him- or herself, guidance may be available through an instruction advance directive. Statutes (variously called natural death, death with dignity, or right to die legislation) that authorize capable adults to execute written declarations or living wills have been enacted in 48 states. These statutes create a mechanism for capable adults to

anticipate future scenarios and instruct their physicians prospectively regarding the use of LSMT. Legal immunity against any form of liability or professional discipline is provided to caregivers who comply with a valid living will, and a physician who chooses for reasons of personal conscience not to comply with the patient's instructions may not interfere with the patient's transfer to a different physician.

A patient's conversations with relatives, friends, and health care providers constitute the most common form of advance directive. Oral statements should be thoroughly documented in the medical record by physicians and other members of the health care team for later reference. Properly verified oral statements carry the same ethical and legal weight as formal written directives, although most physicians feel more confident psychologically in relying on the latter. Physicians and other health professionals should encourage persons who presently have capacity to document their preferences regarding future medical treatment in the form of a written instruction directive or DPOA.

B. Patient Self-Determination Act

The Patient Self-Determination Act (PSDA) of 1990 (Public Law No. 101-508, §§ 4206 and 4751) imposes specific requirements on all hospitals, nursing homes, health maintenance organizations, preferred provider organizations, hospices, and home health agencies that participate in the Medicare and Medicaid programs. Among these mandates are the following:

- The provider develop and disseminate to new patients or their surrogates a written policy on advance directives, consistent with applicable state law.

- The provider inquire at the time of admission or enrollment whether the patient has executed an advance directive.

- If no advance directive has been executed previously and the patient currently retains decisional capacity, the provider give the patient an opportunity to execute an advance directive at that time.

However, the PSDA forbids any provider from requiring a patient to execute an advance directive as a condition of receiving care from that provider. Although the PSDA does not apply expressly to physicians' offices, it in no way precludes discussions from taking place in the primary care setting about patient preferences regarding future medical treatment.

C. Informal Family Decision Making

In the absence of judicial appointment of a guardian or the patient's formal designation of an agent, the long-standing medical custom has been for physicians to turn to family members as surrogate decision makers for incapacitated patients. This practice has been codified in > 30 states by enactment of family consent statutes that expressly authorize specific relatives, in an enumerated priority order, to make particular decisions for their incapacitated family members. This well-established custom and statutory codification are based on the assumption that family members generally know best the basic values and preferences of their relatives (thereby accomplishing substituted judgment) or, at the least, will act as trustworthy advocates for their relatives' best interests. However, health professionals must be alert to possible serious conflicts of interest that can render a relative inappropriate to act as a surrogate decision maker for the patient.

D. "Do Not" Orders

In the critical care context, a physician may issue several kinds of "do not" orders. "Do not" orders are predicated on prospectively made decisions to forgo certain types of LSMT for certain patients under specified circumstances. Most attention has been devoted to "do not resuscitate" (DNR) orders ("no codes") or instructions by the physician to refrain from attempts at cardiopulmonary resuscitation in the event of a cardiac arrest. However, other kinds of prospective orders also may be important, especially within the long-term care environment, such as "do not hospitalize" and "do not treat" orders.

"Do not" orders should be handled according to the same substantive ethical and legal principles and procedural guidelines that apply to other treatment decisions. A capable adult patient has the same right to agree to a "do not" order as to make any other decision about the use of LSMT. For the incapacitated patient, prospective clarification of the medical situation may be available from the patient's previously executed living will or the current instructions of a surrogate. Even without an advance directive, "do not" orders still are permissible for incapacitated patients according to the same general precepts governing other kinds of decisions about LSMT. By allowing and encouraging certain decisions to be made prospectively before a crisis develops, "do not" orders may reduce potential legal risk and should curtail physicians' legal anxieties.

E. Physician-Assisted Death

Forgoing unwanted or disproportionately burdensome LSMT, even when the patient's death is the natural and expected result, is permissible in the United States as an exercise of passive euthanasia in appropriate circumstances. However, affirmative interventions, such as lethal injections, performed for the purpose of hastening a patient's death constitute active euthanasia, which is considered a criminal act of homicide and is opposed by most people on ethical grounds as well.

In contrast to passive or active euthanasia, assisted suicide involves the physician supplying, at the patient's request, the means to actively accelerate the patient's death (eg, a potentially fatal amount of a drug), with the expectation and intention that the patient will use the means so supplied for that purpose. In 1997, the U.S. Supreme Court held that there is no constitutional right entitling people to secure a physician's help to actively hasten their own deaths and that states may continue to criminalize such help by a physician, *Washington v. Glucksberg*, 117 S.Ct. 2302 and *Vacco v. Quill*, 117 S.Ct. 2293. The Court left open the possibility that individual states could decriminalize physician-assisted suicide if they choose to do so. Thus far, only Oregon has exercised its prerogative to do so (by voter referendum).

F. Institutional Ethics Committees

Standards of the Joint Commission on Accreditation of Healthcare Organizations (JCAHO) require that hospitals have a mechanism in place for resolving ethical disputes about patient care. Many, although certainly not all, of those ethical disputes involve disagreements about the use or abatement of LSMT for a particular patient. One mechanism for addressing such disputes is the institutional ethics committee (IEC), variants of which have now been established in many hospitals as well as nursing homes, hospices, and home health agencies. The IEC is an internal, interdisciplinary structure set up to help a facility or agency and its professional staff deal with difficult treatment decisions in an ethically acceptable way.

IECs vary from among institutions or agencies in terms of exact size, composition, structure, processes, activities, and place within the organizational bureaucracy. IECs may be involved in such functions as drafting organizational policies, education of staff and the public, and case consultation on a concurrent or retrospective basis. The involvement of an IEC in a particular case probably has positive legal benefits for the provider organization and its staff in terms of reducing unnecessary guardianship petitions, deterring possible lawsuits against the institution or agency and its staff, and evidencing good faith to bolster the providers' defense against any rare malpractice case that might be brought in this context.

Informed Consent in the Research Context

Whether older individuals, particularly those with cognitive impairment, should be enrolled as participants in biomedical, behavioral, and health services research protocols raises a host of ethical and legal concerns. The issues are particularly pointed when the proposed human participants (until recently usually referred to as subjects) are institutionalized as well as significantly mentally compromised.

Most (but not all) research conducted in the United States is regulated by federal law intended to safeguard the rights and welfare of potential human participants, 45 Code of Federal Regulations Part 46. The Office of Human Research Protection (OHRP) within the Department of Health and Human Services (DHHS) has the authority to suspend an institution's research activities involving human participants for deviation from applicable regulations and has exercised that authority at a number of renowned medical centers in recent years.

No particular legal restrictions apply exclusively to older research participants; therefore, participation by older persons in research protocols occurs under the same legal framework that governs research volunteers of all ages. For decisionally incapacitated individuals, permission for research participation may be obtained from those persons who are authorized to make other kinds of decisions on the older person's behalf. Federal regulations allude to the use of a legally authorized representative under applicable state law for making decisions about participation in research activities.

However, a 1998 report by the National Bioethics Advisory Commission (NBAC) included several recommendations for explicitly protecting potential human research participants (across the age span) who have impaired capacity to personally consent to or refuse their own research participation. Among the other recommendations that NBAC called for were the following:

- Institutional review board (IRB) membership should include at least 2 persons familiar with mental disorders.
- A special standing panel of DHHS (a "super" IRB) should be created to deal with particularly ethically vexing research protocols.
- Research using mentally compromised subjects should be permitted only if the research could not be conducted using mentally healthy volunteers instead.
- For protocols exposing participants to greater than minimal risk, there should be an independent assessment of a potential participant's capacity, and the protocol must detail the process of assessing decisional capacity in each potential participant.

None of these recommendations has been enacted into law yet.

ADULT PROTECTIVE SERVICES

Components

On the basis of their *parens patriae* power to protect those who cannot protect themselves, the states have created a wide variety of programs under the general heading of APS programs. The basic definition of this concept is a system of preventive and supportive services for older persons living in the community to enable them to remain as independent as possible while avoiding abuse and exploitation by others. Good APS programs are characterized by the coordinated delivery of services to adults at risk and the actual or potential authority to provide surrogate decision making regarding those services.

The services ordinarily consist of an assortment of health, housing, and social interventions. Ideally, these services are coordinated by a caseworker/organizer (variously termed a case manager, care manager, or care coordinator), who is responsible for assessing an individual's needs and bringing together the available resources.

The second component of an APS system is authority to intervene on behalf of the person needing help. Ordinarily, that person (if mentally able) will voluntarily grant the helping agency permission to deliver services. However, if that person declines offered assistance despite needing it, the APS agency may turn to the legal system to authorize appointment of a surrogate decision maker over the person's protests. Some states deal with unwilling service recipients through the traditional methods of involuntary commitment or guardianship. Legislation has been enacted in many jurisdictions, however, that creates special procedures to obtain court orders to impose various aspects of APS whether or not the individual wants those services. These legal procedures are either in addition to or in place of the existing guardianship system. Before a court may order APS interventions over a person's objections, that person is entitled to certain due process protections such as notice and a hearing at which there is a right to be represented by legal counsel, present evidence, and examine and cross-examine witnesses.

Physician's Role in Abuse & Neglect Identification, Reporting, & Intervention

In the context of APS, physicians frequently are called on to contribute their expertise and skills in identifying appropriate candidates for services, providing evidence if guardianship or commitment litigation occurs, exploring voluntary alternatives, and service planning and patient placement. Physicians often are in a unique position to identify initially those individuals who satisfy the eligibility criteria for, and could significantly benefit from, the involvement of an APS agency. Notifying a designated APS agency about the existence and identity of such patients is required of the physician in the almost 45 states with mandatory reporting statutes for suspected adult abuse and neglect. Even in the handful of states without mandatory reporting laws, physicians making good faith voluntary reports to APS are immune from any legal liability associated with that reporting.

The definition of elder abuse and neglect is a matter of state law. Each state has enacted its own statutory schema in this sphere, resulting in substantial variation among particular definitions and procedures. The American Medical Association (AMA) has defined elder abuse and neglect as "actions or the omissions of actions that result in harm or threatened harm to the health or welfare of the elderly." These actions or inactions may occur in the older person's home or that of a relative, at the hands of an informal caregiver, or within institutional walls. A single incident may constitute abuse or neglect in most states, but more commonly a repeated pattern is documented, and in some jurisdictions is essential, to satisfy statutory definitions of abuse and neglect. Elder mistreatment may take several forms: physical (eg, assault, forced sexual contact, excessive drug administration, inappropriate imposition of physical restraints); psychological or emotional (eg, threats); denial of basic human needs by the caregiver (eg, withholding needed medical care or food); deprivation of civil rights (eg, freedom of movement and communication); and financial exploitation.

A significant proportion (over half in some states) of reported cases of elder mistreatment fall into the category of self-neglect by older persons living alone, without any informal (ie, unpaid family or friends) or formal (ie, paid) caregivers. Examples of self-neglect include an individual's failure to maintain sufficient nutrition, hydration, or hygiene; failure to use necessary physical aids such as eyeglasses, hearing aids, or false teeth; or failure to maintain a safe environment for him- or herself. Self-neglect may be suspected in the presence of dehydration, malnourishment, decubitus ulcers, poor personal hygiene, or lack of compliance with basic medical recommendations.

Some states have enacted distinct statutes dealing with cases of institutional abuse and neglect of older residents. These statutes may apply to nursing facilities, board and care homes, and assisted-living arrangements. Even if a state does not have such precisely focused legislation, resident mistreatment by long-term care facility staff is prohibited by federal regulations (for nursing facilities) and by state institutional licensure statutes and common law tort standards of care. There are significant legal restrictions on the misuse of involuntary physical and chemical restraints. Also, several states lump together institutional and informal caregiver mistreatment in the same statutes rather than legislatively handling them distinctly.

Patients are entitled to receive reasonable continuity of care from their physicians. If an older person changes placement (eg, moves from a private home to an assisted-living complex or a nursing facility), whether voluntarily or involuntarily, the principle of nonabandonment legally obligates the physician to facilitate continuity of medical care by continuing to treat the patient personally or referring him or her to another competent, willing physician whose services are acceptable to the patient.

CONFIDENTIALITY

General Obligations

As a general ethical and legal precept, health care and human services professionals have a duty to hold in confidence all personal patient information entrusted to them. The patient has a right to expect the fulfillment of that duty. The obligation of confidentiality is reinforced by the AMA's Principles of Medical Ethics as well as the ethical codes of all other health professional organizations.

Most state professional practice (ie, licensing) acts impose an explicit duty of confidentiality. Voluntary, private accrediting bodies, such as JCAHO and the National Committee for Quality Assurance, impose strict standards on accredited service providers regarding the protection of patient privacy. Additionally, courts have allowed patients to impose civil liability on health and human service professionals for violating their duty of confidentiality. Some courts have held that the professional's obligation to maintain confidences is legally enforceable against employees of that professional under the legal principle of *respondeat superior* (literally, "let the master answer").

The Health Insurance Portability and Accountability Act, Public Law No. 104-191 (HIPAA), required DHHS to promulgate rules governing the protection of individually identifiable health information in any form or media including electronic, paper, and oral. In response to this requirement, DHHS issued regulatory Standards for Privacy of Individually Identifiable Health Information (Privacy Rule), which became effective April 2001 with final modifications published August 2002. The Privacy Rule applies to all healthcare settings, providers, and health plans as well as other "covered entities" as defined by DHHS.

U.S. Department of Health and Human Services, Office for Civil Rights: www.hhs.gov/ocr/hipaa

Exceptions to the Duty

The physician's obligation to maintain confidentiality of the patient's disclosures and records is not absolute. There are a variety of circumstances in which the physician is permitted, or even required, to reveal what would otherwise be confidential information about a patient.

First, because it is the patient who owns the right of confidentiality, he or she may waive, or give up, that right as long as this is done in a voluntary, competent, and informed manner. This happens routinely, for example, when the patient authorizes release of personal information to third-party payers or auditors of treatment. Second, the expectation of confidentiality must yield when the physician is mandated or permitted by state law to report to specified public health authorities the existence of certain enumerated conditions known or reasonably suspected in their patients. Such provisions are based on the state's inherent police power to protect and promote the health, safety, and welfare of society as a whole. This rationale would support, for instance, reporting requirements concerning infectious diseases, gunshot wounds, or vital statistics (such as death). Alternatively to the police power, reporting of certain conditions may be mandated or allowed under the state's *parens patriae* power to beneficently protect those individuals who are unable or unwilling to care for their own needs. Mandatory and permissive reporting of elder abuse and neglect was mentioned previously in the context of protective services. Even absent a specific statute or regulation on point, the courts may impose a common law requirement or recognize a common law right for a physician to violate a patient's confidentiality to protect innocent third parties from harm. In most jurisdictions, for instance, a physician is expected to report to the potential victim or to law enforcement officials any express threat made by a dangerously mentally ill patient.

Further, when information is requested about a patient in the context of litigation, ordinarily the physician is precluded from providing that information because specific state statutes create a testimonial privilege between a patient and physicians with whom that patient has formed a professional relationship. However, the physician may be allowed or even compelled to reveal otherwise privileged information when the patient consents to or requests such release. Revelation also may be required by the force of legal process (ie, by a judge's order requiring such information to be released). This may occur when the patient has placed issues pertaining to his or her medical care in issue in the litigation (eg, when the patient is seeking monetary damages for personal injuries), when the communication to the physician was made in the presence of a third party (and, therefore, done without a reasonable expectation of privacy), or the public welfare need for the information outweighs the individual's right to confidentiality in the particular case.

In understanding the ramifications of legal process, it is crucial to distinguish between a subpoena and a court order. A subpoena is a directive from the clerk (administrator) of a court, issued at the request of an attorney in the case, instructing an individual to appear at a specific time and place for the purpose of giving sworn testimony. A subpoena *duces tecum* directs one to bring certain identified tangible items, such as medical records, at the time of testimony. A subpoena may not be ignored, but it may be challenged legally. The court may quash the subpoena if it runs afoul of an applicable testimonial privilege statute. The physician is obligated to comply only if the judge rejects the challenge to a subpoena and orders disclosure over the patient's objection or the patient has been notified about the subpoena and declines to challenge it. Noncompliance with a judge's order constitutes contempt of court and is criminally and civilly punishable.

Impaired Drivers & the Physician

A number of states, either by statute or regulation or as a matter of common law, have addressed the reporting obligations of a physician when a patient's driving abilities have become impaired by age-related neurodegenerative illnesses or sensory impairment. Some states (eg, California) expressly mandate physicians to report to drivers' licensing authorities a medical condition that might be hazardous to driving. Violation of a mandatory reporting requirement may lead to professional discipline. In some cases, it also may give rise to physician liability for injuries to third parties caused by the dangerous driver. However, a physician's failure to obey a mandatory reporting statute will not always make that physician civilly responsible for injuries suffered by a third party when the reporting statute is silent on this point. Even when there is no mandatory reporting statute in their jurisdiction, some physicians have been held civilly liable under a common law negligence theory when they should have foreseen a patient's dangerous driving but did nothing effective to prevent it and the driver then harmed an innocent third party in a motor vehicle accident. Other cases, however, have declined to impose civil liability in such circumstances, finding that the responsibility for safe driving rests exclusively on the driver's shoulders.

The AMA's Code of Medical Ethics §2,24, Impaired Drivers and Their Physicians, provides the following:

1. Physicians should assess patients' physical or mental impairments that might adversely affect driving abilities. Each case must be evaluated individually because not all impairments may give rise to an obligation on the part of the physician. Nor may all physicians be in a position to evaluate the extent or the effect of an impairment (eg, physi-

cians who treat patients on a short-term basis). In making evaluations, physicians should consider the following factors:

- The physician must be able to identify and document physical or mental impairments that clearly relate to the ability to drive.
- The driver must pose a clear risk to public safety.

2. Before reporting (to the state Department of Motor Vehicles), there are a number of initial steps physicians should take. A tactful but candid discussion with the patient and family about the risks of driving is of primary importance. Depending on the patient's medical condition, the physician may suggest that the patient seek further treatment, such as substance abuse treatment or occupational therapy. Physicians also may encourage the patient and family to decide on a restricted driving schedule. Efforts made by physicians to inform patients and their families, advise them of their options, and negotiate a workable plan may render reporting unnecessary.

3. Physicians should use their best judgment when determining when to report impairments that could limit a patient's ability to drive safely. When clear evidence of substantial driving impairment implies a strong threat to patient and public safety, and when the physician's advice to discontinue driving privileges is ignored, it is desirable and ethical to notify the state Department of Motor Vehicles.

4. The physician's role is to report medical conditions that would impair safe driving as dictated by state mandatory reporting laws and standards of medical practice. The determination of the inability to drive safely should be made by the state Department of Motor Vehicles.

5. Physicians should disclose and explain to their patients this responsibility to report.

6. Physicians should protect patient confidentiality by ensuring that only the minimal amount of information is reported and that reasonable security measures are used in handling that information.

7. Physicians should work with their state medical societies to create statutes that uphold the best interests of patients and community and that safeguard physicians from liability when reporting in good faith.

REFERENCES

Frolik LA (editor): Aging and the Law: An Interdisciplinary Reader. Temple University Press, 1999.

Kapp MB: Key Words in Ethics, Law, and Aging—A Guide to Contemporary Usage. Springer, 1995.

Kapp MB: Lessons in Law and Aging: A Tool for Educators and Students. Springer, 2001.

National Bioethics Advisory Commission: Research Involving Persons With Mental Disorders That May Affect Decisionmaking Capacity. U.S. General Printing Office, 1998.

Weisstub DN et al (editors): Aging: Decisions at the End of Life. Kluwer Academic, 2001.

Appendix

Form A. Body mass index (BMI) table.

BMI → Height	19	20	21	22	23	24	25	26	27	28	29	30	35	40
							Weight (in pounds)							
4'10"	91	96	100	105	110	115	119	124	129	134	138	143	167	191
4'11"	94	99	104	109	114	119	124	128	133	138	143	148	173	198
5'	97	102	107	112	118	123	128	133	138	143	148	153	179	204
5'1"	100	106	111	116	122	127	132	137	143	148	153	158	185	211
5'2"	104	109	115	120	126	131	136	142	147	153	158	164	191	218
5'3"	107	113	118	124	130	135	141	146	152	158	163	169	197	225
5'4"	110	116	122	128	134	140	145	151	157	163	169	174	204	232
5'5"	114	120	126	132	138	144	150	156	162	168	174	180	210	240
5'6"	118	124	130	136	142	148	155	161	167	173	179	186	216	247
5'7"	121	127	134	140	146	153	159	166	172	178	185	191	223	255
5'8"	125	131	138	144	151	158	164	171	177	184	190	197	230	262
5'9"	128	135	142	149	155	162	169	176	182	189	196	203	236	270
5'10"	132	139	146	153	160	167	174	181	188	195	202	209	243	278
5'11"	136	143	150	157	165	172	179	186	193	200	208	215	250	286
6'	140	147	154	162	169	177	184	191	199	206	213	221	258	294
6'1"	144	151	159	166	174	182	189	197	204	212	219	227	265	302
6'2"	148	155	163	171	179	186	194	202	210	218	225	233	272	311
6'3"	152	160	168	176	184	192	200	208	216	224	232	240	279	319
6'4"	156	164	172	180	189	197	205	213	221	230	238	246	287	328

Locate height, and then on the same line locate the closest weight in pounds. Use the lower weight, if midpoint. Do not round up. Read to top of the weight column to obtain the BMI value.

Alternative height calculations using knee to heel measurements:
With knee at a 90° angle (foot flexed or flat on floor or bed board), measure from bottom of heel to top of knee.
Men = (2.02 × knee height cm) − (0.04 x age) + 64.19
Women = (1.83 × knee height cm) − (0.24 x age) + 84.88

Body weight calculations in amputees:
For amputations, increase weight by the percentage below for contribution of individual body parts to obtain the weight to use to determine BMI.

Single below knee	6%
Single at knee	9%
Single above knee	15%
Single arm	6.5%
Single arm below elbow	3.6%

Form B. San Francisco VAMC simple geriatric screen.

Patient Name _____ Date _____ Source: Pt _____ Other _____

	Abnormal	Action	Result & Comments
HISTORY ITEMS			
"Have you had any falls in the last year?"	Yes	Tinetti or other gait assessment Further exam, home eval & PT Consider osteoporosis risk	_____
"Do you have trouble with stairs, lighting, bathroom, or other home hazards?"	Yes to any	Home eval &/or PT	_____
"Do you have a problem with urine leaks or accidents?"	Yes	Rule out reversible (DIAPPERS) History (stress, urge), exam, PVR	_____
"Over the past month, have you often been bothered by feeling sad, depressed, or hopeless?" "During the past month, have you often been bothered by little interest or pleasure in doing things?"	Yes to either	GDS or other depression assessment	_____
"Do you ever feel unsafe where you live?" "Does anyone threaten you or hurt you?"	Yes	Explore further, social work, APS	_____
"Is pain a problem for you?"	Yes_____ No_____	Evaluate	_____
Do you have any problems with any of the following areas? Who assists?/Do you use any devices? (for "yes" answers, consider causes, social services, and/or home eval/PT/OT)			
Doing strenuous activities like fast walking/bicycling?	Yes_____ No_____		_____
Cook	Yes_____ No_____		_____
Shop	Yes_____ No_____		_____
Do heavy housework like washing windows	Yes_____ No_____		_____
Do laundry	Yes_____ No_____		_____
Get to a place beyond walking distance by driving or taking a bus	Yes_____ No_____		_____
Manage finances	Yes_____ No_____		_____
Get out of bed/transfer	Yes_____ No_____		_____
Dress	Yes_____ No_____		_____
Toilet	Yes_____ No_____		_____
Eat	Yes_____ No_____		_____
Walk	Yes_____ No_____		_____
Bathe (sponge bath, tub, or shower)	Yes_____ No_____		_____

(continued)

491

Form B. San Francisco VAMC simple geriatric screen. (continued)

	Abnormal	Action	Comments
Review medications that patient brought in	Confusion about meds > 5 meds Doesn't bring in	Consider simplification Medi-set or other aid Consider home visit	
Also ask about herbs, supplements, and nonprescription meds			
PHYSICAL EXAM ITEMS **(performed by nursing staff in some settings)**			
Weight/BMI And ask "have you lost weight?" If so, how much?	BMI <21 Loss of 5% since last visit or 10% over 1 year	Alert provider or nutrition eval Consider medical, dental, social	
Jaeger Card or Snellen eye chart Test each eye (with glasses)	Can't read 20/40	Alert provider or refer	
Whisper short sentence @ 6–12 in. (out of visual view) or audioscopy	Unable to hear Retest/refer/hearing handicap inventory	Cerumen check	
Name three objects/re-ask in 5 min Clock Draw	Remembers <3 or abnormally drawn clock	MMSE or other eval	
"Rise from your chair (do not use arms to get up), walk 10 feet, turn, walk back to the chair and sit down."	Observed problem or unable in <15	Tinetti and/or further exam Home eval & PT	
"Touch the back of your head with your hands." "Pick up the pencil." (Remember to ask about the 3 items!)	Unable to do either	Further exam Consider OP	

Other areas of concern (check those that might apply): Caregiver issues/stress/burnout_____ Social isolation_____ Driving_____

Who is surrogate decision maker?_____ Are advance directives available?_____

Other (eg, ETOH, exercise)_____

Form C. Physical activities of daily living (ADL).

Obtained from Patient	Informant	Activity	Guidelines for assessment
I A D	I A D	**Bathing** (sponge, shower, tub)	I = Able to bathe completely or needs help with only a single body part A = Needs help with more than 1 body part, getting in/out of tub or special tub attachments D = Completely unable to bathe self
I A D	I A D	**Dressing/undressing**	I = Able to pick out clothes, dress/undress self, manage fasteners/braces; tying shoes excluded A = Need assistance as remains partially undressed D = Completely unable to dress/undress self
I A D	I A D	**Personal grooming**	I = Able to comb hair/shave without help A = Needs help to comb hair, shave D = Completely unable to care for appearance
I A D	I A D	**Toileting**	I = Able to get to, on, and off toilet, arrange clothes, clean organs of excretion; uses bedpan only at night A = Needs help getting to and using toilet; uses bed-pan/commode regularly D = Completely unable to use toilet
I A D	I A D	**Continence**	I = Urination/defecation self-controlled A = Partial or total urine/stool incontinence or control by enemas, catheters, regulated use of urinals/bedpans D = Uses catheter or colostomy
I A D	I A D	**Transferring**	I = Able to get in/out of bed/chair without human assistance/mechanical aids A = Needs human assistance/mechanical aids D = Completely unable to transfer; needs lifting
I A D	I A D	**Walking**	I = Able to walk without help except from cane A = Needs human assistance/walker, crutches D = Completely unable to walk; needs lifting
I A D	I A D	**Eating**	I = Able to completely feed self A = Needs help with cutting, buttering bread, etc. D = Completely unable to feed self or needs parenteral feeding

This form may help you assess the functional capabilities of your older patients. The data can be collected by a nurse from the patient or from a family member or other caregiver. I, independent; A, assistance required; D, dependent.

Adapted from Modules in Clinical Geriatrics. Copyright © 1997 by Blue Cross and Blue Shield Association and the American Geriatrics Society. Used with permission.

Form D. Instrumental activities of daily living (IADL).

Obtained from Patient	Informant	Activity	Guidelines for assessment
I A D	I A D	**Using telephone**	I = Able to look up numbers, dial, receive, and make calls without help A = Able to answer phone or dial operator in an emergency but needs special phone or help in getting number, dialing D = Unable to use the phone
I A D	I A D	**Traveling**	I = Able to drive own car or travel alone on buses, taxis A = Able to travel but needs someone to travel with D = Unable to travel
I A D	I A D	**Shopping**	I = Able to take care of all food/clothes shopping with transportation provided A = Able to shop but needs someone to shop with D = Unable to shop
I A D	I A D	**Preparing meals**	I = Able to plan and cook full meals A = Able to prepare light foods but unable to cook full meals alone D = Unable to prepare any meals
I A D	I A D	**Housework**	I = Able to do heavy housework, ie, scrub floors A = Able to do light housework but needs help with heavy tasks D = Unable to do any housework
I A D	I A D	**Taking medicine**	I = Able to prepare/take medications in the right dose at the right time A = Able to take medications but needs reminding or someone to prepare them D = Unable to take medications
I A D	I A D	**Managing money**	I = Able to manage buying needs, ie, write checks, pay bills A = Able to manage daily buying needs but needs help managing checkbook, paying bills D = Unable to handle money

This form may help you assess the functional capabilities of your older patients. The data can be collected by a nurse from the patient or from a family member or other caregiver. I, independent; A, assistance required; D, dependent.

Adapted from Modules in Clinical Geriatrics. Copyright © 1997 by Blue Cross and Blue Shield Association and the American Geriatrics Society. Used with permission.

Form E. Home safety assessment checklist.

Safety item	Yes	No	Comment
1. Are emergency numbers kept by the phone and regularly updated?			
2. Do family members and other caregivers know how to report an emergency?			
3. Are patient, family, and caregivers aware of the dangers of smoking, especially in bed?			
4. If oxygen is used, do patient and caregivers know correct use of equipment, how to operate and clean it correctly?			
5. Are firearms stored unloaded and locked up?			
6. Are all poisons (medications, detergents, insecticides, cleaning fluids, polishes, etc.) kept out of reach of children and discarded when no longer needed?			
7. Is there a fire alarm and extinguisher? Do patient and caregivers know how to use it?			
8. Do the family and caregivers have an escape plan in case of fire or other disaster?			
9. Are throw rugs eliminated or fastened down?			
10. Are all electrical cords in working order, in the open, and not run under rugs or carpets or wrapped around nails?			
11. Are nonslip mats placed in bathtubs and showers?			
12. Are banisters or railings placed along stairways?			
13. Are stairs, halls, and doorways free of clutter?			
14. Are all steps and sidewalks clear of tools, toys, and other articles?			
15. Does adaptive or medical support equipment function adequately?			
16. Do patient and caregivers know safe and effective use of equipment?			
17. Do patient and caregivers know procedures to follow if equipment malfunctions?			

Adapted from Ferrell BA: Home care. In: Cassel CK, et al. (editors), Geriatric Medicine, 3rd ed. Springer Verlag, 1997. Used with permission.

Form F. The confusion assessment method diagnostic algorithm.

Feature 1: Acute onset and fluctuating course	This feature is usually obtained from a family member or nurse and is shown by positive responses to the following questions: Is there evidence of acute change in mental status from the patient's baseline? Did the abnormal behavior fluctuate during the day, that is, tend to come and go or increase and decrease in severity?
Feature 2: Inattention	This feature is shown by a positive response to the following question: Did the patient have difficulty focusing attention, for example, being easily distractible, or having difficulty keeping track of what was being said?
Feature 3: Disorganized thinking	This feature is show by a positive response to the following question: Was the patient's thinking disorganized or incoherent, such as rambling or irrelevant conversation, unclear or illogical flow of ideas, or unpredictable switching from subject to subject?
Feature 4: Altered level of consciousness	This feature is shown by any answer other than "alert" to the following question: Overall, how would you rate this patient's level of consciousness? (alert [normal], vigilant [hyperalert], lethargic [drowsy, easily aroused], stupor [difficult to arouse], or coma [unarousable])

The diagnosis of delirium by the Confusion Assessment Method requires the presence of features and 1 and 2 and either 3 or 4.

Form G. Annotated mini-mental state examination.

THE ANNOTATED MINI MENTAL STATE EXAMINATION (AMMSE)

MiniMentalLLC

NAME OF SUBJECT_____ Age_____

NAME OF EXAMINER _____Years of School Completed_____

Approach the patient with respect and encouragement.   Date of Examination_____
Ask: "Do you have any trouble with your memory?"   ☐ Yes   ☐ No
"May I ask you some questions about your memory?"   ☐ Yes   ☐ No

SCORE	ITEM
5 ( )	**TIME ORIENTATION** Ask: "What is the year_____(1), season_____(1). month of the year_____(1), date_____(1). day of the week_____(1)"?
5 ( )	**PLACE ORIENTATION** Ask: "Where are we now? What is the state_____(1), city_____(1), part of the city_____(1), building_____(1), floor of the building_____(1)?"
3 ( )	**REGISTRATION OF THREE WORDS** Say: "Listen carefully. I am going to say three words. You say them back after I stop. Ready? Here they are. . . PONY (wait 1 second). QUARTER (wait 1 second), ORANGE (wait one second). What were those words?" _____(1) _____(1) _____(1) Give 1 point for each correct answer, then repeat them until the patient learns all three.
5 ( )	**SERIAL 7's AS A TEST OF ATTENTION AND CALCULATION** Ask: "Subtract 7 from 100 and continue to subtract 7 from each subsequent remainder until I tell you to stop. What is 100 take away 7?"_____(1) Say: "Keep Going"_____(1),_____(1), _____(1),_____(1).
3 ( )	**RECALL OF THREE WORDS** Ask: "What were those three words I asked you to remember?" Give one point for each correct answer_____(1), _____(1),_____(1).
2 ( )	**NAMING** Ask: "What is this?" (show pencil)_____(1), "What is this?" (show watch)_____(1).

O   V   E   R

Form G. Annotated mini-mental state examination. (*continued*)

SCORE	ITEM
1 ( )	**REPETITION** Say: "Now I am going to ask you to repeat what I say. Ready? 'No ifs, ands, or buts.' Now you say that."_____(1)
3 ( )	**COMPREHENSION** Say: "Listen carefully because I am going to ask you to do something: Take this paper in your left hand (1), fold it in half (1), and put it on the floor." (1)
1 ( )	**READING** Say: "Please read the following and do what it says, but do not say it aloud." (1)

Close your eyes

1 ( )	**WRITING** Say: "Please write a sentence." If patient does not respond, say: "Write about the weather." (1) _____ _____
1 ( )	**DRAWING** Say: "Please copy this design."

TOTAL SCORE_____Assess level of consciousness along a continuum

	Alert	Drowsy	Stupor	Coma

	YES	NO		YES	NO	FUNCTION BY PROXY
Cooperative:	☐	☐	Deterioration from			Please record date when patient was last
Depressed:	☐	☐	previous level of			able to perform the following tasks.
Anxious:	☐	☐	functioning:	☐	☐	Ask caregiver if patient independently handles.
Poor Vision:	☐	☐	Family History of Dementia:	☐	☐	
Poor Hearing	☐	☐	Head Trauma:	☐	☐	
Native Language:			Stroke:	☐	☐	

FUNCTION BY PROXY:

	YES	NO	DATE
Money/bills:	☐	☐	____
Medication:	☐	☐	____
Transportation:	☐	☐	____
Telephone:	☐	☐	____

Also under "functioning" column: Alcohol Abuse: ☐ ☐, Thyroid Disease: ☐ ☐

SOURCE: Folstein MF, Folstein S, McHugh PR. Mini-Mental State: a practical method for grading the cognitive state of patients for the clinicians. *J Psych Res.* 1975;12(3):189–198. Copyright, 1998. Mini Mental LLC. Reprinted with permission. For more information or additional copies of this exam, call (617)587-4215.

Form H. Median MiniMental State Examination score by age
& educational level.

Age range	Education				
	0–4 years	5–8 years	9–12 years	≥12 years	Total
18–24	23	28	29	30	29
25–29	25	27	29	30	29
30–34	26	26	29	30	29
35–39	23	27	29	30	29
40–44	23	27	29	30	29
45–49	23	27	29	30	29
50–54	22	27	29	30	29
55–59	22	27	29	29	29
60–64	22	27	28	29	28
65–69	22	27	28	29	28
70–74	21	26	28	29	27
75–79	21	26	27	28	26
80–84	19	25	26	28	25
≥ 85	20	24	26	28	25
Total	22	26	29	29	29

Adapted from Crum RM, et al: Population-based norms for the Mini-Mental State Examination by age and educational level. JAMA 1993;269:2386. Used with permission.

Form I. Depression screens.

Geriatric Depression Screen (short form)	
1. Are you basically satisfied with your life?	Yes/**No**
2. Have you dropped many of your activities and interests?	**Yes**/No
3. Do you feel that your life is empty?	**Yes**/No
4. Do you often get bored?	**Yes**/No
5. Are you in good spirits most of the time?	Yes/**No**
6. Are you afraid that something bad is going to happen to you?	**Yes**/No
7. Do you feel happy most of the time?	Yes/**No**
8. Do you often feel helpless?	**Yes**/No
9. Do you prefer to stay at home rather than going out and doing new things?	**Yes**/No
10. Do you feel that you have more problems with memory than most?	**Yes**/No
11. Do you think it is wonderful to be alive now?	Yes/**No**
12. Do you feel pretty worthless the way you are now?	**Yes**/No
13. Do you feel full of energy?	Yes/**No**
14. Do you feel that your situation is hopeless?	**Yes**/No
15. Do you think that most people are better off than you are?	**Yes**/No
	Score: _____

Directions: Score 1 point for each bolded answer. A score of 5 or more is a positive screen for depression.
From Sheikh, JI, Yesavage JA: Geriatric depression scale (GDS): recent evidence and development of a shorter version. Clin Geront 1986;5:165. Used with permission.

Form I. Depression screens. (continued)

Two-Question Case Finding Instrument	
1. During the past month, have you often been bothered by feeling down, depressed, or hopeless?	**Yes**/No
2. During the past month, have you often been bothered by having little interest or pleasure in doing things?	**Yes**/No

Directions: Yes to either question is a positive screen for depression.
From Whooley MA et al: Case-finding instrument for depression: two questions are as good as many. J Gen Intern Med 1997;12:439. Used with permission.

Form J. Functional independence measure.

L E V E L S	7 Complete Independence (Timely, Safely) 6 Modified Independence (Device)	NO HELPER

	Modified Dependence
	   5 Supervision
	   4 Minimal Assist (Subject = 75%+)
	   3 Moderate Assist (Subject = 50%+)
	
	Complete Dependence
	   2 Maximal Assist (Subject = 25%+)
	   1 Total Assist (Subject = 0%+)
		HELPER

	ADMIT	DISCHG	FOL-UP
Self-Care A. Eating B. Grooming C. Bathing D. Dressing-Upper Body E. Dressing-Lower Body F. Toileting	☐	☐	☐
Sphincter Control G. Bladder Management H. Bowel Management	☐	☐	☐
Transfers I. Bed, Chair, Wheelchair J. Toilet K. Tub, Shower	☐	☐	☐
Locomotion L. Walk/wheelchair Walk / Wheelchair / Both M. Stairs	☐	☐	☐
Motor Subtotal Score	☐	☐	☐
Communication Auditory / Visual / Both N. Comprehension Vocal / Non-vocal / Both O. Expression	☐	☐	☐
Social Cognition P. Social Interaction Q. Problem Solving R. Memory	☐	☐	☐
Cognitive Subtotal Score	☐	☐	☐
Total FIM	☐	☐	☐

Note: Leave no blanks; enter 1 if patient not testable due to risk

Form J. Functional independence measure. (*continued*)

FIM (motor)	FIM (cognitive)
Self-care	**Communication**
A. Self-care	N. Comprehension
B. Grooming	O. Expression
C. Bathing	**Social cognition**
D. Dressing upper body	P. Social integration
E. Dressing lower body	Q. Problem solving
F. Toileting	R. Memory
Sphincter control	
G. Bladder management	
H. Bowel management	
Mobility	
Transfer	
I. Bed, chair, wheelchair	
J. Toilet	
K. Tub, shower	
Locomotion	
L. Walk/wheelchair	
M. Stairs	

FIM Scoring: independence:	7, complete independence (timely, safely); 6, modified independence (device used).
Modified dependence:	5, supervision; 4, minimal assistance (subject performs >75% of task); 3, moderate assistance (subject performs 50–74% of task).
Complete dependence:	2, maximal assistance (subject performs 25–49% of task); 1, total assistance (subject performs <25% of task).

Modified from Grander CV, Hamilton BB. The Uniform Data System for Medical Rehabilitation report on first admissions for 1991. Am J Phys Med & Rehabil 1993;72:33. Used with permission.

Form K. Mini nutritional assessment.

Last Name_____ First Name_____ M.I._____ Sex:_____ Date:_____
Age:_____ Weight (kg):_____ Height (cm):_____ Knee Height (cm):_____

Complete the form by writing the numbers in the boxes. Add the numbers in the boxes and compare the total assessment to the Malnutrition Indicator Score.

Anthropometric Assessment	Points		Points

1. Body Mass Index (BMI) (weight in kg)/(height in m^2)
a. BMI < 19 = 0 points
b. BMI 19 to < 21 = 1 point
c. BMI 21 to < 23 = 2 points
d. BMI > 23 = 3 points

2. Mid-arm circumference (MAC) in cm
a. MAC < 21 = 0.0 points
b. MAC 21 ≤ 22 = 0.5 points
c. MAC > 22 = 1.0 points

3. Calf circumference (CC) in cm
a. CC < 31 = 0 points
b. CC ≥ 31 = 1 point

4. Weight loss during last 3 months
a. weight loss greater than 3 kg (6.6 lb) = 0 points
b. does not know = 1 point
c. weight loss between 1 and 3 kg = 2 points
d. no weight loss = 3 points

General Assessment

5. Lives independently (not in a nursing home or hospital)
a. no = 0 points   b. yes = 1 point

6. Takes more than 3 prescription drugs per day
a. yes = 0 points   b. no = 1 point

7. Has suffered psychological stress or acute disease in the past 3 months
a. yes = 0 points   b. no = 1 point

8. Mobility
a. bed or chair bound = 0 points
b. able to get out of bed/chair
   but does not go out = 1 point
c. goes out = 2 points

9. Neuropsychological problems
a. severe dementia or depression = 0 points
b. mild dementia = 1 point
c. no psychological problems = 2 points

10. Pressure sores or skin ulcers
a. yes = 0 points   b. no = 1 point

Dietary Assessment

11. How many full meals does the patient eat daily?
a. 1 meal = 0 points
a. 2 meals = 1 point
a. 3 meals = 2 points

12. Selected consumption markers for protein intake
• At least one serving of dairy products
  (milk, cheese, yogurt) per day   ☐ Yes ☐ No
• Two or more servings of legumes
  or eggs per week   ☐ Yes ☐ No
• Meat, fish, or poultry every day   ☐ Yes ☐ No
a. 0 or 1 yes = 0.0 points
b. 2 yes = 0.5 points
c. 3 yes = 1.0 points

13. Consumes two or more servings of fruits or vegetables per day
a. no = 0 points   b. yes = 1 point

14. Has food intake declined over the past 3 months due to loss of appetite, digestive problems, chewing or swallowing difficulties?
a. severe loss of appetite = 0 points
b. moderate loss of appetite = 1 point
c. no loss of appetite = 2 points

15. How much fluid (eg, water, juice, coffee, tea, milk) is consumed per day? (1 cup = 8 oz.)
a. less than 3 cups = 0.0 points
b. 3 to 5 cups = 0.5 points
c. more than 5 cups = 1.0 points

16. Mode of feeding
a. unable to eat without assistance = 0 points
b. self-fed with some difficulty = 1 point
c. self-fed without any problem = 2 points

Self-Assessment

17. Do they view themselves as having nutritional problems?
a. major malnutrition = 0 points
b. do not know or moderate
   malnutrition = 1 point
c. no nutritional problem = 2 points

18. In comparison with other people of the same age, how do they consider their health status?
a. not as good = 0.0 points
b. do not know = 0.5 points
c. as good = 1.0 points
d. better = 2.0 points

Malnutrition indicator score: ≥ 24 points, well-nourished; 17–23.5 points, at risk of malnutrition; < 17 points, malnourished.
From Vellas B, et al: Nutrition 1999;15:116. Used with permission.

Form L. Hearing handicap inventory for elderly-screening.

Instructions: The purpose of this scale is to identify the problems your hearing loss may be causing you. Answer <u>Yes, Sometimes,</u> or <u>No</u> for each question. <u>Do not skip a question if you avoid a situation because of your hearing loss.</u> It is important that you answer all questions. If you use a hearing aid, please answer the way you hear <u>without</u> the hearing aid.

- -

E S

        (E1) Does a hearing problem cause you to feel embarrassed when meeting new people?

4____   Yes
2____   Sometimes
0____   No

        (E2) Does a hearing problem cause you to feel frustrated when talking to members of your family?

4____   Yes
2____   Sometimes
0____   No

        (S3) Do you have difficulty when someone speaks in a whisper?

4____   Yes
2____   Sometimes
0____   No

        (E4) Do you feel handicapped by a hearing problem?

4____   Yes
2____   Sometimes
0____   No

        (S5) Does a hearing problem cause you difficulty when visiting friends, relatives, or neighbors?

4____   Yes
2____   Sometimes
0____   No

        (S6) Does a hearing problem cause you to attend religious services less often than you would like?

4____   Yes
2____   Sometimes
0____   No

        (E7) Does a hearing problem cause you to have arguments with family members?

4____   Yes
2____   Sometimes
0____   No

        (S8) Does a hearing problem cause you difficulty when listening to a TV or radio?

4____   Yes
2____   Sometimes
0____   No

        (E9) Do you feel that any difficulty with your hearing limits or hampers your personal or social life?

4____   Yes
2____   Sometimes
0____   No

        (S10) Does a hearing problem cause you difficulty when in a restaurant with relatives or friends?

4____   Yes
2____   Sometimes
0____   No

____   Emotional Subscale Total
____   Social Subscale Total
____   **Total Score**

Remember to answer <u>all of the questions</u> and if you wear a hearing aid answer the way you hear <u>without</u> the hearing aid.
S, Social Subscale Question; E, Emotional Subscale Question; yes, 4 points; sometimes, 2 points; no, 0 points. Range of results for total score: 0–8, no hearing handicap; 9–24, mild to moderate hearing handicap; 25–40, severe hearing handicap.
From Ventry I, Weinstein B: The Hearing Handicap Inventory for the Elderly: a new tool. Ear Hear. 1982;83:128. Used with permission.

Form M. Performance-oriented assessment of balance.[a]

Maneuver	Response		
	Normal	Adaptive	Abnormal
Sitting balance	Steady, stable	Holds onto chair to keep upright	Leans, slides down in chair
Arising from chair	Able to arise in a single movement without using arms	Uses arms (on chair or walking aid) to pull or push up; and/or moves forward in chair before attempting to arise	Multiple attempts required or unable without human assistance
Immediate standing balance (first 3–5 s)	Steady without holding onto walking aid or other objects for support	Steady, but uses walking aid or other object for support	Any sign of unsteadiness[b]
Standing balance	Steady, able to stand with feet together without holding object for support	Steady, but cannot put feet together	Any sign of unsteadiness regardless of stance or holds onto object
Balance with eyes closed (with feet as close together as possible)	Steady without holding onto any object with feet together	Steady with feet apart	Any sign of unsteadiness or needs to hold onto an object
Turning balance (360°)	No grabbing or staggering; no need to hold onto any objects; steps are continuous (turn is a flowing movement)	Steps are discontinuous (patient puts one foot completely on floor before raising other foot)	Any sign of unsteadiness or holds onto an object
Nudge on sternum (patient standing with feet as close together as possible, examiner pushes with light even pressure over sternum 3 times; reflects ability to withstand displacement)	Steady, able to withstand pressure	Needs to move feet, but able to maintain balance	Begins to fall, or examiner has to help maintain balance
Neck turning (patient asked to turn head side to side and look up while standing with feet as close together as possible)	Able to turn head at least half way side to side and be able to bend head back to look at ceiling; no staggering, grabbing, or symptoms of lightheadedness, unsteadiness, or pain	Decreased ability to turn side to side to extend neck, but no staggering, grabbing, or symptoms of lightheadedness, unsteadiness, or pain	Any sign of unsteadiness or symptoms when turning head or extending neck
One leg standing balance	Able to stand on one leg for 5 s without holding object for support		Unable
Back extension (ask patient to lean back as far as possible, without holding onto object if possible)	Good extension without holding object or staggering	Tries to extend, but decreased ROM (compared with other patients of same age) or needs to hold object to attempt extension	Will not attempt or no extension seen or staggers

(continued)

Form M. Performance-oriented assessment of balance.[a] (*continued*)

Maneuver	Response		
	Normal	**Adaptive**	**Abnormal**
Reaching up (have patient attempt to remove an object from a shelf high enough to require stretching or standing on toes)	Able to take down object without needing to hold onto other object for support and without becoming unsteady	Able to get object but needs to steady self by holding on to something for support	Unable or unsteady
Bending down (patient is asked to pick up small objects, such as pen, from the floor)	Able to bend down and pick up the object and is able to get up easily in single attempt without needing to pull self up with arms	Able to get object and get upright in single attempt but needs to pull self up with arms or hold onto something for support	Unable to bend down or unable to get upright after bending down or takes multiple attempts to upright
Sitting down	Able to sit down in one smooth movement	Needs to use arms to guide self into chair or not a smooth movement	Falls into chair, misjudges distances (lands off center)

ROM, range of motion.
[a]The patient begins this assessment seated in a hard, straight-backed, armless chair.
[b]Unsteadiness defined as grabbing at objects for support, staggering, moving feet, or more than minimal trunk sway.
From Tinetti ME: Performance-oriented assessment of mobility problems in elderly patients. J Am Geriatr Soc 1986;34:119. Used with permission.

Form N. Performance-oriented assessment of gait.[a]

Components[b]	Observation	
	Normal	**Abnormal**
Initiation of gait (patient asked to begin walking down hallway)	Begins walking immediately without observable hesitation; initiation of gait is single, smooth motion	Hesitates; multiple attempts; initiation of gait not a smooth motion
Step height (begin observing after first few steps: observe one foot, then the other, observe from side)	Swing foot completely clears floor but by no more than 1–2 in	Swing foot is not completely raised off floor (may hear scraping) or is raised too high (> 1–2 in)[c]
Step length (observe distance between toe of stance foot and heel of swing foot; observe from side; do not judge first few or last few steps; observe one side at a time)	At least the length of individual's foot between the stance toe and swing heel (step length usually longer but foot length provides basis for observation)	Step length less than described under normal[c]
Step symmetry (observe the middle part of the patch not the first or last steps; observe from side; observe distance between heel of each swing foot and toe of each stance foot)	Step length same or nearly same on both sides for most step cycles	Step length varies between sides or patient advances with same foot with every step
Step continuity	Begins raising heel of one foot (toe off) as heel of other foot touches the floor (heel strike); no breaks or stops in stride; step lengths equal over most cycles	Places entire foot (heel and toe) on floor before beginning to raise other foot; or stops completely between steps; or step length varies over cycles[c]
Path deviation (observe from behind; observe one foot over several strides; observe in relation to line on floor [eg, tiles] if possible, difficult to assess if patient uses a walker)	Foot follows close to straight line as patient advances	Foot deviates from side to side or toward one direction[d]
Trunk stability (observe from behind; side to side motion of trunk may be a normal gait pattern, need to differentiate this from instability)	Trunk does not sway; knees or back are not flexed; arms are not abducted in effort to maintain stability	Any of proceeding features present[d]
Walk stance (observe from behind)	Feet should almost touch as one passes other	Feet apart with stepping[e]
Turning while walking	No staggering; turning continuous with walking; and steps are continuous while turning	Staggers; stops before initiating turn; or steps are discontinuous

[a]The patient stands with examiner at end of obstacle-free hallway. Patient uses usual walking aid. Examiner asks patient to walk down hallway at his or her usual pace. Examiner observes one component of gait at a time (analogous to heart examination). For some components the examiner walks behind the patient; for other components, the examiner walks next to patient. May require several trips to complete.
[b]Also ask patient to walk at a "more rapid than usual" pace and observe whether any walking aid is used correctly.
[c]Abnormal gait finding may reflect a primary neurological or musculoskeletal problem directly related to the finding or reflect a compensatory maneuver for other, more remote problem.
[d]Abnormality may be corrected by walking aid such as cane, observe with and without walking aid if possible.
[e]Abnormal finding is usually a compensatory maneuver rather than a primary problem.

Form O. Symptom score sheet to assess benign prostatic hyperplasia symptoms.

Variable	Not at all	More than 1 time in 5	Less than half the time	About half the time	More than half the time	Almost always	Patient score
Incomplete emptying: Over the past month, how often have you had a sensation of not emptying your bladder completely after you finished urinating?	0	1	2	3	4	5	
Frequency: Over the past month, how often have you had to urinate again less than 2 h after you finished urinating?	0	1	2	3	4	5	
Intermittency: Over the past month, how often have you found you stopped and started again several times when you urinated?	0	1	2	3	4	5	
Urgency: Over the past month, how often have you found it difficult to postpone urination?	0	1	2	3	4	5	
Weak stream: Over the past month, how often have you had a weak urinary stream?	0	1	2	3	4	5	
Straining: Over the past month, how often have you had to push or strain to begin urination?	0	1	2	3	4	5	
Nocturia: Over the past month, how many times did you most typically get up to urinate from the time you went to bed at night until the time you got up in the morning?	0	1	2	3	4	5	
Total score							

Barry MJ et al: The American Urological Association Symptoms index for benign prostatic hyperplasia. J Urol 1992;148:1549. Used with permission.

Form P. Braden Scale for Predicting Pressure Sore Risk.

Patient's Name _____ Evaluator's Name _____ Date of Assessment _____

SENSORY PERCEPTION Ability to respond meaningfully to pressure-related discomfort	1. Completely Limited: Unresponsive. Does not moan, flinch, or grasp the painful stimuli because of diminished level of consciousness or sedation. OR limited ability to feel pain over most of body surface.	2. Very Limited: Responds only to painful stimuli. Cannot communicate discomfort except by moaning or restlessness. OR has a sensory impairment that limits the ability to feel pain or discomfort over ½ of body.	3. Slightly Limited: Responds to verbal commands, but cannot always communicate discomfort or need to be turned. OR has some sensory impairment that limits ability to feel pain or discomfort in 1 or 2 extremities.	4. No Impairment: Responds to verbal commands. Has no sensory deficit that would limit ability to feel or voice pain or discomfort.
MOISTURE Degree to which skin is exposed to moisture	1. Constantly Moist: Skin is kept moist almost constantly by perspiration, urine, etc. Dampness is detected every time patient is moved or turned.	2. Very Moist: Skin is often, but not always moist. Linen must be changed at least once a shift.	3. Occasionally Moist: Skin is occasionally moist, requiring an extra linen change approximately once a day.	4. Rarely Moist: Skin is usually dry, linen only requires changing at routine intervals.
ACTIVITY Degree of physical activity	1. Bedfast: Confined to bed	2. Chairfast: Ability to walk severely limited or nonexistent. Cannot bear own weight and/or must be assisted into chair or wheelchair.	3. Walks Occasionally: Walks occasionally during day, but for very short distances, with or without assistance. Spends majority on each shift in bed or chair.	4. Walks Frequently: Walks outside the room at least twice a day and inside room at least once every 2 hours during waking hours.
MOBILITY Ability to change and control body position	1. Completely Immobile: Does not make even slight changes in body or extremity position without assistance.	2. Very Limited: Makes occasional slight changes in body or extremity position but unable to make frequent or significant changes independently.	3. Slightly Limited: Makes frequent though slight changes in body or extremity position independently.	4. No Limitation: Makes major and frequent changes in position without assistance.
NUTRITION *Usual* food intake pattern	1. Very Poor: Never eats a complete meal. Rarely eats more than ⅓ of any food offered. Eats 2 servings or less protein (meat or dairy products) per day. Take fluids poorly. Does not take a liquid dietary supplement. OR is NPO and/or maintained on clear liquids or IVs for more than 5 days.	2. Probably Inadequate: Rarely eats a complete meal and generally eats only about ½ of any food offered. Protein intake includes only 3 servings of meat or dairy products per day. Occasionally will take a dietary supplement. OR receives less than optimum amount of liquid diet or tube feeding.	3. Adequate: Eats over half of most meals. Eats a total of 4 servings of protein (meat, dairy products) each day. Occasionally will refuse a meal, but will usually take a supplement if offered. OR is on a tube feeding or TPN regimen that probably meets most of nutritional needs.	4. Excellent: Eats most of every meal. Never refuses a meal. Usually eats a total of 4 or more servings of meat and dairy products. Occasionally eats between meals. Does not require supplementation.

(continued)

509

Form P. Braden Scale for Predicting Pressure Sore Risk.

Patient's Name _____ Evaluator's Name _____ Date of Assessment _____

FRICTION AND SHEAR	1. Problem:	2. Potential Problem:	3. No Apparent Problem:
	Requires moderate to maximum assistance in moving. Complete lifting without sliding against sheets is impossible. Frequently slides down in bed or chair, requiring frequent repositioning with maximum assistance. Spasticity, contractures, or agitation leads to almost constant friction.	Moves feebly or requires minimum assistance. During a move skin probably slides to some extent against sheets, chair, restraints, or other devices. Maintains relatively good position in chair or bed most of the time but occasionally slides down.	Moves in bed and in chair independently and has sufficient muscle strength to life up completely during move. Maintains good position in bed or chair at all times.

A score of less than or equal to 16 = high risk. IVs, intravenous feedings; NPO, nothing by mouth; TPN, total parenteral nutrition. For additional information on administration and scoring refer to the following: Braden BJ, Bergstrom N. Clinical utility of the Braden Scale for predicting pressure sore risk. Decubitus. 1989;2(3):44.
From Barbara Braden and Nancy Bergstrom, 1988. Reproduced by permission.

Index